ORAL AND MAXILLOFACIAL SURGERY SECRETS

ORAL AND MAXILLOFACIAL SURGERY SECRETS

SECOND EDITION

A. Omar Abubaker, DMD, PhD
Professor and Chairman
Department of Oral and Maxillofacial Surgery
Schools of Dentistry and Medicine
Virginia Commonwealth University
Richmond, Virginia

Kenneth J. Benson, DDS
Private Practice
Oral and Maxillofacial Surgery
Apex, North Carolina;
Staff Surgeon, Clinical Instructor
Department of Otolaryngology
Wake Medical Center
Raleigh, North Carolina

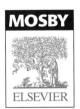

MOSBY

ELSEVIER

MOSBY
ELSEVIER

11830 Westline Industrial Drive
St. Louis, Missouri 63146

ORAL AND MAXILLOFACIAL SURGERY SECRETS,
EDITION 2
Copyright © 2007, 2001 by Elsevier Inc.

ISBN-13: 978-1-56053-615-4
ISBN-10: 1-56053-615-2

Notice

Knowledge and best practice in this field are constantly changing. As new research and experience broaden our knowledge, changes in practice, treatment, and drug therapy may become necessary or appropriate. Readers are advised to check the most current information provided (i) on procedures featured or (ii) by the manufacturer of each product to be administered, to verify the recommended dose or formula, the method and duration of administration, and contraindications. It is the responsibility of the practitioner, relying on his or her own experience and knowledge of the patient, to make diagnoses, to determine dosages and the best treatment for each individual patient, and to take all appropriate safety precautions. To the fullest extent of the law, neither the Publisher nor the Authors assume any liability for any injury and/or damage to persons or property arising out or related to any use of the material contained in this book.

The Publisher

ISBN-13: 978-1-56053-615-4

ISBN-10: 1-56053-615-2

Publisher: Linda Duncan
Senior Editor: John Dolan
Developmental Editor: Courtney Sprehe
Publishing Services Manager: Patricia Tannian
Project Manager: Kristine Feeherty
Design Direction: Andrea Lutes

Printed in the United States of America

Last digit is the print number: 9 8 7 6 5 4 3 2 1

Working together to grow
libraries in developing countries

www.elsevier.com | www.bookaid.org | www.sabre.org

ELSEVIER   BOOK AID International   Sabre Foundation

To all my teachers, especially those in the early years of my education, for planting the seeds of scientific curiosity and thirst for knowledge.

To my mentors, who recognized and nourished the potential in me to learn and teach.

To my students and residents, who taught me by asking me questions.

To my family, who supported me throughout all this.

AOA

To all of my OMFS mentors, for encouraging me to develop and mature in such a diverse and challenging profession.

To my wife, Erin, for all of her continued support and daily motivation.

KJB

CONTRIBUTORS

A. Omar Abubaker, DMD, PhD
Professor and Chairman
Department of Oral and Maxillofacial Surgery
Schools of Dentistry and Medicine
Virginia Commonwealth University
Richmond, Virginia

Shahid R. Aziz, DMD, MD, FACS
Assistant Professor
Department of Oral and Maxillofacial Surgery/Plastic and Reconstructive Surgery
University of Medicine and Dentistry of New Jersey
Newark, New Jersey

Kathy A. Banks, DMD
Department of Oral and Maxillofacial Surgery
University of Medicine and Dentistry of New Jersey
Newark, New Jersey

Timothy S. Bartholomew, DDS
Staff Maxillofacial Surgeon
Centre de Santé l'Espérance de N'Zao
Conakry, Guinea, West Africa

Kenneth J. Benson, DDS
Private Practice
Oral and Maxillofacial Surgery
Apex, North Carolina;
Staff Surgeon, Clinical Instructor
Department of Otolaryngology
Wake Medical Center
Raleigh, North Carolina

Hani F. Braidy, DMD
Assistant Professor
Department of Oral and Maxillofacial Surgery
University of Medicine and Dentistry of New Jersey
Newark, New Jersey

Paul W. Brinser III, DDS
Oral and Maxillofacial Surgeon in Private Practice
Petersburg, Virginia

Corey C. Burgoyne, DMD
Resident
Department of Oral and Maxillofacial Surgery
Virginia Commonwealth University
Richmond, Virginia

Robert E. Doriot, DDS
Adjunct Clinical Professor
Medical College of Virginia;
Director
Northern Virginia Center for Oral, Facial, and Implant Surgery
Fairfax, Virginia

James A. Giglio, DDS, MEd
Professor
Department of Oral and Maxillofacial Surgery
School of Dentistry;
Professor of Surgery
Department of Surgery, Division of Oral and Maxillofacial Surgery
School of Medicine
Virginia Commonwealth University
Richmond, Virginia

Steven G. Gollehon, DDS, MD, FACS
Associate Clinical Professor
Department of Oral and Maxillofacial Surgery
Louisiana State University Health Sciences Center
New Orleans, Louisiana;
Private Practice
Piedmont Oral, Maxillofacial, and Facial Cosmetic Surgery Center
Greensboro, North Carolina

Bradley A. Gregory, DMD
Oral and Maxillofacial Surgeon in Private Practice
Center for Oral and Maxillofacial Surgery
Findlay, Ohio

Hamid Hajarian, MS, DDS, MD
Private Practice
Fountain Valley, California

Alden H. Harken, MD
Professor and Chairman
Department of Surgery
University of California, San Francisco (East Bay);
Chief of Surgery
Department of Surgery
Alameda County Medical Center
Oakland, California

Tabetha R. Harken, MD, MPH
Department of Obstetrics and Gynecology
The University of California, San Francisco
San Francisco, California

Lubor Hlousek, DMD, MD
Private Practice
Annapolis, Maryland

Jason S. Hullett, DMD
Department of Oral and Maxillofacial Surgery
University of Medicine and Dentistry of New Jersey
University Hospital
Newark, New Jersey

Frank P. Iuorno, Jr., DDS, MS
Private Practice
Glen Allen, Virginia

Maria J. Iuorno, MD, MS
Adjunctive Faculty and Clinical Professor of Medicine
Department of Endocrinology and Metabolism
Virginia Commonwealth University;
Physician
Virginia Diabetes and Endocrinology, P.C.
Richmond, Virginia

Jeffrey S. Jelic, DMD, MD
Former Director of Aesthetic Surgery
UNC Department of Maxillofacial Surgery
Chapel Hill, North Carolina;
Private Practice
Durham, North Carolina

John N. Kent, BA, DDS, FACD, FICD
Boyd Professor and Head
Department of Oral and Maxillofacial Surgery
Louisiana State University Health Sciences Center;
Chief, Oral and Maxillofacial Surgery
Medical Center of Louisiana at New Orleans;
Active Staff
Doctor's Hospital of Jefferson and East Jefferson General Hospital
New Orleans, Louisiana

Edward Kozlovsky, DMD
Clinical Assistant Professor
Department of Oral and Maxillofacial Surgery
University of Medicine and Dentistry of New Jersey
Newark, New Jersey;
Private Practice
Oral and Maxillofacial Surgery
Marlboro, New Jersey

Christopher L. Maestrello, DDS
Adjunct Clinical Assistant Professor
Department of Pediatric Dentistry
Medical College of Virginia
School of Dentistry
Virginia Commonwealth University;
Medical Staff—Dentist
Department of Surgery
St. Mary's Hospital; Henrico Doctor's Hospital; Children's Hospital
Richmond, Virginia

Kiki C. Marti, DMD, MD, PhD
Assistant Professor
Department of Oral and Maxillofacial Surgery
University of Athens, School of Dental Medicine
Athens, Greece

Renato Mazzonetto, DDS, PhD
Associate Professor
Department of Oral and Maxillofacial Surgery
Piracicaba Dental School
University of Campinas
Piracicaba, São Paulo, Brazil

Ian McDonald, MD, DMD
Oral and Maxillofacial Surgeon in Private Practice
Escondido, California

Terrence R. Nedbalski, DDS
Chief Resident
Department of Oral and Maxillofacial Surgery
Virginia Commonwealth University
Richmond, Virginia

Gregory M. Ness, DDS
Professor
Department of Oral and Maxillofacial Surgery
Virginia Commonwealth University
Richmond, Virginia

Mark A. Oghalai, DDS
Private Practice, Drs. Bailey, Peoples, and Oghalai
Winston Salem, North Carolina

Esther S. Oh, DDS
Resident
Department of Oral and Maxillofacial Surgery
University of North Carolina
Chapel Hill, North Carolina

Vincent J. Perciaccante, DDS
Assistant Professor and Residency Program Director
Division of Oral and Maxillofacial Surgery
Department of Surgery
School of Medicine
Emory University;
Chief, Division of Oral and Maxillofacial Surgery
Department of Surgery
Grady Memorial Hospital
Atlanta, Georgia

Brenda Price, MD
Obstetrics and Gynecology
Richmond OB/GYN
Richmond, Virginia

Bashar M. Rajab, DDS
School of Medicine
Virginia Commonwealth University
Richmond, Virginia

Noah Sandler, DMD, MD
Midwest Oral Surgery
Shakopee and Savage, Minnesota

Chris A. Skouteris, DMD, PhD
Associate Professor of Oral and Maxillofacial Surgery
Department of Oral and Maxillofacial Surgery
University of Athens, School of Dental Medicine;
Director
Second Oral and Maxillofacial Surgical Service
The Athens Euroclinic
Athens, Greece

Daniel B. Spagnoli, DDS, PhD
Clinical Assistant Professor
Department of Oral and Maxillofacial Surgery
Louisiana State University
University Health Science Center
New Orleans, Louisiana;
Private Practice
University Oral and Maxillofacial Surgery
Charlotte, North Carolina

Gaetano G. Spinnato, DMD, MD
Clinical Assistant Professor
University of Medicine and Dentistry of New Jersey
Private Practice
Bayonne, New Jersey

Robert A. Strauss, DDS, MD
Professor of Surgery
Department of Oral and Maxillofacial Surgery
Virginia Commonwealth University
Richmond, Virginia

Vincent B. Ziccardi, DDS, MD
Associate Professor and Chair
Program Director, Oral and Maxillofacial Surgery Residency Training Program
Department of Oral and Maxillofacial Surgery
New Jersey Dental School
University of Medicine and Dentistry of New Jersey
Newark, New Jersey

Foreword to the Second Edition

When is a secret no longer a secret? When everyone knows about it. *Oral and Maxillofacial Surgery Secrets* is an example of such a phenomenon. The popularity of this book since publication of the first edition in 2001 has clearly established its value as a significant resource for students, residents, and practitioners alike.

This new edition continues the formula so successful in the first edition by providing concise information on a variety of pertinent topics related to the specialty. Because this is a dynamic field, some of the information originally supplied may no longer be applicable and these areas have been carefully updated. Moreover, many new areas have also been added so that, again, the book fulfills its goal of providing answers to clinically relevant questions that may be difficult to find in other sources.

Drs. Abubaker and Benson, as well as the many other contributors to this book, are again to be congratulated for providing so much useful information in such a concise and easy-to-read manner. Who would have thought that learning could be such fun!

Daniel M. Laskin, DDS, MS
Professor and Chairman Emeritus
Department of Oral and Maxillofacial Surgery
Schools of Dentistry and Medicine
Virginia Commonwealth University
Richmond, Virginia

Foreword to the First Edition

Students, residents, and practitioners are constantly bombarded by questions from patients, colleagues, and teachers. When they do not know the answer, they usually turn to their textbooks for the information. However, there are times when textbooks do not provide the appropriate information, the available information is not specific enough, or the correct answer is difficult to find among all of the details that are provided. Thus the need became apparent for another source of concise information on a variety of topics that are specific to a particular area of specialization. Until now, this source has not existed in oral and maxillofacial surgery. Drs. Abubaker and Benson are to be congratulated on filling this niche with *Oral and Maxillofacial Surgery Secrets*.

Following the format used in the other books in this series, *Oral and Maxillofacial Surgery Secrets* covers the broad scope of the specialty, providing precise answers to the most common questions that arise during clinical practice. Therefore it contains information under one cover that ordinarily could be found only by referring to multiple textbooks. In this way, the book makes an important contribution to the field of oral and maxillofacial surgery. Readers will find it valuable as a handy, quick way to obtain answers and also as an excellent review of what is current in the field.

Daniel M. Laskin, DDS, MS
Professor and Chairman
Department of Oral and Maxillofacial Surgery
Schools of Dentistry and Medicine
Virginia Commonwealth University
Richmond, Virginia

Preface to the Second Edition

Since publication of the first edition, we have been very pleased and gratified with the popularity of this book. Here and abroad, we have received favorable comments from students, residents, and practitioners. It is particularly rewarding to hear that the major reasons for the appeal of this book are its applicability to clinical practice and its ease of use. Time is a precious commodity, especially in the life of a resident. We can certainly relate to this, even though our own residencies were quite a few years ago. The rewards to us are even greater when we hear that the book suitably fits into residents' busy schedules, providing ready access to relevant and essential information that enhances their knowledge and training.

It is no secret that oral and maxillofacial surgery is a very complex specialty, encompassing the need for knowledge in many areas, including medicine, general surgery, and anesthesia, as well as oral and maxillofacial surgery. Because of this complexity, in preparation for the new edition, we reviewed several of the other "Secrets" in the series in an attempt to cross-fertilize the information provided. In addition, we have added several new chapters and expanded others to elaborate on those concepts that the readers of the first edition indicated needed more discussion.

New chapters address such areas as treating a pregnant patient, mandibular trauma, midface and frontal sinus fractures, soft tissue injuries, syndromes affecting the craniofacial and oromaxillofacial regions, and the application and interview process to residency programs.

We hope the readers of this edition will find it even more informative and relevant to their daily needs. It should be beneficial to students learning about the specialty, residents training in the specialty and studying for their boards, and practitioners engaged in busy clinical practice. This text, not unlike all the other books in the *Secrets* series, is not intended to be a traditional textbook. Rather, it should be used as a quick reference source for the factual information needed to provide the best care possible for patients.

We are grateful to all of the current chapter authors, to those chapter authors in other *Secrets* series from whom we benefited, and to all those who provided us with the feedback needed to make this edition even better.

A. Omar Abubaker, DMD, PhD
Kenneth J. Benson, DDS

Preface to the First Edition

With the expanding scope of oral and maxillofacial surgery, the breadth of information to be acquired both by the neophyte to the field and by the practicing clinician is increasing daily. Although conventional textbooks contain a great deal of valuable information, it is often difficult, especially for residents and students, to identify and remember the most relevant information. According to the Socratic method, the best way to teach is to question, and this book uses this effective teaching approach to help guide students, residents, and clinicians to acquire and retain the significant knowledge in the field.

Oral and Maxillofacial Surgery Secrets is intended not only to answer questions, but also to provide the additional information an oral and maxillofacial surgeon must have to provide the best care to a patient with a particular problem. With the generous help of the contributors, we have covered the topics that are important for building an adequate knowledge base necessary for supplying appropriate patient care. Of course, no one book can be the source of all the information that a good practitioner needs to know. However, for a quick, concise, and to-the-point way to find the answers to most clinical questions and issues that residents and clinicians face on a daily basis, this part of the *Secrets* series is a valuable first step.

A. Omar Abubaker, DMD, PhD
Kenneth J. Benson, DDS

Contents

Top 100 Secrets, *1*

PART I: PATIENT EVALUATION, 9

Chapter 1: Are You Ready for Your Surgery Rotation?, 9
Tabetha R. Harken, MD, MPH, and Alden H. Harken, MD

Chapter 2: Preoperative Evaluation, 13
James A. Giglio, DDS, MEd, and A. Omar Abubaker, DMD, PhD

Chapter 3: Electrocardiogram, 23
*A. Omar Abubaker, DMD, PhD, Kenneth J. Benson, DDS, and
    Frank P. Iuorno, Jr., DDS, MS*

Chapter 4: Laboratory Tests, 32
Paul W. Brinser III, DDS

Chapter 5: Diagnostic Imaging for the Oral and Maxillofacial Surgery
Patient, 52
*Corey C. Burgoyne, DMD, A. Omar Abubaker, DMD, PhD, and
    James A. Giglio, DDS, MEd*

PART II: ANESTHESIA, 65

Chapter 6: Local Anesthetics, 65
*Christopher L. Maestrello, DDS, A. Omar Abubaker, DMD, PhD, and
    Kenneth J. Benson, DDS*

Chapter 7: Intravenous Sedation, 75
Christopher L. Maestrello, DDS, and A. Omar Abubaker, DMD, PhD

Chapter 8: Inhalational Anesthesia, 82
Christopher L. Maestrello, DDS

PART III: POSTOPERATIVE CARE, 93

Chapter 9: Fluid and Electrolyte Management, 93
*Jason S. Hullett, DMD, Gaetano G. Spinnato, DMD, MD, Lubor Hlousek,
    DMD, MD, and Hamid Hajarian, MS, DDS, MD*

Chapter 10: Nutritional Support, 105
Hani F. Braidy, DMD, and Vincent B. Ziccardi, DDS, MD

Chapter 11: Postoperative Complications, 108
Robert E. Doriot, DDS, James A. Giglio, DDS, MEd, and
A. Omar Abubaker, DMD, PhD

PART IV: MEDICAL EMERGENCIES, 115

Chapter 12: Basic Life Support, 115
Mark A. Oghalai, DDS

Chapter 13: Advanced Cardiac Life Support, 120
Bashar M. Rajab, DDS, and Kathy A. Banks, DMD

Chapter 14: Advanced Trauma Life Support, 134
Edward Kozlovsky, DMD, and Shahid R. Aziz, DMD, MD, FACS

Chapter 15: Tracheostomy and Cricothyrotomy, 140
Timothy S. Bartholomew, DDS, and A. Omar Abubaker, DMD, PhD

Chapter 16: Malignant Hyperthermia, 147
Kathy A. Banks, DMD

PART V: MANAGEMENT CONSIDERATIONS, 153

Chapter 17: Cardiovascular Diseases, 153
A. Omar Abubaker, DMD, PhD, and James A. Giglio, DDS, MEd

Chapter 18: Respiratory Disorders, 172
Robert E. Doriot, DDS, and Kenneth J. Benson, DDS

Chapter 19: Hematology, 178
James A. Giglio, DDS, MEd, and Robert E. Doriot, DDS

Chapter 20: Liver Diseases, 183
Mark A. Oghalai, DDS

Chapter 21: Renal Diseases, 187
Mark A. Oghalai, DDS

Chapter 22: Endocrine Diseases, 192
Maria J. Iuorno, MD, MS

Chapter 23: The Diabetic Patient, 198
Bradley A. Gregory, DMD

Chapter 24: The Immunocompromised Surgical Patient, 208
A. Omar Abubaker, DMD, PhD, and Noah Sandler, DMD, MD

Chapter 25: The Joint Replacement Patient, 219
Kathy A. Banks, DMD

Chapter 26: The Pregnant Oral and Maxillofacial Surgery Patient, 222
Terrence R. Nedbalski, DDS, and Brenda Price, MD

PART VI: MANAGEMENT OF THE ORAL AND MAXILLOFACIAL SURGERY PATIENT, 227

Chapter 27: Applied Orofacial Anatomy, 227
A. Omar Abubaker, DMD, PhD, and Kenneth J. Benson, DDS

Chapter 28: Dentoalveolar Surgery, 248
James A. Giglio, DDS, MEd

Chapter 29: Trigeminal Nerve Injury, 256
Kenneth J. Benson, DDS, and A. Omar Abubaker, DMD, PhD

Chapter 30: Mandibular Trauma, 262
*A. Omar Abubaker, DMD, PhD, Kenneth J. Benson, DDS, Ian McDonald,
     MD, DMD, and Vincent B. Ziccardi, DDS, MD*

Chapter 31: Midfacial Fractures: Fractures of the Nose, Zygoma, Orbit, and Maxilla, 269
*A. Omar Abubaker, DMD, PhD, Vincent B. Ziccardi, DDS, MD, and
     Ian McDonald, MD, DMD*

Chapter 32: Frontal Sinus Fractures, 281
A. Omar Abubaker, DMD, PhD

Chapter 33: Soft Tissue Injuries, 283
Bashar M. Rajab, DDS, and A. Omar Abubaker, DMD, PhD

Chapter 34: Orofacial Infections and Antibiotic Use, 291
A. Omar Abubaker, DMD, PhD

Chapter 35: Temporomandibular Joint Anatomy, Pathophysiology, and Surgical Treatment, 322
*Renato Mazzonetto, DDS, PhD, Steven G. Gollehon, DDS, MD, FACS,
     Daniel B. Spagnoli, DDS, PhD, and Gregory M. Ness, DDS*

Chapter 36: Temporomandibular Disorders and Facial Pain: Biochemical and Biomechanical Basis, 329
*Steven G. Gollehon, DDS, MD, FACS, Daniel B. Spagnoli, DDS, PhD, and
     Gregory M. Ness, DDS*

Chapter 37: Dentofacial Abnormalities, 333
A. Omar Abubaker, DMD, PhD, and Bashar M. Rajab, DDS

Chapter 38: The Cleft Lip and Cleft Palate Patient, 341
A. Omar Abubaker, DMD, PhD

Chapter 39: Craniofacial Syndromes and Syndromes Affecting the Oromaxillofacial Region, 350
A. Omar Abubaker, DMD, PhD, and Kenneth J. Benson, DDS

Chapter 40: Salivary Gland Diseases, 359
Chris A. Skouteris, DMD, PhD

Chapter 41: Oral and Maxillofacial Cysts and Tumors, 365
Chris A. Skouteris, DMD, PhD

Chapter 42: Cancer of the Oral Cavity, 370
Chris A. Skouteris, DMD, PhD, and Kiki C. Marti, DMD, MD, PhD
Chapter 43: Lasers in Oral and Maxillofacial Surgery, 376
Robert A. Strauss, DDS, MD

Chapter 44: Patients Irradiated for Head and Neck Cancer, 380
A. Omar Abubaker, DMD, PhD

Chapter 45: Oral and Maxillofacial Reconstruction, 389
Vincent J. Perciaccante, DDS, and Jeffrey S. Jelic, DMD, MD

Chapter 46: Facial Cosmetic Surgery, 404
Vincent B. Ziccardi, DDS, MD

Chapter 47: Dental Implants, 410
Frank P. Iuorno, Jr., DDS, MS, and Kenneth J. Benson, DDS

Chapter 48: Preprosthetic Surgery, 417
Vincent J. Perciaccante, DDS

Chapter 49: Sleep Apnea and Snoring, 422
Kenneth J. Benson, DDS

Chapter 50: Facial Alloplastic Implants: Biomaterials and Surgical Implementation, 427
Steven G. Gollehon, DDS, MD, FACS, and John N. Kent, BA, DDS, FACD, FICD

Chapter 51: Application and Interview Processes for Oral and Maxillofacial Surgery Residency Programs, 436
Esther S. Oh, DDS

TOP 100 SECRETS

These secrets are the top 100 Board alerts. They summarize the concepts, principles, and most salient details of oral and maxillofacial surgery (OMS).

1. A remittent fever has a diurnal variation of more than 2° F but has no normal readings. Intermittent fever refers to episodes of fever separated by days of normal temperature. A quotidian fever is daily recurring fever often associated with hepatic abscess or acute cholangitis.

2. The fever pattern associated with Hodgkin's disease is called Pel-Ebstein fever. This pattern describes several days of continuous remittent fever followed by remissions for an irregular number of days.

3. Erb's point is on the side of the neck where applied pressure on the roots of the fifth and sixth cervical nerves causes paralysis of the brachial muscles. Muscles involved are of the upper arm (e.g., deltoid, biceps, brachialis anterior).

4. The level of reduced hemoglobin at which a patient becomes cyanotic is 5 g/dL.

5. Anisocoria refers to inequality of the pupils. It is a common normal variation of pupil size but can be an indication of pathology.

6. The four clotting factors synthesized in the liver are factors II, VII, IX, and X.

7. Cone beam computed tomography (CT) differs from a traditional CT scan in that cone beam CT can obtain thinner slices (0.5 mm), reducing the number of artifacts, with a reduced skin dose of radiation.

8. Amide local anesthetics are metabolized mainly by the liver (microsomal enzymes), whereas the ester types are metabolized by the plasma (pseudocholinesterase). An easy way to remember how the most commonly used local anesthetic is metabolized is *l*idocaine and *l*iver.

9. The lipid solubility determines the potency of a local anesthetic. A greater lipid solubility produces a more potent local anesthetic. The degree of protein binding of a local anesthetic agent determines the duration of a local anesthetic. A greater degree of protein binding at the receptor site will create a longer duration of action. The pKa of a local anesthetic determines its speed of onset. The closer the pKa of a local anesthetic is to the pH of tissue (7.4), the more rapid the onset.

10. Benzodiazepines exert their amnestic effect in the central nervous system (CNS) at benzodiazepine receptors, which are found on postsynaptic nerve endings in the CNS. Benzodiazepine receptors are part of the gamma-aminobutyric acid (GABA) receptor complex. The GABA receptor complex consists of two alpha subunits, to which benzodiazepines bind, and two beta subunits, with which GABA binds. A chloride ion channel exists in the middle of the receptor complex. Benzodiazepines enhance the binding of GABA to beta subunits, which opens the chloride ion channel. Chloride ions flow into the neuron, hyperpolarizing it and inhibiting action potentials.

11. Morphine, codeine, and meperidine (Demerol) cause histamine release, resulting in vasodilation and possible hypotension. Fentanyl, sufentanil, and alfentanil do not stimulate histamine release.

12. Tramadol is a unique analgesic with opioid-like activity. The drug also causes catecholamine reuptake inhibition. These properties and its much lower risk for tolerance and addiction allows it to be used as an analgesic for both acute and chronic pain management. Major side effects include sedation and dizziness. One concerning but uncommon adverse side effect is seizures. The drug should therefore be used with caution, if at all, in patients with a history or risk of seizures.

13. Plasma cholinesterase is produced in the liver and metabolizes succinylcholine (SCh) as well as ester local anesthetics and mivacurium, a nondepolarizing neuromuscular blocker (NMB). A reduced quantity of plasma cholinesterase, such as occurs with liver disease, pregnancy, malignancies, malnutrition, collagen vascular disease, and hypothyroidism, may prolong the duration of blockade with SCh.

14. Chvostek's and Trousseau's signs are seen in hypocalcemia. Chvostek's is twitching of the facial muscles as a result of tapping over the facial nerve in the preauricular area, and Trousseau's sign is carpopedal spasm due to occlusion of the brachial artery when a blood pressure cuff is applied above systolic pressure for 3 min.

15. Fluid resuscitation is preferable with 5% dextrose in water (D_5W) over lactated Ringer's solution for symptomatic hypernatremia. Otherwise D_5W is rarely indicated because the glucose load may induce osmotic diuresis.

16. According to the World Health Organization (WHO), malnutrition is "the cellular imbalance between the supply of nutrients and energy and the body's demand for them to ensure growth, maintenance, and specific functions."

17. In pediatric patients younger than ages 10-12, tracheostomy is the preferred emergency surgical airway. The small 3-mm-wide cricothyroid membrane and poorly defined anatomic landmarks make cricothyrotomy all but impossible in children.

18. Malignant hyperthermia (MH) is a hypermetabolic state involving skeletal muscle that is precipitated by certain anesthetic agents in genetically susceptible individuals. The incidence of MH is < 0.5% of all patients who are exposed to anesthetic agents. The major clinical characteristics of MH are (1) acidosis, (2) rigidity, (3) fever, (4) hypermetabolism, and (5) myoglobinuria.

19. Inhalation anesthetic drugs that are known to trigger MH include halothane, enflurane, isoflurane, desflurane, and sevoflurane. Depolarizing neuromuscular blockade agents that can trigger MH include SCh, decamethonium, and suxamethonium.

20. Creatinine is used as a sensitive, indirect measurement of glomerular filtration rate (GFR) because it is filtered by the glomeruli, but minimally secreted or reabsorbed.

21. Nonsteroidal antiinflammatory drugs (NSAIDs) inhibit prostaglandin synthesis and therefore decrease prostaglandin-associated intrinsic renal vasodilatation.

22. Classes of drugs that should be avoided in patients with renal disease are:
    1. Nephrotoxic drugs, including NSAIDs, aminoglycosides, and intravenous (IV) dyes
    2. Drugs that are converted to toxic metabolites, including meperidine and propoxyphene
    3. Drugs that contain excessive electrolytes, including penicillin G and magnesium citrate
    Antibiotics that should be avoided in patients with renal disease are cephalosporins, tetracycline, erythromycin, and aminoglycosides.

23. Analysis of human data shows that fetuses of <16 weeks who had an acute exposure of 0.5 Gy had a higher risk of growth restriction, microcephaly, and mental retardation. During the fetal period, the fetus becomes less sensitive to radiation but retains CNS sensitivity that may lead to growth restriction at term. Diagnostic radiographs that deliver < 0.05-0.1 Gy are not believed to be teratogenic. Virtually all plain film and CT scan irradiation delivers < 0.01 Gy to the fetus.

24. Fresh frozen plasma (FFP) is used for replacement of deficiencies of factors II, V, VII, IX, and XI when specific component therapy is not available or desirable. In an average-size adult, each unit of FFP increases the level of all clotting factors by 2%-3%, and most bleeding can be controlled by transfusion of FFP at a dose of 10 mL/kg of body weight.

25. Heparin is a naturally occurring conjugated polysaccharide formed by many cells, including mast cells located in connective tissue, especially in the lung. Heparin calcium is commercially prepared from porcine intestinal connective tissue, whereas the sodium form is prepared from either porcine intestinal connective tissue or bovine lung. Heparin affects the intrinsic and common pathways of blood coagulation. It prevents the formation of prothrombin activator and inhibits the action of thrombin on fibrinogen. Heparin increases the normal clotting time (4-6 min) to 6-30 min. Its duration of action is 3-4 hr.

26. Cis-atracurium is the best-choice muscle relaxant to use in a patient with liver dysfunction, because it is eliminated by Hofmann elimination and is independent of liver function.

27. HIVs are a group of retroviruses that can be acquired by the transmission of body fluids, including transfusions, and through the infection of infants by infected mothers. The specific target of the virus is the CD4 T-cell lymphocytes. The virus multiplies in the cell and eventually destroys it. Cell-mediated immunity is thereby severely affected.

28. The general categories of HIV-infected patients are:
    1. Asymptomatic patients with evidence of HIV infection demonstrated by the presence of HIV antibodies in the serum or in the secretions of these patients
    2. Patients with AIDS-related complex (ARC), manifested by presence of symptoms including lymphadenopathy, unexplained fever, weight loss, and hematologic and neurologic abnormalities
    3. Patients with AIDS as defined by the Centers for Disease Control and Prevention (CDC) (i.e., HIV infection and CD4 lymphocyte count < 200)

29. *Staphylococcus aureus* and *Staphylococcus epidermidis* are most commonly cultured from infected prosthetic joints because the majority of infections involving prosthetic joints are caused by staphylococcal contamination during the placement of the prosthesis. The bacteria that have been identified in cases of infected prosthetic joints arising by hematogenous spread of infection to the prosthesis from oral sites of infection are *Streptococcus viridans* and *Streptococcus sanguis.*

30. Penicillin affects bacteria by two mechanisms: It inhibits bacterial cell wall synthesis, and it activates endogenous bacterial autolytic processes that cause cell lysis. The bacteria must be actively dividing, and the cell wall must contain peptidoglycans for this action. The penicillin inhibits enzymes necessary for cell wall synthesis.

31. Ludwig's angina is bilateral, brawny, boardlike induration of the submandibular, sublingual, and submental spaces due to infection of these spaces. The term *angina* is used because of the respiratory distress caused by the airway obstruction. This obstruction can occur suddenly owing to the possible extension of the infection from the sublingual space posteriorly to the epiglottis, causing epiglottic edema.

32. Erysipelas is a superficial cellulitis of the skin that is caused by beta-hemolytic streptococcus and by group B streptococcus. It usually presents with warm, erythematous skin and spreads rapidly from release of hyaluronidase by the bacteria. It is associated with lymphadenopathy and fever and has an abrupt onset with acute swelling. It may affect the skin of the face. Treatment consists of parenteral penicillin.

33. Treatment of isolated mandibular deficiency usually involves mandibular advancement. Bilateral sagittal split osteotomy (BSSO) with rigid fixation is the most frequently performed procedure to accomplish this advancement. Augmentation genioplasty procedures using an alloplastic or osteoplastic technique with and without BSSO technique occasionally is used to disguise significant mandibular deficiency. Also, mandibular subapical osteotomy may help in leveling the mandibular arch.

34. Vertical maxillary excess (VME) can be treated with orthodontic intervention early in life (8-12 years) with high-pull head gear or open bite Bionater to control vertical growth of the maxilla. If successful, such treatment may resolve the skeletal abnormalities, and ultimately the soft tissues and other facial structures grow accordingly. However, when an adult presents with this condition, it usually is treated with LeFort I osteotomy and superior repositioning of the maxilla. Recently, with use of skeletal anchorage, skeletal open bite can be closed with orthodontic treatment alone through intrusion of the posterior teeth.

35. Neurosensory deficits of the inferior alveolar nerve following BSSO is one of the most significant concerns with this procedure. Complications occur in 20%-85% of surgeries. However, the incidence is only 9% at 1 year after surgery. This complication is more common in patients older than age 40 and in patients who undergo simultaneous genioplasty.

36. Transverse expansion of the maxilla is the most unstable orthognathic procedure. The greatest relapse is seen in the second molar region with an average of 50% loss of surgical expansion. After 1 year, inferior maxillary positioning and mandibular setbacks were also found to be less predictable than in other surgical techniques.

37. Mandibular prognathism may be present in the following syndromes: basal cell nevus syndrome (Gorlin's syndrome), Klinefelter's syndrome, Marfan's syndrome, osteogenesis imperfecta, and Waardenburg's syndrome. The following syndromes may be associated with midface deficiency: achondroplasia, Apert's syndrome, cleidocranial dysplasia, Crouzon's syndrome, Marshall's syndrome, Pfeiffer's syndrome, and Stickler's syndrome.

38. Surgical repair of cleft lip is generally carried out at 10-14 weeks of age. However, traditionally the time of repair of cleft lip often is based on the Rule of Tens. According to this rule, cleft lip can be closed when the infant is 10 weeks old, the hemoglobin is 10 g/dL, and the infant's weight is 10 lb.

39. Rapid tumor growth or a sudden growth acceleration in a long-standing salivary mass, pain, and peripheral facial nerve paralysis are some of the signs and symptoms suggestive of salivary gland malignancy. However, it has been reported that peripheral facial nerve paralysis can be associated with acute suppurative parotitis, nonspecific parotitis with inflammatory pseudotumor, amyloidosis, and sarcoidosis of the parotid.

40. Sialoliths in the early stage of development are small and not adequately mineralized to be visible radiographically. It has also been reported in the literature that 30%-50% of parotid and 10%-20% of submandibular sialoliths are radiolucent. These radiolucent sialoliths can be visualized indirectly by the imaging defect that they produce on sialography, or directly through sialoendoscopy.

41. Fine-needle aspiration (FNA) biopsy is an efficacious modality in the diagnosis of salivary gland pathology. The specificity of the procedure ranges from 88%-99% and the sensitivity is 71%-93%.

42. Sublingual salivary gland tumors comprise < 1% of all salivary gland neoplasms. These tumors are predominantly malignant (>80%) and are usually adenoid cystic or mucoepidermoid carcinomas.

43. Viral parotitis infection is bilateral and is preceded by prodromal signs and symptoms of 1-2 days' duration, including fever, malaise, loss of appetite, chills, headache, sore throat, and preauricular tenderness. Purulent discharge from Stensen's duct is rare but, if present, might be the result of the development of secondary bacterial sialadenitis. Lab investigations reveal elevated serum titers for mumps or influenza virus, leukopenia, relative lymphocytosis, and high levels of serum amylase.

44. Syndromes that can affect the salivary glands are primary Sjögren's syndrome, which is usually characterized by parotid and lacrimal gland enlargement, xerostomia, and xerophthalmia; secondary Sjögren's syndrome, which involves autoimmune parotitis that occurs with rheumatoid arthritis, lupus, systemic sclerosis, thyroiditis, primary biliary cirrhosis, and mixed collagen disease; and sarcoidosis, which may involve the parotid gland. Sarcoidosis of the parotid gland along with fever, lacrimal adenitis, uveitis, and facial nerve paralysis is called Heerfordt's syndrome. Recently, a sicca syndrome–like condition has been recognized in HIV-positive children. This condition presents with parotid gland enlargement, xerostomia, and lymphadenopathy.

45. Incisional biopsy is indicated for the diagnosis of suspected systemic disease with parotid involvement, particularly when FNA biopsy findings are inconclusive. Systemic conditions in which incisional parotid biopsy can be of great diagnostic value include sarcoidosis, Sjögren's syndrome, lymphoma, and sialosis.

46. The most common benign tumor of minor and major salivary glands is pleomorphic adenoma.

47. The most common malignant tumors of minor and major salivary glands are mucoepidermoid carcinoma in the parotid gland and adenoid cystic carcinoma in the submandibular, sublingual, and minor salivary glands.

48. The methods that have been used for the surgical management of drooling include bilateral submandibular duct relocation to the posterior tonsillar pillar (most preferred); bilateral parotid duct relocation to the posterior tonsillar pillar; bilateral parotid duct diversion with autogenous venous grafts; bilateral submandibular duct relocation plus parotid duct ligation; bilateral submandibular and parotid duct ligation; bilateral submandibular gland excision with parotid duct ligation, if the problem is very severe; and chorda tympani neurectomy (only as an adjunct procedure in carefully selected cases).

49. Evidence suggests that odontogenic keratocysts can be managed effectively by a conservative approach. Good results have been achieved with decompression or marsupialization with or without later cystectomy, enucleation combined with excision of overlying mucosa and Carnoy solution application to the bony defect, and enucleation combined with liquid nitrogen application to the osseous cavity. It appears that although odontogenic keratocysts are notorious for their capricious nature relative to their tendency to recur, block resection of these lesions is hardly justifiable.

50. The incidence of development of cystic lesions around retained, asymptomatic, impacted mandibular third molars is 0.3%-37%.

51. Thyroglossal duct, dermoid, and epidermoid cysts are the most common soft tissue cysts in children. The most common benign soft tissue tumor in children is hemangioma. Odontoma is the most common benign odontogenic intraosseous tumor in children; ossifying fibroma is the most common nonodontogenic tumor in children.

52. A Sistrunk procedure is a surgical procedure used for the excision of thyroglossal duct cysts. In this operation, the central portion of the hyoid bone is always excised. The retrohyoid cyst tract is dissected and excised at the base of the tongue together with the area of the foramen cecum.

53. The most common anatomic sites for oral cancer are the tongue and floor of the mouth. Other sites might be more common in different parts of the world because of certain predisposing ethnic, cultural, or other factors.

54. Carcinoma in situ is an epithelial dysplasia that includes all the layers of the epithelium but does not extend beyond the basal layer. Once the malignant cells have penetrated the basal layer into the lamina propria, early invasive squamous cell carcinoma has been established. If tumor invasiveness extends deeper into the tissues, involving fat, muscle, or other structures, then true invasive squamous cell carcinoma has evolved.

55. The sentinel node is any lymph node receiving direct lymphatic drainage from a primary tumor site.

56. The most common laser used in the OMS practice is carbon dioxide (CO_2) laser. Because of their high affinity for tissue water found in the epidermis and dermis, the CO_2 and Er:YAG lasers are the most common lasers used for skin resurfacing techniques.

57. Wound infections from human bites are frequently caused by *Streptococcus* and *Staphylococcus* organisms. Serious infections may also be associated with *Eikenella*. Prophylactic antibiotic coverage with penicillin or amoxicillin-clavulanic acid is recommended. Unlike human bites, 50%-75% of infections in animal bites are caused by *Pasteurella multocida*. Amoxicillin-clavulanic acid is recommended for prophylaxis in animal bites. Tetanus immunization is required for all bites, and rabies prophylaxis may be required when animals exhibit suspicious behavior.

58. In general, for most oral and maxillofacial bony defects, 10 mL of noncompacted corticocancellous bone is required for every 1 cm of defect to be reconstructed.

59. The seven anatomic structures that attach to the anterior iliac crest are the fasciae latae, inguinal ligament, tensor fasciae latae, sartorius, iliacus, and the internal and external abdominal oblique muscles.

60. Defects of approximately one third of the lower lip and one quarter of the upper lip can be closed primarily without resulting in a significant microstomia.

61. The location of the oral defect determines where a tongue flap is based (whether it should

be an anteriorly based or posteriorly based flap). For defects of the soft palate, retromolar region, and posterior buccal mucosa, a posteriorly based flap is used. Anteriorly based flaps are used for hard palate defects, defects of the anterior buccal mucosa, anterior floor of the mouth, or lips.

62. The measurement of dose of radiation has changed from rads (100 ergs/g) to Grays (Gy; 1 joule/kg): 1 Gy = 100 rads = 100 cGy.

63. The incidence of osteoradionecrosis (ORN) ranges from 1%-44.2% with an overall incidence of 11.8% in most studies published before 1968. Recent studies showed incidences of 5%-15% with an overall incidence of 5.4%. ORN has a bimodal incidence, peaking at 12 months and again at 24-60 months. However, it can occur as late as 30 years later. It is often related to traumatic injuries such as preirradiation extraction (4.4%), postirradiation extraction (5.8%), and denture trauma (<1%). ORN may occur spontaneously (albeit rarely) owing to progression of periapical or periodontal disease.

64. The "new concept" of pathophysiology of ORN is based on a radiation-induced, wound-healing defect. According to this hypothesis, the pathophysiologic sequence is (1) irradiation; (2) hypovascular, hypoxic, and hypocellular tissue (the "3 H's"); (3) tissue breakdown; and (4) a nonhealing wound in which the tissues' metabolic demand exceeds supply.

65. Hyperbaric oxygen therapy is an administration of 100% oxygen via head tent, mask, or endotracheal tube within a special chamber at 2.4 atmospheric absolute (ATA) pressure for 90 min each session. The treatment should be delivered once a day, five times ("dives") a week.

66. Bisphosphonate-related osteonecrosis (BRON) of the jaw is a condition of painful exposure of bone in the mandible and maxilla of a patient receiving various forms of bisphosphonate. Most studies have shown that the largest number of patients reported to have bisphosphonate osteonecrosis are those receiving pamidronate intravenously (Aredia, Novartis Pharmaceutical, East Hanover, NJ) and patients receiving zoledronate (Zometa, Novartis Pharmaceutical, East Hanover, NJ), and the fewest are those receiving alendronate (Fosamax, Merck & Co., West Point, Pa).

67. Submental liposuction is performed at the supraplatysmal plane, a distinct layer of subcutaneous fatty tissue located below the dermis at which the procedure is safely performed in a near bloodless field. The area treated from the submental incision is bounded by the anterior border of the sternocleidomastoid muscle, inferior border of the mandible, and superior border of the thyroid.

68. The chemical properties and interface chemistry of dental implants are determined by the oxide layer and not by the metal of the implant. Therefore the dense oxide film of a titanium implant, for example, is about 100 angstroms (Å) thick. This is considered a normal space between implant and bone in an osseointegrated titanium implant.

69. Torque testing can be done to check for osseointegration at the time of implant uncovering. Ideally, one should be able to place a force of 10-20 N/cm without unscrewing an implant if it is successfully osseointegrated. Other clinical subjective signs of integration are percussion and immobility when placing a fixture mount or impression coping on the implant. When a lateral force of 5 lb is applied, no movement should be seen. Horizontal mobility of > 1 mm or movement < 500 g of force indicates a failed implant.

70. The most useful radiographic sign of implant failure is loss of crestal bone. Early crestal bone loss is a sign of stress at the permucosal site. At least 40% of the trabecular bone must be lost to be detected radiographically. Rapid progressive bone loss indicates failure. This will usually be accompanied by pain on percussion or function.

71. Magnetic resonance imaging (MRI) and CT scans are not contraindicated in patients with pure titanium implants. Most CT scanners can subtract titanium and other metals from the image and eliminate the scatter images.

72. The average size of the maxillary sinus is 14.75 mL, with a range of 9.5-20 mL. On average, the width is 2.5 cm; height, 3.75 cm; and depth, 3 cm.

73. Split-thickness skin grafts (STSGs) can be of varying thickness. An STSG is composed of the epidermis layer and part of the dermis layer. The STSG can be classified as thin, intermediate, or thick, based on the amount of dermis included. STSGs are between 0.010 and 0.025 inch.

74. The thinner a skin graft, the more the contraction. A thin STSG contracts more than an intermediate STSG, which contracts more than a thick STSG. Full-thickness skin grafts hardly contract at all. Primary contraction is caused by elastic fibers in the skin graft as soon as it has been cut. This can be overcome when a graft is sutured in place. Secondary contraction begins about postoperative day 10 and continues for up to 6 months.

75. Plasmic imbibition is the process by which a skin graft absorbs a plasmalike fluid from its underlying recipient bed. It is absorbed into the capillary network by capillary action. This process is the initial means of survival for a skin graft and continues for approximately 48 hr.

76. Obstructive sleep apnea (OSA) is characterized by repetitive, discrete episodes of decreased airflow (hypopnea) or frank cessation of airflow (apnea) for at least 10-sec duration in association with >2% decrease in oxygen hemoglobin saturation. Obstructive events occur during stages III and IV and the rapid eye movement (REM) stage, which are the deeper stages of sleep. Pharyngeal wall collapse is more common during these stages because the muscles are most relaxed.

77. Respiratory disturbance index (RDI) represents the number of obstructive respiratory events/hr of sleep. The RDI, along with oximetry, is the primary clinical indicator in the diagnosis of obstructive sleep apnea syndrome (OSAS). RDI is calculated as RDI = apnea + hypopnea/total sleep time × 60. An RDI of 5 is the upper limit of normal.

78. Virchow's triad is the name given to the three chief causes of deep venous thrombosis (DVT): (1) damage to the endothelial lining of the vessel, (2) venous stasis, and (3) a change in blood constituents attributable to postoperative increase in the number and adhesiveness of the patient's platelets.

79. Homans' sign is pain in the calf that is elicited by forced dorsiflexion of the foot. It was once considered pathognomonic for the presence of DVT, but it is no longer taught because performing this maneuver can increase the risk of movement of an existing thrombus.

80. For every 1° C rise in body temperature, there is a corresponding 9-10 beats/min increase in the patient's heart rate.

81. The most common cause of dysuria in the immediate postoperative period is related to the agents incorporated in the administration of general anesthesia which can inhibit the micturitic reflex, and the patient can suffer bladder distention, which itself may inhibit the ability to micturate. Treatment of postoperative dysuria should begin simply by having the patient stand by or sit on the toilet while running water in the sink. If this does not help and there is no evidence of a hypovolemic state, then the patient should be catheterized. If the residual measures >300 mL, then the catheter should be left in overnight.

82. Some common causes of postoperative nausea and vomiting are hypoxia, hypotension, and narcotics. Postoperative nausea and vomiting occurs more frequently in children than in adults and more commonly in women than in men.

83. A surgical wound infection or *surgical site infection* (SSI) is an infection that occurs typically 12 hr–7 days postoperatively but can occur within 30 days of surgery unless a foreign body is left in situ. In the case of implanted foreign material, 1 year must elapse before surgery can be excluded as causative.

84. The ideal location for applying pressure for external chest compressions in infants is one fingerwidth below the nipple line, with care being taken to stay off the xiphoid process. Use two fingers to perform the compressions.

85. The four conditions other than asystole that can lead to a flat line tracing on electrocardiogram (ECG) are (1) fine ventricular fibrillation, (2) loose electrode leads, (3) no power, and (4) signal gain is turned down.

86. Drugs that can be administered through the endotracheal tube are lidocaine, epinephrine, atropine, and Narcan (L-E-A-N). Administer all tracheal medications at 2-2.5 times the recommended IV dosage, diluted in 10 mL of normal saline or distilled water. Tracheal absorption is greater with distilled water as the diluent than with normal saline, but distilled water has a greater adverse effect on PaO_2.

87. Kiesselbach's plexus of septum arterioles is the source of 90% of nosebleeds. Four anastomosed arteries make up this plexus: the sphenopalatine, anterior ethmoidal, greater palatine, and superior labial arteries. The nasopalatine branch of the descending palatine artery anastomoses with septal branches of the sphenopalatine artery, the anterior ethmoidal artery, and superior lateral branches of the superior labial branch of the facial artery. Traumatic nasal bleeding can be caused by laceration of the nasal mucosa, and any of the nasal vessels can be the source of the bleeding.

88. The nasolacrimal duct lies within the thin, bony wall between the maxillary sinus and the nasal cavity. The duct ends at the inferior nasal meatus through the valve of Hasner. The position of the nasolacrimal duct beneath the inferior turbinate is 11-14 mm posterior to the piriform aperture and 11-17 mm above the nasal floor.

89. The sebaceous glands of the eyelid are called the glands of Zeis. The sweat glands of the eyelid are called the glands of Moll.

90. "Crocodile tears" is a condition that results after injury to the fibers of the facial nerve carrying parasympathetic secretory fibers that normally innervate the salivary gland. The injury causes the fibers to heal in contact with fibers supplying the lacrimal gland, leading to "crying" when the patient eats.

91. All facial muscles except the mentalis, levator angularis superioris, and buccinator receive their innervation along their deep surfaces. However, because these three muscles are located deep within the facial soft tissue and lie deep to the plane of the facial nerve, they receive their innervation along their superficial surfaces. All other facial muscles of expression are located superficial to the plane of the facial nerve and thus receive their innervation along their deep or posterior surfaces.

92. The anulus of Zinn, or common tendinous ring in the orbit, is the fibrous thickening of the periosteum from which the rectus muscles originate.

93. Tenon's capsule is a fascial structure that subdivides the orbital cavity into two halves—an anterior (or precapsular) segment and a posterior (or retrocapsular) segment. The ocular globe occupies only the anterior half of the orbital cavity. The posterior half of the orbital cavity is filled with fat, muscles, vessels, and nerves that supply the ocular globe and extraocular muscles and provide sensation to the soft tissue surrounding the orbit.

94. The inferior alveolar nerve is most often located buccal and slightly apical to the roots of a mandibular third molar. The root of the tooth that is most often dislodged into the maxillary sinus during an extraction procedure is the palatal root of the maxillary first molar. The most reliable signs of a potential nerve injury during extraction of an impacted mandibular third molar are diversion of canal, interruption of canal borders, and darkening of roots.

95. Tinel's sign is a provocative test of regenerating nerve sprouts in which light percussion over the nerve elicits a distal tingling sensation. It is used as a sign of small fiber recovery but is poorly correlated with functional recovery and easily confused with neuroma formation.

96. The incidence of inferior alveolar, lingual, and, less frequently, long buccal nerve injury during mandibular third molar removal ranges between 0.6% and 5.0%. In general, the incidence of inferior alveolar nerve (IAN) injuries is higher than that of the lingual nerve; Factors such as age, surgical technique, and proximity of the nerve to the tooth influence the incidence of these injuries. More than 96% of patients with lingual nerve injuries recover spontaneously.

97. The average rate of an injured axon's forward growth is approximately 1-2 mm/day.

98. Mixed motor and sensory nerves are best treated with the perineural and group fascicular suturing. The sensory IAN can be treated with the epineural suture technique.

99. The sural nerve graft is the best donor site for an interpositional graft for an inferior alveolar nerve defect of approximately 25 mm. The sural nerve can provide up to 30 mm of graft harvest. It provides sensation to the posterior and lateral aspect of the leg and foot. It also has up to 50% fewer axons and smaller axonal size than the inferior alveolar nerve. Because of primary contracture, the length of the harvested nerve should be at least 25% longer than the defect.

100. More than 50% of mandibular fractures are multiple. For this reason, if one fracture is noted along the jaw, the patient should be examined closely for evidence of additional fractures. Radiographic films must be scrutinized carefully for discrete fracture lines. Also, associated injuries are present in 43% of all patients with mandibular fracture, most of whom were involved in vehicular accidents. Cervical spine fractures were found in 11% of this group of patients. It is imperative to rule out cervical neck fractures, especially in patients who are intoxicated or unconscious.

Part I
Patient Evaluation

1. ARE YOU READY FOR YOUR SURGERY ROTATION?*

Tabetha R. Harken, MD, MPH, and Alden H. Harken, MD

Surgery is a participatory, team, and contact sport. Present yourself to patients, residents, and attendings with enthusiasm (which covers a multitude of sins), punctuality (type A people do not like to wait), and cleanliness (you must look, act, and smell like a doctor).

1. Why should you introduce yourself to each patient and ask about his or her chief complaint?

Symptoms are perception, and perception is more important than reality. To a patient, the chief complaint is not simply a matter of life and death—it is much more important. Patients routinely are placed into compromising, uncomfortable, embarrassing, and undignified predicaments. Patients are people, however; they have interests, concerns, anxieties, and a story. As a student, you have an opportunity to place your patient's chief complaint into the context of the rest of his or her life. This skill is important, and the patient will *always* be grateful. You can serve a real purpose as a listener and translator for the patient and his or her family.

Patients want to trust and love you. This trust in surgical therapy is a formidable tool. The more a patient understands about his or her disease, the more the patient can participate in getting better. Recovery is faster if the patient helps. Similarly, the more the patient understands about his or her therapy (including its side effects and potential complications), the more effective the therapy is (this principle is not in the textbooks). You can be your patient's interpreter. This is the fun of surgery (and medicine).

---

*Reprinted from Harken TR, Harken AH: Are you ready for your surgery rotation? In Harken AH, Moore EE (eds): Abernathy's Surgical Secrets, 5th ed. Philadelphia, 2005, Mosby.

2.   What is the correct answer to almost all questions?
Thank you. Gratitude is an invaluable tool on the wards.

3.   Are there any simple rules from the trenches?

- **Get along with the nurses**. The nurses do know more than the rest of us about the codes, routines, and rituals of making the wards run smoothly. They may not know as much about pheochromocytomas and intermediate filaments—but about the stuff that matters, they know a lot. Acknowledge that, and they will take you under their wings and teach you a *ton!*
- **Help out**. If your residents look busy, they probably are. So, if you ask how you can help and they are too busy even to answer, asking again probably wouldn't be very high-yield. Always leap at the opportunity to shag x-rays, track down lab results, and retrieve a bag of blood from the bank. The team will recognize your enthusiasm and reward your contributions.
- **Get scutted**. We all would like a secretary, but one is not going to be provided on this rotation. Your residents do a lot of their own scut work without you even knowing about it. So if you feel like scut work is beneath you, perhaps you should think about another profession (maybe real estate or hair styling).
- **Work hard**. This rotation is an apprenticeship. If you work hard, you will get a realistic idea of what it means to be a resident (and even a practicing doc) in this specialty. (This has big advantages when you are selecting a type of internship.)
- **Stay in the loop**. In the beginning, you may feel like you are not a real part of the team. If you are persistent and reliable, however, soon your residents will trust you with more important jobs.
- **Educate yourself, then educate your patients**. Here is one of the rewarding places (as indicated in question 1) where you can soar to the top of the team. Talk to your patients about everything (including their disease and therapy), and they will love you for it.
- **Maintain a positive attitude**. As a medical student, you may feel you are not a crucial part of the team. Even if you are incredibly smart, you are unlikely to be making the crucial management decisions. So what does that leave? *Attitude.* If you are enthusiastic and interested, your residents will enjoy having you around, and they will work to keep you involved and satisfied. A dazzlingly intelligent but morose complainer is better suited for a rotation in the morgue. Remember, your resident is likely following 15 sick patients, gets paid less than $2/hr, and hasn't slept more than 5 hr in the last 3 days. Simple things such as smiling and saying thank you (when someone teaches you) go an incredibly long way and are rewarded on all clinical rotations with experience and good grades.
- **Have fun!** This is the most exciting, gratifying, rewarding, and fun profession—and is light years better than whatever is second best (this is not just our opinion).

4.   What is the best approach to surgical notes?
Surgical notes should be succinct (Box 1-1). Most surgeons still move their lips when they read.

Box 1-1	*Best Approach to Surgical Notes*

Admission Orders

Admit to 5 West (attending's name)
Condition: Stable
Diagnosis: Abdominal pain; r/o appendicitis
Vital signs: q4h
Parameters: Please call HO for:
               T > 38° C
               160 < BP < 90
               120 < HR < 60
Diet: NPO
Fluids: 1000 LR w 20 mEq KCl @ 100 mL/hr
Med[ication]s: ASA 650 mg PR prn for T > 38.5° C
Thank you.
Sign your name/leave space for resident's signature
(your beeper number)
Key: r/o = rule out, q = every, HO = house officer, T = temperature, BP = systolic blood pressure, HR = heart rate, NPO = nothing by mouth (this includes water and pills), ASA = aspirin, PR = per rectum, prn = as needed. Other useful abbreviations: OOB = out of bed, BRP = bathroom privileges.
Note: You cannot be too polite or too grateful to patients or nurses.

History and Physical Exam (H&P)

Mrs. O'Flaherty is a 55 y/o w/w [white woman] admitted with a cc [chief complaint]: "My stomach hurts." Pt [patient] was in usual state of excellent health until 2 days PTA [prior to admission] when she noted gradual onset of crampy midepigastric pain. Pain is now severe (7/10—7 on a scale of 10) and recurring q5min. Pt described + vomiting (+ bile, – blood) [with bile, without blood].

PMH [*Past Medical History*]
Hosp[italizations]:   Pneumonia (1991)
    Childbirth (1970, 1972)
    Surg[ery]—splenectomy for trauma (1967)
Allergies: Codeine, shellfish
ETOH [alcohol]:   Social
Tobacco: 1 ppd [pack per day] × 25 years

ROS [*Review of Systems*]
Resp[iratory]:   Productive cough
Cardiac: ō chest pain [ō = not observed, noncontributory, or not here]
    ō MI [myocardial infarction]
Renal: ō dysuria
    ō frequency
Neuro[logic]:   WNL [within normal limits]

Physical Exam (PE)
BP: 140/90   *HR:* 100 (regular)
RR [respiratory rate]: 16 breaths/min   *Temp:* 38.2° C

Continued

Box 1-1	*Best Approach to Surgical Notes—cont'd*

WD [well developed], WN [well nourished], mildly obese, 55 y/o in moderate abdominal distress

HEENT [head, eyes, ears, nose, and throat]: WNL

Resp: Clear lungs bilat[erally]
ō wheeze

Heart: ō m [murmur]

Abdomen: RSR [regular sinus rhythm]
Mildly distended, crampy, midepigastric pain
High-pitched rushes that coincide with crampy pain
Tender to palpation (you do not need to hurt the patient to find this out)
ō rebound

Rectal: (Always do—never defer the rectal exam on your surgical rotation)
Hematest—negative for blood
No masses, no tenderness

Pelvic: No masses
No adnexal tenderness
No chandelier sign (if motion of cervix makes your patient hit the chandelier)
No pelvic inflammatory disease (PID; gonorrhea)

Extremities: Full ROM [range of motion]
ō edema
Bounding (3+) pulses

Imp[ression]:   Abdominal pain
r/o SB [small bowel] obstruction 2° [secondary] to adhesions

Rx: NG [nasogastric] tube
IV fluids
Op[erative] consent
Type and hold
[Signature]

Notes on the Surgical H&P

- A surgical H&P should be succinct and focused on the patient's problem.
- Begin with the chief complaint (in the patient's words).
- Is the problem new or chronic?
- PMH: Always include prior hospitalizations and medications.
- ROS: Restrict review to organ systems (lung, heart, kidneys, and nervous system) that may affect this admission.
- PE: Always begin with vital signs (including respiration and temperature)—that is why these signs are vital.
- *Rebound* means inflammatory peritoneal irritation or peritonitis.

Box 1-1   *Best Approach to Surgical Notes—cont'd*

Preop[erative] Note

The preoperative note is a checklist confirming that you and the patient are ready for the planned surgical procedure. Place this note in the Progress Notes:

Preop dx [diagnosis]:	SB obstruction 2° to adhesions
CXR [chest x-ray]:	Clear
ECG [electrocardiogram]:	NSR w/ST-T wave changes
Blood:	Type and crossmatch × 2 u
Consent:	In chart

Operative Note

The operative note should provide anyone who encounters the patient after surgery with all the needed information:

Preop dx:	SB obstruction
Postop dx:	Same, all bowel viable
Procedure:	Exp[loratory] Lap[arotomy] with lysis of adhesions
Surgeon:	Name him/her
Assistants:	List them
Anesthesia:	GEA [general endotracheal anesthesia]
I&O [intake and output]:	In: 1200 mL Ringer's lactate (R/L)
	Out: 400 mL urine
EBL [estimated blood loss]:	50 mL
Specimen:	None
Drains:	None
	[Sign your name]

---

2. PREOPERATIVE EVALUATION

James A. Giglio, DDS, MEd, and A. Omar Abubaker, DMD, PhD

---

1. Which portion of a complete medical history is recorded in the patient's own words?

The chief complaint.

2. What is the review of systems?

This is an outline for review of the patient's medical history that inquires about specific symptoms associated with each organ system of the body.

3. What are the goals of the preoperative evaluation?

The preoperative evaluation consists of gathering information about the patient and formulating an anesthetic and surgical plan. The overall objective is reduction of perioperative morbidity and mortality.

Ideally (and through an interview, physical exam, and review of pertinent current and past medical records), the patient's physical and mental status is determined. All recent medications are recorded, and a thorough drug allergy history is taken. The patient should be questioned about use of cigarettes, alcohol, and illicit drugs. The patient's prior anesthetic experience is of particular interest—specifically, if there is a history of any anesthetic complications, problems with intubation, delayed emergence, malignant hyperthermia, prolonged neuromuscular blockade, or postoperative nausea and vomiting. From this evaluation, a decision can be made whether any preoperative tests or consultations are indicated, and an anesthetic care plan can be formulated. If done well, the preoperative evaluation establishes a trusting doctor-patient relationship that significantly diminishes patient anxiety and measurably influences postoperative recovery and outcome.

4.   What is an informed consent?
Informed consent is communication with the patient so he or she understands the procedures and the possible intraoperative and postoperative complications, including postoperative pain. The alternatives, potential complications, and risks vs. benefits are discussed, and the patient's questions are answered.

5.   What is the American Society of Anesthesiologists' (ASA) physical status classification?
The ASA classification was first established in 1940 for the purposes of statistical studies and hospital records. It is useful for both outcome comparisons and as a convenient means of communicating the physical status of a patient among anesthesiologists. The five classes, as last modified in 1961, are:
- **Class 1:** Healthy patient, no medical problems
- **Class 2:** Mild systemic disease
- **Class 3:** Severe systemic disease, but not incapacitating
- **Class 4:** Severe systemic disease that is a constant threat to life
- **Class 5:** Moribund, not expected to live 24 hr regardless of operation

An *e* is added to the status number to designate an emergency operation. An organ donor is usually designated as a class 6.

6.   What is the difference between a physical sign and a symptom?
In general, a symptom is an abnormal sensation felt by the patient, whereas a sign can be seen, felt, or heard by the examiner.

7.   What are the four vital signs?

1. Pulse   3. Temperature
2. Blood pressure   4. Respiration rate

8.   What are the four methods used in a physical exam?

1. Inspection   3. Percussion
2. Palpation   4. Auscultation

9.   What is the difference between a remittent fever and an intermittent fever?
A *remittent fever* has a diurnal variation of more than 2° F but has no normal readings. *Intermittent fever* refers to episodes of fever separated by days of normal temperature.

10.   What is quotidian fever?
A daily recurring fever often associated with hepatic abscess or acute cholangitis.

11.   What fever pattern is associated with Hodgkin's disease?
Pel-Ebstein fever. This pattern describes several days of continuous remittent fever followed by remissions for an irregular number of days.

12. What are macules, papules, and nodules?

Macules are localized changes in skin color that occur in various shapes, sizes, and colors and are not palpable. Papules are solid and elevated, with a diameter of less than 5 mm. Nodules are also solid and elevated but extend deeper into the skin than papules and usually have diameters greater than 5 mm.

13. What is PERRLA?

PERRLA refers to the eye exam findings of *p*upils *e*qual, *r*ound, and *r*eactive to *l*ight and *a*ccommodation.

14. What is a pterygium?

A raised, yellow plaque, termed the *pinguecula,* is normal and found on a horizontal plane between the canthus and limbus of the eye. In response to chronic irritation, the pinguecula will grow to extend a vascular membrane, termed *pterygium*, over the limbus toward the center of the cornea. Vision may become obstructed.

15. When examining the ear, where is the light reflex normally located and what conditions will alter its location or appearance?

The light reflex is normally noted at about the five o'clock position. Conditions that can alter its appearance include retracted drumhead, serous otitis, bulging drumhead, air bubbles in serous otitis, and a perforated drumhead.

16. What is Darwin's tubercle?

Darwin's tubercle is a fusiform swelling that occasionally develops on the surface of the pinna above the midpoint of the helix on the ear.

17. What is the difference between bone conduction and air conduction when applied to tuning fork tests of hearing?

Air conduction implies sound transmission through the ear canal, tympanic membrane, and ossicle, to the cochlea, and finally to the eighth, or auditory, nerve. Bone conduction relies on the transmission of sound through the skull to the cochlea and to the auditory nerve.

18. What is the difference between the Rinne and Weber tests of auditory function?

The Rinne test makes use of air conduction and bone conduction, whereas the Weber test makes use of bone conduction. A Rinne test is considered normal or positive when sound is heard better by air conduction than by bone conduction. In a Weber test of hearing, a conductive deafness will cause sound to be referred to the side of the deaf ear. The Weber test checks lateralization.

19. What chain of lymph nodes is palpable along the anterior border of the sternocleido-mastoid muscle?

The superior cervical chain, which drains lymph from the skin and neck.

20. Where is Erb's point?

On the side of the neck where applied pressure on the roots of the fifth and sixth cervical nerves causes paralysis of the brachial muscles. Muscles of the upper arm are involved (e.g., deltoid, biceps, brachialis anterior).

21. Which ribs are referred to as "floating" ribs?

The eleventh and twelfth ribs.

22. Where is the angle of Louis?

The angle of Louis is located at the junction between the manubrium and the body of the sternum; it marks the articulation of the second rib on the sternum. It is also known as the angle of Ludwig.

23. What structure lies under the clavicle?
   The first rib.

24. What is Kussmaul breathing?
   Kussmaul breathing is an increase in both rate and depth of respiration and is synonymous with hyperventilation.

25. What is the difference between hyperventilation and hyperpnea?
   Hyperventilation is an increase in both rate and depth of respiration, whereas hyperpnea is an increase in depth only.

26. What is Cheyne-Stokes breathing?
   Cheyne-Stokes breathing is alternating hyperpnea, shallow respiration, and apnea.

27. What is stridor?
   A high-pitched respiratory sound, such as the inspiratory sound heard often in acute laryngeal obstruction.

28. Where is the intercostal angle?
   The inferior margins of the seventh, eighth, and ninth costicartilages meet in the midline (at the infrasternal notch) to form the intercostal angle. It normally measures less than 90 degrees and is increased in obstructive lung disease.

29. At what level of reduced hemoglobin does a patient become cyanotic?
   5 g/dL.

30. What is the diaphragmatic effect on the heart?
   During inspiration, the diaphragm descends, stretching the heart from its anchorage in the fascia surrounding the aorta and pulmonary artery. The vertical cardiac axis becomes elongated, the transverse direction narrowed, and filling of the right ventricle is delayed.

31. When does blood from the coronary arteries perfuse the heart muscle?
   During diastole.

32. What is the PMI?
   The *p*oint of *m*aximum *i*mpulse of the heart. At the beginning of systole the heart is rotated forward toward the chest wall, where the impulse can be felt. The PMI is normally felt at the fifth interspace between the ribs, 1-2 cm medial to the left midclavicular line.

33. What causes the heart sounds?
   At the beginning of systole the ventricles contract, increasing the ventricular pressure and causing the mitral and tricuspid valves to close. Blood rebounds in the ventricles, transmitting vibrations to the chest wall, which can be heard with the stethoscope as S_1. Blood then courses silently through the aorta and pulmonary arteries. The second sound occurs when the ventricles relax in diastole, ventricular pressure decreases, and the aortic and pulmonary valves close. The backflow of blood against these valves sets up another series of vibrations audible as the second heart sound S_2.

34. What is the difference between a physiologic and an organic heart murmur?
   Heart murmurs are caused by disruption of the normal laminar flow of blood. Causes include regurgitation of blood, blood flow through narrowed or stenotic valves or vessels, shunting of blood, increased rate of blood flow, and decreased blood viscosity. An organic

murmur is pathologic and caused by some intrinsic cardiac disease or defect, such as deformed or stenotic heart valves, ventricular septal defects, or a patent ductus arteriosus. Physiologic murmurs are not pathologic and usually result from an altered metabolic state, such as in pregnancy or early childhood.

35. What is a flow murmur?

A flow murmur is induced when the velocity of normal blood is increased as it courses through a normal heart.

36. What are the grades of intensity of heart murmurs?

Intensity of heart murmur is graded on a scale of 1-6. The subjectivity of this scale is minimized by the following guidelines:

- **Grade 1:** Very faint and heard only when paying close attention
- **Grade 2:** Faint, but unmistakably present
- **Grade 3:** Clearly louder than faint, but not associated with a thrill
- **Grade 4:** Loud and associated with a thrill
- **Grade 5:** Very loud but requiring a stethoscope partly on the chest to be heard
- **Grade 6:** Able to be heard with stethoscope off the chest

37. What are Korotkoff sounds?

The sounds produced by the turbulence created when the inflated blood pressure cuff disrupts normal arterial laminar blood flow.

38. How high should the cuff be inflated when measuring blood pressure?

The cuff should be placed over the antecubital fossa and the brachial artery palpated at the lower edge of the cuff. The radial pulse should be palpated while the cuff is being inflated. Inflation should continue to 30 mm of pressure above where the radial pulse is last palpated. This technique is recommended to compensate for the possible presence of an auscultatory gap. This is a period of silence that can occur during the systolic measurement, primarily in hypertensive patients. Arbitrary inflation of the cuff may cause the initial systolic reading to fall somewhere in this gap, or silent period, resulting in an inaccurately (too low) measured systolic pressure.

39. What is the result of using a blood pressure cuff that is too large or too small for the diameter of the patient's arm?

Too large a cuff will result in an erroneously low pressure recording, whereas too small a cuff will result in an erroneously high measurement.

40. When does one use the bell, and when does one use the diaphragm of the stethoscope?

A stethoscope is equipped with bell and diaphragm components on the chest piece. The diaphragm of the stethoscope is best for picking up relatively high-pitched (high-frequency) sounds such as S_1 and S_2, the murmurs of aortic and mitral regurgitation, and pericardial friction rub. The bell is best for hearing low-pitched (low-frequency) sounds such as S_3, S_4, and the diastolic murmur of mitral stenosis.

41. What maneuvers or special positions are used to accentuate abnormalities of heart sounds?

For accentuation of aortic regurgitation, ask the patient to sit up, lean forward and exhale completely, and hold breath in expiration. For accentuating mitral murmurs or S_3, ask the patient to roll onto his or her left side, then listen at the apical area.

42. What is pulse pressure?

Pulse pressure is the numeric difference between the systolic and diastolic blood pressures. The normal pulse pressure is in the range of 30-40 mm Hg. Causes of an increased or widening pulse pressure include hyperkinetic states (anxiety, fever, exercise, hyperthyroidism), aortic regurgitation, and increased aortic rigidity (aging, atherosclerosis). A decrease or narrowing of the pulse pressure can be caused by obstructed ventricular output, as in aortic stenosis or decreased stroke volume from shock or heart failure.

43. If clinical measurement of the blood pressure is not possible in either arm, where are alternative sites to measure blood pressure?

Blood pressure can be auscultated over the dorsal pedis artery with the cuff placed on the lower leg above the malleolus. Pressure measured here is comparable to pressure recorded over the brachial artery. Blood pressure can also be measured over the popliteal artery with a wide (thigh) cuff placed over the femoral artery. Here the blood pressure is higher (10 ± 5 mm Hg) than in the brachial artery.

44. Where in the abdomen is the appendix located?

In the lower right quadrant.

45. Where on the abdomen is the liver percussed?

On the upper right quadrant. A liver span of 6-12 cm in the midclavicular line is considered normal.

46. What is rebound? What is the significance of rebound tenderness during an abdominal exam?

Because the peritoneum is well innervated and exquisitely sensitive, pressure on the abdomen of a patient with an inflamed peritoneum can elicit a distinctive tenderness. During an abdominal exam, if you depress the abdomen gently and release and the patient winces, it is an indication that the peritoneum is inflamed (rebound tenderness).

47. What is the Hering-Breuer reflex?

When the lungs become overly inflated, stretch receptors activate an appropriate feedback response to limit further inspiration. These stretch receptors are located in the walls of the bronchi and bronchioles throughout the lungs that, when overstretched, transmit inhibitory signals through the vagus nerve in the inhibitory center. It seems to be a protective mechanism to prevent overinflation rather than normal control of ventilation.

48. How are deep tendon reflexes graded?

- 0 = no response
- 1+ = diminished; low normal
- 2+ = normal
- 3+ = more brisk than average
- 4+ = hyperactive

49. How is the Babinski sign elicited?

Babinski testing is done by lightly stroking the lateral aspect of the sole of the foot vertically from the heel to the base of the toes. The course of stimulation is changed as you approach the toes by medially directing the path of stimulation along the base of the toes toward the great toe. Normal response is plantar flexion, whereas abnormal response is dorsiflexion of the toe, fanning of the other toes, and dorsiflexion of the ankles.

50. What is anisocoria?

Anisocoria refers to inequality of the pupils. It is a common normal variation of pupil size but can be an indication of pathology.

51. What is the Glasgow Coma Scale?

The Glasgow Coma Scale (GCS) is a quantitative measure of the patient's level of consciousness. The GCS is the sum of scores for three areas of assessment: (1) eye opening, (2) verbal response, and (3) best motor response (Table 2-1). The minimum GCS score that can be obtained is 3, and the maximum is 15.

Table 2-1 *Glasgow Coma Scale*		
AREA OF ASSESSMENT	PATIENT RESPONSE	SCORE
Eye opening	Spontaneous	4
	Responds to verbal command	3
	Responds to pain	2
	No response	1
Motor response	To verbal command	6
	Localizes pain (e.g., moves hand to push yours away)	5
	Withdraws	4
	Flexor response	3
	Extensor response	2
	No response	1
Verbal response	Oriented	5
	Confused conversation	4
	Inappropriate words	3
	Incomprehensible sounds	2
	No response	1

52. What is Homans' sign?
Pain in the calf when the toe is dorsiflexed. This is an early sign of deep venous thrombosis.

53. What are the components of the corneal reflex?
- Sensory limb: fifth cranial nerve (V2)
- Motor response: seventh cranial nerve; look for eye blinking

54. What is the oculocardiac reflex?
The trigeminal-vagal reflex. Pressure applied to the globe or stretching of the extraocular muscles results in 10%-15% reduction in heart rate. It also can cause junctional rhythm and possible premature ventricular contractions (PVCs). Atropine is not useful in treating this situation.

55. What is the direct light reflex?
The direct light reflex occurs when a light is shone into the eye to the retina and the pupil constricts (retina–optic nerve–optic tract).

56. What is the consensual light reflex?
The consensual light reflex occurs when a light is shone into the eye to the retina and the pupil of the opposite eye constricts.

57. What is nystagmus?
Nystagmus is an involuntary, rapid, rhythmic movement of the eyeball, which may be horizontal, vertical, rotatory, or mixed. There are various forms of nystagmus, some of which may be indicative of certain diseases of the vestibular system.

58. What is strabismus?
Strabismus is a deviation of the eye that the patient cannot overcome. The visual axis deviates from that required by the physiologic conditions. There are many forms of strabismus, depending on the direction of the strabismus, whether the condition is affecting one eye or both, and the cause of the condition.

59. What are important features to be aware of during an otoscopic exam?
- Scaling
- Discharge
- Erythema
- Bleeding
- Cerumen
- Lesions
- Foreign bodies

60. What important anatomic feature is noted just beyond the canal hair in an otoscopic exam?
The junction between the lateral cartilaginous canal and the medial bony canal.

61. What descriptors are important in a lymph node exam?
Examination of the lymph nodes should note size, tenderness, shape, and consistency of palpable nodes. It is also important to note if the nodes are fixed, matted, or discrete.

62. What are metabolic equivalent demands (METs) in relation to a preoperative evaluation?
METs are used to evaluate a patient's functional capacity and perioperative cardiac risk. Climbing a flight of stairs is considered a 4-MET activity. Those who cannot meet the demand of a 4-MET activity are considered a high anesthetic risk.

63. Are vital signs really "vital"?
Yes. For example, if heart rate and blood pressure are on the wrong side of 100 (heart rate is > 100 beats/min, systolic blood pressure is < 100 mm Hg), watch out! Also, tachypnea (respiratory rate >16) reflects either pain or systemic acidosis. Temperature, however, is less reliable. Fever may develop late, particularly in the immunosuppressed patient who may be afebrile even in the presence of infection.

64. What is the significance of bowel sounds?
Not unlike other parts of the body, if the part hurts, the patient tends not to use it. Inflamed bowel is less functional and therefore is quiet. Bowel contents squeezed through a partial obstruction produce high-pitched tinkles. However, bowel sounds are not always reliable.

65. What is the significance of abdominal distention?
Abdominal distention may arise from either intraenteric or extraenteric gas or fluid, or from blood. Abdominal distention is always significant and concerning.

66. Is abdominal palpation important?
Yes. Tenderness to palpation leads the examiner to the anatomic zone of the diseased area. It is best to start palpation in an area that does not hurt and proceed toward the painful (tender) region.

67. What are the two key features of the airway exam?
The oropharynx and mental space. The *oropharynx* is examined with the patient in the sitting position, with the neck extended, tongue out, and phonating. The four classes of oropharynx, originally described by Mallampati, are grouped according to visualized structures (Fig. 2-1):

Class I   Class II   Class III   Class IV

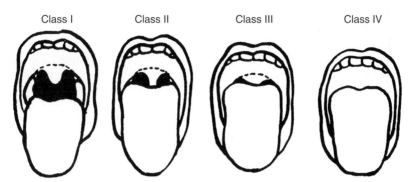

Fig. 2-1 Mallampati classification of the oropharynx. (From Swank KM: Preoperative evaluation. In Duke J [ed]: Anesthesia Secrets, 3rd ed. Philadelphia, 2006, Mosby.)

- **Class I:** Soft palate, fauces, uvula, anterior and posterior tonsillar pillars
- **Class II:** Soft palate, fauces, uvula
- **Class III:** Soft palate, base of uvula
- **Class IV:** Soft palate only

The *mental space* is the distance from the thyroid cartilage to the inside of the mentum, measured while the patient sits with the neck in the sniff position.

A correlation is found between higher oropharyngeal class and decreased glottic exposure at laryngoscopy. The higher oropharyngeal class *combined with* a mental space <2 fingerbreadths better predicts increased difficulty with intubation. Other features include diminished neck extension, decreased tissue compliance, large tongue, overbite, large teeth, narrow high-arched palate, decreased temporomandibular joint mobility, and a short, thick neck.

68. How long should a patient fast before surgery?

Current guidelines for adults with no risk factors for aspiration include no solid food for 6-8 hr; oral preoperative medications may be taken up to 1-2 hr before anesthesia with sips of water.

Current fasting guidelines for pediatric patients are:
- Clear liquids up to 2 hr preoperatively in newborns to age 6 months
- Solid foods, including milk, up to 4 hr preoperatively in newborns to age 6 months; up to 6 hr in children ages 6 months to 3 years; and up to 8 hr in children older than age 3

69. Which patients are at higher risk for aspiration?

Higher-risk patients are those with any degree of gastrointestinal obstruction, a history of gastroesophageal reflux, diabetes (gastroparesis), recent solid-food intake, abdominal distention (obesity, ascites), pregnancy, depressed consciousness, or recent opioid administration (decreased gastric emptying). In addition, nasooropharyngeal or upper gastrointestinal bleeding, airway trauma, and emergency surgery are high-risk settings.

70. Which conditions identified at preoperative evaluation most commonly result in changes in the anesthetic care plan?

The conditions identified at preoperative evaluation that most commonly result in changes in the anesthetic care plan are gastric reflux, insulin-dependent diabetes mellitus, asthma, and suspected difficult airway.

71. What is the significance of runny nose and postnasal drip in a child before an elective surgery with general anesthesia or deep sedation? Should you postpone surgery?

It has been shown that viral upper respiratory tract infections (URIs) are associated with intraoperative and postoperative bronchospasm, laryngospasm, and hypoxia because of their effect on the quality and quantity of airway secretions and increased airway reflexes to mechanical, chemical, or irritant stimulation. In addition, there is evidence that the risk of pulmonary complications may remain high for at least 2 weeks, and possibly 6-7 weeks, after a URI. Accordingly some recommend avoiding anesthesia whenever possible for at least several weeks after a URI. However, in most children, it is generally agreed that chronic nasal discharge poses no significant anesthesia risk. In contrast, children with severe URI or lower respiratory tract infections almost always have their elective surgery postponed. Probably most anesthesiologists will proceed to surgery with a child with a resolving, uncomplicated URI, unless the child has a history of asthma or other significant pulmonary disease.

72. What particular medical and anesthetic problems are associated with obesity?[*]

Obesity is defined as excess body weight >20% over the predicted ideal body weight. Obese patients have a higher incidence of diabetes, hypertension, and cardiovascular disease. There is a higher incidence of difficulty with both mask ventilation and intubation. They have a decreased functional residual capacity, increased O_2 consumption and CO_2 production, and often, diminished ventilation ranging from mild ventilation-perfusion mismatch to actual obesity-hypoventilation and obstructive sleep apnea (pickwickian syndrome). These changes result in more rapid apneic desaturation. If the patients are pickwickian, they may have pulmonary hypertension with or without right ventricular failure. Increased intraabdominal pressure is associated with hiatal hernia and reflux. Because of their higher gastric volume and lower pH, obese patients are at greater risk for aspiration. Pharmacokinetics for many anesthetic agents are altered in them. Finally, regional anesthesia is more difficult and more often unsuccessful.

73. What comprises the preoperative evaluation of a diabetic patient?[*]

How long has the patient had diabetes mellitus? How good is the glycemic control? Patients with frequent insulin reactions and episodes of ketoacidosis (i.e., "brittle" diabetics) are more likely to be metabolically unstable perioperatively. Diabetics with a long history of poor control are also more likely to have end-organ disease. Specifically, the anesthesiologist should look for evidence of coronary disease (often "silent"), hypertension, autonomic neuropathy (check for orthostatic changes in vital signs), renal insufficiency, cardiomyopathy, and gastroparesis (ask about reflux and early satiety). Find out what medications the patient takes for the diabetes, the most recent dose, and current blood sugar. Some diabetics may have diminished neck extension owing to atlantooccipital involvement with the stiff joint syndrome.

Serious preoperative metabolic derangements are seen more often in insulin-dependent diabetic patients, especially in the setting of trauma or infection. Look for high or low glucose levels, electrolyte abnormalities, ketoacidosis, hypovolemia, and hyperosmolarity.

Preoperative testing should include, at a minimum, glucose, electrolytes, blood urea nitrogen, creatinine, urinalysis, and electrocardiogram. Additional lab work might include arterial blood gas, ketones, osmolarity, calcium, phosphorus, and magnesium.

BIBLIOGRAPHY

1. Bates B, Bickley L, Hoekelman R: A Guide to Physical Examination and History Taking, 6th ed. Philadelphia, 1995, J.B. Lippincott.
2. DeGowin E, DeGowin R: Bedside Diagnostic Examination, 2nd ed. London, 1965, Macmillan.
3. Handler B: History and physical examination. In Kwon PH, Laskin DM (eds): Clinician's Manual of Oral and Maxillofacial Surgery, 2nd ed. Carol Stream, Ill, 1997, Quintessence.
4. Peterson SL: Surgical wound infection. In Harken AH, Moore EE (eds): Abernathy's Surgical Secrets, 5th ed, Philadelphia, 2005, Mosby.

*Reprinted from Role PA, Galloway FM: The preoperative evaluation. In Duke J (ed): Anesthesia Secrets, 2nd ed. Philadelphia, 2000, Hanley & Belfus.

5. Role PA, Galloway FM: The preoperative evaluation. In Duke J (ed): Anesthesia Secrets, 2nd ed. Philadelphia, 2000, Hanley & Belfus.
6. Sarin EL, Moore JB: Initial assessment. In Harken AH, Moore EE (eds): Abernathy's Surgical Secrets, 5th ed. Philadelphia, 2005, Mosby.
7. Seidel HM, Ball JW, Dains JE et al: Mosby's Guide to Physical Examination, 6th ed. St Louis, 2006, Mosby.
8. Swank KM: Preoperative evaluation. In Duke J (ed): Anesthesia Secrets, 3rd ed. Philadelphia, 2006, Mosby.

3. ELECTROCARDIOGRAM

A. Omar Abubaker, DMD, PhD, Kenneth J. Benson, DDS, and
Frank P. Iuorno, Jr., DDS, MS

1. What are the components of an electrocardiogram (ECG)? How do they relate to the physiology of the myocardium?

The ECG tracing is a recording of the summed electrical vectors produced during depolarization and repolarization of the heart. Electrical forces directed toward an electrode are represented as positive forces (upward deflections), whereas forces directed away from an electrode are represented as negative forces (downward deflections).

The standard representation of the cardiac cycle is seen in the ECG as the P wave, the QRS complex, and the T wave. These waves and complexes are separated by regularly occurring intervals.

The **P wave** represents atrial depolarization and contraction. It originates in the sinoatrial (SA) node. Usually, depolarization is noted on an ECG with repolarization usually too small or obscured by other waves. Normal is < 0.12 sec. The **PR interval** represents conduction of an impulse through the atrioventricular (AV) node. Normal is < 0.2 sec. The **QRS complex** represents the electrical activity of ventricular depolarization and contraction. Normal is < 0.12 sec. The **ST segment** represents the maintenance depolarization of the ventricles. The **T wave** represents electrical repolarization of the ventricles and is not associated with any physical event.

2. What do the various types of PR interval indicate?

The *normal* PR interval (<0.2 sec) represents the lag in electrical conduction through the AV node. It allows time for ventricular filling. A *narrow* PR interval (<0.12 sec) may reveal accelerated AV conduction (as in Wolff-Parkinson-White syndrome) or premature junctional complexes. *Wide* PR intervals (>0.2 sec) indicate first-degree AV block. *Progressively lengthening* PR intervals indicate second-degree AV block or multifocal atrial tachycardia.

3. What are the intrinsic automatic firing rates of the sinus node, the AV node, and the ventricles?

The sinus node fires at an intrinsic rate of 60-100 beats/min. The AV node and the ventricles fire intrinsically at about 60 and 30-40 beats/min, respectively.

4. What disorders can be evaluated perioperatively by the ECG?

Preoperative ECG, when indicated, can be used to evaluate and help diagnose the following conditions:

- Conduction abnormalities (AV blocks, premature atrial contractions [PACs], premature ventricular contractions [PVCs])
- Myocardial ischemia
- Myocardial infarctions
- Ventricular and atrial hypertrophy

- Pacemaker function
- Preexcitation (e.g., Wolff-Parkinson-White syndrome)
- Drug toxicity (digitalis, antiarrhythmics, tricyclic antidepressants)
- Electrolyte abnormalities (e.g., disturbances in calcium, potassium)
- Various medical conditions (e.g., pericarditis, hypothermia, pulmonary emboli, cor pulmonale, cerebrovascular accidents, increased intracranial pressure)

5.   What is the normal route of conduction?
Via sinus node $\rightarrow$ AV node $\rightarrow$ HIS-Purkinje fibers.

6.   What are the markings of an ECG?
- 1 small square (light lines) = 1 mm = 1 mV = 0.04 sec
- 1 large square (dark lines) = 5 mm = 5 mV = 0.2 sec
- Normal paper speed = 25 mm/sec

7.   How do I determine the heart rate from an ECG (Fig. 3-1, *A* and *B*)?

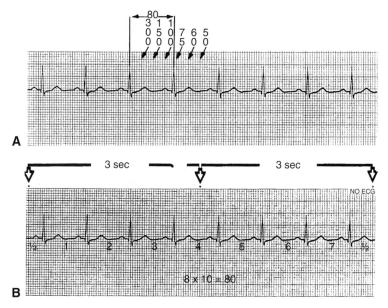

Fig. 3-1   **A,** Grid method for determining rate. Note that next R wave falls between dark lines representing 75 beats/min (or approximately 80 beats/min). **B,** Scan method for determining rate. (From Strauss RA: ECG interpretation. In Kwon PH, Laskin DM: Clinician Manual of Oral and Maxillofacial Surgery, 3rd ed. Chicago, 2001, Quintessence.)

The distance between the heavy lines represents 1/300 min. So two 1/300-min units = 2/300 min = 1/150 min (or 150/min rate), and three 1/300 units = 3/300 min = 1/100 min (or 100/min rate). So to determine the actual rate, find the R wave nearest the dark line and then count the dark lines until the next R wave. If the R wave falls on the next dark line, the rate is 300; if it falls on the second dark line, the rate is 150; if it falls on the third dark line, the rate is 100; and so on (Fig. 3-1, *A*). Alternatively, the rate can be determined by multiplying the number of beats in 6-sec strips (two 3-sec marks) by 10 (Fig. 3-1, *B*).

8. How are leads placed to determine the direction of the cardiac impulse in the frontal plane?

An ECG measures the electrical impulse between two leads. By measuring these impulses using several leads at different angles, the axis (or overall vector) of the impulse can be derived. The limb leads are used to determine the impulse direction in the frontal plane. Leads are placed on the right arm, left arm, and left leg. Impulses that travel toward the positive lead have a positive deflection on the ECG. Using a common ground, two leads may be averaged to yield three more vectors named **aVR, aVL,** and **aVF.**

9. How are leads placed to determine the axis of the cardiac impulse in the axial or horizontal plane?

Chest leads V1-V6 are used to determine the direction of an impulse in the axial plane. They are placed sequentially: V1 (right of sternum in fourth intercostal space), V2 (left of sternum), V3 (midway between V2 and V4), V4 (midclavicular line in fifth intercostal space), V5 (midway between V4 and V6), and V6 (lateral chest in fifth intercostal space).

10. When analyzing ECGs, what are the five factors to consider?

1. Rate
2. Rhythm
3. Axis
4. Hypertrophy
5. Infarction

11. What are tachycardia and bradycardia?

Sinus tachycardia indicates a rate >100 beats/min, and bradycardia is a rate <60 beats/min.

12. How do I determine the axis of the heart's electrical impulse?

Consider leads I and aVF. Remember that the more positive deflection in each lead indicates the axis following in the same direction. Lead I flows from right to left, and lead aVF flows from superior to inferior. A normal axis shows positive deflections in both leads I and aVF. Left axis deviation shows positive in lead I and negative in aVF, and the patient may have left ventricular hypertrophy or bundle branch block. Right axis deviation shows negative in lead I and positive in aVF, and the patient may have right ventricular hypertrophy or bundle branch block. Extreme right axis deviation is negative in both leads I and aVF and is rare.

13. How do potassium and calcium affect the ECG?

Hypokalemia causes U waves (small, positive deflections following T waves). Hypokalemia may also be seen as ST depression and flat T waves. Hyperkalemia causes tall, narrow, peaked T waves, QRS widening, and P-wave flattening and can progress to ventricular fibrillation. Hypocalcemia causes prolonged QT intervals. Finally, hypercalcemia causes shortened QT intervals.

14. What is the following rhythm (Fig. 3-2)?

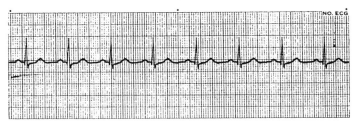

Fig. 3-2 (From Strauss RA: ECG interpretation. In Kwon PH, Laskin DM: *Clinician Manual of Oral and Maxillofacial Surgery*, 3rd ed. Chicago, 2001, Quintessence.)

Sinus rhythm. The rate is normally 60-100 beats/min. The PR interval is 0.12-0.2 sec. The QRS complex is 0.04-0.12 sec. The rhythm is regular.

15. What is the following rhythm (Fig. 3-3)?

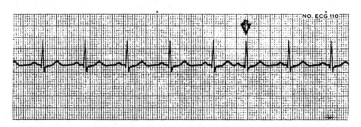

Fig. 3-3   (From Strauss RA: ECG interpretation. In Kwon PH, Laskin DM: Clinician Manual of Oral and Maxillofacial Surgery, 3rd ed. Chicago, 2001, Quintessence.)

Premature atrial contractions. Here the rate varies depending on the number of these contractions. A different P wave (originating from an ectopic focus in the atrium) and a shortened PR interval are evident. The QRS complex is normal, however, and the rhythm is basically normal, with the exception of occasional prematurities (arrow indicates premature wave).

16. What is the following rhythm (Fig. 3-4)?

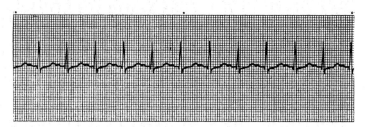

Fig. 3-4   (From Strauss RA: ECG interpretation. In Kwon PH, Laskin DM: Clinician Manual of Oral and Maxillofacial Surgery, 3rd ed. Chicago, 2001, Quintessence.)

Sinus tachycardia. By definition, the rate at rest is >100 beats/min. The P waves, PR intervals, and QRS complexes are normal. The rhythm is regular.

17. What is the following rhythm (Fig. 3-5)?

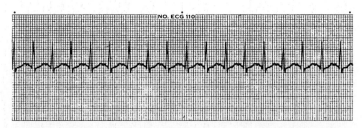

Fig. 3-5   (From Strauss RA: ECG interpretation. In Kwon PH, Laskin DM: Clinician Manual of Oral and Maxillofacial Surgery, 3rd ed. Chicago, 2001, Quintessence.)

Supraventricular tachycardia. Generally, the rate is 150-250 beats/min. The P waves differ from normal and may be coincident with the previous T waves, with a noticeable lack of PR interval. The QRS complexes are normal.

18. What is the following rhythm (Fig. 3-6)?

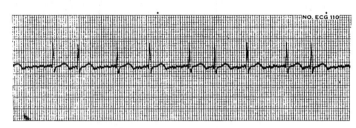

Fig. 3-6 (From Strauss RA: ECG interpretation. In Kwon PH, Laskin DM: Clinician Manual of Oral and Maxillofacial Surgery, 3rd ed. Chicago, 2001, Quintessence.)

Atrial fibrillation. Commonly remembered as an irregularly irregular rhythm, the rate is usually 300-500 beats/min, with a ventricular capture rate of 150-180 beats/min. P waves are not usually discrete, and PR intervals are virtually impossible to distinguish. The QRS complexes are normal.

19. What is the following rhythm (Fig. 3-7)?

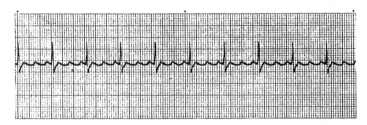

Fig. 3-7 (From Strauss RA: ECG interpretation. In Kwon PH, Laskin DM: Clinician Manual of Oral and Maxillofacial Surgery, 3rd ed. Chicago, 2001, Quintessence.)

Atrial flutter. The "sawtooth" rhythm. The atrial rate averages 220-350 beats/min; the ventricular rate is also variable at 100-220 beats/min. P waves give the characteristic sawtooth appearance to this rhythm (flutter or "F" waves). PR intervals are usually regular, and the QRS complexes are normal.

20. What is the following rhythm (Fig. 3-8)?

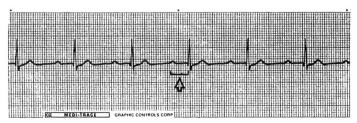

Fig. 3-8 (From Strauss RA: ECG interpretation. In Kwon PH, Laskin DM: Clinician Manual of Oral and Maxillofacial Surgery, 3rd ed. Chicago, 2001, Quintessence.)

First-degree AV block. The only unusual finding on this ECG is a prolonged PR interval (>0.2 sec; see arrow).

21. What is the following rhythm (Fig. 3-9)?

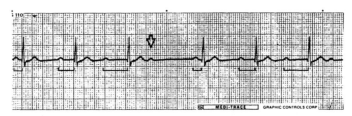

Fig. 3-9   (From Strauss RA: ECG interpretation. In Kwon PH, Laskin DM: Clinician Manual of Oral and Maxillofacial Surgery, 3rd ed. Chicago, 2001, Quintessence.)

Second-degree AV block, Mobitz type I (Wenckebach). The atrial rate is usually fixed, but the ventricular rate is slower. Here the P waves are normal, but the PR intervals lengthen until eventually a QRS complex is dropped. The QRS complexes are normal. Brackets indicate increasing PR intervals; arrow indicates P wave that is not conducted to ventricles ("dropped beat").

22. What is the following rhythm (Fig. 3-10)?

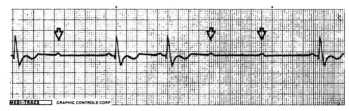

Fig. 3-10   (From Strauss RA: ECG interpretation. In Kwon PH, Laskin DM: Clinician Manual of Oral and Maxillofacial Surgery, 3rd ed. Chicago, 2001, Quintessence.)

Second-degree AV block, Mobitz type II. The rate is usually normal in the atrium, but the ventricular rate is slower by a factor of two (2:1) or three (3:1). Here the P waves are normal, and when conducted, the PR interval is usually normal. There are simply missed QRS complexes for P waves. Arrows indicate intermittent nonconducting P waves.

23. What is the following rhythm (Fig. 3-11)?

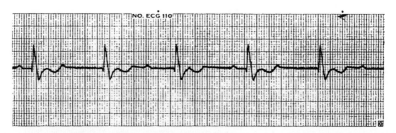

Fig. 3-11   (From Strauss RA: ECG interpretation. In Kwon PH, Laskin DM: Clinician Manual of Oral and Maxillofacial Surgery, 3rd ed. Chicago, 2001, Quintessence.)

Third-degree AV block. There is total dissociation of the atrium and the ventricles. Thus the P waves and QRS complexes are regular but do not coincide, leaving a rate of 20-60 beats/min. The QRS complexes may be normal to wide.

24. What is the following rhythm (Fig. 3-12)?

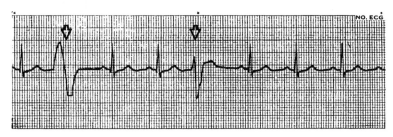

Fig. 3-12   (From Strauss RA: ECG interpretation. In Kwon PH, Laskin DM: Clinician Manual of Oral and Maxillofacial Surgery, 3rd ed. Chicago, 2001, Quintessence.)

Premature ventricular contractions. The overall rate is normal, but the P waves are usually indistinguishable from the QRS complex. The PR interval is not measurable, and the QRS complex is prolonged (>0.12 sec). Arrows indicate premature complexes.

25. What is the following rhythm (Fig. 3-13)?

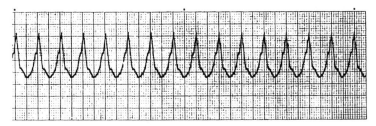

Fig. 3-13   (From Strauss RA: ECG interpretation. In Kwon PH, Laskin DM: Clinician Manual of Oral and Maxillofacial Surgery, 3rd ed. Chicago, 2001, Quintessence.)

Ventricular tachycardia. P waves and PR intervals are not seen. The rate is usually >100 beats/min, and the QRS complexes are wide (>0.12 sec).

26. What is the following rhythm (Fig. 3-14)?

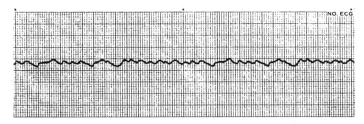

Fig. 3-14   (From Strauss RA: ECG interpretation. In Kwon PH, Laskin DM: Clinician Manual of Oral and Maxillofacial Surgery, 3rd ed. Chicago, 2001, Quintessence.)

Ventricular fibrillation. The rate is not calculable because there are no actual QRS complexes. There are no P waves or PR intervals to speak of. The patient is usually without a pulse.

27. What is the following rhythm (Fig. 3-15)?

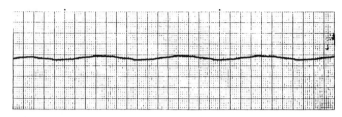

Fig. 3-15   (From Strauss RA: ECG interpretation. In Kwon PH, Laskin DM: Clinician Manual of Oral and Maxillofacial Surgery, 3rd ed. Chicago, 2001, Quintessence.)

Asystole. Commonly referred to as flat line. No discernable waves are present.

28. What arrhythmia may occur with prolonged QT interval?
Torsades de pointes. This arrhythmia may lead to ventricular fibrillation.

29. What are typical ECG signs of ischemia, injury, and infarction?
Ischemia shows inverted T waves in the leads nearest the part of the affected myocardium most easily identified in the chest leads. ST depression may also be seen. *Injury* to heart muscle is indicated by ST elevation and tall, positive T waves. *Infarction* shows Q waves that are 0.04 sec or longer, or > one third the size of the entire QRS complex. Location can be determined from the lead. Anterior leads show Q waves in V1 and V2; inferior leads in II, III, and aVF; and lateral leads in I, aVL, V5, and V6.

30. What is Wolff-Parkinson-White (WPW) syndrome?
WPW syndrome is a preexcitation syndrome caused by conduction from the SA node to the ventricle through an accessory pathway that bypasses the AV node. Early depolarization of the ventricles produces a short PR interval and a delta wave (a delay in initial deflection of the QRS complex) on ECG just before normal ventricular depolarization is initiated. Clinically, this syndrome is manifested as tachyarrhythmias.

31. How is digitalis toxicity seen on ECG?
Digitalis toxicity has several ECG manifestations, including SA and AV node blocks, tachycardia, premature ventricular contractions, ventricular tachycardia, atrial fibrillation, and possible sloping of the ST segment.

32. What is the ECG manifestation of hypothermia?
Hypothermia is seen on ECG as sinus bradycardia, AV junctional rhythm, or ventricular fibrillation. Typically there is an elevated J point, and there may be an intraventricular conduction delay and prolonged QT interval.

33. Who should have a preoperative 12-lead ECG?
For the most part, this depends on many factors, including the clinical presentation of the patient and the individual hospital regulations. However, it is generally agreed that the following patients may benefit from a preoperative 12-lead ECG to fully assess the surgical and anesthetic risks of these patients:

- Any patient older than age 50, or any patient older than age 40 when risk factors are present
- Any other patient who has signs or symptoms of cardiac disease
- Patients with prior history of cardiac ischemia, dysrhythmias, or pacemaker placement
- Patients with history of cocaine use who are to undergo procedure under general anesthesia

34. What artifacts can alter the ECG monitor intraoperatively?*

Artifacts on the ECG monitor may lead to inaccurate diagnosis. The following conditions may produce artifacts on the ECG:

- Loose or misplaced ECG wires or electrodes
- Improper electrode placement or adhesion (e.g., electrodes placed on hair or burned tissue, inadequate skin preparation, surgical scrub, loose electrodes, or use of dry electrode gel)
- Motion (e.g., shivering, tremor, hiccuping, surgical preparation, or diaphragmatic movement)
- Operating room (OR) equipment (e.g., electrocautery, cardiopulmonary bypass pump, OR lasers, irrigation/suction devices, evoked potential monitoring, and surgical drills and saws)
- Patient contact by surgeons, nurses, or anesthesia personnel

35. What two leads would you select as primary ECG monitors?*

Studies of patients with known coronary artery disease who were monitored for ischemia during anesthesia and surgery showed that 75% of the ischemic events occurred in lead V5. Combining leads V4 and V5 resulted in detection of approximately 85% of all the detected events. Lead II is usually best for monitoring P waves, enhancing diagnosis of dysrhythmias, and detecting inferior wall ischemia. Lead V5 is most sensitive for detection of anterior and lateral ischemia. By monitoring leads II and V5 simultaneously, the most information can be obtained.

36. After orthotopic heart transplantation, what changes can be seen on the ECG tracing?*

During orthotopic heart transplantation, the patient's original heart is removed except for the posterior walls of the atria for anastomosis to the donor heart. The patient's original SA node often remains with the original atria, and two P waves can be seen on ECG tracing.

37. Do all wide-complex beats derive from the ventricles?†

No, but most do. An impulse of supraventricular origin that is conducted with aberrancy through the ventricle can take enough time to make it a wide-complex beat.

38. What are the steps in calling a dysrhythmia by name?†
- **Bradycardia:** <60 beats/min
- **Tachycardia:** 100-250 beats/min
- **Flutter:** atrial or ventricular rate 250-400 beats/min
- **Fibrillation:** atrial or ventricular rate >400 beats/min

39. Are cardiac dysrhythmias and cardiac arrhythmias the same?†

Yes. Some purists will tell you that an arrhythmia can be only the absence of a cardiac rhythm. But these are the same purists who use the word *iatrogenic* to mean "caused by a physician," when, of course, the only thing that can truly be "iatrogenic" is a physician's parents.

40. How do you distinguish supraventricular from ventricular origin?†

Supraventricular origin: When an impulse originates above the AV node (supraventricular),

---

*Reprinted from Rosher JW: Electrocardiography. In Duke J (ed): Anesthesia Secrets, 2nd ed. Philadelphia, 2000, Hanley & Belfus.
†Reprinted from Harken AH: Evaluation and treatment of cardiac dysrhythmias. In Harken AH, Moore EE (eds): Abernathy's Surgical Secrets, 5th ed. Philadelphia, 2005, Mosby.

it can access the ventricles only through the AV node. The AV node connects with the endocardial Purkinje system, which conducts impulses rapidly (2-3 m/sec). A supraventricular impulse activates the ventricles rapidly (<0.08 sec, 80 msec, or two little boxes on the ECG paper), producing a narrow-complex beat.

Ventricular origin: When an impulse originates directly from an ectopic site on the ventricle, it takes longer to access the high-speed Purkinje system. A ventricular impulse activates the entire ventricular mass slowly (>0.08 sec, 80 msec, or two little boxes on the ECG paper), producing a wide-complex beat.

BIBLIOGRAPHY

1. Baker WA, Lewkowiez L: Electrocardiography. In Duke J (ed): Anesthesia Secrets, 3rd ed. Philadelphia, 2006, Mosby.
2. Dubin D: Rapid Interpretation of EKG, 5th ed. Tampa, Fla, Cover Publishing, 1997.
3. Gomella LG: Basic ECG reading. In Clinician Pocket Reference, 7th ed. Norwalk, Conn, Appleton & Lange, 1993.
4. Harken AH: Evaluation and treatment of cardiac dysrhythmias. In Harken AH, Moore EE (eds): Anesthesia Secrets, 2nd ed. Philadelphia, 2000, Hanley & Belfus.
5. Harken AH: Cardiac dysrhythmias. Evaluation and treatment of cardiac dysrhythmias. In Wilmore DW, Cheung L, Harken AH et al (eds): Scientific American Surgery. New York, 1999, Scientific American.
6. Rosher JW: Electrocardiography, dysrhythmias. In Harken AH, Moore EE (eds): Anesthesia Secrets, 2nd ed. Philadelphia, 2000, Hanley & Belfus.
7. Steeling C: Simplified EKG Analysis. Philadelphia, 1992, Hanley & Belfus.
8. Strauss R: ECG interpretation. In Kwon PH, Laskin DM (eds): Clinician Manual of Oral and Maxillofacial Surgery, 2nd ed. Chicago, 1996, Quintessence.

4. LABORATORY TESTS

Paul W. Brinser III, DDS

1. What is included in a complete blood count (CBC), and how are the results charted?
The CBC or heme 8 typically includes the items described in Table 4-1 and Fig. 4-1.

2. What information does a white blood cell (WBC) differential provide?
The total WBC count is made up of neutrophils (50%-70%), lymphocytes (20%-40%), monocytes (0%-7%), basophils (0%-1%), and eosinophils (0%-5%). Most labs also provide the absolute number of each cell type as well as percentage. Differentials for alterations in the WBC fractions are described in Box 4-1.

3. What is a "left shift," and how is it significant?
Polymorphonuclear neutrophils (PMNs) are subdivided morphologically on the blood smear into segmented neutrophils ("segs" or "polys") and band forms ("bands"), based on the nuclear lobes and their chromatin connections. The segs are more mature neutrophils, having 2-5 nuclear lobes and thin strands of chromatin and comprising 50%-70% of total PMNs. The bands are immature neutrophils, make up 0%-5% of total PMNs, and have a thick band of chromatin connecting 1-2 nuclear lobes. On the early manual neutrophil counting machines, the keys that represented the bands were on the left side and the keys representing segs were on the right. If the bands increased to more than 20% of the WBC total, or the PMNs were more than 80% of the WBC total, the result was said to have a "left shift." This shift increases the likelihood of bacterial infection, sepsis, or hemorrhage as the etiology of an elevated WBC count.

Table 4-1 *Complete Blood Cell Count*

	DEFINITION	NORMAL RANGE
White blood cell count		$4\text{-}11 \times 10^3$ cells/mm^3
RBC count		$4.5\text{-}6 \times 10^6$ cells/mm^3
Hgb		Men: 14-18 g/dL
		Women: 12-16 g/dL
Hematocrit	Percentage of RBC mass in blood volume	Men: 40%-54% Women: 37%-47%
Platelets		$150\text{-}400 \times 10^3$/mm^3
RBC indices:		
Mean corpusclular volume	Average RBC volume in fL	80-100 fL
Mean corpuscular hemoglobin	Estimates weight of Hgb in average RBC	27-31 pg
Mean corpuscular hemoglobin concentration	Estimates average concentration of Hgb in average RBC	32%-36%

fL, Femtoliters; *Hgb,* hemoglobin; *RBC,* red blood cell.

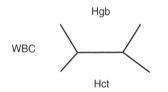

Fig. 4-1. Demonstrates method of recording values in patient chart. The charting method allows universal communication with the patient progress notes.

Box 4-1 *Differentials for Alterations in the White Blood Cell Fractions*

Polymorphonuclear Neutrophils (PMNs)

INCREASED:	DECREASED:
Bacterial infection	Aplastic anemia
Tissue damage (myocardial infarction, burn, or crush injury)	Viral infection
Leukemia	Drugs
Uremia	Radiation
Diabetic ketoacidosis (DKA)	Kidney dialysis
Acute gout	
Eclampsia	
Physiologic:	
Severe exercise	
Late pregnancy	
Labor	
Surgery	
Newborn	

Continued

Box 4-1	*Differentials for Alterations in the White Blood Cell Fractions—cont'd*

Lymphocytes (Lymphs)

INCREASED (LYMPHOCYTOSIS):

DECREASED:

Viral infections	Uremia
Acute or chronic lymphocytic leukemia	Stress
Tuberculosis (TB)	Burns
Mononucleosis	Trauma
	Steroids
	Normal in 20% of population

Monocytes

INCREASED (MONOCYTOSIS):

DECREASED:

Subacute bacterial endocarditis	Aplasia of bone marrow
TB	
Protozoal infection	
Leukemia	
Collagen disease	

Basophils

INCREASED (BASOPHILIA):

DECREASED:

Chronic myeloid leukemia	Acute rheumatic fever
Polycythemia	Lobar pneumonia
After recovery of infection or	Steroid treatment
hypothyroidism (rarely)	Stress
	Thyrotoxicosis

Eosinophils

INCREASED (EOSINOPHILIA):

DECREASED:

Allergy	Steroids
Parasite	Stress (infection, trauma, and burn)
Malignancy	Increased adrenocorticotropic hormone
Drugs	(ACTH)
Asthma	Cushing's syndrome
Addison's disease	
Collagen vascular diseases	

4. How are the red blood cell (RBC) indices used clinically?

The indices are used to diagnose and classify anemia, which is defined as a decreased RBC mass or hemoglobin (Hgb) content below physiologic needs. The mean corpuscular volume (MCV) and mean corpuscular hemoglobin concentration (MCHC) are the most useful in determining the etiology of the anemia.

$$MCV = (Hematocrit [Hct] \times unit\ constant)/RBC$$

- Macrocytic (>100 fL): megaloblastic anemia (B_{12} or folate deficiency), chronic liver disease, alcoholism, reticulocytosis, physiologic in the newborn
- Microcytic (<80 fL): iron deficiency, thalassemia, chronic disease (cancer, renal, infection), or lead toxicity

$$MCH = Hgb/RBC$$

MCH helps to diagnose chromaticity of cells because cells with increased Hgb content will have more pigment (hyperchromic) and will be hypochromic in the reverse situation. This tends to parallel changes in MCV in that macrocytic cells are usually hyperchromic and microcytic, or hypochromic cells have low MCH.

$$MCHC = Hgb/Hct$$

This is increased with prolonged severe dehydration, heavy smoking, intravascular hemolysis, and spherocytosis. The MCHC will be decreased in overhydration, iron deficiency anemia, thalassemia, and sideroblastic anemia.

5. What does the reticulocyte count mean?

Reticulocytes are immature RBCs. These cells are larger, continue Hgb synthesis, and are bluer in color on smears than mature erythrocytes. The normal count is 1% of total RBCs but will increase if the need for erythrocytes rises. A "corrected count" is made by multiplying the reticulocyte count by the measured Hct divided by 45; the result should be <1.5%. If the count is increased, then erythropoiesis is usually caused by bleeding, hemolysis, and correction of iron, folate, or B_{12} deficiencies. Decreased reticulocyte counts are often the result of transfusions or aplastic anemia.

6. What information is obtained from the Hgb and Hct values?

The Hgb concentration is an indicator of oxygen-carrying capacity of blood. It is dependent primarily on the number of RBCs and much less significantly (or treatably) on the amount of Hgb per cell. Additionally, Hgb is known to vary by as much as 1 g/dL diurnally, with peaks in the morning. Studies have also shown a 1 g/dL variation between Hgb values drawn on admission and those taken following one night of bed rest. The relation between Hgb and Hct is given by:

$$Hgb \times 3^* = Hct$$
$$RBC \text{ (millions)} \times 3 = Hgb$$
$$RBC \times 9 = Hct$$

Increased Hgb and Hct values may result from polycythemia, dehydration, heart disease, increased altitude, heavy smoking, or birth physiology. *Decreased* levels may indicate anemia, hemorrhage, dilution, alcohol, drugs, or pregnancy.

7. Are Hgb and Hct primary indicators of blood loss and the need for transfusion?

No! These are poor early measures of bleeding because one loses plasma and RBCs in equal measures. It takes 2-3 hr after fluid resuscitation before the Hgb/Hct will reflect blood loss. Previously, surgical transfusion guidelines were 10 g/dL or 33% Hct, then 9 g/dL or 25%-30% Hct. Today most patients are transfused for Hgb <7 g/dL, but the best guidelines are the vital signs and symptoms such as shortness of breath and exercise tolerance. Initially low Hct values suggest chronic blood loss, which should be supported by low MCV and a high reticulocyte count.

---

*This varies between 2.7 and 3.2 based on the MCHC.

8. What are some common terms and significant morphologic changes on smears?

- Poikilocytosis: Irregularly shaped RBCs
- Anisocytosis: Irregular RBC size
- Sickled cells: Crescent or sickle-shaped RBCs seen with decreased oxygen (O_2) tension
- Howell-Jolly bodies: Large RBC basophilic inclusions (megaloblastic anemia, splenectomy, hemolysis)
- Basophilic stippling: Small RBC blue inclusions (lead poison, thalassemia, heavy metals)
- Spherocytes: Spherical RBCs (autoimmune hemolytic anemia, hereditary)
- Burr cells: Spiny RBCs (liver disease, anorexia, ↑ bile acids)
- Schistocyte: Helmet RBCs (severe anemia, hemolytic transfusion reaction)
- Döhle's inclusion bodies: PMNs (burns, infection)
- Toxic granulation: PMNs (burns, sepsis, fever)
- Auer bodies: Acute myelogenous leukemia
- Hypersegmentation: PMNs with six to seven lobes (megaloblastic anemia, liver disease)

9. What is clinically useful about the platelet count?

Thrombocytopenia (low platelet count) that is < 50,000/mm^3 is an absolute contraindication to elective surgical procedures because of the possibility of significant bleeding. Patients with <10,000-20,000 platelets have been known to bleed spontaneously. Platelet counts between 50,000 and 100,000 have not been associated with significant bleeding, provided platelet function is normal. Possible etiologies for low platelet counts are idiopathic thrombocytopenic purpura (ITP), disseminated intravascular coagulation (DIC), marrow invasion or aplasia, hypersplenism, drugs, cirrhosis, transfusions, and viral infections (mononucleosis).

10. How is platelet function assessed, and what drug most commonly affects the test?

Bleeding time is a screening test that assesses platelet number and function. The test is performed by inflating a blood pressure cuff to 40 mm Hg, making a standard incision in the patient's forearm, and recording the time until the bleeding stops (Ivy method). It has been recommended that this test be used to diagnose specific hemorrhagic diseases and to monitor therapy of these diseases, but not to screen preoperative patients who have no history of bleeding or abnormal coagulation studies. The bleeding time is increased by platelet counts <100,000 and by the presence of aspirin, antibiotics (synthetic penicillins), uremia, alcoholism, chronic liver disease, vasculitis, Ehlers-Danlos syndrome, and von Willebrand's disease. There is an undefined risk of bleeding with elevated test times until about double the control time. Aspirin irreversibly blocks cyclooxygenase function, inhibiting platelet aggregation for their 7- to 10-day life span. Because approximately 10% of platelets are replaced each day, it takes an average of 2-3 days for bleeding time to normalize, but most experts recommend allowing 7 days without aspirin before surgery. Other nonsteroidal antiinflammatory drugs (NSAIDs) will alter platelet function only temporarily, usually <24 hr. Capillary fragility is also assessed in bleeding time values.

11. How are platelet abnormalities categorized?

Platelet disorders can be either quantitative or qualitative in nature:

Quantitative platelet disorders include thrombocytopenia; dilution, as after massive blood transfusion; decreased platelet production owing to malignant infiltration (aplastic anemia, multiple myeloma); drugs (chemotherapy, cytotoxic drugs, ethanol, hydrochlorothiazide); radiation exposure; or bone marrow depression after viral infection. Other examples are increased peripheral destruction due to hypersplenism, DIC, extensive tissue and vascular damage after extensive burns, or immune mechanisms (idiopathic thrombocytopenic purpura, drugs such as heparin, autoimmune diseases).

Qualitative platelet disorders include inherited (e.g., von Willebrand's disease) and acquired (uremia; cirrhosis, particularly after ethanol; drugs, such as aspirin, NSAIDs) disorders.

12. **Which clotting factors are synthesized in the liver?**
    Four clotting factors are synthesized in the liver: factors II, VII, IX, and X.

13. **Which vitamin deficiency can affect coagulation and extrinsic pathway coagulation lab values?**
    Vitamin K deficiency.

14. **What is an acceptable preoperative platelet count?**[*]
    A normal platelet count is 150,000-440,000/mm^3. *Thrombocytopenia* is defined as a count of <150,000/mm^3. Intraoperative bleeding can be severe with counts of 40,000-70,000/mm^3, and spontaneous bleeding usually occurs at counts <20,000/mm^3. The minimal recommended platelet count before surgery is 75,000/mm^3. Although prophylactic preoperative platelet transfusion is generally advocated to treat preexisting thrombocytopenia, the methods of evaluating clinical need are imprecise. Qualitative differences in platelet function make it unwise to rely on platelet number as the sole criterion for transfusion. Thrombocytopenic patients with accelerated destruction but active production of platelets have relatively less bleeding than patients with hypoplastic disorders at a given platelet count.
    Assessment of preoperative platelet function is further complicated by lack of correlation between bleeding time or any other test of platelet function and a tendency to increased intraoperative bleeding. However, normal bleeding times range from 4-9 min, and a bleeding time >1$\frac{1}{2}$ times normal (>15 min) is considered significantly abnormal.

15. **How does aspirin act as an anticoagulant?**[*]
    Primary hemostasis is controlled by the balance between the opposing actions of two prostaglandins, thromboxane A2 and prostacyclin. Depending on the dose, salicylates produce a differential effect on prostaglandin synthesis in platelets and vascular endothelial cells. Lower doses preferentially inhibit platelet cyclooxygenase, impeding thromboxane A2 production and inhibiting platelet aggregation. The effect begins within 2 hr of ingestion. Platelets lack a cell nucleus and cannot produce protein. Aspirin's effect therefore lasts for the entire life of the platelet (7-10 days). NSAIDs have a similar but more transient effect than aspirin, lasting for only 1-3 days after cessation of use.

16. **What are the differences between the coagulation tests?**[*]
    The basic difference between the intrinsic and extrinsic pathways is the phospholipid surface on which the clotting factors interact before union at the common pathway. Either platelet phospholipid (for the intrinsic pathway) or tissue thromboplastin (for the extrinsic pathway) can be added to the patient's plasma, and the time taken for clot formation is measured. Less than 30% of normal factor activity is required for the tests to be sensitive to decreased levels. The tests are also prolonged in cases of decreased fibrinogen concentration (<100 mg/dL^{-1}) and dysfibrinogenemias.

Measurement of the Intrinsic and Common Pathways

1. Partial thromboplastin time (PTT)
   - Partial thromboplastin is substituted for platelet phospholipid and eliminates platelet variability.
   - PTT measures the clotting ability of all factors in the intrinsic and common pathways except factor XIII.
   - Normal PTT is about 40-100 sec; more than 120 sec is abnormal.

---

[*]Reprinted from Katz JJ: Coagulation. In Duke J (ed): Anesthesia Secrets, 2nd ed. Philadelphia, 2000, Hanley & Belfus.

2. Activated PTT (aPTT)
   - An activator is added to the test tube before addition of partial thromboplastin.
   - Maximal activation of the contact factors (XII and XI) eliminates the lengthy natural contact activation phase and results in more consistent and reproducible results.
   - Normal aPTT is 25-35 sec.
3. Activated clotting time (ACT)
   - Fresh whole blood (providing platelet phospholipid) is added to a test tube already containing an activator.
   - The automated ACT is widely used to monitor heparin therapy in the operating room.
   - Normal range is 90-120 sec.

Measurement of the Extrinsic and Common Pathways

1. Prothrombin time (PT)
   - Tissue thromboplastin is added to the patient's plasma.
   - Test varies in sensitivity and response to oral anticoagulant therapy whether measured as PT in seconds or simple PT ratio ($PT_{patient}/PT_{normal}$) (normal = the mean normal PT value of the lab test system).
   - Normal PT is 10-12 sec.
2. International normalized ratio (INR)
   - Developed to improve the consistency of oral anticoagulant therapy.
   - Converts the PT ratio to a value that would have been obtained using a standard PT method.
   - INR is calculated as $(PT_{patient}/PT_{normal})^{ISI}$. (ISI is the international sensitivity index assigned to the test system.)
   - The recommended therapeutic ranges for standard oral anticoagulant therapy and high-dose therapy, respectively, are INR values of 2.0-3.0 and 2.5-3.5.

17. What are the current indications for transfusion of fresh frozen plasma (FFP)?*

A task force of the American Society of Anesthesiologists (ASA) recommends the use of FFP in the following circumstances:
- Urgent reversal of warfarin therapy
- Correction of known anticoagulation deficiencies for which specific concentrates are unavailable
- Correction of microvascular bleeding in the presence of elevated (>1.5 times normal) PT or PTT
- Correction of microvascular bleeding secondary to coagulation factor deficiencies in patients transfused with more than one blood volume, when a PT or PTT cannot be obtained in a timely fashion

The dose given should be calculated to achieve a minimum of 30% of plasma factor concentration (usually about 10-15 mL/kg of FFP).

18. What are the indications for the use of platelets?*

The ASA recommends the following:
- Prophylactic platelet transfusion is ineffective and rarely indicated when thrombocytopenia is caused by increased platelet destruction.
- For surgical patients with thrombocytopenia caused by decreased platelet production and surgical and obstetric patients with microvascular bleeding, platelet transfusion is rarely indicated when the count is $> 100 \times 10^9$/L and usually indicated if the count is $< 50 \times 10^9$/L. With intermediate values, platelet therapy should be based on the risk of bleeding.

19. What is DIC?*

DIC is not a disease entity, but rather a manifestation of disease associated with various well-defined clinical entities:

- Obstetric conditions (amniotic fluid embolism, placental abruption, retained fetus syndrome, eclampsia, saline-induced abortion)
- Intravascular hemolysis (hemolytic transfusion syndromes, minor hemolysis, massive transfusion)
- Septicemia (gram-negative: endotoxin; gram-positive: mucopolysaccharides)
- Viremias (cytomegalovirus, hepatitis, varicella, HIV)
- Disseminated malignancy
- Leukemia
- Burns
- Crush injury and tissue necrosis
- Liver disease (obstructive jaundice, acute hepatic failure)
- Prosthetic devices (LeVeen shunt, aortic balloon)

DIC usually is seen in clinical circumstances in which the extrinsic or intrinsic coagulation pathway or both are activated by circulating phospholipid, leading to generation of thrombin, but the usual mechanisms preventing unbalanced thrombus formation are impaired. After systemic deposition of intravascular fibrin thrombi, consumption of factors V and VIII, and loss of platelets, the resulting circulating level of clotting factors and platelets represents a balance between depletion and production. The fibrinolytic system is activated, and plasmin begins to cleave fibrinogen and fibrin into fibrinogen and fibrin degradation products (FDPs). Recognizing and understanding the syndrome are made difficult by the occurrence of both acute and chronic forms and by a clinical spectrum varying from diffuse thrombosis to diffuse bleeding or both.

20. What tests are used for the diagnosis of DIC?[*]

There is no one pathognomonic test for the diagnosis of DIC. In acute DIC, the PT is elevated in about 75% of patients, whereas PTT is prolonged in 50%-60%. Platelet count is typically greatly reduced. Hypofibrinogenemia is common. The D-dimer test is a newer diagnostic test. The D-dimer is a neoantigen formed by the action of thrombin in converting fibrinogen to cross-linked fibrin. It is specific for fibrin degradation products formed from the digestion of cross-linked fibrin by plasmin. In 85%-100% of patients, FDPs are elevated. Elevated levels are not diagnostic of DIC but indicate the presence of plasmin and plasmin degradation of fibrinogen or fibrin.

21. What is the treatment for DIC?[*]

The treatment for DIC is confusing and controversial. The triggering process should be identified and treated accordingly. If bleeding continues, heparin is used to stop the consumption process before administration of specific coagulation products. If these measures fail, specific blood components may be depleted and should be replaced after identification. If bleeding still continues, antifibrinolytic therapy with epsilon aminocaproic acid should be considered, but only if the intravascular coagulation process is shown to have stopped and residual fibrinolysis to continue.

22. What factors increase and decrease prothrombin time (PT)?

PT will be increased by warfarin, vitamin K deficiency, fat malabsorption, liver disease, DIC, and, artificially, increased tourniquet time. Warfarin blocks vitamin K use, whereas broad-spectrum antibiotics elevate PT by killing normal bowel flora, which decreases vitamin K absorption. Heparin in high doses also will increase PT by altering factor X. In dental extractions, few bleeding effects are seen with PT ≤2.5 control. FFP will reverse warfarin effects immediately, whereas vitamin K requires 12-24 hr to begin decreasing the PT.

23. How does heparin work?

Heparin's primary effect is to activate antithrombin III, which blocks coagulation by inhibiting mostly IX and X factors. Antithrombin III amounts are significantly decreased in severe malignancy, severe liver disease, nephrotic syndrome, deep venous thrombosis (DVT), septicemia, major surgery, malnutrition, and DIC. Low-molecular-weight heparin (Enoxaparin) also works on antithrombin III. Heparin's peak effect is at 30 min–1 hr after intravenous use and 3-4 hr after subcutaneous dose. Its duration of effect is approximately 3-4 hr when given intravenously and 6 hr subcutaneously.

24. Why are FDPs and fibrin "split" products (FSPs) important?
  The result of the clotting cascade is an insoluble polymeric fibrin meshwork. Naturally occurring fibrinolysin (plasmin) attacks and breaks down fibrinogen and fibrin leaving split products behind. Physiologically, this occurs after trauma or surgery and is quickly regulated. Pathologically, plasmin may be activated in DIC, DVT, malignancy, emboli, infections (especially gram-negative sepsis), necrosis, or infarctions. This will result in an elevated fibrin split product assay. Fibrinogen assays will be decreased (<150 mg/dL) in DIC, burns, surgery, neoplasia, severe acute bleeding, snakebites, and some hematologic diseases. Protamine sulfate and D-dimer (a specific FSP) are other tests that look for abnormal clotting activity. Though not very specific, the D-dimer assay is used to screen for DVT in the emergency department because a normal value virtually excludes the possibility of this clotting problem.

25. What is measured in a blood chemistry test (also called basic metabolic, chem 7, or SMA 7), and how they are charted?
  The basic electrolytes, renal function evaluation, and blood glucose are tested (Fig. 4-2).

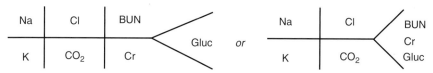

Fig. 4-2. Demonstrates method of recording values in the patient chart. This charting method allows universal communication within the patient progress notes.

	Normal Ranges
1. Sodium (Na)	136-145 mEq/L
2. Potassium (K)	3.5-5.2 mEq/L
3. Chloride (Cl)	95-108 mEq/L
4. Carbon dioxide (CO_2)	24-30 mEq/L
5. Blood urea nitrogen (BUN)	6-20 mg/dL
6. Creatinine	0.7-1.4 mg/dL
7. Glucose	65-110 mg/dL (fasting)

26. What are common causes of basic electrolyte disturbances (Box 4-2)?

Box 4-2	*Common Causes of Basic Electrolyte Disturbances*	
	INCREASE	DECREASE
Sodium (Na)	Dehydration Glycosuria Diabetes insipidus	Diuretics CHF Renal failure

CHF, Congestive heart failure; *DKA,* diabetic ketoacidosis; *SIADH,* syndrome of inappropriate secretion of diuretic hormone.

Box 4-2	Common Causes of Basic Electrolyte Disturbances—cont'd	
	INCREASE	DECREASE
	Cushing's syndrome	Vomiting
	Excessive sweating	Diarrhea
		Liver failure
		Nephrotic syndrome
		SIADH
		Hypothyroidism
		Pancreatitis
		Hyperlipidemia
		Multiple myeloma
		Hyperglycemia—corrected Na = $1.6 \times$ 1/100 g glucose over 100 g/dL
Potassium (K)	Factitious (sample hemolysis, probably most common cause)	Diuretics
		Nasoastric suctioning
		Vomiting
	Dehydration	Alkalosis
	Renal failure	Mineral corticoid excess
	Acidosis	Zollinger-Ellison syndrome
	Addison's disease	Vomiting
	Iatrogenic	Excessive sweating
Chloride (Cl)	Dehydration	CHF
	Metabolic acidosis (nonanion gap)	Chronic renal failure
		Diuretics
	Diarrhea	DKA
	Diabetes insipidus	SIADH
	Medications	Aldosterone excess
	Aldosterone deficiency	
Carbon dioxide (CO_2)	Dehydration	Metabolic acidosis
	Respiratory acidosis	Respiratory alkalosis
	Vomiting	Renal failure
	Emphysema	Diarrhea
	Metabolic alkalosis	Starvation

27. What tests are used as markers for liver function or disease?

Serum albumin, total protein, bilirubin, aspartate aminotransferase (AST = SGOT), alanine aminotransferase (ALT = SGPT), alkaline phosphatase (ALP), gamma-glutamyl transferase (GGT), lactate dehydrogenase (LDH), PT, bile acids, and blood ammonia.

28. How is the synthetic function of the liver evaluated?

Serum levels of albumin, total protein, PT, bile acids, conjugated bilirubin, BUN, and ammonia are used to examine liver function. Although not widely used, the most sensitive test for liver or bile tract abnormality is for bile acids. These are water-soluble compounds produced from cholesterol metabolism in the liver. This test is best done 2 hr after eating and will show abnormalities in inactive cirrhosis and resolving hepatitis when other tests are normal. More commonly used is the albumin level, which is decreased with liver damage as well as starvation, inflammatory bowel disease, nephrotic syndrome, leukemia, and hemorrhage or burns. Albumin is produced almost exclusively by the liver and makes up almost 75% of the total protein in serum, so these tests usually parallel each other. Prothrombin is synthesized by the liver using vitamin K and will be abnormal in severe, most often end-stage, chronic liver disease. The absence of conjugated bilirubin in the blood with severely elevated unconjugated bilirubin could indicate severely decreased liver function. The ammonia level is used to diagnose and follow hepatic encephalopathy when failure of the liver is already known.

29. What is the clinical significance of liver enzymes?

Any increase of "hepatic" enzymes indicates cellular damage. AST is made in the liver, heart, skeletal muscle, and RBCs so elevations may be due to liver disease, acute myocardial infarction (AMI), pancreatitis, muscle trauma, hemolysis, congestive heart failure (CHF), surgery, burns, or renal infarction. Increased specificity for liver damage occurs with elevation of ALT, GGT, or 5′nucleotidase. ALP is found in liver cells, bile duct epithelium, and osteoblasts. Therefore, elevations of ALP should be confirmed to involve the liver or bile ducts by checking a liver specific fraction (GGT, ALT, or 5′nucleotidase level). These tests will help rule out bone diseases, bone growth, healing of fractures, pregnancy, or childhood physiology as the cause of ALP elevation. Lastly, LDH also is increased in liver cell damage with the LDH_5 subfraction showing about the same sensitivity and somewhat greater specificity as AST.

30. What are the causes of bilirubin abnormalities?

Bilirubin is produced by the breakdown of hemoglobin in the reticuloendothelial system. This newly formed bilirubin (indirect or unconjugated) circulates through the bloodstream bound to albumin. Liver cells extract the bilirubin and conjugate it to a water-soluble pigment (direct or conjugated bilirubin) that is excreted in bile. Elevations of total bilirubin in the blood cause jaundice (yellowing of skin and sclera, and pruritus) and may be caused by bile obstruction or excessive hemolysis. Elevation of indirect bilirubin occurs with obstruction and hepatocellular disease, and hemolytic anemia and physiologically in newborns. The direct bilirubin increases primarily with obstruction to bile flow and should be associated with an increase in ALP.

31. What are common lab trends in liver disorders (Table 4-2)?

Table 4-2   *Lab Trends in Liver Disorders*

	AST	ALT	ALP	BILIRUBIN TOTAL	CONJU-GATED	UNCONJU-GATED	GGT	BILE ACID
Acute viral hepatitis	↑↑↑↑	↑↑↑↑	↑	↑ varies	↑↑	↑	↑-↑	↑↑↑
Chronic-resolving hepatitis	N-↑	N-↑	N-↑	N	—	—	N-↑	↑↑
Cirrhosis (active)	↑↑↑	↑↑	↑	N-↑	—	—	↑↑	↑↑↑
Cirrhosis (inactive)	N-↑	N-↑	N-↑	N-↑	—	—	N-↑	↑↑↑
ETOH hepatitis	↑↑↑	↑-↑↑	↑	N-↑	—	—	↑↑↑	↑↑
Obstruction (intrahepatic)	↑↑	N-↑↑	↑↑-↑↑↑	↑↑	↑↑	↑↑	↑↑↑	↑↑↑
Obstruction (extrahepatic)	N-↑	N-↑	↑↑↑	↑↑↑	↑↑↑	N-↑	↑↑↑	↑↑
Metastatic disease	N	N	↑↑	±↑	—	—	↑↑	↑↑

ETOH, Ethyl alcohol.

32. What tests monitor calcium (Ca) in the body?

Ca is the fourth most common extracellular cation and plays a vital role in membrane permeability. The metabolically active Ca in the body is the ionized Ca^{2+} portion, which represents approximately 50% of total serum Ca. The range that is considered normal covers only 0.44 mg/dL, an indication of its physiologic importance. The other half of serum Ca is bound by albumin (45%) and complexed with anions. So the total Ca level will be lowered by decreases in albumin such that for each 1 mg/dL drop of albumin, Ca will decrease by 0.8 mg/dL. That is, "corrected" total Ca = 0.8 × (normal albumin − measured albumin) + measured Ca. Possible causes of hypercalcemia include hyperparathyroidism, Paget's disease, metastatic bone tumor, hyperthyroidism, hypervitaminosis D, multiple myeloma, osteoporosis, immobilization, thiazide drugs, and parathyroid-secreting tumors (lung, breast). Causes of hypocalcemia include hypoparathyroidism (commonly after thyroid surgery), insufficient vitamin D, chronic renal failure, hypomagnesemia, seizures, acute pancreatitis, and inaccurate reading as a result of hypoalbuminemia.

33. What two body elements are commonly linked to Ca metabolism?

Magnesium (Mg) and phosphorus (P) play important nutritional roles in the body and are associated with Ca metabolism (Box 4-3). Mg is the second most abundant intracellular cation and is found mostly in muscle, soft tissues, and bones (50%). Less than 5% of Mg circulates in the blood, and 30% of this is bound to albumin. P is used interchangeably with phosphate because much of the body's store is as the anion compound. About 80%-85% of P is found in bones and 10% in muscle, and it is the most common intracellular anion.

Box 4-3	*Common Causes of Calcium Metabolism Abnormalities*	
	INCREASED LEVELS	DECREASED LEVELS
Magnesium (Mg)	Renal failure	Alcoholism
	Mg antacid overdose	Malnutrition
	Specimen hemolysis	Severe diarrhea
	DKA	Hypercalcemia
	Lithium intoxication	Hemodialysis
	Hypothyroidism	Loop/thiazide diuretics
		Hypoalbuminemia
		Nasogastric suction
		Pancreatitis
		Acidosis compensation
Phosphorus (P)	Hypoparathyroidism	Hyperparathyroidism
	Chronic renal failure	Alcoholism
	Bone diseases	Vitamin D deficiency
	Healing fracture	Glucose or insulin administration
	Childhood	Hypomagnesemia
	Hemolysis	Diuretics
		Antacids
		Nasogastric suction
		Alkalosis
		Hypokalemia
		Gram-negative sepsis

DKA, Diabetic ketoacidosis.

34. What blood tests are used to follow renal function?

BUN (normal: 6-20 mg/dL) and creatinine (normal: 0.7-1.4 mg/dL) blood levels are the products of protein and muscle metabolism, respectively, that are excreted by the kidneys. Decreased levels of creatinine are rarely significant, whereas drops in BUN may be due to liver failure (site of urea production), starvation, protein deficiency, overhydration, nephrotic syndrome, or late pregnancy. Elevations of these compounds indicate severely decreased glomerular or tubular function. This can be the result of reduced blood volume to kidneys (dehydration, shock, pump failure), increased protein intake, or catabolism. It can also be the result of direct parenchymal damage (glomerulonephritis, chronic pyelonephritis, acute tubular necrosis, acute glomerular damage) or obstruction of urine flow (stones, strictures, tumor). These etiologies are often grouped as "prerenal," "renal," and "postrenal," respectively, and may be responsible, separately or in combination, for elevations of the BUN or creatinine.

35. Are there more sensitive indicators of kidney dysfunction?

Yes. Urine clearance of creatinine, specific gravity, osmolality, electrolyte excretion, and free water clearance are tests used to evaluate kidney function. Clearance studies are most sensitive at defining mild-to-moderate, diffuse glomerular disease by providing an estimate of glomerular filtration rate (GFR). Creatinine is most often used because it estimates GFR with approximately 90% accuracy, whereas urea only approximates to 60%. These studies are very difficult to perform because they require a 24-hr collection, and all urine needs to be obtained accurately. In addition, the creatinine clearance must be corrected for variation in muscle mass, age, and sex. Urine specific gravity and osmolality tests measure the renal tubules' ability to concentrate urine and involve protracted preparation and collection times. All the above tests give more sensitive information regarding both glomerular and tubular function than BUN or creatinine; however, all are more expensive and difficult to obtain.

36. What information is obtained from a urinalysis?

- **pH** (4.5-8.0): Provides little useful information.
- **Specific gravity** (1.001-1.035): Provides spot view of kidney tubule concentrating ability.
- **Osmolality** (500-1200 mOsm/L): Provides similar information as specific gravity.
- **Blood or hemoglobin:** Results may indicate stone, trauma, tumor, infection, or menstruation.
- **Glucose/acetone:** Positive results may indicate diabetes mellitus, pancreatitis, tubular disease, or shock.
- **Bilirubin:** Normal is negative; positive results may indicate hepatitis or obstructive jaundice.
- **Protein:** Normal is negative; positive results might indicate fever, hypertension, glomerulonephritis, nephrotic syndrome, myeloma, or heavy exercise.
- **Nitrite:** Normal is negative; positive results indicate infection.
- **Leukocyte esterase:** Normal is negative; positive results indicate infection.
  Ketones: Normal is negative; positive results may indicate starvation, diabetic ketoacidosis (DKA), vomiting, diarrhea, or pregnancy.
- **Microscopic:**
  Squamous epithelial cells: Normal is none; any may indicate contamination.
  RBC: Normal is none; any may indicate tumor, stone, or pyelonephritis.
  WBC: Count <5/hpf indicates infection.
  Casts indicate tubular kidney disease or crystals/stones.

37. What lab studies are used to evaluate the pancreas?

Because the pancreas is vital for digestion and maintenance of homeostasis, the effects of pancreatic disease are seen in many tests. However, serum levels of amylase (starch digestion), lipase (fat digestion), and trypsin (protein digestion) allow a direct indication of pancreatic cell damage. Amylase levels peak about 29 hr after the onset of acute pancreatitis, as does lipase; however, once active cell damage has stopped, the amylase returns to normal within 72 hr, whereas lipase does not normalize for 7-10 days. Amylase levels also may be elevated because of common bile duct lithiasis, cholecystitis, tumor, peritonitis, peptic ulcer, intraabdominal hemorrhage, intestinal obstruction or infarction, acute salivary gland disease, DKA, pregnancy, burns, and renal failure. Lipase shows an increased specificity to the pancreas because lipase levels are elevated in pancreatitis, pancreatic duct obstruction, renal failure, and, much less significantly, intestinal obstruction or infarction and cholangitis. Trypsin is the most pancreatic-specific exocrine enzyme, but this assay is not widely available. Lastly, Ca levels also are followed in acute pancreatitis because it decreases with lipase's digestion of peritoneal fat (fat necrosis) and provides prognostic information.

38. How is blood glucose regulation monitored by the lab?

Glucose is regulated primarily by the liver in response to hormones released from structures such as the pancreas (insulin, glucagon), adrenal medulla (epinephrine), and adrenal cortex (cortisol/cortisone). Blood glucose is used most commonly to diagnose diabetes mellitus and to explain altered mental status. A fasting level above 140 mg/dL or nonfasting glucose >200 mg/dL is indicative of diabetes. A glucose tolerance test provides a more accurate assessment of the patient's ability to process glucose but may be inaccurate in cases of fever, stress, afternoon testing, inactivity, advancing age, trauma, or myocardial infarction. Glycosylated hemoglobin or HgbA1c (normally 6%-7% of total Hgb) is used to monitor patient compliance and treatment effectiveness. The amount of Hgb glycosylated is a function of degree and duration of RBC exposure to glucose and illustrates average blood glucose over a 2- to 4-month period.

An *increase* in glucose levels may indicate diabetes mellitus (type I or II), acute pancreatitis, hyperthyroidism, Cushing's syndrome, acromegaly, epinephrine (e.g., exogenous, pheochromo-cytoma, stress, burn), advancing age, or sample drawn above intravenous access.

A *decrease* in glucose levels may indicate oral hypoglycemics or exogenous insulin, pancreatitis, starvation, liver disease, sepsis, hypothyroidism, or postprandial "reactive" hypoglycemia (after gastric surgery).

39. What is measured by a "blood gas"?

This test is drawn from an artery (usually radial or femoral) and is sent to the lab in ice with the patient's temperature and current oxygen supplementation recorded (Table 4-3).

Table 4-3 *Blood Gas Measurements*

	DEFINITION	NORMAL RANGE
pH	Negative logarithm of hydrogenion concentration	7.35-7.45
P_{CO_2}	Partial pressure of CO_2 gas in blood that is proportional to the amount of dissolved CO_2	34-45 mm Hg
HCO_3^-	Concentration of bicarbonate in serum	20-28 mEq/L
Base difference or excess/deficit	The "normal" base amount is calculated using measured Hgb and normal values for pH and HCO_3^-, then this is compared with measured amount of blood base	$^{+}2-^{-}2$

Continued

Table 4-3   *Blood Gas Measurements—cont'd*

	DEFINITION	NORMAL RANGE
Po_2	Blood oxygen tension or dissolved O_2 content of plasma	80-95 mm Hg If patient is younger than age 60, the lower limit is dropped 1 mm Hg/year until age 60 is reached
$\%Sao_2$	Amount of Hgb bound with O_2 compared with the amount of Hgb available	Should be >90%

Hgb, Hemoglobin.

40. What components of the blood gas are used in determining acid-base status?

The essential test values are the pH, Pco_2, HCO_3^-, base difference, and anion gap (AG) from the basic metabolic formula:

$$AG = [Na^+] - ([Cl^-] + [HCO_3^-])$$

with a normal value of 8-12 mEq/L. The major buffering system of the blood is bicarbonate-carbonic acid:

$$CO_2 + H_2O \rightleftharpoons H_2CO_3 \rightleftharpoons H^+ + HCO_3^-$$

where H_2CO_3 = carbonic anhydrase, which is found in RBCs and kidney tubule epithelium. pH is determined as follows:

$$pH = pKa + \log (base/acid) = pKa + \log ([HCO_3^-]/0.03 \times Pco_2)$$

The normal $HCO_3^-/CO_2 = 20/1$.

The lung is the major regulator of Pco_2 with an increase of 10 mm Hg in hypoventilation corresponding to a pH drop of 0.08 U. The kidney regulates $[HCO_3^-]$ with response to acid-base abnormalities, taking 1-2 days for correction. Hemoglobin accounts for 75% of nonbicarbonate-based buffering of blood, whereas phosphate and other extracellular proteins account for the rest.

41. How are acid-base abnormalities determined and classified?

The first step is to evaluate pH. If pH < 7.35, then the finding is **acidosis.** A pH >7.45 indicates **alkalosis.** The next step uses Pco_2 and HCO_3^- to classify the primary abnormality as **respiratory** or **metabolic,** respectively. Metabolic acidosis is then further classified as an anion gap or nonanion gap problem. There will be a response to the primary disturbance by the opposite component in an attempt to compensate or normalize the pH. Any pH changes beyond 6.8-7.8 are incompatible with life. If the blood gas does not match the calculated compensation, then a **mixed acid-base disorder** should be suspected; that is, a respiratory acidosis and metabolic acidosis occurring simultaneously.

42. What are the common causes and compensations in the primary acid-base disorders?

Respiratory acidosis (hypoventilation): Pco_2 >45 mm Hg; HCO_3^- increase = change $Pco_2/10$ (acute) or $4 \times \Delta Pco_2/10$ (chronic 2-5 days). Possible etiology: chronic obstructive pulmonary disease (COPD), asthma, cardiac arrest, severe pulmonary edema or pneumonia, injury to airway or chest wall, cerebrovascular accident (CVA), drugs (narcotics, sedatives), foreign body, muscular dystrophy, or myasthenia gravis.

Respiratory alkalosis (hyperventilation): P_{CO_2} <35 mm Hg; HCO_3^- decrease = 2 × $\Delta P_{CO_2}/10$ (acute), 5 × $\Delta P_{CO_2}/10$ (chronic). Possible etiology: anxiety, pain, fever, pulmonary embolus, mechanical overventilation, head injury, hypoxia, increased altitude, interstitial lung disease, pregnancy, hyperthyroidism, hepatic insufficiency, aspirin overdose, or early sepsis.

Metabolic acidosis: HCO_3^- <20 mEq/L; P_{CO_2} decrease = 8 + (1.5 × HCO_3^-). Possible etiology:

- Anion gap normal: diarrhea, fistula, renal tubular acidosis
- Anion gap increased = extra acid:
  Exogenous: aspirin, methanol, ethylene glycol, ETOH ketoacidosis, hyperalimentation
  Endogenous: lactic acidosis, DKA or starvation ketoacidosis, uremia, severe dehydration

Metabolic alkalosis: HCO_3^- > 28 mEq/L, CO_2 increase = 0.6 × $\Delta[HCO_3^-]$. Possible etiology: nasogastric suction, vomiting, diuretics, cystic fibrosis, posthypercapnia, Cushing's syndrome, hyperaldosteronism, exogenous steroids, or hypoparathyroidism.

43. What components of the blood gas evaluate oxygenation?

The P_{O_2} and $\%SaO_2$ are used to monitor oxygenation. The P_{O_2} gives an estimate of the alveolar gas exchange with inspired air, so that the patient likely has normal ventilation if the P_{O_2} is normal. The amount of oxygen available to cells is given by the $\%SaO_2$, which may also be obtained using pulse oximetry. The "pulse ox" has been shown to measure Hgb O_2 saturation accurately between 70% and 100%, or P_{O_2} > 35-40 mm Hg. The oxygen saturation is influenced by temperature, pH, level of 2,3-diphosphoglycerate (2,3-DPG), and P_{O_2} as seen on the sigmoid-shaped O_2 dissociation curve. Hgb's affinity for O_2 is decreased by acidosis, fever, elevated 2,3-DPG, and hypoxia, which causes a shift of the curve to the right, and is increased with alkalosis, hypothermia, decreased 2,3-DPG, and banked blood, which causes a shift to the left.

44. How is an AMI ruled in or ruled out by the lab?

Much like the liver and pancreas, the heart has enzymes and proteins that are released from its cells in damage or death. A single measure alone of these substances is not adequate to rule out an AMI, and they should be checked at least twice in a 12-hr timeframe.

AST (SGOT) is found to increase in 90%-95% of AMIs, begins elevation in 8-12 hr, peaks at 1-2 days, and is normal in 3-8 days. There is a rough correlation between degree of elevation and extent of damage to the heart but low specificity for heart muscle.

LDH levels are elevated in 92%-95% of AMIs with slightly increased sensitivity over AST. LDH begins to rise at 24-48 hr, peaks at 2-3 days, and is normal at 5-10 days. Fractionating of isoenzymes shows improved specificity. LDH_1/LDH_2 >1 is seen in 80%-85% of AMIs. LDH_1 is found in RBCs, the heart, and the kidney, and normal values at 24 and 48 hr effectively rule out AMI.

Creatine kinase (CK) is increased in 90%-93% of AMIs. Levels begin to rise in 3-6 hr, peak at 12-24 hr, and are normal in 1-2 days. Fractionated isozymes are MM (skeletal muscle, 94%-100% of total), BB (brain and lung, usually 0% of total), and MB (heart fraction, usually <6% of total) and allow greater test specificity. There is a rough correlation with size of increase and amount of heart infarcted. Levels are usually checked at 0, 12, and 24 hr or 0, 8, 16, and 24 hr.

Troponin-T: An antibody that detects the cardiac-specific regulatory proteins. It has approximately the same specificity and sensitivity as CK-MB but rises in 4-6 hr, peaks at 11 hr, and is normal in 4 days.

Troponin-I: Same as above, but its timing is different; it begins to rise after 4-6 hr, peaks at 10-24 hr, and is normal after 10 days or more.

45. What tests are used to evaluate possible collagen vascular diseases?

Several nonspecific lab tests are used to help diagnose these enigmatic diseases:

- **Rheumatoid factor:** Positive in collagen vascular diseases, rheumatoid arthritis (RA), systemic lupus erythematosus (SLE), Sjögren's syndrome, scleroderma, polyarteritis nodosa, infections, CHF, inflammation, subacute bacterial endocarditis, MI, and lung disease

- **Lupus erythematosus (LE) preparation:** No cells = normal; positive in SLE, RA, scleroderma, and drug-induced lupus
- **Antinuclear antibody (ANA):** Negative result = normal; positive in SLE, scleroderma, drug-induced lupus, mixed connective tissue disease, RA, polymyositis, and juvenile RA
- **Antimicrosomal:** Detects Hashimoto's thyroiditis
- **Anticentromere:** Tests for scleroderma; Raynaud's disease; and *c*alcinosis, *R*aynaud's phenomenon, *e*sophageal involvement, *s*clerodactyly, and *t*elangiectasia (CREST) syndrome
- **Anti-SCL 70:** Detects scleroderma
- **Anti-DNA:** Detects SLE, mononucleosis, chronic active hepatitis

46. What are C-reactive protein (C-RP) and erythrocyte sedimentation rate (ESR) tests used to evaluate?

The C-RP and ESR are nonspecific but very sensitive markers for infections and inflammatory diseases. The ESR measures changes in plasma proteins (mainly fibrinogen) and is evaluated using several scales (zeta sedimentation ratio, Wintrobe method, Westergren method). The ESR is increased by any infection, inflammation, rheumatic fever, endocarditis, neoplasm, or AMI. The C-RP is a glycoprotein produced by acute inflammation and tissue destruction. Its levels are noted to begin elevating 4-6 hr after onset of inflammation and should be normal 5-7 days postoperatively or at least decreasing by day 3 after surgery; otherwise, an infection is likely. Other than inflammation or infection, the C-RP is also increased by pregnancy, oral contraceptives, and malignancies.

47. What tests are used to screen for thyroid disease?

The most sensitive screening test for thyroid disease is the thyroid stimulating hormone (TSH) level. It is elevated in hypothyroidism and low in hyperthyroidism. The thyroxine total (T_4 Tot) screens for hyperthyroidism with 95% sensitivity but is less accurate for hypothyroidism. Triiodothyronine (T_3) resin uptake (RU) is an indirect measurement of T_4. The test measures the protein thyroid-binding sites that are unbound and is elevated in hyperthyroidism, as a result of low thyroid-binding globulin (TBG), or if the patient is taking medications that bind TBG (e.g., phenytoin, aspirin, steroids, heparin). The T_3 RU is 80% sensitive for hyperthyroidism but only 40% for hypothyroidism. The free thyroxine index (FTI) is determined by multiplying the T_4 Tot by the T_3 RU and has a 95% sensitivity for hyperthyroidism and 90%-95% sensitivity for hypothyroidism. The FTI attempts to balance the TBG effects on T_4 measurement. TBG is elevated in pregnancy, estrogen use, liver disease, and hypothyroidism. Total serum T_3 (T_3-RIA) is also measured in some labs and is equivalent to T_4 Tot measurements.

48. What tests can be used to evaluate possible bone disease?

The Ca and P levels (discussed previously). Alkaline phosphatase also can be used and is elevated in hyperparathyroidism, Paget's disease, osteoblastic bone tumors, osteomalacia, rickets, pregnancy, childhood, healing fractures, hyperthyroidism, and liver disease. The liver disorders may be ruled out using fractionated enzyme levels or checking GGT or 5'nucleotidase.

49. What procedures are done to evaluate body fluids and pathology specimens for organisms?

The most definitive test to isolate infectious agents is culturing, but this requires 24 hr at minimum. Staining allows for rapid screening identification to assist in selecting empiric antibiotics. The most common stains are:

- **Gram:** "Positive" organisms turn a violet color because the microorganisms' thick cell walls of peptidoglycan and teichoic acid resist decolorization. "Negative" organisms have a thin cell wall and outer lipoprotein or lipopolysaccharide coat that decolorize in alcohol and pick up the counterstain (red).

- **Acid-fast:** These organisms do not decolorize in strong acid and are usually mycobacterium species.
- **Potassium hydroxide (KOH):** 10% KOH dissolves most cellular elements except for fungus species.
- **Wayson:** Used for general bacteria screening.
- **India ink:** Identifies mostly fungi in cerebrospinal fluid (CSF).
- **Giemsa:** Stains intracellular organisms (chlamydia, malaria) and viral inclusion bodies.
- Newer technology with DNA/polymerase chain reaction (PCR) probes and enzyme-linked immunosorbent assay (ELISA) tests allows rapid detection of organisms (e.g., *Gonozyme*, *Streptozyme*) or monospot tests.

50. What tests are used to evaluate viral hepatitis?

Hepatitis A: Oral/fecal hepatitis is usually self-limited. Acute infection tests positive for immunoglobulin M (IgM) ± IgG. Old infection or convalescence tests negative for IgM but positive for IgG. The antigen may be detected in stool but usually is gone before symptoms appear.

Hepatitis B: Blood-borne disease with 1% acute fatality; 5%-15% develop chronic disease and 3% develop hepatoma:
- HBsAg: Surface antigen from viral outer envelope indicates current or active hepatitis B virus (HBV) infection; DNA PCR probe is most accurate indicator of activity, infectivity, and progression to chronicity.
- Anti-HBs: Indicates immunity and end of acute HBV.
- Anti-HBcAg (presence of antibody to core viral protein): Indicates a recent or acute infection and is present during "core window" while HBsAg and anti-HBs are negative; drops out after 3-6 months.
- Anti-HBc Tot: Stays positive for life; shows old infection if HBsAg and HBc-IgM are negative.
- HBeAg/Anti-HBe: Indicate infectivity, because as anti-HBe increases, the infectivity decreases.
- Chronic hepatitis B states:
  Carrier-positive HBsAg but negative biopsy and liver function tests (LFTs).
  Persistent hepatitis B: As above, with negative biopsy and abnormal LFTs.
  Active hepatitis B: As above, with positive biopsy and abnormal LFTs.

Hepatitis C: Posttransfusion transmission; low severity acutely but 60% for chronic disease. Hepatitis C virus (HCV) nucleic probe shows current infection, but this is still investigational, and anti-HC indicates current, convalescing, or old HCV infection.

Hepatitis D: Requires HBV infection to be present, parenteral transmission, 5% acute fatality, 5% chronic. HDAg indicates infection; may follow with antibody levels.

51. What tests are used to detect and monitor HIV infection?

HIV antigen detection is used by blood banks because they may detect viral presence as early as 1-2 weeks. Antibodies are used to detect core proteins p24 or p55 and envelope glycoproteins gp41, 120, or 160. They are about 80%-90% sensitive if patients have symptoms but 60%-65% without. Nucleic acid probe with PCR amplification is also being used with 98% sensitivity at 3 months but 40%-60% at 1-2 weeks. More commonly, patients are screened for the presence of antibodies in their serum, which take an average of 6-10 weeks to develop or "seroconvert." The ELISA test screens the patient's blood for antibodies. A positive ELISA test is confirmed by Western blot, which looks for the most specific antibodies to gp41 and p24 or group-specific antigen (gag) core protein. Once HIV infection is determined, the CD4 T-cell count, viral load, and beta$_2$-microglobulin levels are followed for infection severity, prognosis, and activity, and to direct therapy. The CD4 count (normal 600-1600 cells/mm^3) is a useful indicator of immune system damage and ability to respond effectively to pathogens. Immune suppression occurs with counts below 500 cells/mm^3 denoting an advanced risk of opportunistic infections and need for prophylactic antibiotics. Viral load assays appear to be the best prognostic marker for a patient's long-term clinical outcome and are used in conjunction with CD4 counts to direct antiviral therapy. Beta$_2$-microglobulin is a soluble marker for immune system activation and can be used to evaluate disease progression or exacerbation.

52. What tests screen for or assist diagnosis of cancer?

Alpha-fetoprotein (AFP): Elevated in hepatoma, testicular tumors, occasionally benign hepatic disease (hepatitis, alcoholic cirrhosis) and in pregnancy: neural tube defects, multiple gestation, or fetal death.

Cancer antigen 19-9 (CA 19-9): Elevated in 80%-85% pancreatic adenocarcinoma, 40%-50% gastric adenocarcinoma, 30%-40% colorectal cancer, 50% hepatoma, 16%-20% lung cancer, and 14%-27% breast cancer.

CA 125: Increased in ovarian, endometrial, and colon cancers; also in endometriosis, inflammatory bowel disease, pelvic inflammatory disease, pregnancy, breast lesion, and teratomas.

Carcinoembryonic antigen (CEA): Not used to screen but is a good monitor of recurrence and response to treatment (if checked before started). Elevated in colon, pancreas, lung, and stomach cancers, as well as in smokers and those with Crohn's disease, liver disease, and ulcerative colitis.

Prostate specific antigen (PSA): Good for screening and monitoring after treatment. Levels above 10 mg/dL are associated with cancer >90%. Also, a "velocity" of 0.75 mg/mL/year indicates high suspicion for cancer. Differential diagnosis for elevation includes prostate cancer, acute prostatitis, benign prostate hypertrophy, prostate surgery, and vigorous prostate massage. Normal rectal exam has no influence.

53. What basic tests are used to evaluate CSF?

Opening pressure: Normal is 100-200 mm Hg; most significantly elevated in bacterial infections (meningitis) and subarachnoid hemorrhage (SAH).

Color or appearance: Normal is clear and colorless, but bloody or xanthochromic (yellow from Hgb breakdown) after 2-8 hr in SAH and white or cloudy in bacterial infections.

Glucose: Normal is $\frac{1}{2}$ serum glucose (45-80 mg/dL) but will be < 20 mg/dL in meningitis and between 20 and 40 mg/dL in granulomatous infection (tuberculosis or fungal).

Protein: Normal range is 15-45 mg/dL, but the upper limit is debated. Levels will be 50-1500 mg/dL in meningitis and will be increased but <500 mg/dL in granulomatous disease.

Cell count: Normal is up to 5/mm^3 with all being lymphocytes; any condition that affects the meninges will cause CSF leukocytosis, the degree being determined by type, duration, and severity of irritation. The highest counts are seen in meningitis with PMNs dominating, whereas viral and granulomatous disease cause elevations to 10-500 cells, with lymphocytes predominant. SAH and traumatic taps will have increased cell counts made up of RBCs and WBCs in a ratio about equal to blood (1 WBC per 500-1000 RBCs). However, no good formulas exist to confirm that the WBC elevation is an artifact from a traumatic tap vs. infective or inflammatory increase. Gram's stain and culture are performed in all suspected infective taps.

54. What tests can be done to verify or exclude a CSF leak in craniofacial trauma?

Confirmation of CSF otorrhea or rhinorrhea in trauma can be challenging. Typically, one looks for a colorless fluid, glucose about 45 mg/dL (nasal secretions < 30 mg/dL and blood > 80 usually), and low protein and potassium compared with nasal secretions or serum. Trauma patients, however, often exhibit a complex mixture of these body fluids, blocking chemical analysis. The most sensitive and specific test requires about 2-10 µL of fluid, protein electrophoresis, and about 3 hr to complete in a modern lab. The beta$_2$-transferrin isozyme will be isolated correctly in the presence of any mixture of fluid, and a beta$_1$ subset allows reduction of cirrhotic false-positive results. This test helps prevent the need for more invasive radiologic studies to rule out CSF leak.

55. Is a complete blood count of value in making a diagnosis?

Yes, but mostly in certain diagnoses. For example, if the Hct is high (>45%), the patient is most likely dehydrated or may have chronic obstructive pulmonary disease (emphysema). If it is low (<30%), the patient may have a more chronic disease associated with blood loss.

Similarly, for WBC count it takes hours for inflammation to release cytokines and cause elelvation of the WBC count. Accordingly, a normal WBC count is not entirely inconsistent with infection.

56. How is urinalysis useful?

WBCs in the urine should direct attention to the diagnosis of pyelonephritis or cystitis. Hematuria may indicate renal or ureteral stones. RBCs and WBCs may be found in the urine of patients with appendicitis.

BIBLIOGRAPHY

1. Aziz N, Detels R, Fahey JL et al: Prognostic significance of plasma markers of immune activation, HIV viral load and CD4 T-cell measurements. AIDS 12:1581-1590, 1998.
2. Burns ER, Lawrence C: Bleeding time. A guide to its diagnostic and clinical utility. Arch Pathol Lab Med 113:1219-1224, 1989.
3. Fauci A (ed): Harrison's Principles of Internal Medicine, 14th ed. New York, 1997, McGraw-Hill.
4. Gomella LG (ed): Clinician's Pocket Reference, 8th ed. Stamford, Conn, 1997, Appleton & Lange.
5. Harken AH: Priorities in evaluation of the acute abdomen. In Harken AH, Moore EE (eds): Abernathy's Surgical Secrets, 5th ed. St Louis, 2005, Mosby.
6. Harken AH, Moore EE (eds): Abernathy's Surgical Secrets, 5th ed. St Louis, 2005, Mosby.
7. Jacobs DS, DeMott WR, Grady HJ et al (eds): Laboratory Test Handbook, 4th ed. Hudson, Ohio, 1996, Lexi-Corp.
8. Kaiser R, Kupfer B, Rockstroh JK et al: Role of HIV-1 phenotype in viral pathogenesis and its relation to viral load and CD4+ T-cell count. J Med Virol 56:259-263, 1998.
9. Krutsch JP: Coagulation. In Duke J (ed): Anesthesia Secrets, 3rd ed. Philadelphia, 2006, Mosby.
10. Kwon P, Laskin D (eds): Clinical Manual of Oral and Maxillofacial Surgery, 2nd ed. Chicago, 1997, Quintessence.
11. Little JW, Falace DA, Miller CS et al: Dental Management of the Medically Compromised Patient, 6th ed. St Louis, 2002, Mosby.
12. Malley WJ: Clinical Blood Gases: Assessment and Intervention, 2nd ed. Philadelphia, 2005, Saunders.
13. Miller-Keane, O'Toole MT: Miller-Keane Encyclopedia & Dictionary of Medicine, Nursing, & Allied Health, 7th ed. Philadelphia, 2005, Saunders.
14. Patton LL, Shugars DC: Immunologic and viral markers of HIV-1 disease progression: implications for dentistry. J Am Dent Assoc 130:1313-1322, 1999.
15. Peacock MK, Ryall RG, Simpson DA: Usefulness of beta$_2$-transferrin assay in the detection of cerebrospinal fluid leaks following head injury. J Neurosurg 77:737-739, 1992.
16. Ravel R: Clinical Laboratory Medicine, 6th ed. St Louis, 1995, Mosby.
17. Schwarz SI, Shires GT, Spencer FC (eds): Principles of Surgery, 7th ed. New York, 1998, McGraw-Hill.
18. Wu AHB: Tietz Clinical Guide to Laboratory Tests, 4th ed. St Louis, 2006, Saunders.
19. Zaret DL, Morrison N, Gulbranson R et al: Immunofixation to quantify beta$_2$-transferrin in cerebrospinal fluid to detect leakage of cerebrospinal fluid from skull injury. Clin Chem 38:1908-1912, 1992.

5. DIAGNOSTIC IMAGING FOR THE ORAL AND MAXILLOFACIAL SURGERY PATIENT

Corey C. Burgoyne, DMD, A. Omar Abubaker, DMD, PhD, and James A. Giglio, DDS, MEd

1. What are the basic units of radiation?

The units of absorbed radiation:
- Gray (Gy)
- Rads

The units of biologically effective radiation:
- Rem
- Sieverts (Sv)

Conversion between units:
- 1 Gy = 100 rad
- 1 mSv = 0.001 Gy

2. What are the radiographic patterns of disease on an x-ray exam of the chest?

The patterns of disease on a chest radiograph are limited. The three most common patterns are:

1. **Alveolar.** Pulmonary alveolar disease is the most common pattern and appears as a localized, homogeneous, fluffy density. It can represent water, blood, pus, or tumor within the alveoli.
2. **Interstitial.** The interstitial pattern may be reticular (linear), nodular, or a combination of the two (reticulonodular). The reticular pattern usually is bilateral and diffuse.
3. **Nodular.** The nodular pattern of disease appears as discrete, well-circumscribed, radiopaque masses in the lung field.

3. What is the diagnostic value of posteroanterior (PA) chest films (Fig. 5-1)?

A PA chest film is taken by directing an x-ray beam from posterior to anterior on the chest. This radiograph is useful to evaluate the soft tissue and bony tissues of the chest, the diaphragm, the heart and mediastinum, the hila of the lungs, and the entire PA view of the lung fields.

4. What are the main uses of a lateral chest film (Fig. 5-2)?

- Localizing lesions to a specific area of the lungs or mediastinum
- Diagnosing small pleural effusions (blunting of the posterior costophrenic angles)
- Diagnosing vertebral and sternal abnormalities

5. What is the chest x-ray appearance of a pneumothorax (Fig. 5-3)?

Pneumothorax is usually represented by a thin, linear density that parallels the chest wall. No long markings should be seen peripheral to this line. In tension pneumothorax, a shift in the mediastinum is seen, especially with a large tension pneumothorax.

6. What radiographic changes are associated with chronic obstructive pulmonary disease (COPD)?

- Hyperexpanded lung fields
- Flattening of the diaphragm
- A large, radiolucent zone behind the sternum
- Elongated heart

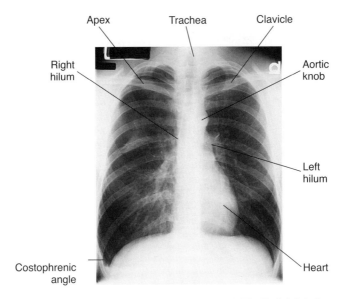

Fig. 5-1   Posteroanterior chest projection. (From Long BW, Frank ED, Ehrlich RA: Bony thorax, chest, and abdomen. In Long BW, Frank ED, Ehrlich RA: Radiography Essentials for Limited Practice, 2nd ed. St Louis, 2006, Saunders.)

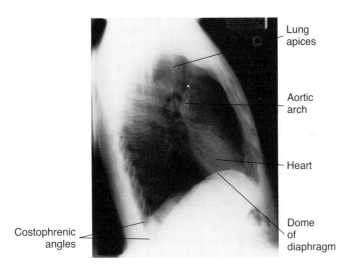

Fig. 5-2   Lateral chest projection. (From Long BW, Frank ED, Ehrlich RA: Bony thorax, chest, and abdomen. In Long BW, Frank ED, Ehrlich RA: Radiography Essentials for Limited Practice, 2nd ed. St Louis, 2006, Saunders.)

7.   What radiographic changes are associated with chronic bronchitis?

Chest radiographs of chronic bronchitis show increased bronchiovascular markings at the base of the lungs. In patients with emphysema, chest radiographs show overdistention of the lungs, flattening of the diaphragm, and emphysematous bullae.

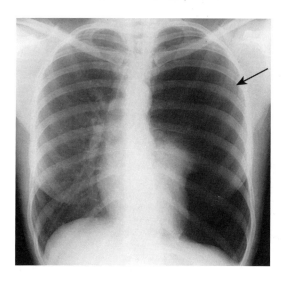

Fig. 5-3 Posteroanterior chest film showing a left pneumothorax (*arrow*). (From Bosker JI, Powers MP, Bosker H: Management of nonpenetrating chest trauma. In Fonseca RJ, Walker RV, Betts NJ [eds]: Oral and Maxillofacial Trauma, 3rd ed. St Louis, 2005, Saunders.)

8. How do lung masses show up on chest films?

Lung masses usually follow the nodular pattern of disease. Masses within the lung fields can be divided into **cavitary** and **noncavitary lesions** and represent either tumor or infection. Other causes of masses include vascular malformations, but these are far less common than tumor and infection.

9. What is a lordotic chest radiograph used for?

A lordotic chest radiograph permits better visualization of the apices of the lung. This view should be obtained when a questionable lesion is seen in these areas on a standard chest radiograph.

10. What is the common chest radiographic finding in AIDS patients?

Infectious pulmonary disease. *Pneumocystis carinii* pneumonia, the most common infection, usually has the pattern of a fine, diffuse reticular process.

11. Which views are included in an acute abdominal series? When are they used?

• Supine and upright abdominal films (to view the kidneys, ureter, and bladder)
• Chest radiograph
  These views are used for the initial evaluation of acute abdominal pain or trauma.

12. What is a KUB?

KUB is a radiographic view to evaluate the *k*idneys, *u*reters, and *b*ladder. The series, which is also known as a **supine abdominal radiograph,** is useful in the initial work-up of abdominal pain, distention of the bowel, and change of bowel habits. It also is used for evaluation of urinary tract problems. Renal stones and 10%-20% of gallstones are visualized by a KUB. Evaluation of the KUB views involves examining the bowel gas pattern and looking for calcifications and radiopaque foreign bodies. The psoas; renal, liver, and splenic shadows; flank stripes; vertebral bodies; and pelvic bones also are examined.

13. What is a barium swallow (esophagram)?

An esophagram, usually performed with barium, a water-soluble contrast agent, is used to evaluate the swallowing mechanism and to look for esophageal lesions or abnormal peristalsis. No preparation is required for this study.

14. What is the upper gastrointestinal series (UGI)?

UGI, which includes an esophagram, is used to study the stomach and duodenum. This double-contrast study uses barium and air and is useful for detection of gastritis, ulcers, masses, hiatal hernias, and gastrointestinal reflux. It is also an important part of the work-up of heme-positive stools and upper abdominal pain.

15. What is an intravenous pyelogram (IVP)?

This imaging technique uses intravenous (IV) contrast to evaluate the kidneys, ureters, and bladder. This test is indicated for patients with hematuria, kidney stones, urinary tract infection, and suspected malignancy of the kidney or bladder and is used for the work-up of patients with flank pain.

16. What are the different nuclear scans and their uses?

In nuclear scans, or nuclear medicine studies, radionuclides are injected intravenously, and results are based on detection of the tissue uptake of these radionuclides, specifically the degree of uptake, the time intervals between the studies, and the injection of the radionuclides.

Bone scan is a nuclear scan study that uses radioactive tracers, such as technetium 99, to detect areas of increased or decreased bone **metabolism** (turnover). Areas that absorb little tracer appear as dark or "cold" spots, which may indicate a lack of blood supply to the bone or the presence of certain types of cancer. Areas of rapid bone growth or repair absorb increased amounts of the tracer and show up as bright or "hot" spots in the pictures, which indicate the presence of a tumor, a fracture, or an infection. Bone scans are used in metastatic work-ups, especially in patients with cancer that has a predilection to metastasize to bone (e.g., breast, prostate, kidney, lung, thyroid). It is also used as a screening test for primary tumors, osteomyelitis, avascular necrosis, and stress fractures.

Gallium scan is used to locate abscesses that are more than 5-10 days old. When used in combination with a bone scan, the gallium scan is very specific for osteomyelitis. **Indium 111 white blood cell scans** can be substituted for gallium scanning to detect osteomyelitis.

Cardiac scan has become increasingly popular in recent years and is used for many purposes, including detection of myocardial infarction and ischemia, stress testing, and evaluation of ejection fractions, cardiac output, and ventricular aneurysms.

Liver-spleen scan is used to estimate parenchymal disease, abscess, tumors, and cysts in these organs. The current preference for computed tomography (CT) scanning has significantly decreased the use of the liver-spleen scan.

Ventilation-perfusion lung scan is used principally for the evaluation of pulmonary emboli. Although not as sensitive or specific as a pulmonary angiogram or spiral CT, the ventilation-perfusion scan is less invasive and often is obtained following a chest radiograph when the diagnosis of pulmonary embolus is suspected.

17. What (plain film) views are included in a facial series, and what are they used for?

A facial series usually includes Caldwell's view, Waters' view, lateral skull view, and submentovertex view (view of the zygomatic arches). These studies are used for the initial work-up of facial trauma.

18. What plain film views are included on a mandible series, and what are they used for?

A mandibular series includes a Towne's view, a PA skull view, both oblique views of the mandible, and a panoramic view. This series is used mainly for evaluation of the mandible following facial trauma.

19. What views are included in a nasal bone series?

Nasal bone series includes an anteroposterior (AP) skull view and both lateral views of the nasal bones. This series is used for evaluation of trauma to the nose.

20. **What are the normal anatomic radiographic landmarks on a Panorex and plain facial film (Fig. 5-4)?**

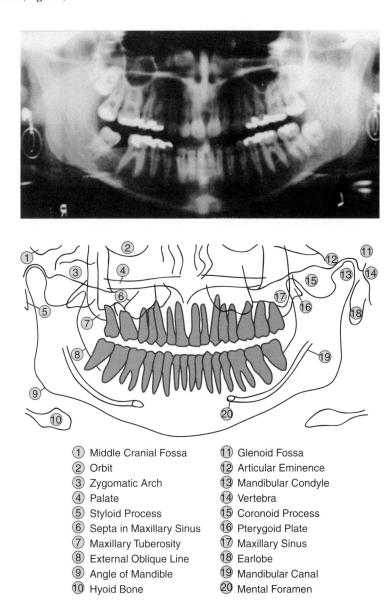

① Middle Cranial Fossa	⑪ Glenoid Fossa
② Orbit	⑫ Articular Eminence
③ Zygomatic Arch	⑬ Mandibular Condyle
④ Palate	⑭ Vertebra
⑤ Styloid Process	⑮ Coronoid Process
⑥ Septa in Maxillary Sinus	⑯ Pterygoid Plate
⑦ Maxillary Tuberosity	⑰ Maxillary Sinus
⑧ External Oblique Line	⑱ Earlobe
⑨ Angle of Mandible	⑲ Mandibular Canal
⑩ Hyoid Bone	⑳ Mental Foramen

Fig. 5-4   Panoramic radiograph and tracing showing numbered anatomic landmarks. (Courtesy KaVo Dental Corporation, Lake Zurich, Ill.)

21. **What is a sinus series?**

A sinus series is used for evaluating the paranasal sinuses, including the frontal, ethmoid, maxillary, and sphenoid sinuses. The views taken usually include a Caldwell's, Waters', lateral, and submentovertex. This series is used for the initial evaluation of sinusitis or sinus masses.

22. What views are included in the cervical spine series?
   The cervical spine series usually includes PA and lateral views, both oblique views, and odontoid views of the cervical spine. This series is useful for evaluating traumatic injury, neck pain, and neurologic symptoms referable to the upper extremities. All seven cervical vertebrae must be seen for the exam to be considered acceptable.

23. What views are included in airway films?
   Airway films include AP and lateral views of the neck to provide good visualization of the airways and adjacent soft tissues. It is used as the initial step in the work-up of masses, foreign bodies, and infections of the airway.

24. What are the uses and advantages of plain film tomography?
   With the advent of CT, plain film tomography now has only limited utility in the evaluation of problems within the head and neck. Its principal advantage is that it does not show the metallic artifact that often obscures the CT evaluation of postoperative patients. It also has the advantage of allowing three-plane evaluation of bony structures, which can only be accomplished with CT scans by reconstruction of axial views. In evaluating temporomandibular joints (TMJs), sagittal tomography frequently provides more information about the bony architecture of this joint than axial CT scans do.

25. When are CT scans of the head and neck indicated?
- **Head CT:** Head trauma to rule out intracranial injury or pathology and to evaluate for skull fractures
- **MaxFace CT:** Head or facial trauma to evaluate midface and/or orbital fractures
- **MaxFace CT with extension through the mandible:** Head or facial trauma to evaluate midface and/or orbital fractures, with suspected mandible fracture also
- **Neck CT:** To evaluate the mandible and/or airway for trauma and/or infection
- **C-spine CT:** When a cervical spine series is deemed inadequate

26. When is contrast indicated/contraindicated for head and neck CT scans?
   Contrast agents are used in CT exams and in other radiology procedures to illuminate details of anatomy more clearly. Some contrasts are natural, such as air or water. Iodine or barium sulfate oral or rectal contrast is usually given when examining the abdomen or cells, but not when scanning the brain or chest. Iodine is the most widely used IV contrast agent and is given through an IV needle.
Indications: To illuminate anatomy via enteral or parenteral contrast
Contraindications: Allergic reaction, renal failure, elevated creatinine

27. What prophylactic measures may be taken for patients who have a previous allergy to IV contrast?
   Anaphylactic reactions to contrast agents used during endoscopic retrograde cholangiopancreatography (ERCP) are rare. Nevertheless, a history of sensitivity to iodine contrast or drug should always be considered in the preprocedure assessment and in the informed consent process. In patients with prior allergy to contrast media, prophylactic measures adopted by most endoscopists include:
- Use of nonionic/low osmolarity contrast media
- Premedication with oral steroids starting the day before ERCP, or IV steroids when allergy is discovered just before the procedure. Some endoscopists also give an IV antihistamine in combination with the steroids.

28. What is sialography?
   Sialography is an imaging study used for the radiographic demonstration of the salivary gland ductal system. It is accomplished by cannulating the ducts of the submandibular and parotid glands and injecting a radiopaque contrast medium.

29. When is sialography indicated?

- To detect or confirm small radiopaque or radiolucent sialoliths or foreign bodies
- To evaluate damage secondary to recurrent inflammation
- To provide a more detailed evaluation of suspected neoplasms, such as size, location, and extension into adjacent tissues
- To evaluate fistulas, strictures, and diverticula of the ductal system, especially in posttraumatic cases
- To detect chronic sialadenitis and chronic stricture (rarely used)

30. When is sialography contraindicated?

- In patients with known sensitivity to iodine compounds
- In acute salivary inflammation

31. What does the obstructive form of salivary gland disease look like on a sialogram?

In the acute form of obstructive salivary gland disease and acute sialadenitis, sialography is rarely performed and mostly contraindicated. However, a sialogram performed during a clinically quiescent period of the disease in a patient with the obstructive form of the disease usually shows a focal narrowing (stricture) of the main duct and a central dilatation (sialectasia), with these ducts tapering dramatically to normal peripheral ducts. If the acini are compressed and destroyed by the cellular infiltrate, the peripheral ducts and acini are not visualized, even on a technically good sialogram.

32. What is the appearance of Sjögren's syndrome on a sialogram?

Sjögren's syndrome initially involves only the peripheral intraglandular ducts and acini. Accordingly, the early stages of the disease are manifested on a sialogram as normal central duct system and numerous, uniform, peripheral punctate collections of contrast material throughout the gland. These changes are the earliest sialographic features and are diagnostic of the disease. As the disease progresses, the sialogram is said to resemble a leafless fruit-laden tree or a mulberry tree. The advanced form of the disease is seen on a sialogram as dilatation of the central ducts and, eventually, a large peripheral collection of the contrast material and the associated changes of sialadenitis superimposed on the punctate and globular findings of Sjögren's syndrome.

33. What is the best imaging technique to diagnose TMJ disc displacement (Fig. 5-5)?

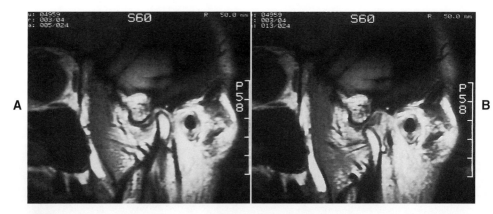

Fig. 5-5   Magnetic resonance imaging of open (**A**) and closed (**B**) views of right temporomandibular joint with early anterior disc displacement with reduction. (From Quinn PD: Diagnostic imaging of the temporomandibular joint. In Quinn PD: Color Atlas of Temporomandibular Joint Surgery. St Louis, 1998, Mosby.)

Currently magnetic resonance imaging (MRI) is the imaging of choice to show disc displacement with and without reduction. Dynamic MRI techniques are also used to enhance the diagnostic quality of the image. Although an arthrogram was used in the past to make such diagnosis, it is currently rarely used for such purpose.

34. How are disc perforations of the TMJ diagnosed?

Although MRI is usually the first choice for soft tissue imaging of the TMJ in most clinical situations, the best imaging modality available to diagnose disc perforations is arthrography. Because of the recent decrease in use of arthrography, diagnosis of disc perforation currently is based on clinical exam.

35. What is arthrography?

A major limitation of plain radiography is the poor visualization of soft tissues. To overcome this problem, intraarticular contrast agents—standard 60% iodinated contrast is the usual choice—may be used to highlight soft tissue structures by coating their surfaces with radiopaque liquid and/or air. This allows for a better identification of loose bodies, ligament or tendon injuries, synovial or cartilage pathology, sinus tracts or cavities, and loosening of joint prostheses. Although arthrography can also be performed using either CT or MRI, standard arthrography is still helpful for the evaluation of joint replacements because of the presence of metal in the implant.

Arthrography is performed using fluoroscopic guidance. Following the administration of local anesthesia, the joint space is entered and contrast, and occasionally air (to produce a double contrast image), are injected through a 20-gauge spinal needle. Synovial fluid may be aspirated for diagnostic and/or therapeutic purposes. Selected radiographs are obtained immediately and after manipulation of the joint.

Complications of arthrography are few, the most common being synovial irritation (chemical synovitis) induced by the iodinated contrast agent. Infection is very rare.

36. What are the main disadvantages to arthrography?

TMJ arthrography is an invasive imaging modality that requires a skilled, well-trained, and knowledgeable radiologist. It also can be associated with some degree of pain and discomfort.

37. What are the advantages and disadvantages of MRI for the diagnosis of TMJ pathology?

Advantages

- Provides an image of both hard and soft tissue structures of the TMJ in multiple planes
- Does not use radiation
- Is not technically demanding

Disadvantages

- Is expensive for patients
- Is not well tolerated by patients suffering from claustrophobia

38. What are indications and contraindications for MRI? What are T1 and T2 images?

Magnetic resonance images are based on proton density and proton relaxation dynamics due to magnetic fields. These vary according to the tissue under examination and reflect its physical and chemical properties. There is no radiation exposure during MRI.

In the detection, localization, and treatment planning of head and neck tumors, MRI offers an advantage over CT because of its multiplanar capabilities, tissue characterization potential, and the absence of bone and teeth artifacts. MRI affords ready distinction of vessels from lymph nodes. MRI also depicts the contents of the orbit.

T1 weighted images: DARK = water, cerebrospinal fluid (CSF), edema, calcium
LIGHT = lipid, gadolinium
T2 weighted images: DARK = calcium, bone
LIGHT = water, CSF, edema

MRI is absolutely contraindicated in patients with cerebral aneurysm clips and cardiac pacemakers. However, it should be noted that titanium in bone plates and dental implants do not affect the MRI exam. Remember that MRI machines are large magnets that never turned off!

39. How can CT assist in dental implant treatment planning?

Historically, implant patients were evaluated with panoramic, intraoral, and cephalometric films to determine the location of the inferior alveolar nerve, sinus location, and ridge height. However, exact measurements are not possible, and these films do not allow assessment of the average width of the ridge. Hence, a CT program was developed (DentaScan) that provides direct axial images of the mandible and maxilla to permit accurate measurements for implant length and width and visualization of internal anatomy.

40. How does cone beam imaging differ from a traditional CT scan?

Cone beam imaging can obtain thinner slices (0.5 mm vs. 1.0 mm), reducing the number of artifacts, with a reduced skin dose of radiation.

41. How is diagnostic and interventional angiography used by the oral and maxillofacial surgeon?

Diagnostic and interventional angiography assists the oral and maxillofacial surgeon in the diagnosis and delineation of uncontrollable hemorrhage and vascular tumors in the maxillofacial region. When coupled with CT and MRI exams, the surgical approach and definitive treatment can be planned. The use of interventional angiography for embolization of vascular tumors before or instead of surgical resection has become a popular modality in the management of these tumors.

42. What is the role of radionuclide scintigraphy in oral and maxillofacial surgery?

Oral and maxillofacial surgeons use radionuclide scintigraphy to evaluate bone and joint diseases because it provides more sensitive bone imaging than conventional radiologic techniques. Specifically, scintigraphy or bone scanning can assist in the evaluation of arthritic changes to the TMJ, condylar hyperplasia, idiopathic condylar resorption (active and inactive), metabolic disorders, viability of bone grafts, trauma, dental disorders, osteomyelitis, and malignancies. However, it should be noted that scintigraphy has a low specificity for abnormal findings, and 20%-50% of patients referred for routine bone scan may have abnormal activity in the mandible or face.

43. What diagnostic imaging modalities are useful for the diagnosis of cysts and benign odontogenic tumors of the jaw?

Most pathologies in the oral and maxillofacial region can be demonstrated through conventional radiographs. The panoramic radiograph is still the primary screening film for the oral and maxillofacial surgeon, but CT and MRI have proved to be useful adjuncts, especially when planning surgical intervention. CT is extremely helpful for illustrating cysts and tumors of the mandible and maxilla, especially if the lesion extends beyond the bony cortex with encroachment on the adjacent soft tissue structures. MRI is useful in differentiating cysts from solid tumors and differentiating fluid within the cystic lumen from other cystic components such as keratin and blood degradation products.

44. What diagnostic imaging modalities are used for evaluation of malignant diseases of the jaws?

- CT
- Polycycloidal tomography

- MRI
- Panoramic radiography
- Radionuclide scanning techniques

Radiologic evaluation of jaw lesions requires an image that accurately differentiates bone and soft tissue. CT permits the accurate assessment of tumor size, location, and extent of spread and detects subtle bony involvement and calcifications. However, MRI provides high-resolution, thin tomographic images with superior soft tissue contrast. In addition, MRI allows visualization of blood vessels without IV contrast agents and some information regarding tissue composition.

45. What are the uses of the different imaging techniques for mandibular fractures?

Plain films are the most cost-effective and adequate means to image mandibular injuries. The panoramic radiograph is still the primary imaging modality used by the oral and maxillofacial surgeon to evaluate mandibular fractures. AP, lateral skull, Waters', and Towne's views also can be helpful. Additionally, CT exam in the axial and coronal planes can assist in the diagnosis of mandibular fractures, especially in the condylar-subcondylar region.

46. Which imaging modalities are used to diagnose midfacial fractures?

The initial radiographic survey of patients with midface trauma should include Waters', Towne's, AP, lateral skull, and submentovertex views. However, because the facial bone diverges in a posterior-to-anterior direction, AP views distort bone anatomy and produce magnified and overlapping structural images. Hence, CT is the definitive means of imaging midfacial trauma. Generally, axial views are easily obtained and very useful, but they should be supplemented with views in the coronal plane. Direct coronal views are obtained to appreciate the orbital roof, floor, palate, and maxillary alveolar processes. However, direct coronal views are attainable only after the patient's cervical spine is clear, because the patient must assume a position with the neck in hypertension. If direct coronals are not possible, reconstruction data from axial images may be used to obtain coronal images. These reconstructed images are usually somewhat deformed and misleading because the pixel edges of each slice give a serrated appearance to bone surfaces; they will, however, demonstrate gross discrepancies in position or size of structures.

47. What imaging techniques are used for evaluation of maxillary sinus pathology?

Radiographic examination of the maxillary sinus is routinely conducted as a standard sinus series in three imaging planes with the patient in the upright position, allowing fluid and air to be separated horizontally. The standard sinus series generally includes Waters', Caldwell, lateral skull, and submentovertex views, but it can be supplemented with panoramic radiography. If indicated by the plain film examination, a CT can be performed to allow visualization of both bony and soft tissues. In addition, CT allows visualization of the extent of bone destruction and soft tissue reactions to disease including infiltrations. Recently, MR tomography has proved to be a useful imaging modality for the sinuses owing to its superior soft tissue imaging and ability to demonstrate edematous and inflammatory changes with great clarity. Furthermore, MRI is not affected by the beam-hardening artifacts from dental amalgam or dense cortical bone.

48. What imaging modalities are used for diagnosis of inflammatory disorders of the jaw?

Most inflammatory disorders of the jaw can be evaluated by plain radiographs, but plain films may require supplementation by CT, MRI, or radionuclide scanning techniques. MRI and CT are helpful in determining the extent of the pathology and any localized destruction and invasion, especially in cases of osteomyelitis. Scintigraphy or radionuclide imaging is the most definitive way of demonstrating bone changes and clinical activity caused by inflammation or suspected osteomyelitis.

49. Which imaging techniques will reveal soft tissue infection in the head and neck regions (Fig. 5-6)?

The primary imaging modalities to evaluate infection in the head and neck are CT and MRI.

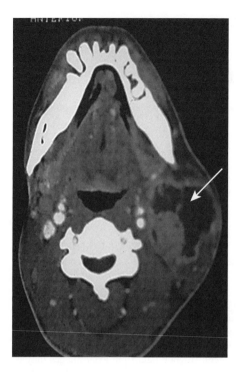

Fig. 5-6 Computed tomography scan of an abscess collection and gas posterior to the mandible (*arrow*).

CT and MRI both differentiate abscess from cellulitis, indicate the presence of venous thrombosis and airway compromise, and show the exact location and extent of the infectious process. CT is better than MRI in evaluating the integrity of cortical bone, and CT takes less time, costs less, and is more readily available than MRI. MRI, on the other hand, allows imaging in the sagittal, coronal, and axial planes with the patient supine, does not use radiation, and is not affected or degraded by artifacts from dental amalgam. Overall, CT with contrast with a very high diagnostic quality in all stages of oral and facial infections is most commonly used for this purpose.

BIBLIOGRAPHY

1. Abrams JJ: CT assessment of dental implant planning. Oral Maxillofac Surg Clin North Am 4:1-18, 1992.
2. Barsotti JB, Westesson PL, Ketonen LM: Diagnostic and interventional angiographic procedures in the maxillofacial region. Oral Maxillofac Surg Clin North Am 4:35-50, 1992.
3. Conway WF: Diagnostic imaging. In Kwon PH, Laskin DM (eds): Clinical Manual of Oral and Maxillofacial Surgery, 2nd ed. Chicago, 1996, Quintessence.
4. Dolan KD, Ruprecht A: Imaging of mandibular and temporomandibular joint fractures. Oral Maxillofac Surg Clin North Am 4:113-124, 1992.
5. Dolan KD, Ruprecht A: Imaging of midface fractures. Oral Maxillofac Surg Clin North Am 4:125-152, 1992.
6. Hashimoto K, Arai Y, Iwai K et al: A comparison of a new limited cone beam computed tomography machine for dental use with a multidetector row helical CT machine. Oral Surg Oral Med Oral Pathol Oral Radiol Endod 95:371-377, 2003.
7. Holliday RA, Prendergast NC: Imaging inflammatory processes of the oral cavity and suprahyoid neck. Oral Maxillofac Surg Clin North Am 4:215-240, 1992.
8. Little JW, Falace DA, Miller CS et al: Dental Management of the Medically Compromised Patient, 6th ed. St Louis, 2002, Mosby.

9. Miles DA: Imaging inflammatory disorders of the jaw: simple osteitis to generalized osteomyelitis. Oral Maxillofac Surg Clin North Am 4:207-214, 1992.
10. O'Mara RE: Scintigraphy of the facial skeleton. Oral Maxillofacial Surg Clin North Am 4:51-60, 1992.
11. Som PM, Brandweir M: Salivary glands. In Som PM, Curtin HD (eds): Head and Neck Imaging, vol 2. St Louis, 1996, Mosby.
12. Sune, Ericson: Conventional and oral computerized imaging of maxillary sinus pathology related to dental problems. Oral Maxillofac Surg Clin North Am 4:153-182, 1992.
13. U.S. Nuclear Regulatory Commission, http://www.nrc.gov/reading-rm/doc-collections/cfr/part020/part020-1004.html
14. van Rensburg LJ, Nortje CJ: Magnetic resonance imaging and computed tomography of malignant disease of the jaws. Oral Maxillofac Surg Clin North Am 4:75-112, 1992.
15. Virginia Commonwealth University, http://www.utdol.com.proxy.library.vcu.edu/application/topic.asp?file=biliaryt/11141&type=A&selectedTitle=1~4
16. Wandtke JC: Chest imaging for the oral and maxillofacial surgeon. Oral Maxillofac Surg Clin North Am 4:241-252, 1992.
17. Weber AL: Imaging of cysts and benign odontogenic tumors of the jaw. Oral Maxillofac Surg Clin North Am 4:61-74, 1992.
18. WebMD, http://www.webmd.com/hw/health_guide_atoz/hw200283.asp
19. Westesson P: Magnetic resonance imaging of the temporomandibular joint. Oral Maxillofac Surg Clin North Am 4:183-206, 1992.
20. White SC: Computer-assisted radiographic differential diagnosis of jaw lesions. Oral Maxillofac Surg Clin North Am 4:261-272, 1992.

Part II
Anesthesia

6. LOCAL ANESTHETICS

*Christopher L. Maestrello, DDS, A. Omar Abubaker, DMD, PhD,
and Kenneth J. Benson, DDS*

1. **What is the maximum amount of 2% lidocaine with 1:100,000 epinephrine (in milligrams) that can be administered to a healthy 150-lb man?**
   477 mg. The maximum dose of 2% lidocaine with 1:100,000 epinephrine for the adult patient is 7 mg/kg (Table 6-1). Convert pounds to kilograms by dividing by 2.2.

$$150 \text{ lb} \div 2.2 \text{ lb/kg} = 68 \text{ kg}$$
$$68 \text{ kg} \times 7 \text{ mg/kg} = 477 \text{ mg}$$

Table 6-1 *Adult Dosages for Commonly Used Local Anesthetics in Dentistry*

AGENT	CARTRIDGE SIZE (mg)	MAXIMUM DOSE mg/kg	mg/lb	MAXIMUM DOSE
2% lidocaine	36	4.5	2	300
2% lidocaine with 1:100,000 epinephrine	36	7	3.3	500
3% mepivacaine	54	5.5	2.6	400
2% mepivacaine with 1:20,000 levonordefrin	36	5.5	2.6	400
4% prilocaine	72	8	4	600
4% prilocaine with 1:200,000 epinephrine	72	8	4	600
0.5% bupivacaine with 1:200,000 epinephrine	9	1.3	0.6	90
1.5% etidocaine with 1:200,000 epinephrine	27	5.5	2.6	400
4% articaine* with 1:100,000 epinephrine	68	7	3.2	500

Maximum dosages are based on an adult weight of 150 lb or 70 kg and taken from the following manufacturers: Astra (Xylocaine, prilocaine, Citanest, Duranest), Cook-Waite (Marcaine), and Septodont (Septocaine).
*Articaine (Septocaine) dosages are based on a 1.7-mL cartridge.

2. **In the above scenario, how many dental cartridges does this equal?**
   13 cartridges. One dental cartridge of 2% lidocaine with 1:100,000 epinephrine contains 20 mg/mL of lidocaine. A 1.8-mL cartridge contains 36 mg of lidocaine.

477 mg ÷ 36 mg/cartridge = 13.25 cartridges

Outside the United States, anesthetic manufacturers also provide 2.2-mL dental cartridges of 2% lidocaine with 1:100,000 epinephrine, with the total amount of comparable local anesthetic being 44 mg. *Note:* Articaine is packaged as a 1.7-mL cartridge in the United States.

3. **How many dental cartridges of lidocaine or mepivacaine can be administered to a 30-lb child? What should be considered when selecting a local anesthetic for children?**
The pharmaceutical industry generally is not required to perform drug testing on the pediatric population; therefore definitive maximum drug dosages are often unknown. In addition, pharmaceutical manufacturers are reluctant to recommend maximum pediatric dosages of a drug because of variations in age and weight. Two standard formulas can be used to calculate pediatric drug dosages: Young's rule, which is based on the child's age, and Clark's rule, which is based on the child's weight. Clark's rule, the preferred formula, is:

Maximum pediatric dose = (weight of child in lb ÷ 150) × (maximum adult dose in mg)

The maximum number of cartridges has been calculated for the following local anesthetics:
2% lidocaine with 1:100,000 epinephrine	2.7 cartridges
2% lidocaine	1.6 cartridges
2% mepivacaine with 1:20,000 levonordefrin	2.2 cartridges
3% mepivacaine	1.5 cartridges

It is easy to exceed the maximum dose of local anesthetics with the pediatric patient. The practitioner needs to be especially careful if, for example, a child requires extraction of four abscessed teeth that are located in different quadrants. If all four teeth are to be extracted in one appointment, the practitioner has to be very careful with the amount of local anesthetic administered in each quadrant. Vasoconstrictors are another consideration. They limit the uptake of local anesthetic by the vasculature and thereby decrease systemic effects, allowing for an increase in dosage. Therefore the solution concentration and the use of a vasoconstrictor will change the maximum dose of local anesthetic that can be administered.

The safest local anesthetic to use in the pediatric patient is 2% lidocaine with 1:100,000 epinephrine. A simple method for remembering the pediatric dose of 2% lidocaine with or without vasoconstrictor is to use one cartridge for every 20 lb of the child's weight.

4. **What effect does narcotic sedation have on the maximum pediatric dose of local anesthetic?**
Amide local anesthetics and narcotics have an additive effect, thereby increasing the chance of a toxic reaction. Lowering the calculated pediatric maximum dose (e.g., 4.4 mg/kg of 2% lidocaine with 1:100,000 epinephrine) is recommended to prevent possible respiratory depression or acidosis that may decrease the seizure threshold. Opioids (fentanyl, meperidine, and morphine) may cause this amide local anesthetic additive effect because of their similar chemical structures (both are basic lipophilic amines) and a first-pass pulmonary effect. The lungs may serve as a reservoir for these drugs with a subsequent release back into the system.

5. **How are local anesthetics classified?**
All local anesthetics contain an aromatic ring linked to amide groups. The link is either an amide or an ester and thus determines the classification (Fig. 6-1).
An easy way to identify amide local anesthetics is to remember that the drug name contains an *i* plus *-caine* (lid*i*caine, mep*i*vacaine, and bup*i*vacaine). Esters such as Novocain, procaine, benzocaine, and tetracaine contain no *i*.
A new local anesthetic, articaine, was approved for use in the United States in April 2000, although it has been used in other countries for some time. This local anesthetic contains both an amide and an ester link, although it is classified as an amide.

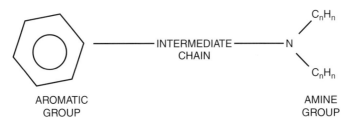

Fig. 6-1   Structure of esters and amides. (Modified from Kumar S: Local anesthetics. In Duke J [ed]: Anesthesia Secrets, 3rd ed. Philadelphia, 2006, Mosby.)

6.   How are local anesthetics metabolized?

Amide local anesthetics are metabolized mainly by the liver (microsomal enzymes), whereas the ester types are metabolized by the plasma (pseudocholinesterase). An easy way to remember how the most commonly used local anesthetic is metabolized is *l*idocaine and *l*iver.

7.   What is the mechanism of action of local anesthetics?

Once injected into the tissue, local anesthetics exist in both an ionized and a nonionized form. The nonionized base is able to penetrate many layers of tissue. The base, guided by its lipophilic aromatic ring, passes through the lipid nerve sheath and membrane. Reequilibration between the ionized and nonionized forms occurs once passage is completed. While in the nerve axon, the ionized form is able to block sodium (Na^+) channels, prevent the inflow of Na^+, slow the rate of depolarization, and thus prevent an action potential from occurring (Fig. 6-2).

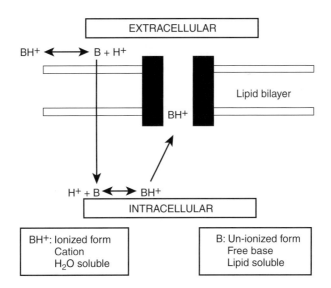

Fig. 6-2   Mechanism of action of local anesthetics. (Modified from Kumar S: Local anesthetics. In Duke J [ed]: Anesthesia Secrets, 3rd ed. Philadelphia, 2006, Mosby.)

8.   How is a nerve impulse transmitted on the cellular and microanatomic level?

A nerve impulse is generated when an electrical gradient occurs across the nerve membrane. An initial stimulus with sufficient intensity (−90 mV to −60 mV) must occur to allow depolarization of the nerve, propagation of the impulse, and restoration of the Na^+-K^+ pump to equilibrium. During depolarization, Na^+ flows from the extracellular to the intracellular space. Repolarization occurs when K^+ flows from the intracellular to the extracellular space (Fig. 6-3).

The electrical gradient generated across the nerve membrane is initiated at the outermost surface of the nerve (mantle) and continues toward the center of the nerve (core). The outer surface is responsible for innervating the proximal structures, whereas the core is responsible for innervating distal structures. Proximal structures are innervated more rapidly than distal structures. After a mandibular inferior alveolar injection, one notices an almost immediate local anesthetic effect at the site of injection, whereas a delayed effect is noticed at the peripheral tissues (tongue, then lip).

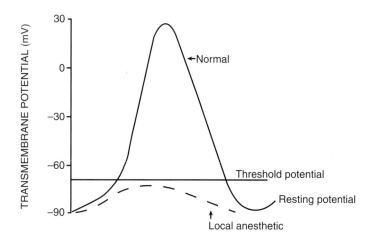

Fig. 6-3   Local anesthetics slow the rate of depolarization of the nerve action potential such that the threshold potential is not reached. (Modified from Stoelting RK, Miller RD: Local anesthetics. In Stoelting RK, Miller RD [eds]: Basics of Anesthesia, 3rd ed. New York, 1994, Churchill Livingstone.)

9. **How does the onset of anesthesia proceed in a peripheral nerve block? What is the clinical relevance with regard to an inferior alveolar nerve block?**

Conduction blockade caused by local anesthetics proceeds from the outermost (mantle) of the nerve to the innermost (core) nerve bundles. Generally speaking, mantle fibers innervate structures supplied by proximal nerves and core fibers innervate distal nerves.

With regard to the inferior alveolar nerve, the innermost (core) part of the nerve supplies the lower lip and anterior teeth and the outermost (mental) supplies posterior structures of the oral cavity (molars, premolars). Accordingly, when the lower lip is anesthetized, that is a very good indication that the structures supplied by the mantle of the nerve (posterior teeth) are also anesthetized.

10. **After a local anesthetic injection, anesthetic effects will disappear and reappear in a definite order. What are the sensations in increasing order of resistance to conduction?**

*   Pain
*   Cold
*   Warm
*   Touch
*   Deep pressure
*   Motor

11. **What are the causes and clinical manifestations of local anesthetic toxicity?**

Local anesthetic toxicity is caused by elevated plasma levels of the anesthetic. This may be caused by an inadvertent vascular injection or by iatrogenically violating the maximum milligram/kilogram dose. A classic sign of systemic local anesthetic toxicity is circumoral numbness. However, if circumoral numbness is the desired effect of a nerve blockade, additional signs need to be recognized. Toxicity involves the cardiovascular and central nervous systems. Initial signs include tachycardia, hypertension, drowsiness, confusion, tinnitus, and a metallic taste. Progressive signs include tremors, hallucinations, hypotension, bradycardia, and decreased cardiac output. Late signs include unconsciousness, seizures, ventricular dysrhythmias, and respiratory and circulatory arrest.

12. Who is at greatest risk for local anesthetic toxicity?

The potential for local anesthetic toxicity is greatest in geriatric and pediatric patients. Older individuals generally metabolize drugs at a slower rate. A geriatric patient who takes multiple medications may experience adverse drug reactions when lidocaine is administered. Cimetidine (Tagamet), a histamine H_2-receptor antagonist, inhibits the hepatic oxidative enzymes needed for metabolism, thereby allowing lidocaine to accumulate in the circulating blood. This adverse reaction is seen only with cimetidine and not with other H_2-receptor antagonists. Propranolol (Inderal), a beta-adrenergic blocker, can reduce both hepatic blood flow and lidocaine clearance. Therefore a local anesthetic toxic reaction would not be expected with a routine injection of lidocaine in a patient who takes cimetidine or propranolol, but it may result if high doses of lidocaine are given.

In addition, a possible additive adverse drug reaction exists with the administration of local anesthetics and opioids in the geriatric and pediatric populations.

13. What is methemoglobinemia, what are its causes and clinical manifestations, and how can it be treated?

A hemoglobin deficiency occurring when hemoglobin has been oxidized to methemoglobin. Oxidized hemoglobin cannot bind or carry oxygen. Excessive doses of prilocaine (above 600 mg) or articaine (above 500 mg) may result in the accumulation of an oxidized metabolite, ortho-toluidine, that is capable of allowing this conversion. Clinical manifestations include a decreased pulse oximeter reading, cyanosis, and chocolate-colored blood in the surgical field. This condition can be reversed with intravenous administration of 1-2 mg/kg of methylene blue over a 5-min period.

Benzocaine also has the potential to cause methemoglobinemia. Benzocaine can be found in certain topical liquids, gels, ointments, and sprays (e.g., Hurricaine, Cetacaine). Methemoglobinemia formation can occur with benzocaine doses of 15-20 mg/kg. Benzocaine gels typically contain 18%-20% benzocaine. Sprays containing 14%-20% benzocaine can deliver 45-60 mg of benzocaine in 1 sec.

Prilocaine is marketed as a 4% solution. A 4% solution contains 72 mg of prilocaine, with eight cartridges needed to obtain 600 mg. The use of a benzocaine topical along with prilocaine will reduce the maximum amount of injectable local anesthetic that can be used. In some countries other than the United States and Canada, prilocaine is marketed as a 3% solution. A 3% solution is less likely to cause an excessive delivery of this local anesthetic.

EMLA (eutectic mixture of local anesthetic) cream, used preoperatively before venous access, contains both lidocaine and prilocaine. EMLA cream should be used with caution in children, and it is not recommended for use in children younger than age 12 months because of potential methemoglobinemia development.

14. Why are epinephrine and levonordefrin added to local anesthetics?

These substances are added to local anesthetics because of their vasoconstrictive properties. Vasoconstriction at the site of injection is beneficial because it limits the uptake of the anesthetic by the vasculature, thereby increasing the duration of the anesthetic and diminishing systemic effects.

15. What is the maximum amount of epinephrine or levonordefrin that can be administered to a 70-kg patient with a history of coronary artery disease?

An average adult patient with a history of coronary artery disease should receive no more than 0.04 mg (40 µg) of epinephrine or 0.20 mg (200 µg) of levonordefrin. Each dental cartridge of 1:100,000 epinephrine contains 0.01 mg/mL of epinephrine; therefore no more than two cartridges (3.6 mL) should be administered. Each dental cartridge of 1:20,000 levonordefrin contains 0.5 mg/mL of levonordefrin; therefore no more than two cartridges (3.6 mL) should be administered. If the patient is also being sedated, then additional epinephrine could be administered (Table 6-2).

Table 6-2 *Maximum Allowable Vasoconstrictor for the Cardiac Patient*

VASOCONSTRICTOR CONCENTRATION AND TYPE	VASOCONSTRICTOR (mg/mL)	STANDARD DENTAL CARTRIDGE (mg/1.8 mL)	MAXIMUM ALLOWED CARTRIDGES
1:20,000 levonordefrin	0.5	0.09	2
1:50,000 epinephrine	0.02	0.036	1
1:100,000 epinephrine	0.01	0.018	2
1:200,000 epinephrine	0.005	0.009	4

When treating a patient with coronary artery disease, the objective is to prevent increases in heart rate. Increases in heart rate can decrease stroke volume and thereby decrease cardiac output. A decreased cardiac output will diminish the amount of oxygenated blood flowing to poorly perfused areas of the damaged pericardium.

Electing to perform a sedation procedure on a patient with coronary artery disease for minor outpatient surgical procedures (e.g., surgical extraction of a tooth) is often good treatment planning. The idea is to sedate a cardiac patient not for anxiolytic purposes but to control heart rate. The amount of epinephrine used can be titrated to the patient's heart rate.

16. What adverse drug effects are associated with vasoconstrictor use?

Possible adverse drug reactions exist between vasoconstrictors and tricyclic antidepressants (TCAs), beta-adrenergic antagonists, volatile anesthetics, cocaine, and other vasoconstricting products.

TCAs (e.g., amitriptyline) increase the availability of endogenous norepinephrine, which could create an exaggerated heart rate or blood pressure response with the use of sympathomimetics (e.g., epinephrine, ephedrine, phenylephrine). Additionally, TCAs block muscarinic and alpha$_1$-adrenergic receptors that directly depress the myocardium. The potential for this adverse reaction is greatest during the first 14-21 days of drug administration, probably because of downregulation of the norepinephrine receptors as treatment continues. This same type of exaggerated response was originally thought to exist with monoamine oxidase (MAO) inhibitors, but now that appears not to be the case. This adverse reaction appears to have the greatest adverse effect with the use of levonordefrin and imipramine (Tofranil).

Epinephrine has the potential to counteract vasodilating beta$_2$ receptors, thus allowing epinephrine to act vascularly as a pure alpha-adrenergic stimulant. It is therefore prudent to limit the amount of vasoconstrictors used in these patients and to aspirate to prevent any intravascular injections.

The potential for dysrhythmic effects exists between the inhalational anesthetic halothane (Fluothane) and epinephrine or levonordefrin by stimulation of both alpha$_1$ and beta receptors. It is recommended that 2 μg/kg of epinephrine be used when halothane is administered. The greatest potential exists for an adverse reaction during the first 10 min of halothane administration, so it is prudent to wait this amount of time before injecting the local anesthetic.

Cocaine also potentiates the effects of adrenergic vasoconstrictors. The dysrhythmic results of this interaction can be life threatening. Unfortunately, obtaining a factual health history from a cocaine user may be difficult. All suspected drug users should be made aware of these lethal side effects, especially if cocaine has been used recently.

17. What types of local anesthetics have the greatest allergic potential?

Esters have a greater allergic potential than amides. Procaine (Novocain) was, at one time, the most commonly used ester local anesthetic in dentistry. Although procaine is no longer available in dental cartridges, practitioners still need to be aware of ester allergies. Patients often give a history of rapid heart rate after the administration of a local anesthetic. The vasoconstrictor in the local anesthetic or an intravascular injection is often the cause. Practitioners are often quick to attribute a history of "allergy to Novocain" to the effects of the vasoconstrictor. A careful history taking may reveal that the patient did indeed have an allergic reaction to procaine when the anesthetic was available (before 1996).

Other topical esters are still commonly used in the practice of dentistry. Most topical local anesthetic ointments and gels contain benzocaine (an ester). Intraoral topical sprays may contain benzocaine and tetracaine (an ester). It is not uncommon for an oral and maxillofacial surgeon to use topical cocaine solutions (4%) as topical applications to the nasal mucosa to control hemostasis.

The newest local anesthetic, articaine, is classified as an amide but has both amide and ester linkages. Therefore it has the potential to cause an ester allergic reaction as well.

18. To what components of a local anesthetic are patients most likely to be allergic?

Methylparaben, a bacteriostatic preservative, is found in multidose vials of local anesthetics. Many oral and maxillofacial surgeons use multidose vials in their offices, the emergency room, or the operating room and need to be cautious of potential allergic reactions. Methylparaben is no longer added to dental cartridges (since 1984). Because the cartridge is intended to be used as a single-dose vial, a preservative is not required.

Bisulfites are food and drug preservatives. They are commonly used as preservatives at salad bars and in wines. Any local anesthetic cartridge containing a vasoconstrictor will have metabisulfite added as a preservative for the vasoconstrictor. Patients with known bisulfite allergies need to be given local anesthetics without vasoconstrictors. Interestingly, one of the new manufacturers of propofol also uses bisulfite as a preservative.

Sulfa drug allergies are common among our patient population. Articaine contains a small amount of sulfa and should not be administered to these patients.

Latex allergies should also be considered with the use of local anesthetics. The local anesthetic itself contains no latex, but its container may. The needle-puncture diaphragm of dental cartridges and multidose vials contains latex. The dental plunger of a dental cartridge may also contain latex. A disposable, latex-free syringe is recommended for the latex-allergic patient. The anesthetic solution may be drawn using a filtered needle or by removing the rubber diaphragm.

19. What determines the potency of a local anesthetic?

The lipid solubility determines the potency of a local anesthetic. A greater lipid solubility produces a more potent local anesthetic (Table 6-3). Bupivacaine is a more potent local anesthetic than lidocaine, for example. Therefore only a 0.5% solution is required to obtain comparable local anesthesia, instead of a 2% solution.

20. What determines the duration of a local anesthetic?

The degree of protein binding of a local anesthetic agent determines the duration of the anesthetic. A greater degree of protein binding at the receptor site will create a longer duration of action (see Table 6-3). Because bupivacaine, tetracaine, and etidocaine are all highly protein bound, they are long-acting local anesthetics Vasoconstrictors will also determine the duration of a local anesthetic, but for different reasons.

21. What determines the onset time of a local anesthetic agent?

The pKa of a local anesthetic determines its speed of action. The closer the pKa of a local anesthetic is to the pH of tissue (7.4), the more rapid the onset (see Table 6-3). The pKa of a local anesthetic is the pH at which equal concentrations of ionized and un-ionized forms exist. It is the un-ionized form that must cross the axonal membrane to initiate neural blockade.

Table 6-3 *Properties of Local Anesthetics*

AGENT	LIPID SOLUBILITY	PROTEIN BINDING	DURATION	pKa	ONSET TIME
Mepivacaine	1	75	Medium	7.6	Fast
Lidocaine	4	65	Medium	7.7	Fast
Bupivacaine	28	95	Long	8.1	Moderate
Tetracaine	80	85	Long	8.6	Slow
Etidocaine	140	95	Long	7.7	Fast

22. Why are local anesthetics often ineffective when injected into an area of infection?

Local anesthetics exist in both an ionized (cation) and un-ionized (base) form. If an acidic tissue infection exists, then the un-ionized form may be neutralized. The base form is necessary for passage of the anesthetic into the nerve membrane.

23. Why does inflammation impede the onset of local anesthesia?

Products of inflammation in the tissues lower the pH of the affected tissue and limit the formation of free base (the reaction shifts to the left). Inflammatory exudates also enhance nerve conduction, making the blockage of nerve impulses more difficult.

24. How does lidocaine toxicity affect the central nervous system (CNS)?

Lidocaine usually has a sedative effect on the brain. Initially, lidocaine toxicity depresses brain function in the form of drowsiness and slurred speech. It can progress to unconsciousness and even coma.

25. What cardiovascular effects does lidocaine toxicity exhibit?

Lidocaine has a depressor effect on the myocardium. Toxic doses of lidocaine cause sinus bradycardia, because lidocaine increases the effective refractory period relative to the action potential duration and lowers cardiac automaticity. If a very high dose has been administered, impaired cardiac contractibility, arteriolar dilation, and profound hypotension and circulatory collapse can result.

26. What is the mechanism of degradation epinephrine?

The action of epinephrine is terminated primarily by its reuptake by the adrenergic nerves. Epinephrine that is not taken up again is rapidly metabolized and inactivated in the blood by the enzymes catechol-O-methyltransferase (COMT) and by MAO, both of which are present in the liver. One of the final products is vanillylmandelic acid (VMA). Only a small percentage (1%) of epinephrine is excreted unchanged in the urine.

27. How do you calculate the amount, in milligrams, of any anesthetic and vasoconstrictor in a given solution?

For local anesthetics, for every 1% solution there is 10 mg/mL. Therefore:

$$\text{Total milligrams} = \% \text{ of the solution} \times 10 \times \text{total milliliters}$$

For vasoconstriction, for every 1:100,000 there is 0.01 mg/mL. Therefore:

$$\text{Total milligrams} = \text{ratio} \times \text{total milliliters}$$

28. What is the effect and importance of pKa of a local anesthetic?

Because only the base form can diffuse rapidly into the nerve, drugs with a high pKa tend to have a slower onset (bupivacaine: pKa 8.1) than similar agents with more favorable dissociation constants (lidocaine: pKa 7.9).

29. **A healthy, afebrile 70-kg man has been referred to your office for extraction of a symptomatic, abscessed mandibular molar. You have made two attempts to anesthetize the inferior alveolar nerve, the long buccal nerve, and the lingual nerve and have given an intraligament injection. Adequate soft tissue anesthesia has been obtained, but the patient complains when you attempt to luxate the tooth. What are 10 ways that may help achieve adequate anesthesia?**

   1. Allow adequate time for the anesthetic to take effect. Sit the patient in an upright position and wait an additional 5-10 min. This is difficult for the oral and maxillofacial surgeon who is inherently impatient.
   2. Consider readministering the local anesthetic at a higher level on the ramus.
   3. Consider innervation from the mylohyoid nerve and anesthetize accordingly (lingual to the mandibular second molar).
   4. Administer another cartridge of anesthetic at the highest level possible by using the Gow-Gates technique (intraoral condylar injection).
   5. Administer an intraosseous injection or use an intraosseous system (e.g., Stabident).
   6. Consider using a higher pH anesthetic solution (one without a vasoconstrictor) to help overcome the acidity created by the infection.
   7. Alkalinize (buffer) your anesthetic by adding sodium bicarbonate to your local anesthetic just before injecting.
   8. Use a larger amount (but do not exceed the maximum recommended dose) of local anesthetic to overcome the acidity created by the infection.
   9. Sedate the patient with a small amount of narcotic or nitrous oxide and proceed.
   10. Consider placing the patient on antibiotics and reschedule the procedure.

30. **A healthy 60-kg woman has been referred to your office for extraction of an infected posterior molar. The patient presents with trismus and has been on antibiotics and analgesic medication for a week with little relief. What can you do to help her?**

   Administer local anesthesia using an extraoral approach or using the closed-mouth mandibular block (Vazirani block, Akinosi block, or Vazirani-Akinosi block).

   An **extraoral block** is performed by first preparing the epidermis (i.e., with povidone-iodine [Betadine]) adjacent to the lateral portion of the zygomatic arch. A lateral approach to the nerve can be accomplished by using a short-length needle and injecting just below the sigmoid notch of the zygomatic arch.

   A **closed-mouth block** can be performed by retracting the buccal tissues away from the dentition and inserting a long needle at the medial border of the ramus and adjacent to the mucogingival junction of the maxillary posterior molars. Then insert the needle to the approximate middle portion of the ramus and deposit the local anesthetic.

31. **What types of local anesthetics can be used in the pregnant and lactating patient?**

   Category B (see the following list) local anesthetics are recommended for the pregnant and lactating patient. Local anesthetics can cross the placental barrier but are generally not harmful unless excessive amounts are administered. A mother's normal tissue pH is 7.4, whereas the fetus has a pH of approximately 7.2. An excessive amount of local anesthetic could dangerously lower the fetus's pH (ion trapping).

Category B	**Category C**
Lidocaine	Articaine
Prilocaine	Bupivacaine
Etidocaine	Mepivacaine

32. **During delivery of an inferior alveolar injection, you know that you have directly contacted the nerve (bull's-eye) because the patient jumps. Should you deliver the local anesthetic at this location?**

Although definitive anesthesia will be obtained, one should never directly inject a local anesthetic within the nerve sheath, to avoid traumatizing (lacerating) the nerve or causing the development of a neuroma. More importantly, the administration of a fluid bolus within the nerve sheath can physically damage the nerve and cause indefinite facial pain. Injecting anesthetic directly into a foramen (e.g., mental) also carries the risk of traumatizing the nerve. Additionally, paresthesia has been reported with the use of 4% solutions of local anesthetics. Thus additional care should be taken when injecting prilocaine or articaine near a foramen.

33. **What profession uses local anesthetics most frequently on a daily basis?**

With the possible exception of obstetric anesthesiologists, dental practitioners, specifically oral and maxillofacial surgeons, use local anesthetics most frequently. Therefore a thorough understanding of the pharmacokinetics and pharmacodynamics of local anesthetics is essential.

34. **How does a patient become toxic from local anesthetics? What are the clinical manifestations of local anesthetic toxicity?**

Systemic toxicity is the result of elevated plasma levels of local anesthetics. It is usually a manifestation of overdose or inadvertent intravascular injection. Toxicity from local anesthetics involves mostly the CNS and cardiovascular system. Because the CNS is generally more sensitive to the toxic effects of local anesthetics, it is usually affected first. The manifestations are presented below in chronologic order.

CNS

- Lightheadedness, tinnitus, perioral numbness, confusion
- Muscle twitching, auditory and visual hallucinations
- Tonic-clonic seizure, unconsciousness, respiratory arrest

Cardiac

- Hypertension, tachycardia
- Decreased contractility and cardiac output, hypotension
- Sinus bradycardia, ventricular dysrhythmias, circulatory arrest

35. **Is there an easy way to remember important data about lidocaine?**

Yes. Because lidocaine is one of the safest and most commonly used local anesthetics, it is useful to commit to memory certain information about this drug. Its molecular weight is 234, its protein binding is 56%, and its pKa is 7.8, so just remember 2, 3, 4, 5, 6, 7, 8.

36. **What should a dentist do if a patient states that he was told he is "allergic" to Novocain, which he received for a tooth extraction? Should the dentist avoid using local anesthetics in this patient?**

Novocain is the trade name for procaine, an ester local anesthetic. Esters are derivatives of *para*-aminobenzoic acid (PABA), reactions to which, although rare, do occur. A thorough history will reveal whether the patient experienced the symptoms of a true allergic reaction—hives, wheezing, tachycardia, shock. Symptoms of palpitations and nervousness may represent a response to a local anesthetic additive, such as epinephrine, *not* an allergic reaction.

Additionally, the patient may be describing the sequelae of an accidental intravascular injection or overdose of local anesthetic. If a true allergy is suspected, another class of local anesthetic may be used because cross-reactivity between local anesthetics is rare. If the offending allergen remains unidentified, skin testing followed by a subcutaneous challenge injection may be warranted but is not without hazard.

BIBLIOGRAPHY

1. Bennett CR: Monheim's Local Anesthesia and Pain Control in Dental Practice, 6th ed. St Louis, 1978, Mosby.
2. Braverman B, McCarthy RJ, Ivankovich AD: Vasopressor challenges during chronic MAOI or TCA treatment in anesthetised dogs. Life Sci 40:2587-2595, 1987.
3. Fitzpatrick K: Local anesthetics. In Duke J (ed): Anesthesia Secrets, 2nd ed. Philadelphia, 2000, Hanley & Belfus.
4. Haas DA, Lennon D: A 21-year retrospective study of reports of paresthesia following local anesthetic administration. J Can Dent Assoc 61:319-330, 1995.
5. Kumar S: Local anesthetics. In Duke J (ed): Anesthesia Secrets, 3rd ed. Philadelphia, 2006, Mosby.
6. Local Anesthetics for Dentistry: Prescribing Information. Westborough, Mass, 1995, Astra USA, Inc.
7. Malamed SF: Handbook of Local Anesthetics, 5th ed. St Louis, 2004, Mosby.
8. Moore PA: Preventing local anesthetic toxicity. J Am Dental Assoc 123:61-64, 1992.
9. Moore PA: Adverse drug interactions in dental practice: interactions associated with local anesthetics, sedatives and anxiolytics. J Am Dental Assoc 130:541-554, 1999.
10. Roering DL, Kotrly KJ, Vucins EJ et al: First pass uptake of fentanyl, meperidine, and morphine in the human lung. Anesthesiology 67:466-472, 1987.
11. Samdal F, Arctander K, Skolleborg KC et al: Alkalisation of lignocaine-adrenaline reduces the amount of pain during subcutaneous injection of local anesthetic. Scand J Plast Reconstr Hand Surg 28:33-37, 1994.
12. Stoelting RK, Miller RD: Local anesthetics. In Stoelting RK, Miller RD (eds): Basics of Anesthesia, 4th ed. New York, 2000, Churchill Livingstone.
13. Wilburn-Goo D, Lloyd LM: When patients become cyanotic: acquired methemoglobinemia. J Am Dental Assoc 130:826-831, 1999.
14. Yagiela JA: Adverse drug interactions in dental practice: interactions associated with vasoconstrictors. J Am Dent Assoc 130:701-709, 1999.

7. INTRAVENOUS SEDATION

Christopher L. Maestrello, DDS, and A. Omar Abubaker, DMD, PhD

1. How is an intravenous (IV) anesthetic agent used in anesthesia?

An IV anesthetic is a drug that is intravenously injected to induce unconsciousness at the beginning of general anesthesia. At the same time, it allows rapid recovery after termination of its effect.

2. What are the properties of an ideal induction agent?

- The drug should be soluble in water, have IV fluid compatibility, and be stable in aqueous solution.
- It should elicit rapid onset and recovery of anesthesia (within 1 arm-brain circulation time).
- It should not possess any unwanted cardiovascular or neurologic side effects or produce any unwanted movements.
- It should retain anticonvulsant, antiemetic, analgesic, and amnestic properties.
- It should not impair renal or hepatic function or steroid synthesis.

3. What are barbiturates?

Barbiturates are a derivative of barbituric acid. They exhibit a dose-dependent central nervous system (CNS) depression with hypnosis and amnesia. Barbiturates are very lipid soluble, which results in a rapid onset of action. They are used most often for induction of anesthesia because they produce unconsciousness in less than 30 sec.

4.   What are the pharmacologic effects of barbiturates?

Barbiturates decrease the rate of dissociation of gamma-aminobutyric acid (GABA) from its receptors. GABA, an inhibitory neurotransmitter, causes an increase in chloride concentration within the membranes of postsynaptic neurons resulting in hyperpolarization. Barbiturates are capable of depressing the reticular activating system, which is important in maintaining wakefulness and medullary ventilatory centers to decrease responsiveness to ventilatory stimulant effects of carbon dioxide. In addition, barbiturates induce depression of the medullary vasomotor center, causing decreased sympathetic nervous system impulses from autonomic ganglia. This results in decreases in blood pressure (10-20 mm Hg) secondary to peripheral vasodilation. Finally, barbiturates are potent cerebral vasoconstrictors resulting in decreases in cerebral blood flow, cerebral blood volume, and intracranial pressure (ICP).

5.   What are the pharmacokinetics of barbiturates?

Maximal uptake of barbiturates by the brain occurs within 30 sec after IV administration. This accounts for the rapid (1 arm-brain circulation) induction of anesthesia. The redistribution of these drugs from the brain to inactive tissues, especially skeletal muscle and fat, results in prompt awakening. The elimination of barbiturates is dependent on hepatic function because less than 1% of the administered dose is cleared unchanged by the kidneys.

6.   What are the most commonly used barbiturates for induction of anesthesia?

Thiopental sodium (Pentothal) is a thiobarbiturate usually prepared as a 2.5% solution. The pH of thiopental is 10.5. When injected intravenously, it can be irritating. An induction dose of 3-5 mg/kg produces a loss of consciousness within 30 sec and recovery in 5-10 min. Because the elimination half-life is 6-12 hr, patients may experience a slow recovery. After 24 hr, approximately 28%-30% may be detectable in the body. Thiopental is not used to maintain anesthesia because of accumulation in inactive tissues with repeated doses.

Methohexital (Brevital) is somewhat less lipid soluble and less ionized at physiologic pH than thiopental. The pH is 10.5. An induction dose of 1-2 mg/kg produces loss of consciousness in less than 20 sec and recovery in 4-5 min. The elimination half-life of methohexital is 3 hr, which allows a clearance rate that is three to four times faster than that of thiopental. In addition, methohexital activates epileptic foci, facilitating their identification during surgery to ablate these sites.

7.   What is propofol?

Propofol (Diprivan), a substituted isopropylphenol, is an IV sedative-hypnotic agent used for induction and maintenance of anesthesia. It also can be used during conscious sedation. Propofol is highly lipophilic, which increases its ability to cross the blood-brain barrier.

8.   What are the pharmacokinetics and pharmacologic effects of propofol?

An intravenous induction dose of 2.0-2.5 mg/kg produces unconsciousness in less than 30 sec, followed by recovery in 4-8 min. A rapid elimination half-life of 0.5-1.5 hr results in prompt hepatic metabolism to inactive metabolites. In addition, redistribution to inactive tissue sites plays a significant role in early awakening. Because propofol exhibits awakening with minimal residual CNS effects more quickly than any other IV anesthetic, it is the most widely used agent for ambulatory anesthesia. Anesthesia is maintained with a continuous infusion of 0.1-0.2 mg/kg/min or intermittent doses. Propofol causes a 20%-30% decrease in blood pressure and heart rate. The cardiovascular effects are due to rapid arterial and venous vasodilation and mild negative inotropic effects. Propofol has a low incidence of postoperative nausea and vomiting. Pain on injection may be related to release of local kininogens, although the exact cause remains unknown. Awake patients are likely to experience pain at the injection site; the pain may be decreased with administration of lidocaine before injection.

9.   What are the pharmacologic properties and side effects of etomidate?

Etomidate (Amidate) is a carboxylated imidazole derivative. An induction dose of 0.2-0.4 mg/kg IV produces rapid induction of anesthesia that lasts 3-12 min. The CNS effects are dose dependent, and recovery of psychomotor skills is equal to that of thiopental. Rapid awakening results from redistribution and nearly complete hydrolysis to inactive metabolites. Because etomidate produces no noticeable cardiovascular changes, it is used in patients with limited cardiac reserve. In addition, etomidate decreases cerebral blood flow and ICP. Like methohexital, it activates seizure foci.

Side effects include venoirritation with rapid infusion, involuntary skeletal muscle movements, and a high incidence of nausea and vomiting. Also, etomidate suppresses adrenocortical function for up to 8 hr after administration. During this time, the adrenal cortex is unresponsive to adrenocorticotropic hormone (ACTH).

10.   What is ketamine, and how does it exert its physiologic action?

Ketamine, a phencyclidine (PCP) derivative, is 10 times more lipid soluble than thiopental, enabling it to cross the blood-brain barrier quickly. It produces dissociative anesthesia, which can be seen on electroencephalogram (EEG) as dissociation between the thalamus and limbic system. Rapid CNS depression with hypnosis, sedation, amnesia, and intense analgesia occurs in 30-60 sec after IV administration. The anesthetic induction doses are 1-2 mg/kg IV, with effects lasting 5-10 min, or 10 mg/kg intramuscular (IM), which acts in 2-4 min. A ketamine dart of 4 mg/kg IM can be administered to uncooperative patients to facilitate completion of short procedures.

11.   What are the pharmacologic effects and side effects of ketamine?

Ketamine is highly lipid soluble, is rapidly redistributed to muscle and fat, and undergoes extensive hepatic metabolism to a weakly active metabolite, norketamine. Ketamine stimulates the cardiovascular system, increasing the heart rate, blood pressure, and cardiac output. In patients with ischemic heart disease, ketamine may adversely increase myocardial oxygen requirements. In addition, ketamine produces bronchial smooth muscle relaxation because of sympathetic stimulation, which may be beneficial in patients with bronchospasm or asthma. Airway secretions are increased by ketamine, creating the need for anticholinergics such as glycopyrrolate in the preoperative period. Ketamine is a potent cerebral vasodilator and will increase ICP in patients with intracranial lesions. Finally, emergence from ketamine anesthesia may be associated with unpleasant auditory, visual, and out-of-body illusions that can progress to delirium. It is recommended that benzodiazepines or droperidol be administered either preoperatively or after induction to decrease the incidence of emergence delirium.

12.   What are the clinical uses for benzodiazepines?

- Preoperative medication
- Intravenous sedation
- Induction of anesthesia
- Maintenance of anesthesia
- Suppression of seizure activity

Anterograde amnesia, minimal depression of ventilation and the cardiovascular system, and sedative properties make benzodiazepines favorable preoperative medications.

13.   What is the IV sedation dose for ketamine?

The dose ranges between 0.25 mg/kg and 0.75mg/kg.

14.   Where in the CNS do benzodiazepines exert their amnestic effect?

These effects occur at benzodiazepine receptors, which are found on postsynaptic nerve endings in the CNS. Benzodiazepine receptors are part of the GABA receptor complex. The GABA receptor complex consists of two alpha subunits, to which benzodiazepines bind, and two beta subunits, to which GABA binds. A chloride ion channel exists in the middle of the receptor complex. Benzodiazepines enhance the binding of GABA to beta subunits, which opens the chloride ion channel. Chloride ions flow into the neuron, hyperpolarizing it and inhibiting action potentials.

15. What clinical properties make benzodiazepines good preoperative medications?

At lower doses, only anxiolysis is obtained. Anterograde amnesia, sedation, and anxiolysis are produced at higher concentrations. At this concentration, patients are conscious and can maintain their own airway but will not remember events during surgery. Finally, at even higher concentrations, benzodiazepines will produce unconsciousness, although they are not complete anesthetics. A complete general anesthetic produces the effects already mentioned plus analgesia, control of the autonomic nervous systems, and occasionally muscle relaxation. Benzodiazepines do not provide analgesia, and they should not be used alone to produce general anesthesia. They are best used in low doses to supplement inhaled or intravenous anesthetics to provide amnesia.

16. What benzodiazepines are most commonly used as amnestics in anesthesiology?

- Midazolam (most common)
- Lorazepam
- Diazepam

17. What are the properties and pharmacokinetics of midazolam?

Midazolam is prepared as a water-soluble compound that is transformed into a lipid-soluble compound by exposure to the pH of blood upon injection. This unique property of midazolam improves patient comfort when administered by the IV or IM route. This prevents the need for an organic solvent such as propylene glycol, which is required for diazepam and lorazepam. Midazolam is the most lipid soluble of the three and, as a result, has a rapid onset and a relatively short duration of action. The elimination half-life is 1-4 hr. A dose of 1-2.5 mg administered intravenously is useful for anxiolysis, amnesia, and conscious sedation. Induction of anesthesia can be produced by the administration of 0.1-0.2 mg/kg IV. Unconsciousness will occur within 60-90 sec. This is more rapid than diazepam but slower than the barbiturates. Benzodiazepines are not used often for induction because of the potential for delayed awakening, particularly with diazepam and lorazepam.

18. What are the properties and actions of diazepam?

Diazepam is a water-insoluble benzodiazepine and requires the organic solvent propylene glycol to dissolve it. Propylene glycol is most likely responsible for the venoirritation and thrombophlebitis that may occur during injection. At the same time, it is less lipid soluble than midazolam. A dose of 5-10 mg given intravenously will provide amnestic, calming, and sedative effects; however, midazolam will have a quicker onset and greater amnestic effect than diazepam. The induction dose of diazepam is 0.3-0.5 mg/kg, and onset is slightly slower than that of midazolam. In addition, diazepam (0.1 mg/kg IV) is effective at abolishing the seizure activity that is produced by local anesthetics, alcohol withdrawal, and status epilepticus. The elimination half-life of diazepam is 21-37 hr, which may account for the delayed awakening after induction doses. Diazepam undergoes hepatic metabolism to active desmethyldiazepam and oxazepam that can produce sedation 6-8 hr after its initial administration.

19. What are the properties and actions of lorazepam?

- Lorazepam is the least lipid soluble of the three main benzodiazepines, resulting in a slow onset of action but long duration of action.
- Lorazepam requires propylene glycol to dissolve it, which increases its venoirritation.
- Lorazepam is a more powerful amnestic agent than midazolam, but its slow onset and long duration of action limit its usefulness for preoperative anesthesia.

20. What is the antagonist for benzodiazepines?

Flumazenil, a competitive antagonist, given in increments of 0.2 mg IV every 60 sec, will reverse unconsciousness, sedation, respiratory depression, and anxiolysis. Flumazenil has a rapid onset with the peak effect occurring in about 1-3 min. The effect of flumazenil lasts for about 20 min, and resedation may occur.

21. What is the mechanism of action of opioids?

Opioids act as agonists through complex interactions with mu, delta, and kappa receptors in the CNS. Supraspinally, mu receptors are responsible for analgesia, euphoria, miosis, nausea and vomiting, urinary retention, depression of ventilation, and bradycardia. Delta and kappa receptors are active at the spinal level mediating spinal analgesia, sedation, and miosis. In addition, opioids may act presynaptically to interfere with the release of neurotransmitters such as acetylcholine, dopamine, norepinephrine, and substance P.

22. How are opioids used clinically?

Uses include provision of analgesia before or after surgery, synergistic effects with inhaled anesthetics being used for maintenance of anesthesia, induction and maintenance of anesthesia (particularly in patients with severe cardiac dysfunction), and inhibition of reflex sympathetic nervous system activity. Usually, opioids are administered intermittently in lower doses during maintenance of anesthesia or as continuous infusions to augment inhaled anesthetics. Often, small doses of fentanyl, sufentanil, or alfentanil are administered just before direct laryngoscopy and tracheal intubation to attenuate blood pressure and heart rate responses evoked by these stimuli.

23. What are the pharmacologic effects of opioids?

Opioids are cardiac-stable drugs. In many settings, opioids are used as the principal anesthetic agent for cardiac anesthesia because of their hemodynamic stability; however, they do lack an amnestic effect. At the same time, opioids can cause a dose-dependent bradycardia resulting from vagal stimulation in the medulla. In contrast, meperidine will cause tachycardia because it is structurally similar to atropine and elicits atropine-like effects. Opioids act on the medullary ventilatory centers to produce rapid and sustained dose-dependent depression of ventilation. This is characterized by increases in the resting $PaCO_2$ and decreased responsiveness to the ventilatory stimulant effects of carbon dioxide. In the CNS, opioids do not produce unconsciousness reliably. They do, however, stimulate dopamine receptors in the chemoreceptor trigger zone of the medulla, causing nausea and vomiting. Finally, rapidly administered high doses can cause spasm of the thoracoabdominal muscles, resulting in hypoventilation.

24. What are the properties and adverse effects of the opioid IV induction agents?

Fentanyl (Sublimaze) is 100 times more potent than morphine. Its onset of action is quicker than that of morphine, its duration of action is shorter than that of morphine, and its elimination half-life is longer than that of morphine. Anesthetic doses of 30-100 µg/kg produce an onset of action in 1-2 min. Because it is very lipid soluble, it is rapidly redistributed to inactive tissues. It is slowly released into the plasma and made available for clearance.

Sufentanil (Sufenta) is structurally similar to fentanyl but is five to seven times more potent. It is more lipid soluble, which results in faster onset of action. Its elimination half-life (2-3 hr) is somewhat shorter than that of fentanyl, resulting in more rapid awakening and less postoperative respiratory depression. Induction doses range from 5-13 µg/kg.

Alfentanil (Alfenta) is one fifth to one third as potent as fentanyl. Because it is more lipid soluble than fentanyl, alfentanil has a rapid onset and short duration of action. Alfentanil often causes nausea and vomiting.

25. Which opioids stimulate the release of histamine?

Morphine, codeine, and meperidine (Demerol) cause histamine release, resulting in vasodilation and possible hypotension. Fentanyl, sufentanil, and alfentanil do not stimulate histamine release.

26. What opioid antagonist is most commonly used in clinical anesthesia?

Naloxone is the pure mu-receptor antagonist that is used to reverse the effects of opioids.

Naloxone will reverse overdoses and respiratory depressant effects; however, at the same time, it reverses the analgesic effects. Normal dosages may cause abrupt reversal, which can result in tachycardia, hypertension, pulmonary edema, and cardiac dysrhythmias. To avoid these adverse effects, naloxone should be given in doses of 40 μg (0.1 mL), repeated every few minutes.

27. Why is propofol the best agent for outpatient anesthesia?
- Rapid induction and recovery
- Lower incidence of nausea and vomiting
- Patients regain cognitive function quickly, which leads to a shorter recovery period

28. Which intravenous induction agents are recommended for use in major trauma or other hypovolemic states?
Etomidate is an agent commonly used because of its cardiac stability in patients with limited cardiac reserve. Ketamine is recommended for patients who are hypovolemic because of the direct stimulation of sympathetic outflow from the CNS. However, patients with depleted endogenous catecholamines may not be able to respond to the stimulation, resulting in more hypotension. The induction dose of etomidate is 2-3 mg/kg and that of ketamine is 1-2 mg/kg.

29. Which induction agents alter ICP?
Thiopental, propofol, etomidate, and fentanyl reduce ICP because they cause decreases in cerebral blood flow and cerebral metabolic consumption of oxygen. Ketamine increases cerebral blood flow, cerebral metabolism, and ICP.

30. What effect does age have on dosing of induction agents?
With increasing age, elimination time and renal clearance time increase, resulting in longer-lasting drug effects. Elderly patients are more sensitive to intravenous anesthetics; therefore dose reductions are necessary in this group of patients.

31. What are three commonly used anticholinergics?
Atropine, scopolamine, and glycopyrrolate.

32. What are the key values of the oxyhemoglobin dissociation curve?
- P50 (the Pao_2 at which hemoglobin is 50% saturated, called the P50) is approximately 27 mm Hg.
- The saturation of mixed venous blood (in the pulmonary artery) is about 75%, which occurs at a Po_2 of 40 mm Hg.
- A Pao_2 of 30 mm Hg produces 60% SaO_2, and a Pao_2 of 60 mm Hg produces 90% SaO_2.
- A Pao_2 of 75 mm Hg produces an SpO_2 of 95%.

33. What is the most commonly used opioid antagonist?[*]
Naloxone is the pure mu-receptor antagonist used to treat opioid overdose and to reverse opioid-induced ventilatory depression. However, reversing the ventilatory depressant effects also reverses analgesia. Abrupt reversal of analgesia may also produce a catecholamine surge, resulting in tachycardia, hypertension, pulmonary edema, and cardiac dysrhythmias. To avoid the abrupt reversal of analgesia, naloxone should be administered in doses of about 40 μg (0.1 mL), repeated in a few minutes, if necessary. Because naloxone has a short duration of action, it is often necessary to repeat the dosage or to give a continuous infusion to avoid further recurrence of narcotic-related depression of ventilation.

---

[*]Reprinted from Hatheway JA: Opioids. In Duke J (ed): Anesthesia Secrets, 2nd ed. Philadelphia, 2000, Hanley & Belfus.

34. What is tramadol?*

Tramadol is a unique analgesic with opioid-like activity. The drug also causes catecholamine reuptake inhibition. These properties and its much lower risk for tolerance and addiction allows it to be used as an analgesic for both acute and chronic pain management. Major side effects include sedation and dizziness. One concerning but uncommon adverse side effect is seizures. The drug should therefore be used with caution, if at all, in patients with a history or risk of seizures.

35. What is the preoperative management of a morbidly obese patient with a difficult airway? (Assume that the patient is otherwise healthy.)†

A morbidly obese patient is similar to a patient with a full stomach. Therefore H_2 blockers given the evening before and the morning of surgery, preoperative metoclopramide, and oral nonparticulate antacids are in order. Glycopyrrolate is useful for planned fiberoptic bronchoscopy. It improves visualization by drying secretions, increases the effectiveness of the topical anesthesia, and decreases airway responsiveness. Sedation with narcotics, benzodiazepines, and droperidol should be judiciously titrated, using supplemental oxygen and close observation to ensure an awake, appropriately responding patient who can protect his or her own airway.

36. What is the normal SpO_2?‡

Saturation measured by pulse oximetry is denoted by SpO_2 ("p" is for pulse oximetry). Partial pressure of oxygen in arterial blood (PaO_2), and hence SpO_2, varies with age, altitude, and health. Identifying abnormal values is helpful for screening people for cardiopulmonary disease, but perioperative assessment of SpO_2 has a different motive. In general, the SpO_2 should be above the "cliff" of the oxyhemoglobin dissociation curve (Fig. 7-1). At and below the cliff, which appears at a saturation of approximately 90%, a small decrease of PaO_2 results in swift desaturation. For example, on the steep part of curve, as PO_2 changes by 1 mm Hg, SaO_2 changes by 3%. In the effort to keep the SpO_2 in the safe zone, supplemental oxygen is usually administered to patients who are receiving or recovering from general anesthesia.

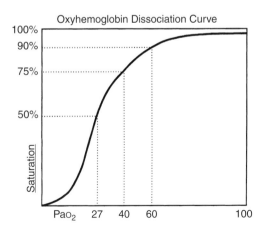

Fig. 7-1 The oxyhemoglobin dissociation curve describes the nonlinear relationship between PaO_2 and percentage saturation of hemoglobin with oxygen (SaO_2). In the steep part of the curve (50% region), small changes in PaO_2 result in large changes in SaO_2. The converse is true when PaO_2 rises above 60 mm Hg. Three regions of the curve have been marked. (From Edwards RK: Pulse oximetry. In Duke J [ed]: Anesthesia Secrets, 3rd ed. Philadelphia, 2006, Mosby.)

---

†Reprinted from Nabonsal J: Preoperative medications. In Duke J (ed): Anesthesia Secrets, 2nd ed. Philadelphia, 2000, Hanley & Belfus.
‡Reprinted from Goldman JM: Pulse oximetry. In Duke J (ed): Anesthesia Secrets, 2nd ed. Philadelphia, 2000, Hanley & Belfus.

37. Why is SpO_2 such a big deal? ‡

One reason, of course, is that SpO_2 can be measured inexpensively and noninvasively. The second reason requires an understanding of oxygen carriage in the blood. The amount of oxygen carried by a sample of blood depends on the SaO_2 and hemoglobin concentration. If hemoglobin concentration remains constant, blood that is 50% saturated with oxygen binds half as much oxygen as a sample that is 100% saturated. Examination of the oxyhemoglobin dissociation curve tells the rest of the story because it illustrates the nonlinear relationship between SaO_2 and PaO_2. For example, as PaO_2 increases from 60 to 100 mm Hg, SaO_2 increases only about 6%. In contrast, as PaO_2 increases 33 mm Hg, from 27 to 60 mm Hg, SaO_2 increases by 25%.

BIBLIOGRAPHY

1. Allen DM: Intravenous anesthetics and benzodiazepines. In Duke J (ed): Anesthesia Secrets, 3rd ed. Philadelphia, 2006, Mosby.
2. Hatheway J: Opioids. In Duke J (ed): Anesthesia Secrets, 2nd ed. Philadelphia, 2000, Hanley & Belfus.
3. Hudson RJ, Stanski DR, Burch PG: Pharmacokinetics of methohexital and thiopental in surgical patients. Anesthesiology 59:215-219, 1983.
4. McDowell G: Intravenous induction agents. In Duke J (ed): Anesthesia Secrets, 2nd ed. Philadelphia, 2000, Hanley & Belfus.
5. Nabonsal J: Preoperative medications. In Duke J (ed): Anesthesia Secrets, 2nd ed. Philadelphia, 2000, Hanley & Belfus.
6. Reves JG, Fragen RJ, Vinik HR et al: Midazolam: pharmacology and uses. Anesthesiology 62:310-324, 1985.
7. Stoelting RK, Miller RD: Intravenous anesthetics. In Stoelting RD, Miller RD (eds): Basics of Anesthesia. New York, 1999, Churchill Livingstone.
8. Swank KM: Preoperative evaluation. In Duke J (ed): Anesthesia Secrets, 3rd ed. Philadelphia, 2006, Mosby.
9. Winkelmann G: Benzodiazepines. In Duke J (ed): Anesthesia Secrets, 2nd ed. Philadelphia, 2000, Hanley & Belfus.

8. INHALATIONAL ANESTHESIA

Christopher L. Maestrello, DDS

1. What inhalational anesthetics are currently available, and how are they delivered in clinical use?

Five volatile liquids (desflurane, enflurane, halothane, isoflurane, and sevoflurane) and one gas (nitrous oxide) are used clinically. Enflurane is used infrequently and is not discussed in this chapter. The volatile liquids require a vaporizer for inhalational administration. Additionally, the desflurane vaporizer has a heating component to allow delivery at room temperature.

These inhalation agents can be administered in a hospital operating room or in a clinical situation, provided adequate scavenging and ventilation exists. Many oral and maxillofacial procedures require a nonsurgical field; therefore anesthetic delivery systems can be used in an office setting. Inhalational anesthetic delivery systems exist for the delivery of one or multiple gases. These delivery systems have mandatory scavenging and fail-safe mechanisms to optimize safety.

2. How long can oxygen at 2 L/min be delivered from an E cylinder with a reading of 500 psi?

A full E cylinder of oxygen (O_2) contains approximately 600 L at a pressure of 2000 psi.

At 2 L/min, a full E cylinder will deliver O_2 for approximately 300 min, or 5 hr. A reading of 500 psi will therefore give you approximately 1 hr and 15 min of O_2.

3. How long can nitrous oxide (N_2O) at 2 L/min be delivered from an E cylinder that reads 750 psi?

N_2O has a pressure of 750 psi and contains approximately 1600 L in an E cylinder. N_2O is a compressed liquid and not a compressed gas like O_2. A compressed liquid does not show a linear correlation between volume and pressure as does a compressed gas. N_2O pressure will remain at 750 psi until all the liquid has been vaporized. Therefore an estimated time cannot be determined.

4. Why is N_2O use contraindicated in patients with conditions involving closed gas spaces?

N_2O has a low blood-to-gas partition coefficient (0.46) and therefore low solubility. It can leave the blood and enter air-filled cavities 34 times more quickly than nitrogen can leave the cavity to enter the blood. The use of N_2O can increase the expansion of compliant cavities, such as a pneumothorax, bowel gas in a bowel obstruction, and an air embolism. An increase in pressure will occur when N_2O is used with noncompliant cavities, such as the middle ear or sinuses.

The oral and maxillofacial surgeon needs to be cautious when treating the recent trauma patient (e.g., motor vehicle accident victim). An asymptomatic, undiagnosed closed pneumothorax can double in size in 10 min after the administration of 70% N_2O. Nitrous oxide–oxygen sedation should be postponed in patients with gastrointestinal obstructions, middle ear disturbances, and, possibly, sinus infections.

5. Should a patient with an upper respiratory infection (URI) be given N_2O via a nasal hood?

Because a patient with a URI has nasal blockage, the delivery of the N_2O is limited and the potential for leakage of N_2O around the hood is more likely. In addition, patients with a URI are also more likely to have associated middle ear and sinus infections. Therefore the use of N_2O with patients with URI is unwise.

6. Can inhalational anesthetics be administered to patients with chronic obstructive pulmonary disease (COPD)?

Administration of volatile anesthetics (desflurane, enflurane, halothane, isoflurane, and sevoflurane) is not a concern for COPD patients (asthmatic bronchitis, emphysema, and chronic bronchitis). All volatile anesthetics are bronchodilators and therefore are beneficial to patients with COPD.

N_2O-O_2, however, should be used cautiously. Patients with mild to moderate COPD should be administered a supplemental inspired oxygen concentration (FiO_2) of no greater than 40. N_2O-O_2 sedation without any additional intravenous sedation is generally safe. Remember, 4 L through a nasal cannula equals 36% O_2.

Nasal cannula (3-6 L/min): $FiO_2 = 20 + 4 \times L/min$
Face mask with reservoir (6-10 L/min): $FiO_2 = 10 \times L/min$

During deep sedation, keep patients breathing spontaneously and do not take away their respiratory drive. O_2 supplementation should be avoided or used only with extreme caution in patients with severe COPD. These patients have an increased incidence of pulmonary bullae or blebs (combined alveoli). Because of N_2O's low blood solubility, it can increase the volume and pressure of these lung defects, which could create an increased risk of barotrauma and pneumothorax.

Carbon dioxide (CO_2) is a respiratory stimulus for patients with normal respiratory physiology. Patients with COPD retain larger amounts of CO_2 in their lungs and, over time, lose this respiratory drive. COPD patients thus develop a hypoxic drive. The potential for the hypoxic drive to cease with the severe chronic patient exists when O_2 is > 21% room air (i.e., N_2O-O_2 at 70/30%).

Asthmatic bronchitis patients may be of any age and could easily be encountered in the office. Patients with debilitating emphysema and chronic bronchitis are often chronically ill and are not seen commonly in an office setting. They may, however, be encountered in nursing homes and hospitals.

7.   When is administration of N_2O-O_2 sedation contraindicated in an asthmatic patient?

There are no contraindications for the use of N_2O-O_2 sedation in asthmatic patients. Because anxiety is a stimulus for an asthmatic attack, N_2O-O_2 sedation is actually beneficial for these patients.

There have been no reported allergies to N_2O. The potential for an allergic reaction does exist, however, in the latex-allergic individual who receives N_2O-O_2 via a nasal hood.

8.   What is the second gas effect?

This occurs when one gas speeds the rate of increase of the alveolar partial pressure of a second gas. This effect is normally associated with an inhalational induction involving a large volume of N_2O and a volatile anesthetic. N_2O's low blood solubility allows it to be absorbed quickly by the alveoli, thus causing an increase in the alveolar concentration of the volatile anesthetic. In theory, a high concentration of one gas (e.g., 70% N_2O) could speed the induction of a second, less soluble gas (e.g., halothane).

Inhalational inductions are normally used in energetic pediatric patients. Obtaining intravenous access in children who cannot sit still is difficult, and a quick induction is desirable. The rate of induction of halothane should be increased when it is used concurrently with 70% N_2O.

9.   What is minimal alveolar concentration (MAC)?

MAC is the concentration of an inhaled anesthetic at 1 atm that prevents skeletal muscle movement's response to a painful stimulus (e.g., surgical skin incision) in 50% of patients (Table 8-1). A MAC of 1.3 prevents skeletal movement in approximately 95% of individuals undergoing surgery. The potency of anesthetic gases can be compared using MAC.

Table 8-1   *Minimal Alveolar Concentration (MAC) of Commonly Used Agents*

AGENT	MAC
Nitrous oxide	104
Isoflurane	1.15
Halothane	0.77
Desflurane	6.0
Sevoflurane	1.71

10.   What factors affect MAC?

Factors That *Decrease* MAC:

Higher altitudes (↓ barometric pressure)
Pregnancy
Hypothermia
Hyponatremia
Alcohol (acute use)
Barbiturates
Calcium channel blockers
Opioids

Factors That *Increase* MAC:

Increased central neurotransmitter levels (MAOIs, cocaine, ephedrine, levodopa)
Hyperthermia
Alcohol (chronic use)
Hypernatremia

11. How can MAC values be used to gauge awareness during surgery?

Intraoperative patient awareness is a concern with all patients undergoing a deep sedation or general anesthesia. Volatile anesthetics have amnestic properties at an adequate MAC. Intravenous medications are often used in conjunction with volatile anesthetics, which often cause a decrease in MAC. This decreased MAC may prevent an amnestic state. Although specific concentrations of volatile agents have not been established for the elimination of intraoperative recall, clinical studies show that awareness is eliminated between 0.4 and 0.6 MAC for isoflurane. Attaining a MAC of 0.8 has been recommended to guarantee unconsciousness.

Awareness precautions need to be taken with certain anesthetic techniques. An anesthetist may be tempted to decrease the concentration of a volatile anesthetic when a paralytic has been used because surgical stimulation has been eliminated. The addition of midazolam, an amnestic benzodiazepine, can be used in situations where MAC has been reduced below 0.8. MAC is often reduced in patients who develop intraoperative hypotension because of volatile inhalational vasodilating properties. Vasopressors, such as ephedrine and phenylephrine, may be necessary in order to maintain a MAC of 0.8 when additional amnestic medications are not being used.

12. Why are additive values of MAC for inhalational anesthetics beneficial?

Additive values are beneficial when a decrease in ventilatory and circulatory effects of volatile anesthetics is desired. MAC values are additive; therefore the simultaneous administration of N_2O with a volatile anesthetic will decrease the MAC of both agents. For example, using 0.5 MAC N_2O (approximately 50%) with 0.5 MAC isoflurane (approximately 0.6%) results in a MAC of 1.0.

The only inhalational anesthetics that would be administered simultaneously would be a volatile anesthetic (desflurane, halothane, isoflurane, and sevoflurane) and N_2O. Fail-safe mechanisms exist on anesthetic machines to prevent the simultaneous administration of two volatile agents.

N_2O has a MAC >100% and therefore cannot be used as a sole anesthetic agent, because a minimum of 21% O_2 is required at 1 atm. Typically, N_2O concentrations of 20%-70% are used.

13. What are the hemodynamic effects of volatile anesthetics?

Volatile anesthetics depress the cardiovascular system, and this depression results in a reduced mean arterial pressure. Halothane primarily causes a reduction in heart rate and contractility. Desflurane, isoflurane, and sevoflurane cause primarily a decrease in systemic vascular resistance, which is reflected by a reduced blood pressure.

14. What are the hemodynamic considerations of the combined use of a volatile anesthetic and the intravenous anesthetic propofol?

The inhalational anesthetics desflurane, isoflurane, and sevoflurane and the intravenous agent propofol are potent vasodilators. Additive effects causing hypotension from a decrease in systemic vascular resistance occur with simultaneous administration of these two anesthetic groups. Combining these agents should be done cautiously in elderly patients and patients taking hypertensive medications. Noting preoperative blood pressures is extremely important. Selection of an alternative intravenous anesthetic agent may be indicated. If propofol is used along with a volatile anesthetic, then vasopressors (e.g., ephedrine, phenylephrine) should be diluted properly and made readily available.

15. What are the ventilatory effects of volatile anesthetics?

Volatile anesthetics will cause a dose-dependent decrease in ventilation. Volatile anesthetics cause a decrease in tidal volume (TV) with a compensatory increase in respiratory rate (RR) but a net decrease in minute ventilation (mV).

Ventilatory effects of volatile anesthetics: net $\downarrow$mV = $\uparrow$RR × $\downarrow$TV

This decreased minute ventilation causes an increase in CO_2. An increase in CO_2 stimulates the respiratory drive in the unanesthetized patient. Inhalational anesthetics, however, shift the CO_2 response curve to the right and lessen the ventilatory response to hypercarbia and hypoxia (Fig. 8-1).

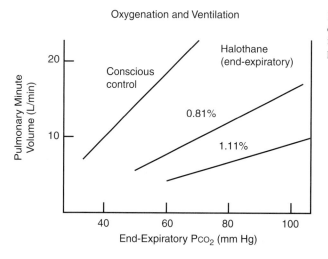

Oxygenation and Ventilation

Fig. 8-1 The CO_2 response curve. Note the effects of inhalational anesthetics on the pulmonary minute volume.

16. What adverse reaction can occur if halothane and epinephrine are combined?

The potential for life-threatening dysrhythmic effects exists between inhalational anesthetics and vasoconstrictors. The combination creating the greatest adverse effect is between halothane and epinephrine. The addition of thiopental (Pentothal), an ultra short-acting barbiturate, further enhances these dysrhythmic effects. The true mechanism of action creating these dysrhythmic disturbances is not completely understood, but it appears to involve stimulation of both alpha- and beta-adrenergic receptors.

The potential for this adverse reaction is greatest when anesthesia and surgery have just begun. If anesthesia is induced with thiopental and maintained with halothane, and local anesthesia involving epinephrine is used by the surgeon, then an adverse reaction may ensue. Several recommendations have been proposed to prevent such reactions. Do not inject a local anesthetic with epinephrine immediately after the induction of anesthesia with halothane or thiopental; it is prudent to wait for 10 min. Use 2 μg/kg of epinephrine if either halothane or thiopental is being administered and 1 μg/kg if halothane and thiopental are being used. Remember, a local anesthetic with 1:100,000 epinephrine contains 10 μg/mL of epinephrine.

17. What is partition coefficient? How can it influence the speed of induction?

A partition coefficient is defined as a distribution ratio of a volatile anesthetic as it distributes itself between two phases at equilibrium when the temperature, pressure, and volume are the same (Table 8-2). A blood-to-gas coefficient therefore describes the distribution of anesthetic between blood and gas. A high blood solubility requires a greater concentration of inhaled anesthetic to be dissolved in the blood before equilibrium with the gas phase can occur. The blood acts as an inactive reservoir that prevents the anesthetic from reaching the site of action, thereby slowing induction.

The difference in blood-to-gas partition coefficients between halothane and sevoflurane explains why sevoflurane is a more rapid induction agent. With all other factors being equal (e.g., alveolar concentration, cardiac output), the lower solubility of sevoflurane will make it more readily available as an anesthetic.

Table 8-2   *Partition Coefficients for Inhaled Anesthetics*

	DESFLURANE	HALOTHANE	ISOFLURANE	N_2O	SEVOFLURANE
Blood:gas	0.42	2.4	1.4	0.46	0.68
Brain:blood	1.3	2.9	1.6	1.1	1.7
Muscle:blood	2.0	3.4	2.9	1.2	3.1
Fat:blood	27	51	45	2.3	48
Oil:blood	18.7	224	90.8	1.4	47.2

18. **Which volatile anesthetic has the quickest wake-up potential after a long (>5 hr) surgical procedure?**

Anesthetic takes awhile to be distributed from the blood to the tissues (e.g., muscle, fat). As the length of time of a surgery increases and tissues become increasingly saturated with anesthetic, wake-up times increase. The fat-to-blood partition coefficient for desflurane is the lowest for all volatile anesthetics, and it provides the quickest wake-up. A common misconception is that sevoflurane has a quick wake-up time because it has a quick onset. For short surgeries this is true, because tissue saturation has not had time to occur. For long surgeries, however, sevoflurane does not provide a quick wake-up (check sevoflurane's tissue:blood coefficients in Table 8-2).

19. **What is diffusion hypoxia?**

Although its existence has been questioned, diffusion hypoxia is postulated to occur when the administration of N_2O has been discontinued with the spontaneous breathing of room air. The theory holds that N_2O's low blood solubility allows it to leave the blood rapidly and enter the alveoli. Excessive N_2O in the alveoli dilutes the O_2 and makes the patient hypoxic. This phenomenon has been refuted by many studies. Nonetheless, because of side effects such as headaches, nausea, vomiting, and lethargy, administering O_2 for 3-5 min following N_2O use is prudent.

20. **What are the concerns to administration of N_2O-O_2 sedation to an obstetric patient?**

N_2O crosses the placenta and therefore has the potential to cause teratogenic effects to the fetus. The greatest potential for problems exists during the first trimester when organs are forming. Significant exposure during the first 6 weeks can inhibit DNA synthesis. Consequently, female surgeons and staff who aren't aware that they are pregnant may be at greater risk than patients.

Recent research has refuted the claim that N_2O is dangerous to the fetus. Although N_2O has been used safely for years in obstetrics, it would be wise to obtain a medical consult before its administration in pregnant women who are in their second or third trimesters. Even if N_2O-O_2 sedation is approved by the patient's obstetrician, it should be used only for short procedures, and no more than 50% N_2O should be administered.

21. **How long does it take before changes in oxygen saturation are reflected in pulse oximeter readings?**

Approximately 20 sec. It takes time for O_2 delivered to the lung to influence oxygenation at the fingertip. Pulse oximeter signals are also averaged over different periods. This is mainly to reduce spurious pulse oximeter readings, such as those caused by patient movement. The trade-off is that true reductions in pulse oximeter readings are delayed (a patient desaturating faster than the pulse oximeter indicates). Similarly, once adequate delivery of oxygen is restored, there will be a delay in recovery of the pulse oximeter readings. The period of signal averaging can often be changed in commonly used pulse oximeters.

22. What are neuromuscular blocking agents (NMBs)?[*]

NMBs, commonly called muscle relaxants, are drugs that interrupt transmission at the neuromuscular junction. These drugs provide skeletal muscle relaxation and, consequently, can be used to facilitate tracheal intubation, assist with mechanical ventilation, and optimize surgical conditions. Occasionally, they may be used to reduce the metabolic demands of breathing; in the management of status epilepticus (although they do not diminish central nervous system [CNS] activity), status asthmaticus, or tetanus; and to facilitate the treatment of raised intracranial pressure.

These drugs are very dangerous and inhibit the function of all skeletal muscle, including the diaphragm, and must be administered only by personnel skilled in airway management. NMBs should never be given without preparation to maintain the airway and ventilation. The concomitant use of sedative-hypnotic or amnestic drugs is indicated, because NMBs alone achieve complete paralysis while allowing the patient complete awareness.

23. How are NMBs classified?[*]

These drugs are classified into two groups according to their actions at the neuromuscular junction:

Depolarizing NMB (succinylcholine [SCh]): SCh mimics the action of acetylcholine by depolarizing the postsynaptic membrane at the neuromuscular junction. Because the postsynaptic receptor is occupied and depolarized, acetylcholine has no effect.

Nondepolarizing NMBs: These agents act by competitive blockade of the postsynaptic membrane, so that acetylcholine is blocked from the receptors and cannot have a depolarizing effect.

24. What is the mechanism of action of SCh?[*]

SCh is the only depolarizing agent to be used widely in clinical anesthetic practice. The depolarizing agent mimics the action of acetylcholine. However, because SCh is hydrolyzed by plasma cholinesterase (pseudocholinesterase), which is present only in the plasma and not at the neuromuscular junction, the length of blockade is directly related to the rate of diffusion of SCh away from the neuromuscular junction. Consequently, the resultant depolarization is prolonged when compared with acetylcholine. Depolarization gradually diminishes, but relaxation persists as long as SCh is present at the postsynaptic receptor.

25. What are the indications for using SCh?[*]

In clinical situations in which the patient has a full stomach and is at risk for regurgitation and aspiration when anesthetized, rapid paralysis and airway control are priorities. Such situations include diabetes mellitus, hiatal hernia, obesity, pregnancy, severe pain, and trauma.

SCh provides the most rapid onset of any NMB currently available. In addition, the duration of blockade induced by SCh is only 5-10 min. Respiratory muscle function returns quickly should the patient prove difficult to intubate (see question 11).

26. What is the breakdown and elimination process of nondepolarizing NMBs?[*]

Atracurium is unique in that it undergoes spontaneous breakdown at physiologic temperatures and pH (Hoffmann elimination), as well as ester hydrolysis, and thus it is ideal for use in patients with compromised hepatic or renal function. Mivacurium, like SCh, is metabolized by pseudocholinesterase.

Aminosteroid relaxants (pancuronium, vecuronium, pipecuronium, and rocuronium) are deacetylated in the liver, and their action may be prolonged in the presence of hepatic dysfunction. Vecuronium and rocuronium also have significant biliary excretion, and their action may be prolonged with extrahepatic biliary obstruction.

[*]Reprinted from Warnecke DE: Neuromuscular blocking agents. In Duke J (ed): Anesthesia Secrets, 2nd ed. Philadelphia, 2000, Hanley & Belfus.

Relaxants with significant renal excretion include tubocurarine, metocurine, doxacurium, pancuronium, and pipecuronium.

27. Is it possible to reverse the effects of the nondepolarizing NMBs?[*]
Just as competition at the receptor sites of the neuromuscular junction allows the relaxant to overcome the effects of acetylcholine, medications that increase the amount of acetylcholine at the neuromuscular junction facilitate reversal of relaxation. Reversal agents are **acetylcholinesterase inhibitors** and include neostigmine, pyridostigmine, and edrophonium (Table 8-3). These drugs inhibit the enzyme that breaks down acetylcholine, making more of this neurotransmitter available at each receptor. Physostigmine, another acetylcholinesterase inhibitor, crosses the blood-brain barrier and is not used for reversal of muscle relaxants. Pyridostigmine is used in the management of patients with myasthenia gravis. The acetylcholinesterase inhibitors possess positively charged quaternary ammonium groups, are water-soluble, and are renally excreted.

Table 8-3   *Neuromuscular Blocking Reversal Agents*

DRUG	DOSE (mg/kg)	ONSET (min)	DURATION (min)
Edrophonium	0.5-1.0	2	45-60
Neostigmine	0.035-0.07	7	60-90
Pyridostigmine	0.15-0.25	11	60-120

28. NMB reversal agents cause an increase in available acetylcholine. Is this a problem?[*]
It is important to remember that the muscarinic effects of these drugs at cholinergic receptors in the heart must be blocked by atropine or glycopyrrolate to prevent bradycardia. The degree of bradycardia may be significant. Even asystole has been noted. The most common doses used for this purpose are 0.01 mg/kg of atropine and 0.005-0.015 mg/kg of glycopyrrolate.
To prevent bradycardias associated with the anticholinesterases it is important to administer an anticholinergic with a similar onset of action. Atropine is administered with edrophonium and glycopyrrolate with neostigmine.

29. The heart is a muscle. Do muscle relaxants decrease contraction of the myocardium?[*]
The NMBs have their primary effect at nicotinic cholinergic receptor sites. The myocardium is a muscle with nerve transmission accomplished via adrenergic receptors using norepinephrine as the transmitter. Consequently, muscle relaxants have no effect on cardiac contractility. NMBs also have no effect on smooth muscle.

30. How do we make muscle relaxants work faster if we need to secure the airway sooner?[*]
By overwhelming the sites of action (receptors in the neuromuscular junction), one can provide a competitive advantage for the blocking drug over acetylcholine. This is exactly what is done with the standard intubating dose of a nondepolarizing relaxant. The usual intubating dose is approximately three times the ED95 (the dose expected to show 95% reduction in twitch height on electrical stimulation). For relaxants with cardiovascular stability, further increases in initial dose can provide some decrease in onset time without producing side effects. However, with the exception of the nondepolarizing NMB *rocuronium*, and possibly the new drug *rapacuronium*, it is very difficult to decrease the onset time to that of SCh. For drugs with side effects such as histamine release, increases in dose usually increase side effects as well.

Another method of decreasing onset time is the **priming technique.** By giving one third of the ED95 at 3 min before the intubating dose, one can decrease onset time by as much as 1 min. However, sensitivity to the paralyzing effects of these agents varies greatly among patients, and some patients may become totally paralyzed with a priming dose. Other patients may experience distressing diplopia, dysphagia, or the sensation of not being able to take a deep breath. For this reason, the practice of administering "priming" doses of relaxants is discouraged by many anesthesiologists. Once relaxants are administered at any dose, the caregiver should be in the position to assist ventilation.

31. What is plasma cholinesterase (pseudocholinesterase)?[*]

Plasma cholinesterase is produced in the liver and metabolizes SCh as well as ester local anesthetics and mivacurium, a nondepolarizing NMB. A reduced quantity of plasma cholinesterase, such as occurs with liver disease, pregnancy, malignancies, malnutrition, collagen vascular disease, and hypothyroidism, may prolong the duration of blockade with SCh.

32. What is the importance of a dibucaine number?[*]

Plasma cholinesterase can have qualitative as well as quantitative effects, the most common being dibucaine-resistant cholinesterase deficiency. Dibucaine inhibits normal plasma cholinesterase by 80%, whereas atypical plasma cholinesterase is inhibited by only 20%. A patient with normal SCh metabolism will have a dibucaine number of 80. If a patient has a dibucaine number of 40-60, then that patient is heterozygous for this atypical plasma cholinesterase and will have a moderately prolonged block with SCh. If a patient has a dibucaine number of 20, the patient is homozygous for atypical plasma cholinesterase and will have a very prolonged block with SCh.

It is important to remember that a dibucaine number is a qualitative, and not quantitative, measurement. Consequently, a patient may have a dibucaine number of 80 but have prolonged blockade with SCh related to decreased levels of normal plasma cholinesterase.

33. Are clinicians accurate in determining arterial desaturation by "visual oximetry" (how red is the blood)?[†]

No. Pulse oximetry should be regarded as the fifth vital sign.

34. Can any other environmental or clinical conditions result in inaccurate pulse oximetry values?[†]

Reliability depends on a strong arterial pulse plus good light transmission. Inaccuracy results with hypotension (mean arterial pressure < 50 mm Hg), hypothermia (<35° C), vascular disease (poor peripheral perfusion), and vasopressor therapy (vasoconstriction). Bright lights, intravenous dyes, nail polish, and excessive motion each may produce bad information.

35. What is the relationship between oxyhemoglobin saturation (SaO_2) and partial pressure of oxygen (PaO_2)?[†]

Proper interpretation of pulse oximetry requires recall of the oxyhemoglobin dissociation curve. A rightward shift (decreased hemoglobin affinity for oxygen) facilitates oxygen unloading at the tissue level. Increasing temperature, increasing $PaCO_2$, increasing 2,3-diphosphoglycerate, and increasing hydrogen ion concentration—all "increases"—shift the curve to the right. When the PaO_2 is > 100 mm Hg, however, the curve is virtually flat. Consequently, a large drop in PaO_2 (e.g., from 200-100 mm Hg) may occur with no discernible change in SaO_2.

[†]Reprinted from Haenel J, Johnson JL: Oxygen monitoring and assessment. In Harken AH, Moore EE (eds): Abernathy's Surgical Secrets, 5th ed. Philadelphia, 2005, Mosby.

36. How should a hypoxic event be managed?[†]

Before you even start trying to make the diagnosis, give oxygen. The first maneuver for intubated patients is to hand-ventilate with an Ambu bag. A ruptured endotracheal tube cuff is self-evident, whereas difficult bagging implies airway obstruction, bronchospasm, or tension pneumothorax. Inability to pass a suction catheter confirms endotracheal tube obstruction. If the obstruction is not reversible by changing head position or by cuff deflation, the endotracheal tube must be replaced immediately. If there is difficulty with bagging and no evidence of airway obstruction, listen to the chest for breath sounds to exclude a tension pneumothorax. The mechanical ventilator and breathing circuit must be examined for malfunction. Send arterial blood gases to confirm hypoxia (low P_{O_2}) and rule out hypoventilation (high P_{CO_2}).

Next, get a chest x-ray (to rule out a pneumothorax and to confirm the correct position of the endotracheal tube) and review recent medications, interventions (e.g., suctioning, position changes, nursing care), and changes in clinical status. Most acute hypoxic events in the intensive care unit are the result of easily identified and reversible mechanical problems, such as disconnects from oxygen delivery systems or mucus plugging that requires suctioning.

BIBLIOGRAPHY

1. Adamson DT: Oxygenation and ventilation. In Duke J (ed): Anesthesia Secrets, 2nd ed. Philadelphia, 2000, Hanley & Belfus.
2. Browne MD: Volatile anesthetics. In Duke J (ed): Anesthesia Secrets, 3rd ed. Philadelphia, 2006, Mosby.
3. Cahalan MK, Lurz FW, Eger EI 2nd et al: Narcotics decrease heart rate during inhalation anesthesia. Anesth Analg 66:166-170, 1987.
4. Christensen LQ, Bonde J, Kampmann JP: Drug interactions with inhalational anaesthetics. Acta Anesthesiol Scand 37:231-244, 1993.
5. Clark MS, Brunick AL: Handbook of Nitrous Oxide and Oxygen Sedation, 2nd ed. St Louis, 2003, Mosby.
6. Duke J: Airway management. In Duke J (ed): Anesthesia Secrets, 3rd ed. Philadelphia, 2006, Mosby.
7. Eger EI 2nd, Saidman LJ: Hazards of nitrous oxide anesthesia in bowel obstruction and pneumothorax. Anesthesiology 26:61-66, 1965.
8. Foltz B, Benumof J: Mechanisms of hypoxia and hypercarbia in the perioperative period. Crit Care Clin 3:269-286, 1987.
9. Haenel JB, Johnson JL: Oxygen monitoring and assessment. In Duke J (ed): Anesthesia Secrets, 2nd ed. Philadelphia, 2000, Hanley & Belfus.
10. Hayashi Y, Kamibayashi T, Sumikawa K et al: Adrenoreceptor mechanism involved in thiopental-epinephrine-induced arrhythmias in dogs. Am J Physiol 265:H1380-H1385, 1993.
11. Johnston RR, Eger EI 2nd, Wilson C: A comparative interaction of epinephrine with enflurane, isoflurane, and halothane in man. Anesth Analg 55:709-712, 1976.
12. Kamibayashi T, Hayashi Y, Takada K et al: Adrenoreceptor mechanism involved in thiopental-induced potentiation of halothane-epinephrine arrhythmias in dogs. Res Comm Mol Pathol Pharmacol 93:225-234, 1996.
13. Katz RL, Matteo RS, Papper EM: The injection of epinephrine during general anesthesia with halogenated hydrocarbons and cyclopropane in man. 2. Halothane. Anesthesiology 23:597-600, 1962.
14. Leichliter C: Awareness during anesthesia. In Duke J (ed): Anesthesia Secrets, 3rd ed. Philadelphia, 2006, Mosby.
15. Malamed SF: Sedation: A Guide to Patient Management, 4th ed. St Louis, 2003, Mosby.
16. Miller HJ: Chronic obstructive pulmonary disease. In Duke J (ed): Anesthesia Secrets, 3rd ed. Philadelphia, 2006, Mosby.
17. Rosen MA: Management of anesthesia for the pregnant surgical patient. Anesthesiology 91:1159-1163, 1999.
18. Stoelting RK, Miller RD: Effects of inhaled anesthetics on ventilation and circulation. In Stoelting RK, Miller RD (eds): Basics of Anesthesia, 3rd ed. New York, 1994, Churchill Livingstone.
19. Warnecke DE: Neuromuscular blocking agents. In Duke J (ed): Anesthesia Secrets, 2nd ed. Philadelphia, 2000, Hanley & Belfus.

Part III
Postoperative Care

9. FLUID AND ELECTROLYTE MANAGEMENT

Jason S. Hullett, DMD, Gaetano G. Spinnato, DMD, MD,
Lubor Hlousek, DMD, MD, and Hamid Hajarian, MS, DDS, MD

1. What is the percentage of total body water (TBW), and how would you describe the composition of the two main fluid compartments?

TBW is 60% of body weight in the average male.

Water occupies two main fluid compartments:

- Intracellular fluid (ICF): about two thirds by volume, contained in cells
- Extracellular fluid (ECF): one third; consists of two major subdivisions:
  - Intravascular: the fluid portion of the blood ($\frac{1}{3}$)
  - Interstitial fluid (IF): fluid in spaces between cells ($\frac{2}{3}$)

2. What are the mechanisms by which TBW is maintained?

The main mechanisms are neural (hypothalamic thirst center), renin-angiotensin-aldosterone, atrial natriuretic hormone (ANH), and antidiuretic hormone (ADH). Changes in osmolarity and sodium concentration have physiologic effects on the hypothalamus to cause secretion of ADH (vasopressin) from the posterior pituitary. ADH is also secreted through the renin-angiotensin-aldosterone pathway. Low blood pressure stimulates secretion of renin by the kidney. Then renin stimulates production of angiotensin I, which in turn, is converted to angiotensin II in the lungs. Angiotensin II stimulates ADH (vasopressin) from the pituitary gland acting on the kidney to increase sodium and water reabsorption, increasing blood pressure. In the face of elevated blood pressure, ANH is produced in the right atrium, which increases sodium and water loss in the form of urine.

3. What are the major extracellular and intracellular cations?

The major extracellular cation is sodium, and it is responsible for most of the osmotic force that maintains the size of the ECF volume (ECFV). The concentration is usually kept within a narrow range (135-145 mEq/L). Potassium is the major intracellular cation. The intracellular concentration is about 130-140 mEq/L, and the extracellular concentration is 3.5-5.0 mEq/L. A stable plasma concentration is essential for normal cellular function, cardiac rhythm, and proper neuromuscular transmission.

4. What is the effect of decreased renal perfusion that results from ECFV depletion?

With decreased renal perfusion, the juxtaglomerular cells of the kidney release renin. Renin converts angiotensinogen to angiotensin I. This in turn is converted to angiotensin II by angiotensin-converting enzyme. Angiotensin II causes sodium retention and the release of aldosterone from the adrenal cortex, which in turn promotes sodium retention by the distal nephron.

5.   What is body fluid osmolality?

This is the ratio of solute (particles) to water in all compartments. Because water can move freely between compartments, changes in ECF osmolality cause reciprocal changes in the intracellular volume.

6.   What are the main solutes of the ECFV?

The main solutes of the ECFV are sodium, glucose, and urea.

7.   What is the importance of solutes in the ECFV for calculated and measured osmolality?

By calculating the serum osmolality based on the main solutes present in that compartment, the ECF osmolality can be approximated:

$$\text{Calculated osmolality} = 2\,[Na^+] + [glucose]/18 + [BUN]/2.8$$

Usually the measured and the calculated osmolality are equal unless there are osmotically active substances present, which do not enter into the calculation of osmolality. This difference is called the osmolal gap (OSM GAP).

$$\text{OSM GAP} = \text{OSM (meas)} - \text{OSM (calc)}$$

The presence of drugs such as ethylene glycol, methanol, and ethanol can cause values to be > 10 mOsm/L because sodium, glucose, and urea do not increase the osmol gap. These solutes affect both the calculated and the measured osmolalities.

8.   What is tonicity (effective osmolality)?

Tonicity is the ability of solutes to generate an increase in osmotic pressure, when they are restricted to a compartment, causing water to move from an intracellular compartment to an extracellular one to establish osmotic equilibrium. These solutes are termed effective osmoles. Sodium, glucose, mannitol, and sorbitol are effective osmoles. An increase in tonicity is the main stimulus for thirst and the release of ADH to help water regulation.

9.   What does the kidney require to maintain fluid balance?

For the kidney to regulate water excretion and keep the sodium concentration of the ECFV constant, the following are required:

- The glomerular filtration rate must be adequate.
- The glomerular filtrate delivered to the concentrating and diluting segments of the loop of Henle and the distal nephron must be sufficient.
- The tubular concentrating and diluting mechanisms must be intact.
- The kidney must respond to ADH.
- The mechanism for turning ADH on and off must be functioning appropriately.

10. What is the difference between syndrome of inappropriate antidiuretic hormone (SIADH) and diabetes insipidus (DI)?

In SIADH, there is an increase in ADH secretion, resulting in increased water retention and hyponatremia. In DI, there is a decrease in ADH secretion, causing large volumes of dilute urine, dehydration, and hypernatremia.

11. What are the initial signs of severe hypokalemia?

Hypokalemia can be defined as plasma potassium concentration <3.5 mEq/L. Usually, skeletal muscle weakness or cramping is the first sign; however, paralysis; paresthesias; palpitations; constipation; nausea or vomiting; abdominal cramping; polyuria, nocturia, or polydipsia; psychosis, delirium, or hallucinations; and depression also can be early signs.

12. **What is central DI?**

In the absence or lack of ADH, the kidney is unable to concentrate urine. This can lead to excessive loss of water from the kidney and hypernatremia. This is manifested by polyuria and polydipsia.

13. **What is nephrogenic DI?**

In this syndrome, there are adequate levels of circulating ADH; however, water is not absorbed because the permeability of collecting tubules is not increased. This results in hypernatremia because of excessive water loss.

14. **What is the difference between loop and thiazide diuretics?**

Both types of diuretics block the reabsorption of sodium in the kidney, causing a loss of both sodium and water and a decrease in the size of the ECFV. However, loop diuretics block sodium reabsorption in the ascending loop of Henle, where 20%-30% of filtered sodium is reabsorbed. Thiazides work in the distal tubule, where only 5%-10% of filtered sodium is reabsorbed. Therefore loop diuretics cause a greater loss of both sodium and water than the thiazides. Because the loss is proportional, thiazides cause a relatively lesser amount of water to be excreted than sodium. This relative retention of water can cause ECF concentration of sodium to be lower, resulting in hyponatremia.

15. **A healthy, 32-year-old patient with Ludwig's angina has a low potassium level of 3.1 mEq/L because of decreased oral intake and trismus. How many doses of 10 mEq of KCl should bring the potassium up to 3.5 mEq/L?**

For each single dose of 10 mEq of KCl, potassium should increase by 0.1 mEq/L. Therefore four doses of 10 mEq KCl each over 1 hr should be sufficient to raise the potassium to 3.5 mEq/L.

16. **In the surgical patient, what is the most common volume change?**

The most common volume change is volume deficit, which is due to loss of electrolytes and fluid.

17. **What is the water exchange process like in the normal person?**

The average person has a daily intake of water amounting to about 2500 mL. Most of it (1500 mL) is obtained orally by drinking. The balance of water requirements is extracted from solid foods and endogenous metabolism. Water is excreted from the body mostly through the kidneys as urine (500-1500 mL daily). Other ways that water is excreted are through the gastrointestinal (GI) tract in the form of stools (250 mL) and through the skin and lungs (insensible losses, 600 mL). Insensible losses can be affected by ambient temperature, an increase in the respiratory rate, elevated body temperature, and hypermetabolism. For each degree of increased body temperature, there is an additional 100-150 mL water loss/day.

18. **What approach to the patient is taken to make a diagnosis of fluid and electrolyte disorders?**

A history should be taken to determine if there is an increased dietary sodium intake or use of medications such as angiotensin-converting enzyme (ACE) inhibitors, calcium channel blockers, or mineralocorticoids or neurologic symptoms. Evaluation can be made of recent weight gain or loss. A physical exam should also evaluate whether the patient has jugular venous distention or other circulatory symptoms. Effective circulating volume changes can also be assessed by pulmonary wedge pressure, central venous pressure, and ultrasonography to measure the diameter of the inferior vena cava. Other evaluations should include urinalysis, serum osmolality, and serum electrolytes.

19. What are some of the causes, signs, and symptoms of volume depletion?

GI causes of volume depletion are vomiting, diarrhea, nasogastric suctioning, upper and lower GI bleeding, and drainage from fistulas.

Volume depletion can be due to fluid being lost from skin and lungs because of high fever, sweat, increased respiratory rate, an unhumidified tracheostomy with hyperventilation, and burns.

Renal losses can occur because of diuretic use, adrenal insufficiency, postobstructive diuresis, the recovery phase of acute tubular necrosis, osmotic diuresis, and DI.

Other causes can be third spacing, such as in soft tissue injuries, infections, peritonitis, rhabdomyolysis, pancreatitis, and intestinal obstruction.

Initial signs of mild volume depletion can be tachycardia and orthostatic hypotension. As depletion worsens, patients can become sleepy and/or anorexic, have decreased skin turgor, exhibit xerostomia, and have cool extremities, distant heart sounds, absent peripheral pulses, hypotension, and diminished urine output.

20. When does volume excess occur? What are some causes, and how is it treated?

Volume excess can occur when water and sodium intake and retention are greater then renal and extrarenal losses. Some causes of volume expansion are acute renal failure, nephrotic syndrome, Cushing's syndrome, primary hyperaldosteronism, cirrhosis of the liver, and congestive heart failure (CHF) with pulmonary edema. Limitation of sodium intake along with the use of diuretics is the usual treatment for this condition.

21. What is the most common electrolyte disorder in hospitalized patients? What are general considerations?

Hyponatremia is the most common electrolyte disorder in hospitalized patients. It is defined as having a serum sodium concentration <130 mEq/L. It is usually caused by a water imbalance because of increased water intake or a decrease in excretion by the kidney. The most common type is a hypoosmolar form in which the serum osmolarity is reduced to <280 mOsm/kg. Two other types must be ruled out. One is an isotonic form, in which the serum osmolality is normal (280-295 mOsm/kg) and is caused by hyperproteinemia, hyperlipemia, and posttransurethral resection (TUR) prostatectomy. The other is a hyperosmolar form with a serum osmolality >295 mOsm/kg caused by hyperglycemia, mannitol, and radiocontrast agents.

22. What is hypoosmolar hyponatremia?

Hypoosmolar hyponatremia can occur with normal TBW (euvolemic hyponatremia), excess TBW (hypervolemic hyponatremia), and low TBW (hypovolemic hyponatremia). The most common cause of hyponatremia with euvolemia is SIADH. Other causes of this can be drugs (nonsteroidal antiinflammatory drugs, Diabinese, Tegretol, cytotoxin), diuretics, pulmonary infection, meningitis, and oat cell carcinoma. Hypervolemic hyponatremia is a depletion of the effective circulating volume with no restriction of water intake (CHF, hepatic cirrhosis, nephrotic syndrome). Hypovolemic hyponatremia can be nonrenal in origin (vomiting, diarrhea, sweating) when the urine sodium concentration is < 10 mEq/L, or renal (diuretics, a salt-losing renal disease or adrenal insufficiency) when the urine sodium concentration is > 20 mEq/L. Rapid correction can lead to irreversible central nervous system (CNS) damage.

23. When can D$_5$W be used, and why?

One liter of D$_5$W contains 1 L of free water and 50 g of glucose. Because it contains no sodium, it is used in patients with hypernatremia. Free water will distribute evenly between the ICFV and the ECFV, and the glucose will move into the cell. Pure water is not given because it can cause hemolysis. It is not used in diabetics because it can cause hyperglycemia, so in nondiabetics it is used to give medications. It should not be used in patients with depletion of ECFV because it is a hypotonic solution and its use could cause hyponatremia. It can be used in patients with ECFV overload as a KVO (keep vein open) solution.

24. What is edema?

Edema is a condition of volume excess that occurs in the interstitial or extracellular space and is not evident until 3-4 L of fluid have accumulated.

25. What is hypernatremia?

Hypernatremia is the result of water loss being greater than sodium loss. It rarely occurs if there is an intact thirst mechanism. Mostly the cause is iatrogenic and is seen often in institutionalized patients who have no access to water. It can also be seen in patients on total parenteral nutrition with uncontrolled hyperglycemia and in patients with water loss from DI, osmotic diuretics, burns, and high-output renal failure. Some signs of hypernatremia are dehydration, fever, oliguria, delirium, and coma.

26. What are the causes, signs, and symptoms of hyperkalemia?

Renal failure with oliguria is the most common cause of true hyperkalemia. Potassium can be released because of massive cell death from crush injuries, arterial emboli, and hemolysis. Hyperkalemia can be released from the ICF to the ECF with acidosis. Drugs used for CHF and renal insufficiency, such as ACE inhibitors and angiotensin receptor blockers, can also cause hyperkalemia. Hypernatremia can result from excessive potassium intake and can be seen in HIV-infected patients on pentamidine or Bactrim and in organ transplant patients on immuno-suppressive drugs such as tacrolimus or cyclosporine. Some signs and symptoms include nausea, vomiting, diarrhea, and ventricular fibrillation leading to cardiac arrest. Calcium chloride is given to stabilize the cardiac membrane, and insulin and/or bicarbonate is given to shift potassium into the cell. It can also be treated by withholding potassium administration of diuretics and cation exchange resins (polystyrene sulfonate—Kayexalate) by mouth or enema. In cases of severe renal impairment and massive cell death, potassium may have to be removed by hemodialysis or peritoneal dialysis.

27. What are some of the signs and symptoms of hypokalemia?

In cases in which the potassium levels are below 2.5 mEq/L, arrhythmias, tetany, rhab-domyolysis, flaccid paralysis, and hyporeflexia can be seen.

28. What are the electrocardiogram (ECG) changes that can occur with abnormal levels of potassium and calcium?

With hyperkalemia, the most striking feature is peaked T waves. The QRS complex becomes wider because ventricular depolarization takes longer as the P wave flattens and becomes wider or almost disappears, causing the rhythm to look like a sine wave. In moderate cases of hypokalemia, T waves begin to flatten and U waves appear. As the condition worsens, T waves become inverted and U waves become more prominent.

29. What are the causes, signs, and symptoms of hypocalcemia?

Patients with hypocalcemia have an ionized calcium level below 2.0 or serum calcium concentration lower than 9 mg/dL. Some of the most common causes are renal failure and hypoalbuminemia. Other causes are vitamin D deficiency, hypoparathyroidism, pancreatitis, rhabdomyolysis, severe hypomagnesemia, multiple citrated blood transfusions, and drugs (anti-neoplastic agents, antimicrobials, agents used to treat hypercalcemia). Chronic hypocalcemia can be asymptomatic. Clinical manifestations are paresthesias of the lips and extremities due to increased excitability of nerves, tetany, cramps and abdominal pain due to spasm of skeletal muscle, and convulsions.

30. How is the true serum calcium concentration determined in patients with hypo-albuminemia?

The most common cause of hypocalcemia is hypoalbuminemia. For every 1 g/dL decrease in albumin below 4 g/dL, the total serum calcium is corrected by adding 0.8 mg/dL. Thus for a patient with a measured calcium of 8.0 mg/dL and an albumin of 2 g/dL, the corrected calcium is 9.6 mg/dL.

31. What are Chvostek's and Trousseau's signs?

These are seen in hypocalcemia. Chvostek's is twitching of the facial muscles as a result of tapping over the facial nerve in the preauricular area, and Trousseau's sign is carpopedal spasm due occlusion of the brachial artery when a blood pressure cuff is applied above systolic pressure for 3 min.

32. What is the mnemonic for symptoms of hypercalcemia?

- **Stones**—renal calculi
- **Bones**—bone destruction
- **Moans**—confusion, lethargy fatigue, weakness
- **Abdominal groans**—abdominal pain, constipation, polyuria, and polydipsia

33. What are some of the signs that should alert you to a patient having an acid-base disorder?

A patient who has a change in mental status; tachypnea; Kussmaul breathing; cyanosis; respiratory failure; severe fluid loss from vomiting, diarrhea, or shock; and a history of an endocrine disorder, renal problems, or drug ingestion should be suspected of having an acid-base problem.

34. What are the mnemonic MUD PILES and USED CARP for?

MUD PILES is the mnemonic for increased anion gap metabolic acidosis:

M—Methanol	**P**—Paraldehyde
U—Uremia	**I**—Infection
D—Diabetic ketoacidosis	**L**—Lactic acidosis
	E—Ethylene glycol
	S—Salicylates

USED CARP is the mnemonic for normal anion gap metabolic acidosis:

U—Ureterostomy	**C**—Carbonic anhydrase inhibitors
S—Small bowel fistulas	**A**—Adrenal insufficiency
E—Extra chloride	**R**—Renal tubular acidosis
D—Diarrhea	**P**—Pancreatic fistula

35. When is a hypotonic saline solution used?

A hypotonic saline solution such as 0.45% saline is used to expand the ECFV in someone who is volume depleted and to correct hypertonicity in someone who is hyperglycemic or hypernatremic.

36. What is the TBW, the ECFV, the total ECF sodium, and the K^+ in the ECFV in a 70-kg man?

- TBW: $6 \times 70 = 42$ L
- FV is approximately one third of TBW: $42 \div 3 = 14$ L
- Total ECF sodium: 14 L $\times$ 140 mEq/L = 1960 mEq
- Total potassium in ECFV: 14 L $\times$ 4.0 mEq/L = 56 mEq

37. What is respiratory alkalosis?

Respiratory alkalosis occurs when there is a reduction in the arterial P_{CO_2} and an increase in the pH because of hyperventilation. Some causes are hyperventilation syndrome, hypoxia from high altitudes, severe anemia, CNS-mediated disorders, gram-negative septicemia, pulmonary disease, pulmonary embolism, and mechanical overventilation. Some symptoms include anxiety and lightheadedness. Other symptoms include paresthesias such as circumoral numbness and tingling in the extremities. Severe cases can result in tetany. Treatment is directed toward the cause. Rebreathing into a paper bag, in cases in which hyperventilation is caused by anxiety, usually increases the PCO_2 and stops the attack.

38. **Which commonly used parenteral fluid most closely resembles ECF? How does its composition differ from 5% dextrose in half normal saline (D_5-$\frac{1}{2}$ NS) (Table 9-1)?**

Table 9-1 *Commonly Used Parenteral Fluids*

	ELECTROLYTE CONTENT (mEq/L)						
	SODIUM	POTASSIUM	CALCIUM	MAGNESIUM	CHLORIDE	HCO$_3$	OSMOLARITY (IN OSM)
Lactated Ringer's	130	4	3	—	109	28 (as lactate)	273
ECF	142	4	5	3	103	27	280-310
D_5-$\frac{1}{2}$ NS	77	—	—	—	77	—	407

ECF, Extracellular fluid; *OSM*, osmoles.

39. **In which condition is fluid resuscitation preferable with 5% dextrose in water (D_5W) over lactated Ringer's solution?**
    Symptomatic hypernatremia. Otherwise D_5W is rarely indicated because the glucose load may induce osmotic diuresis.

40. **What are the critical levels of hyponatremia, and how can this condition be corrected?**
    Symptoms usually occur during an acute, sudden decrease of sodium levels to <130 mEq/L or during a chronic, gradual decrease to <120 mEq/L. Treat the underlying cause or restrict free water intake first. Treat only acutely hyponatremic and profoundly symptomatic patients, and raise serum sodium levels by 2 mEq/L/hr but no higher than 125 mEq/L, with 3% NaCl.

$$\frac{2 \text{ mEq/L} \times 0.6 \times (\text{body weight in kg}) \times 1000}{513 \text{ mEq/L}} = \text{mL/hr of 3\% NaCl}$$

For example, for a 70-kg patient:

$$\frac{2 \times 0.6 \times 70 \times 1000}{513} \cong 160 \text{ mL/hr of 3\% NaCl}$$

41. **What are the risks of rapid correction of hyponatremia or hypernatremia?**
    Rapid correction of hyponatremia with hypertonic solution may lead to permanent brain damage, seizures, and pontine myelinolysis. Rapid expansion of the ECF compartment can also worsen preexisting conditions, such as CHF. Rapid correction of hypernatremia and a severe decrease in serum osmolarity can cause convulsions, coma, and death.

42. **How is water deficit in hypernatremia calculated and replaced?**
    Slowly replace the lost water after calculating the water deficit.

$$\text{Water deficit} = 0.6 \times (\text{body weight in kg}) \times [(\text{Na}/140) - 1]$$

For example, in a 70-kg patient with a serum sodium of 150 mEq/L:

$$\text{Water deficit} = 0.6 \times 70 \times [(150/140) - 1] = 42 \text{ L of body water} \times (1.07 - 1) = 3 \text{ L}$$

43. What is normal plasma osmolarity, and how is it calculated?
Normal plasma osmolarity is 290-310 mOsm/L. It can be calculated as:

$$\text{Plasma osmolarity} = 2[\text{Na}^+] + (\text{glucose}/18) + (\text{BUN}/2.8)$$

Discrepancies between measured and calculated plasma osmolarity may indicate the presence of other osmotically active substances, such as ketone bodies.

44. How can low serum sodium concentration be an artifact of measurement?
Hyperlipidemia and hyperproteinemia cause exclusion of sodium from a water-free space in the plasma sample. Therefore apparent hyponatremia can be an artifact in the presence of either one of these conditions.

45. What is the significance of anion gap, and how is it calculated?
Anion gap can be calculated quickly from results of the basic metabolic panel (BMP). Concentration of two major cations in ECF (and plasma) approximately equals the concentration of the three major anions:

$$[\text{Na}^+] + [\text{K}^+] = [\text{Cl}^-] + [\text{HCO}_3^-] + [\text{anion gap}]$$

Anion gap normally ranges from 8-12 mmol/L. It becomes significant in the presence of metabolic acidosis, which can be due to an increase in anion gap (anion gap acidosis) or to a drop in bicarbonate with normal anion gap (nonanion gap acidosis). The quick estimate may help differentiate the two.

46. What are the most common causes of anion gap acidosis?
The anion gap will increase in renal failure, lactic acidosis (decreased perfusion or intense exercise), or ketoacidosis (diabetes mellitus or starvation) and after ingestion of ethylene glycol, salicylates, methanol, and paraldehyde.

CLINICAL APPLICATIONS: CASE SCENARIOS

47. The postoperative BMP received for a patient who just underwent lengthy composite resection of intraoral malignant tumor reveals a potassium level of 6.5 mEq/L. What is the sequence of further management of this patient?
First, repeat the study to rule out an artifact. Then, obtain a 12-lead ECG and look for peaked T waves, prolonged PR interval, decreased P wave, or widened QRS complex. If positive for ECG changes, give 10 mL of 10% calcium gluconate intravenously to stabilize myocardial membranes and prevent ventricular fibrillation. Also administer 10-15 U of regular insulin (which drives potassium intracellularly) in 50-100 mL of $D_{50}W$ intravenously and 20-60 g of potassium trapping resin (Kayexalate) in 100-150 g of sorbitol orally or as an enema. If the ECG is normal, stop administration of potassium and repeat the study in several hours.

48. What is the estimated blood volume in a typical patient?
The estimated blood volume is 5.5 L in a 70-kg patient, or approximately 75 mL/kg.

49. A patient presents to the emergency room after ingesting a bottle of aspirin. Lab results reveal a metabolic acidosis with an increased anion gap. However, the expected decrease in PCO_2 is lower than expected. What mixed disorder is present?

The expected compensation in PCO_2 in metabolic acidosis is determined by $1.5 \times HCO_3^- + 8$ (+2). If there is a significant difference between the expected and measured compensation in either direction, this indicates a coexisting respiratory disorder. If the PCO_2 is higher than expected, there is a coexisting respiratory acidosis, as in this case. If the PCO_2 is lower than expected, there is a coexisting respiratory alkalosis.

50. What is a desirable parenteral fluid level in a sickle cell crisis patient who weighs 150 lb?

$\frac{1}{2}$ NS will create an osmotic gradient to distribute water intracellularly. This is thought to cause cellular swelling and reduce sickling of red blood cells.

$$kg = lb - 10/2 \qquad 150 - 10/2 = kg \qquad 70 \text{ kg}$$

"4, 2, 1 method": 40 mL first 10 kg/hr + 20 mL second 10 kg/hr + 10 mL for each additional 10 kg/hr. Therefore the 70-kg patient will receive 110 mL/hr of $\frac{1}{2}$ NS.

51. What is the maintenance fluid requirement of a healthy 72-kg adult who is restricted from oral intake (NPO) while awaiting surgery?

Maintenance fluid should be replaced with lactated Ringer's solution or D_5-$\frac{1}{2}$ NS with 20 mEq KCl/L in the following amount:

40 mL/hr for the first 10 kg of body weight + 20 mL/hr for second 10 kg + 10 mL/hr for each additional 10 kg

Therefore for a 72-kg patient, the fluid requirement is:

40 mL/hr + 20 mL/hr + 52 mL/hr = 112 mL/hr (for practical purposes, 115 mL/hr)

52. How will the same situation be managed in a patient with end-stage renal disease?

Intravenous (IV) fluids will be restricted to minimal level, usually 30 mL/hr of D_5-$\frac{1}{2}$ NS regardless of weight. Potassium usually will be avoided.

53. What is the drug therapy for an unconscious patient who develops DI after extensive panfacial and cranial fractures? How does therapy differ for a patient who is conscious and alert?

Unconscious patients may receive 5 U of the ADH analogue desmopressin (1-deamino-8-D-arginine vasopressin; DDAVP) subcutaneously every 4 hr along with slow replacement of free water. Patients who are alert and have sufficient oral intake of water may receive 2-4 μg of intranasal DDAVP twice a day.

54. How is the true serum calcium level calculated in a patient with a lab calcium concentration of 7.5 mg/dL and an albumin level of 2.0 g/dL? What other lab value might be helpful?

Most serum calcium is bound to albumin, and therefore hypoalbuminemia will give a false reading of hypocalcemia. The minimal normal albumin level is 3.5 g/L, and the corrected calcium level is calculated as:

(3.5 g/dL – albumin level) × 0.8 + calcium level (mg/dL)
(3.5 – 2.0) × 0.8 + 7.5 = 8.7 mg/dL of corrected calcium level

The measurement of ionized calcium (iCa) in serum will give a true level of available calcium in serum.

55. An 11-month-old infant who underwent palatoplasty had minimal blood loss but is refusing any type of feeding and will be temporarily started on parenteral fluids. She weighs 22 lb. What is her TBW? What is her minimal acceptable urine output? What maintenance parenteral fluids should be prescribed?

TBW in infants represents 75%-80% of the kilogram body mass (in comparison to 50%-60% in adults). Adequate urinary output in children younger than age 1 is 2.0 mL/kg/hr (in comparison to 0.5-1.0 mL/kg/hr in adults).

Maintenance IV fluids would be D_5-$\frac{1}{4}$ NS + 20 mEq KCl/L in the amount of 40 mL/hr. The amount of fluids is calculated the same way as in adults. The sodium and potassium intake requirements for infants are 3 mEq/kg/day and 2 mEq/kg/day, respectively.

56. A young, healthy woman who was hospitalized and treated for Ludwig's angina is unable to have any oral intake and is currently running a fever of 39.4° C. She weighs 60 kg, and her electrolytes are within normal limits. How should her parenteral fluids be managed?

Two to 2.5 mL/kg/day per each degree above 37.0° C are added to the appropriate maintenance fluid requirement to compensate for insensible losses due to fever. This patient's baseline would be 100 mL/hr of lactated Ringer's solution, and 12 mL/hr would be added according to the formula:

$$\frac{2 \times 6 \ (kg)}{24 \ hr} \times 2.4 \ (^\circ C) = 12 \ mL/hr$$

57. A 65-year-old man sustained severe facial trauma and underwent reconstructive surgery that lasted 12 hr. His medical history reveals chronic renal disease, and his preoperative chest radiograph is suggestive of left ventricular hypertrophy (LVH). The patient is managed on parenteral fluids in the intensive care unit. On the third postoperative day, his SaO_2 is difficult to maintain above 90% on 35% oxygen (O_2) administered by endotracheal tube. What is the possible cause? What diagnostic and therapeutic measures can you take?

This patient is manifesting symptoms of pulmonary edema, possibly due to fluid overload. It can be escalated by mobilization of fluid from the third space, which frequently starts on the third postoperative day. Therefore lung auscultation, chest radiograph, and BMP with electrolyte level would be appropriate. Fluid restriction and possible administration of a loop diuretic (e.g., 10 mg of furosemide intravenously) would be the first line of action. Some patients with severely compromised cardiac function may require placement of a Swan-Ganz catheter to monitor ECF and central venous pressure.

58. A patient has hyposmolar, hypervolemic hyponatremia 24 hr after surgery. What is the initial treatment?

Restrict oral fluid intake (usually to about 1000 mL/24 hr). This patient most likely has been overhydrated with hypotonic IV fluid. If the sodium level is not in the range that needs emergent correction, the patient will mobilize the fluid, and the sodium level will be corrected slowly on its own.

59. A trauma patient who has undergone repair of maxillofacial fractures develops oliguria with a serum osmolarity of 1000 mOsm/dL. What is the most likely diagnosis?

SIADH, probably due to trauma.

60. **A patient who has been on IV antibiotics for 7 days develops diarrhea. The patient is hemodynamically stable. What is the most appropriate fluid to administer initially?**

This patient is suffering from insult to normal intestinal function. Thus the patient is losing sodium, potassium, and, to a lesser extent, other ions (e.g., calcium, magnesium). Lactated Ringer's solution is the best fluid for this situation because it contains sodium, potassium, calcium, lactic acid, and sodium bicarbonate, which resemble the fluid lost from the small intestine.

61. **A patient with a history of CHF is on loop diuretics and digoxin. He is admitted for maxillofacial surgery. Perioperatively, what is the most important electrolyte to check and adjust?**

Potassium. Loop diuretics (e.g., furosemide) are potassium-wasting drugs. Digoxin is an inotrope, which blocks Na/K channels. The serum potassium level of patients who take digoxin and loop diuretics should be safely above 4.0 mEq/L to prevent arrhythmia. This patient has the potential to develop hypokalemia because of the loop diuretic. Thus paying close attention to the serum potassium level is critical for prevention of cardiac dysfunction.

62. **A patient manifests signs and symptoms of muscle twitching and prolonged QT on ECG. What electrolyte should be checked?**

Calcium. Hypocalcemia increases excitation of the neuromuscular system, causing cramps and tetany. Chvostek's sign and Trousseau's sign (carpopedal spasm following occlusion of arterial blood supply to the arm for 3 min) are clinically important indications of hypocalcemia. Prolonged QT may lead to arrhythmias and subsequent heart failure if not treated.

63. **A trauma patient develops polyuria with low osmolarity on day 1 of hospital admission. What is the most likely diagnosis, and what is the initial management?**

DI is the most likely diagnosis. The initial management would be IV $\frac{1}{2}$ NS and DDAVP. In DI, ADH is not adequately released from the posterior pituitary. In this patient, trauma to the stalk in the pituitary gland is probably the cause. Therefore the patient is losing free water. The patient requires IV fluid to keep him hemodynamically stable and prevent hyperosmolar hypovolemic hypernatremia. This is best accomplished with a hypotonic solution, such as $\frac{1}{2}$ or $\frac{1}{4}$ NS. The patient also needs exogenous replacement of ADH. Thus DDAVP needs to be administered intravenously to prevent free water loss.

64. **After a motor vehicle accident, a patient is on a ventilator, receives appropriate fluid, has a Foley catheter, and has no oral intake. What is the source of his insensible fluid loss?**

Perspiration. Sensible losses are through the kidneys and feces. Insensible losses are through the skin and lungs. When a patient is on a closed-system ventilator, there is really no insensible loss through the lungs. Thus the only insensible loss that needs to be replaced is the evaporated sweat.

65. **A patient who has a past medical history significant for chronic renal failure is put on a regular diet. The next day, the patient develops flaccid muscles and decreased urine output. His magnesium is normal. Which electrolyte is the most likely cause?**

Potassium. Hyperkalemia is characterized by flaccid muscle, fatigue, and ECG abnormalities in severe cases. Considering the patient's history, he might have hypermagnesemia or hyperkalemia, but the magnesium is reported as normal. Therefore the potassium level must be checked and treated accordingly.

66. **A patient with a history of insulin-dependent diabetes mellitus and buccal space infection has a fever of 38° C and is responding to treatment very slowly. She**

progresses into diabetic ketoacidosis. Her potassium is 6.2 in a nonhemolyzed serum, and her glucose is 400 mg/dL. How should her potassium be corrected?

IV insulin in D_5-$\frac{1}{2}$ NS. True severe hyperkalemia is a serious condition that needs to be treated urgently. Initial treatment is administration of insulin with glucose to force the potassium ions into intracellular compartments. This could be followed by administration of calcium gluconate to protect myocardium against hyperpolarization, IV administration of appropriate sodium bicarbonate, and an oral chelating agent (EDTA). In life-threatening situations, or if the patient is refractory to the above treatment, plasmapheresis is the treatment of choice.

67. **Twenty-four hours after an elderly patient underwent oral maxillofacial surgery, she develops tonic-clonic seizures. Her lab results indicate that her serum sodium is 119 mEq/L and her serum osmolarity is 250 Osm. The patient is euvolemic with stable vital signs. What is the appropriate fluid management of the patient?**

Fluid restriction and very slow replacement with hypertonic saline solution (usually 3% NaCl). Many conditions can cause hypotonic, euvolemic hyponatremia. This patient is symptomatic (seizure), which should be treated first (e.g., with Valium). Sodium must be replaced very slowly to prevent CNS damage.

BIBLIOGRAPHY

1. Ahya SN: Washington Manual of Medical Therapeutics, 30th ed. Philadelphia, 2001, Lippincott.
2. Andreoli TE: Cecil Essentials of Medicine, 6th ed. Philadelphia, 2004, Saunders.
3. Arieff AL, Ayus JC: Treatment of symptomatic hyponatremia: neither haste nor waste [editorial]. Crit Care Med 19:748-751, 1991.
4. Awde NE, Davison JK, Bailin MT et al: Clinical Anesthesia Procedures of the Massachusetts General Hospital, 6th ed. Philadelphia, 2002, Lippincott Williams & Wilkins.
5. Cline DM: Just the Facts in Emergency Medicine. New York, 2001, McGraw-Hill.
6. Condon RE: Manual of Surgical Therapeutics. Boston, 1996, Little, Brown and Company.
7. Dorland's Illustrated Medical Dictionary, 30th ed. Philadelphia, 2003, Saunders.
8. Dubin D: Rapid Interpretation of EKGs. Tampa, Fla, 2000, COVER Publishing.
9. Lyerly HK, Gaynor JW (eds): Handbook of Surgical Intensive Care: Practices of the Surgical Residents of the Duke University Medical Center, 3rd ed. St Louis, 1992, Mosby.
10. Narins EG (ed): Maxwell and Kleemnan's Clinical Disorders of Fluid and Electrolyte Metabolism, 5th ed. New York, 1994, McGraw-Hill.
11. Oh MS, Carroll HJ: Disorders of sodium metabolism: hypernatremia and hyponatremia. Crit Care Med 20:94-103, 1992.
12. Preston RA: Acid-Base, Fluids and Electrolytes Made Ridiculously Simple. Miami, 2002, MedMaster.
13. Roberts JP, Roberts JD, Skinner C et al: Extracellular fluid deficiency following operation and its correction with Ringer's lactate: a reassessment. Ann Surg 202:1-8, 1985.
14. Schwartz S: Principles of Surgery, 7th ed. New York, 1999, McGraw-Hill.
15. Shires GT, Canizaro PC, Shires GT III et al: Fluid, electrolyte, and nutritional management of the surgical patient. In Schwartz SI (ed): Principles of Surgery, 5th ed. New York, 1989, McGraw-Hill.
16. Tierney LM, Jr, McPhee SJ, Papadakis MA: Lange Current Medical Diagnosis and Treatment, 44th ed. New York, 2005 McGraw-Hill.
17. Whang R, Ryder KW: Frequency of hypomagnesemia and hypermagnesemia: requested vs. routine. JAMA 263:3063-3064, 1990.
18. Wrenn KD, Slovis CM, Slovis BS: The ability of physicians to predict hyperkalemia from the ECG. Ann Emerg Med 20:1229-1232, 1991.

10. NUTRITIONAL SUPPORT

Hani F. Braidy, DMD, and Vincent B. Ziccardi, DDS, MD

1. When is enteral feeding/nutrition indicated?
- Inability to ingest food normally because of maxillofacial trauma
- Protein-energy malnutrition
- Normal functioning bowel

2. What are the indications for nutritional support?
- Inadequate intake for more than 5 days
- Malnourished patients undergoing surgery
- Major trauma (burn victims, blunt or penetrating injury, etc.)

3. What are the causes of malnutrition?
- Neglect (e.g., severe alcoholics, extreme of ages)
- Inadequate food intake
- Dysphagia
- Vomiting
- Digestive problems
- Chronic illness
- Stress and trauma

4. What is the definition of malnutrition according to the World Health Organization (WHO)?
According to the WHO, malnutrition is "the cellular imbalance between supply of nutrients and energy and the body's demand for them to ensure growth, maintenance, and specific functions."

5. What are the two forms of protein-energy malnutrition?
Marasmus and kwashiorkor.

6. What is marasmus?
Marasmus is a form of protein malnutrition in the presence of inadequate total calorie intake. It is endemic in third world countries and characterized by decreased weight, decreased body fat, loss of muscle mass, hypothermia, apathy, and dehydration.

7. What is kwashiorkor?
Kwashiorkor is a form of protein malnutrition in the presence of near-normal total calorie intake. It is endemic in third world countries and characterized by hypoalbuminemia, edema, muscle wasting, immunosuppression, fatty liver, and distension of the abdomen. Patients with marasmus undergoing major surgery or stress may suffer subsequently from kwashiorkor.

8. If a patient is at risk for aspiration, which short-term feeding route is indicated?
If a patient is at risk for aspiration, the nasoduodenal and nasojejunal (postpyloric) routes are best. The technique of nasoduodenal feeding can overcome problems of gastric retention. There are fewer problems with gastroesophageal reflux and subsequent risk of tracheobronchial aspiration. The technique of nasojejunal feeding bypasses an obstructive lesion or motor abnormalities involving the gastrointestinal (GI) tract proximal to the jejunum.

9.   What route of administration is indicated for long-term enteral feedings?

For long-term enteral feeding, enterostomies are the preferred access route. Percutaneous endoscopic gastrostomy (PEG) involves placement of a 16- to 18-gauge latex or silicone catheter through the abdominal wall and directly into the stomach.

10. Which feeding route is preferred when a patient is at risk for aspiration?

If a patient is at risk for aspiration, the feeding tube should be placed in the small intestine either surgically via a jejunostomy or nonsurgically via a percutaneous jejunostomy tube.

11. Where does a nasogastric tube (NGT) extend, and what are some advantages to its use?

The NGT extends from the nose into the stomach. NGTs are advantageous because:
- The NGT tolerates high osmotic loads without cramping, distention, vomiting, diarrhea, or fluid and electrolyte shifts.
- It allows intermittent or bolus feedings because the stomach has a large reservoir capacity.
- It is easier to position a tube into the stomach than into the jejunum.
- The presence of hydrochloric acid in the stomach may help prevent infection.

12. Where does a nasoduodenal tube (NDT) extend, and when is it indicated?

The NDT extends from the nose through the pylorus and into the duodenum. NDT feedings are indicated in:
- Patients at risk for aspiration
- Patients who are debilitated, demented, stuporous, or unconscious
- Patients with gastroparesis or delayed gastric emptying

13. What is meant by continuous feeding, and what are its advantages and disadvantages?

Continuous feeding allows a patient to receive a constant infusion of enteral feedings. The advantages of continuous feeding are decreased risk of aspiration, bloating, distention, and osmotic diarrhea with improved patient tolerance. The disadvantages of continuous feeding are that it requires the patient to be physically connected to the apparatus during infusion and the expense associated with the purchase of volumetric infusion pumps.

14. What three macronutrients are required when infusing total parenteral nutrition (TPN)?

1. Glucose
2. Protein
3. Lipids

15. What parameters should be monitored in patients receiving TPN?

- Metabolic parameters: sodium, potassium, chloride, CO_2, blood urea nitrogen (BUN), creatinine, glucose, hematocrit, hemoglobin, white blood cell (WBC) count, calcium, magnesium, phosphorus, and platelets
- Nutrition: daily weight evaluations, albumin, and prealbumin
- Fluid status
- Infection: If WBC count is increasing or the patient is febrile, a blood culture should be obtained and consideration given to changing the central line.

16. What are some of the physical findings clinically seen in malnutrition?

- Temporal wasting, decreased skin fold (pinch test)
- Glossitis, cheilosis, decreased taste
- Hair loss, dry skin, edema
- Confusion, gait abnormalities, loss of tactile sense, peripheral neuropathies

17. What are the lab values typically assessed when evaluating a patient for malnutrition?
- Albumin (20 days half-life, 3.5-5.0 g/dL)
- Transferrin (7-10 days half-life, 200-400 mg/dL)
- Prealbumin (2 days half-life, 16.0-35.0 mg/dL)
- Vitamin and mineral levels

18. What is the Harris-Benedict equation?
This equation is an estimation of the daily calorie requirement at rest (expenditure) in relation to a patient's weight, height, and age. It usually overestimates by 20%-60%.

$$\text{Males: } 66.5 + 13.8 \times weight + 5 \times height - 6.8 \times age$$
$$\text{Females: } 655.1 + 9.5 \times weight + 1.8 \times height - 4.7 \times age$$

This estimation can be adjusted to various level of stress. For instance, in a patient who sustained severe trauma, this equation can be multiplied by 1.6.

19. Other than the Harris-Benedict equation, what other method can be used to estimate the daily total calorie requirement?
30 cal/kg is a gross estimation of the total daily calorie requirement in a nonstressed patient.

20. How many calories are provided by different organic fuels (glucose, protein, fat)?

Glucose	3.7 cal/g
Protein	4.0 cal/g
Fat	9.1 cal/g

21. How much carbohydrates, fat, and protein are required in the diet of the surgical patient?
The bulk of the energy requirement should be provided by carbohydrates (70%) and lipids (30%). Proteins are calculated in relation to a patient's catabolic state. Normally, 0.8-1.0 g/kg is necessary, whereas 1.2 g-1.6 g/kg are required in the stressed patient.

22. What is enteral nutrition?
Enteral nutrition is a technique to provide nutrition to a patient through the gut using a tube placed in the GI tract. An orogastric tube (OGT) or NGT can be used to deliver special liquid formulas. These formulations are especially useful in patients who have undergone oral and maxillofacial surgical procedures and in malnourished patients. Long-term enteral feedings are best achieved through a percutaneous gastrostomy tube inserted endoscopically (PEG).

23. What are the contraindications for enteral nutrition?
Enteral nutrition is possible only if the gut is functioning. In patients with intestinal ischemia, ileus, or bowel obstruction, enteral nutrition is contraindicated, as well as in patients in shock and those with severe pancreatitis.

24. What are some of the problems associated with enteral nutrition?
Insertion of the tube into the trachea is possible and potentially fatal due to aspiration pneumonia. Sometimes, tube occlusion can occur. Pulmonary aspiration (80% occurrence), nausea, and vomiting can ensue if the infusion rate is too high. Diarrhea is a common side effect. When the carbohydrate intake is too high, a hyperosmolar state or diabetes can complicate the feedings. Most of the issues associated with enteral nutrition can be rectified by changing the rate or the osmotic content of the enteral solution.

25. What are the main components of enteral feeding formulas?

Protein	Usually 35-40 g/L
Calories	Between 1-2 cal/mL
Osmolality	Usually between 280-1100 mOsm/L, a value that is directly related to the amount of carbohydrates

26. What is parenteral nutrition?

Parenteral nutrition is a way to feed the patient intravenously. It can be delivered centrally through a central venous catheter, most commonly in the superior vena cava or peripherally (PPN) via a peripheral vein.

27. What is total parenteral nutrition (TPN)?

TPN is the delivery of all the required nutrients parenterally. It is a solution containing proteins, carbohydrates, fat, vitamins, and minerals. Because of the high osmolarity of the solution and the risk of phlebitis, it is usually given centrally rather than peripherally. Consequently, solutions delivered peripherally need to be diluted and may not meet the complete nutritional requirements of the patients.

28. When are TPN and PPN indicated?

TPN is indicated when patients need long-term nutritional support but are not able to receive enteral feedings (nonworking GI tract, shock, pancreatitis, bone marrow transplant, etc.). PPN is indicated in patients requiring short-term nutritional support (<10 days) to restrict protein breakdown.

29. What are the complications of parenteral nutrition?

Hyperglycemia, fatty liver, hypercapnia, acute respiratory distress syndrome, GI mucosal atrophy (predisposing the gut for bacterial translocation and septicemia). Catheter-related complications include infections and pneumothorax.

BIBLIOGRAPHY

1. Kasper DL, Braunwald E, Fauci A et al.: Harrison's Principles of Internal Medicine, 16th ed. New York, 2004, McGraw-Hill.
2. Marino PL: The ICU Book, 2nd ed. Philadelphia, 1998, Lippincott Williams & Wilkins.
3. Rolandelli RH, Bankhead R, Boullata J et al: Clinical Nutrition: Enteral and Tube Feeding, 4th ed. Philadelphia, 2005, Saunders.
4. Souba WW: Nutritional support. N Engl J Med 336:41-48, 1997.

11. POSTOPERATIVE COMPLICATIONS

*Robert E. Doriot, DDS, James A. Giglio, DDS, MEd,
and A. Omar Abubaker, DMD, PhD*

1. What are the most common causes of fever in the first 24 hr after surgery?
• Aspiration pneumonia
• An ill-defined response to the surgery itself

2. What are the most common causes of postoperative fever in the first 24-72 hr?
• Bacterial pneumonia   • Thrombophlebitis

3. What are the most common causes of fever 72 hr after surgery?
- Pneumonia
- Pulmonary emboli
- Intravenous (IV) catheter infection
- Wound infection
- Urinary tract infection

4. What are the "five Ws" of postoperative fever?
The five Ws are the possible causes of any postoperative fever: *w*ind, *w*ater, *w*ound, *w*alking, and *w*onder drugs.

5. When can the surgical site be considered the source of postoperative fever?
Typically, the surgical site should not be considered the primary source of postoperative fever until at least 48-72 hr after surgery. However, surgical wound infection occurs between 12 hr–7 days postoperatively.

6. How often should IV catheter sites be changed to avoid infection?
In general, IV access sites should be changed every 72 hr.

7. What are the common signs and symptoms of phlebitis?
- Pain
- Tenderness
- Edema
- Erythema
- Streaking of the limb

8. What is the treatment for phlebitis?
- Remove the IV catheter.
- Elevate the affected limb.
- Apply warm, moist packs to the infected site.
- Initiate IV antibiotics (preferably cefazolin [Ancef], 1 g IV bolus push every 8 hr), for appropriate staphylococcus coverage.

9. What are the most frequent respiratory complications following oral and maxillofacial surgery?
- Pulmonary atelectasis
- Aspiration pneumonia
- Pulmonary embolus

10. Which group of patients is predisposed to the development of postoperative atelectasis?
Postoperative atelectasis occurs more often in smokers than in any other subset of patients.

11. Where is the most common site for aspiration pneumonia to develop?
If aspiration pneumonia occurs, it is most likely to manifest itself initially in the patient's right lung.

12. Where do most postoperative pulmonary emboli originate?
In the deep venous systems of the lower extremities, especially in nonambulatory patients.

13. What is Virchow's triad?
Virchow's triad is the name given to the three chief causes of deep venous thrombosis (DVT): (1) damage to the endothelial lining of the vessel, (2) venous stasis, and (3) a change in blood constituents attributable to postoperative increase in the number and adhesiveness of the patient's platelets.

14. What are the classical clinical features of DVT?
- Calf swelling and tenderness
- Fever
- Chest pain
- Sudden dyspnea
- Tachypnea

15. What is Homans' sign?

Homans' sign is pain in the calf that is elicited by forced dorsiflexion of the foot. It was once considered pathognomonic for the presence of DVT, but this test is no longer taught because performing this maneuver can increase the risk of movement of an existing thrombus.

16. What is the immediate treatment of DVT?

A patient who has developed DVT should be started immediately on systemic anticoagulation with elevation of the affected limb. Subcutaneous heparin and low-molecular-weight heparin are choices to consider.

17. How are the development of fever and the patient's heart rate interrelated?

For every 1° C rise in body temperature, there is a corresponding 9-10 beats/min increase in the patient's heart rate.

18. What are some common causes of postoperative bleeding?
- Incompletely ligated or cauterized vessels
- Wound infection
- Coagulopathy
- Rebound effect of hypotensive anesthesia

19. What are some common causes of postoperative hypotension?

A good differential diagnosis for the development of hypotension should include intravascular hypovolemia, rewarming vasodilation, myocardial depression, and hypothyroidism.

20. What are the most common causes of postoperative hypertension?
- Pain and anxiety
- Overdistention of the bladder
- Hypoxia
- Hypercapnia

21. What are some possible treatment options for postoperative hypotension?
- Elevation of the lower extremities
- Administration of carefully monitored fluid boluses
- Administration of vasopressors (e.g., ephedrine)

22. What is the most common cardiac arrhythmia observed in the postoperative period? Why?

The most common postoperative arrhythmia is the development of ventricular complexes or premature ventricular contractions (PVCs). Hypoxia, pain, or fluid overload, all of which are common in the postoperative period, can precipitate PVCs.

23. What is the most common cause of dysuria in the immediate postoperative period?

The agents incorporated in the administration of general anesthesia can inhibit the micturitic reflex, and the patient can suffer bladder distention, which itself may inhibit the ability to micturate.

24. What are some other causes of dysuria in the postoperative period?
- Positional inhibition (many patients find it difficult to pass urine while supine)
- Preexisting prostatism
- Inadequate fluid replacement during surgery, which creates a hypovolemic state

25. What are the treatment options for postoperative dysuria in a patient with suprapubic pain and an obviously distended bladder elicited by palpation in the first 4-6 hr after surgery?

Treatment of postoperative dysuria should begin simply by having the patient stand by or sit on the toilet while running water in the sink. If this does not help and there is no evidence of a hypovolemic state, then the patient should be catheterized. If the residual measures >300 mL, then the catheter should be left in overnight.

26. What are some common causes of postoperative nausea and vomiting?

Hypoxia, hypotension, and narcotics.

27. What types of patients are more likely to develop postoperative nausea and vomiting?

Postoperative nausea and vomiting occurs more frequently in children than in adults and more commonly in women than in men.

28. What is a seroma, and how can it be prevented?

A seroma is fluid (other than pus or blood) that has collected in the wound. Seromas often appear after surgical procedures that involve elevation of skin flaps and transection of numerous lymphatic channels. The incidence of seromas can be decreased if proper pressure dressing is applied to the wound after surgery.

29. What is the treatment for seroma?

Seromas should be evacuated either by needle aspiration or by incision and drainage because they can delay healing and provide an excellent medium for bacterial growth. A pressure dressing should be placed immediately after drainage to help seal lymphatic leaks and prevent additional accumulation of fluids.

30. How can aspiration be prevented?

Aspiration can be prevented by avoiding general anesthesia in patients who have recently eaten, positioning the patient correctly before endotracheal intubation, and using high-volume, low-pressure cuffs on the endotracheal tube. If the risk of aspiration is high, metoclopramide should be administered before surgery to minimize the incidence of aspiration pneumonia.

31. Which surgical patients are predisposed to aspiration?

Tracheostomy patients. Incidence as high as 80% has been reported.

32. Why does postoperative pneumonia develop?

After surgery, a patient's host defense against pneumonia is compromised. This impairment is likely caused by several factors: The cough mechanism may be impaired and may not effectively clear the bronchial tree, the mucociliary transport mechanism may be damaged by endotracheal intubation, and the alveolar macrophage may be compromised by a number of factors that may be present during and after surgery (e.g., hypoxia, pulmonary edema, aspiration, or corticosteroid therapy). All these factors may decrease the patient's immune response to infection with pneumonia and increase the incidence of postoperative pneumonia.

33. What is the primary pathogen in postoperative pneumonia?

Approximately half the pulmonary infections that follow surgery are caused by gram-negative bacilli, which are usually acquired by aspiration of oropharyngeal secretions.

34. What is the treatment for postoperative pneumonia?

Appropriate antibiotic therapy, which can be determined through sputum culture, and sensitivity and clearing of secretions through aggressive suctioning and chest physical therapy.

35. What are the common causes of postoperative cardiac arrhythmias?
Postoperative arrhythmias are generally related to reversible factors such as hypokalemia, hypoxemia, alkalosis, and digitalis toxicity, but they could be the first sign of postoperative myocardial infarction. Postoperative myocardial infarction is rare, with an incidence of 0.7% for patients without preexisting cardiac disease. However, incidence increases to 6% for patients with preexisting cardiac disease.

36. Why is postoperative myocardial infarction difficult to diagnose?
More than one third of postoperative myocardial infarctions are asymptomatic as a result of the residual effects of anesthesia and analgesics administered postoperatively.

37. What is a surgical wound infection?
Surgical wound infections or *surgical site infections* (SSIs) occur within 30 days of surgery unless a foreign body is left in situ. In the case of implanted foreign material, 1 year must elapse before surgery can be excluded as causative.

38. What are the types of surgical wound infection?
Depending on the depth of tissue involvement, SSIs can be subdivided into three categories:
1. **Superficial incisional SSIs,** involving only the skin and subcutaneous tissue
2. **Deep incisional SSIs,** involving deep soft tissue layers, such as fascial or muscle layers of the incision
3. **Organ space SSIs,** involving any anatomic structure opened or manipulated during the operative procedure

39. What are the classic signs of superficial incisional SSI?
Signs of superficial incisional infection are calor (heat), rubor (redness), tumor (swelling), dolor (pain), and purulent drainage.

40. What are the signs of deep-space SSIs?
Deep-space infection should be suspected in the presence of systemic signs and symptoms: fever, ileus, and shock. Definitive diagnosis of deep-space SSIs may require imaging studies.

41. What is a fever?[*]
A fever is a pathologic state reflecting a systemic inflammatory process with a core temperature of >38° C but rarely >40° C.

42. What causes fever?[*]
Macrophages are activated by bacteria and endotoxin. Activated macrophages release interleukin-1, tumor necrosis factor, and interferon, which reset the hypothalamic thermoregulatory center.

43. Can fever be treated?[*]
Yes. Aspirin, acetaminophen, and ibuprofen are cyclooxygenase inhibitors that block the formation of prostaglandin E_2 in the hypothalamus and effectively control fever.

44. Should fever be treated?[*]
This is controversial. No evidence suggests that suppression of fever improves patient outcome. Patients are more comfortable, however, and the surgeon receives fewer calls from the nurses.

---

[*]Reprinted from Harken AH: What does postoperative fever mean? In Harken AH, Moore EE (eds): Abernathy's Surgical Secrets, 5th ed. Philadelphia, 2005, Mosby.

45. Should fever be investigated?*

Yes. Fever indicates that something (frequently treatable) is going on. The threshold for inquiry depends on the patient. A transplant patient with a temperature of 38° C requires scrutiny, whereas a healthy young person with an identical temperature of 38° C 24 hr after an appendectomy can be ignored.

46. What are the components of a fever work-up?*

- Order blood cultures, urine Gram stain and culture, and sputum Gram stain and culture.
- Look at the surgical incisions.
- Look at old and current IV sites for evidence of septic thrombophlebitis.
- If breath sounds are worrisome, obtain a chest x-ray.

47. What are the most common late causes of postoperative fever?*

Septic thrombophlebitis (from an IV line) and occult (usually intraabdominal) abscesses tend to present 2 weeks after surgery.

48. Should atelectasis be treated with incentive spirometry?*

Yes, but not to avoid fever.

49. Are certain wounds prone to infection?*

Each milliliter of human saliva contains 10^8 aerobic and anaerobic, gram-positive and gram-negative bacteria. Therefore, all human bite wounds must be considered contaminated. Animal bite wounds typically are less contaminated.

50. Do incisions become infected early after surgery?*

The incision must be examined in a patient with a fever (39° C) <12 hr after surgery. Look for a foul-smelling, serous discharge in a particularly painful wound (all incisions hurt) with or without crepitus. Gram stain of the serous discharge for gram-positive rods confirms or excludes the diagnosis of clostridial infection.

51. When do urinary tract infections (UTIs) occur?*

The longer the urethral (Foley) catheter is in place, the more likely the infection. Urologic instrumentation at the time of surgery may accelerate the process considerably. Germs crawl up the outside of the urethral catheter, and by 5-7 days after surgery most patients harbor infected urine.

52. How is a UTI diagnosed?*

Urine culture with >10^5 bacteria/mL defines a UTI. White blood cells on urinalysis are highly suspicious.

53. What is the most common cause of fever during the early postoperative period (1-3 days)?*

Many surgical textbooks state that atelectasis is the usual cause of postoperative fever in the first 48 hr, but a number of physicians challenge this theory. It may be assumed that, because pulmonary atelectasis is common postoperatively, it is the cause of fever, but there is no data to support this assumption. In fact, there is evidence that fever occurring in patients with atelectasis indicates concurrent pulmonary infection. Many authors have asked, why does a little atelectasis cause fever, whereas a lot of atelectasis (pneumothorax) does not? The most likely explanation is that sterile atelectasis (and early postoperative lung collapse typically is not infected) has nothing to do with fever (an edited answer).

Experimental studies have been performed in animals in which induced atelectasis did not produce fever unless there was a coexisting pulmonary infection. Recent prospective clinical studies have also weakened the link between atelectasis and postoperative fever. Both showed that there was no significant association between atelectasis and fever.

BIBLIOGRAPHY

1. Barie PS: Modern surgical antibiotic prophylaxis and therapy: less is more. Surg Infect 1:23-29, 2000.
2. Harken AH: What does postoperative fever mean? In Harken AH, Moore EE (eds): Abernathy's Surgical Secrets, 5th ed. Philadelphia, 2005, Mosby.
3. Hollingsworth JW, Govert JA: Fever in the critical care patient. In Jafek BW, Murrow BW (eds): ENT Secrets, 3rd ed. Philadelphia, 2005, Hanley & Belfus.
4. Kluytmans J, Voss A: Prevention of postsurgical infections: some like it hot. Curr Opin Infect Dis 15:427-432, 2002.
5. Leigh JM: Postoperative care. In Rowe NL, Williams IL (eds): Maxillofacial Injuries, vol II. New York, 1985, Churchill Livingstone.
6. Meyer LE: Postoperative problems. In Kwan PH, Laskin DM (eds): Clinical Manual of Oral and Maxillofacial Surgery, 2nd ed. Carol Stream, Ill, 1997, Quintessence.
7. Myles PS, Iacono GA, Hunt JO et al: Risk of respiratory complications and wound infection in patients undergoing ambulatory surgery. Anesthesiology 97:842-847, 2002.
8. Pellegrini CA: Postoperative complications. In Way L (ed): Current Surgical Diagnosis and Treatment, 6th ed. Los Altos, Calif, 1983, Lange.
9. Peterson SL: Surgical wound infection. In Harken AH, Moore EE (eds): Abernathy's Surgical Secrets, 5th ed. Philadelphia, 2005, Mosby.
10. Singer AJ, Quinn JV, Thode HC Jr et al: Trauma Seal Study Group: determinants of poor outcome after laceration and surgical incision repair. Plast Reconstr Surg 110:429-435, 2002.

Part IV
Medical Emergencies

12. BASIC LIFE SUPPORT
Mark A. Oghalai, DDS

1. **What maneuver should the rescuer first use to open the airway in an otherwise uninjured patient?**
    Head tilt with chin lift.

2. **What is the most frequent cause of airway obstruction in an unconscious person?**
    The tongue.

3. **What are the ABCDs of basic life support (BLS)?**
    *A*irway, *b*reathing, *c*irculation, and *d*efibrillation.

4. **A victim whose heart and breathing have stopped has the best chance for survival if emergency medical services (EMS) are activated and cardiopulmonary resuscitation (CPR) is begun within how many minutes?**
    4 min.

5. **At what point should EMS be activated with adult victims?**
    Immediately, when an adult is found to be unresponsive. Most adults in cardiac arrest are in ventricular fibrillation (V-fib); therefore the time from collapse until defibrillation is the single greatest factor in survival. Survival from V-fib decreases by 7%-10% every minute without defibrillation, and by 12 min the survival rate is only 2%-5%. This provides the rationale for immediate EMS activation in adults. This is termed a "phone-first" response.

6. **At what point should EMS be activated with infant and children victims in a one-person rescue?**
    After 1 min or 5 cycles of CPR. In infancy and childhood, most out-of-hospital cardiac arrests are characterized by a progression of hypoxia to respiratory arrest and bradycardia followed by asystole. Because V-fib is uncommon in this age group, immediate CPR is indicated. This is termed a "phone-fast" response. If a child collapses suddenly, the provider should activate the emergency response system first.

7. **What is the length of time recommended to deliver each breath to an adult victim?**
    At least 1 sec/breath. This time reflects a change to the upper range of inspiratory time compared with the 1992 guidelines. The new recommendation is designed to decrease the risk of gastric inflation. It is also important to allow a full exhalation between breaths.

8. **What is the length of time recommended to deliver each breath to an infant or child victim?**
    Time is not as critical with the new guidelines. Now it is most important to deliver breaths that make the victim's chest rise.

9. **What is the best indicator of effective ventilation?**
    Seeing the chest rise when delivering breaths.

10. **What length of time is used when assessing for a pulse?**
    5-10 sec. The brachial pulse is assessed in infants, whereas the carotid pulse should be assessed in children and adults.

11. **When an adult victim has a pulse but is breathless, what is the recommended rate of rescue breathing?**
    Once every 5-6 sec (10-12 breaths/min).

12. **When a child or infant has a pulse but is breathless, what is the recommended rate of rescue breathing?**
    Once every 3 sec (20 breaths/min).

13. **What should be done after each rescue breath?**
    Watch the victim's chest fall as you allow time for the lungs to empty. This will decrease the chance of exceeding the esophageal opening pressure and lead to less regurgitation and aspiration.

14. **In a victim with a pulse, how often should the pulse be checked during rescue breathing?**
    Once every 2 min.

15. **What happens if chest compressions are interrupted?**
    Blood flow and blood pressure will drop to zero.

16. **In a pulseless victim, how often should the pulse be checked during CPR?**
    After the first minute and every few minutes thereafter. The goal is to minimize interruption during compressions.

17. **What are the two primary indicators of effective CPR?**
    - Seeing the chest rise when rescue breathing is delivered
    - Presence of a pulse during chest compressions

18. **What are the three main categories of airway obstructions?**
    - Partial airway obstruction with good air exchange
    - Partial airway obstruction with poor air exchange
    - Complete airway obstruction

19. **In the initial assessment, how is the presence or absence of breathing determined?**
    Look for movement of the chest while listening and feeling for air movement at the nose and mouth (*Look, Listen, Feel*).

20. **Where is the correct location for applying pressure for external chest compressions in adult and children victims?**
    The center of the breast bone, between the nipples. In adults, use both hands, with one stacked on the other to perform the compressions. In children ages 1-8, use the heel of one hand.

21. **Where is the ideal location for applying pressure for external chest compressions in infants?**
    One fingerwidth below the nipple line, with care being taken to stay off the xiphoid process. Use two fingers to perform the compressions.

22. What is the depth of external chest compressions in adults?
1.5-2 inches.

23. What is the depth of external chest compressions in children?
Approximately one third to one half the depth of the child's chest, which should correspond to 1-1.5 inches.

24. What is the depth of external chest compressions in infants?
Approximately one third to one half the depth of the infant's chest, which should correspond to 0.5-1 inch.

25. What is the rate of external chest compressions for adults?
100/min. Studies have shown that optimal forward flow of blood takes place at 100 compressions/min, so the American Heart Association (AHA) changed its recommendation to this rate in adults.

26. What is the rate of external chest compressions for children?
100/min.

27. What is the rate of external chest compressions for infants?
At least 100/min.

28. What is the ratio of external chest compressions to breaths for one or two rescuers with an adult victim?
30 compressions for every two breaths. Evidence has shown that an increase in the number of compressions/min will increase adult survival despite a decrease in the number of ventilations. The increased number of uninterrupted compressions leads to increased coronary perfusion pressures.

29. What is the rate of external chest compressions to breaths for one or two rescuers with a pediatric victim age 1 year old to puberty?
10 compressions for every two breaths for one rescuer CPR, and 15 compressions for every two breaths for two rescuer CPR.

30. What is the rate of external chest compressions to breaths for one or two rescuers with an infant victim?
The same rate for pediatric victims age 1 year to puberty.

31. What is the recommended method of clearing foreign body airway obstructions in infants?
A combination of back slaps and chest thrusts. Five back slaps followed by five chest thrusts, repeated until the object is dislodged. Do not use the Heimlich maneuver because an infant's liver is not well protected by the ribs and is at risk for injury with this technique.

32. What is the recommended method of clearing foreign body airway obstructions in responsive children and adults?
The Heimlich maneuver abdominal thrusts are used in responsive victims.

33. Why should blind finger sweeps not be used in children and infants?
The object may be pushed deeper in the airway.

34. After successful defibrillation, what is done with the patient?
If signs of circulation and breathing return, place patient in recovery position. Leave automated external defibrillator (AED) electrodes on the patient and turned on while monitoring the patient.

35. What are five conditions that require you to change how to use an AED?
1. Victim is younger than age 8 (do not use on a patient who is younger than age 8).
2. Victim is in water (remove to dry area and dry off chest).
3. Victim has implanted pacemaker or defibrillator (place electrodes away from device).
4. Victim has transdermal patch (remove and clean area).
5. Victim has a hairy chest.

36. What are the major initial differences between resuscitation efforts for pediatric patients vs. adult patients?
Two rescuers must open the pediatric victim's airway and give rescue breaths before phoning the emergency response team ("phone fast").

37. Where should you check for a pulse in an infant? In a child?
The brachial pulse in an infant and the carotid pulse in a child.

38. What age ranges delineate infants and children?
An infant is younger than age 1 and a child is age 1 year old to puberty.

39. What are the four universal steps of AED operation?
1. Power on AED.
2. Attach AED to victim's chest.
3. Clear victim and analyze heart rhythm.
4. Clear victim and deliver shock if indicated.

40. What are three major signs of cardiac arrest?
1. No response
2. No adequate breathing
3. No signs of circulation

41. What three actions must occur at the scene of cardiac arrest?
1. Activate emergency response system (set AED).
2. Perform CPR.
3. Use AED.

42. What are exceptions to "phone first"/"phone fast" rules for adults and children?
- Near drowning: Provide 1 min CPR for *all* victims, then phone 911.
- Cardiac arrest with injury: Provide 1 min CPR for *all* victims, then phone 911 (emergency response).
- Drug overdose: Rescue support for *all* victims, then phone 911.
- Children at risk for sudden cardiac arrest: Phone first when a child predisposed to cardiac arrest collapses suddenly.

43. What is the predominant determinant of successful CPR?*
Time to restoration of spontaneous circulation, which itself is a function of the time to effective chest compression and time to defibrillation of V-fib. The chance of a good outcome decreases by 10%/min. Successful outcomes are more likely if CPR is initiated promptly and if preexisting hypothermia is present.

44. How do you establish an airway, even in a patient with suspected neck injury?*
The three basic maneuvers are **head tilt, chin tilt, and jaw thrust.** In an unconscious patient,

*Reprinted from Paradis NA, Harken AH: Cardiopulmonary resuscitation. In Harken AH, Moore EE (eds): Abernathy's Surgical Secrets, 5th ed. Philadelphia, 2005, Mosby.

the jaw muscles relax. The jaw thrust subluxes the mandible, pulling the tongue and epiglottis anteriorly off the upper airway (with minimal cervical hyperextension).

45. Is endotracheal intubation mandatory?*
   No.
- Mouth-to-mouth ventilation delivers 16% inspired oxygen.
- Bag-mask ventilation delivers 21% oxygen.
- Bag-mask ventilation with an oxygen supply can deliver close to 100% oxygen.

46. What are the advantages of endotracheal intubation?*
   A relatively secure airway. Mouth-to-mouth or bag-mask ventilation can deliver significant amounts of air to the stomach. Gastric distention impairs diaphragmatic movement and may predispose to aspiration.

47. Does an endotracheal tube (even with the cuff up) prevent aspiration?*
   No. If you place a couple of drops of methylene blue on the tongue of an intubated patient, you can suction "blue" from the other end of the tube (beyond the cuff) within 90 sec.

48. Which size endotracheal tube should you use?*
   Select a tube with an internal diameter equal to the width of the patient's little finger. The average size of a tube for a 70-kg adult is 7.5-mm. Do not delay ventilation by trying to locate or place an ideal-size endotracheal tube. Adequate ventilation can be achieved through smaller tubes.

49. How do you confirm that the endotracheal tube is in the proper position?*
- Listen to both lung fields.
- Observe symmetric chest excursion with each tidal breath.
- Listen over the epigastrium (you do not want to hear gurgles from the stomach).

   These physical findings are not fully reliable, however. In patients with spontaneous circulation, it is now standard to confirm tube placement with end-tidal CO_2 ($ETCO_2$) measurement. In cardiac arrest, even $ETCO_2$ may be unreliable. You should confirm tube position as soon as possible by chest x-ray.

50. Which is preferred—oral or nasal intubation?*
   Oral intubation. You can watch the tube pass directly through the vocal cords, ensuring proper placement. Nasal intubation is a blind technique, relatively contraindicated in patients with maxillofacial trauma (because of the risk of intracranial placement of the tube through an anterior fossa fracture) and in patients with known or suspected coagulopathy (because nasal mucosa is well vascularized, intubation may cause major epistaxis). Oral endotracheal intubation with "in-line" neck stabilization is preferred, even in patients with suspected neck injury.

51. What is the role of an esophageal obturator airway (EOA)?*
   None. At present, the EOA is not indicated because alternative techniques (mask or endotracheal tube) are safer and more effective.

52. What should be your first consideration if you are unable to ventilate or intubate a patient?*
   Foreign body airway obstruction. Attempt to visualize the foreign body directly, then remove it with either suction or Magill forceps.

53. What are the essentials of external chest compression?*
   Even performed properly, external chest compression produces only a fraction of normal vital organ blood flow. Coronary blood flow occurs only during the release phase. Most providers

do not use adequate force. Make sure that the chest is compressed at least 2 inches in adults. Interruption in chest compression (to check the ECG rhythm or pulse) significantly reduces the efficacy of CPR.

54. What are the complications of external chest compression?*

Complications are common, but not important. Rib and sternal fractures occur 80% of the time. Major cardiac or pericardial injuries (lacerations) are rare. Bone marrow and fat emboli are common (80% in one series). Do not let fear of complications interfere with effective chest compression.

55. What are the indicators that effective CPR is being performed?*

Real-time indicators of vital organ perfusion are lacking. Effective CPR and pressor drugs should cause the V-fib waveform amplitude to increase—so-called coarsening. Improved cerebral perfusion may result in gasping. During CPR, $ETCO_2$ >15 mm Hg predicts return of spontaneous circulation. Switch chest compression providers if the $ETCO_2$ begins to fall because this may indicate fatigue of the rescuer.

BIBLIOGRAPHY

1. Efferon DM: Cardiopulmonary Resuscitation, 4th ed. Tulsa, Okla, 1993, CPR Publishers.
2. Malmed SF: Medical Emergencies in the Dental Office, 5th ed. St Louis, 1999, Mosby.
3. Paradis NA, Halperin HR, Nowak RM (eds): Cardiac Arrest: The Science and Practice of Resuscitation Medicine. Baltimore, 1996, Williams & Wilkins.
4. Paradis NA, Harken AH: Cardiopulmonary resuscitation. In Harken AH, Moore EE (eds): Abernathy's Surgical Secrets, 5th ed. Philadelphia, 2005, Mosby.
5. Paradis NA, Martin GB, Rivers EP et al: Coronary perfusion pressure and the return of spontaneous circulation in human cardiopulmonary resuscitation. JAMA 263:1106-1113, 1990.
6. Sanders AB, Kern KB, Otto CW et al: End-tidal carbon dioxide monitoring during cardiopulmonary resuscitation: a prognostic indicator for survival. JAMA 262:1347-1351, 1989.
7. Strauss RA: Managing medical emergencies. In Kwon P, Laskin D (eds): Clinical Manual of Oral and Maxillofacial Surgery, 2nd ed. Chicago, 1997, Quintessence.

13. ADVANCED CARDIAC LIFE SUPPORT

Bashar M. Rajab, DDS, and Kathy A. Banks, DMD

1. What are the primary and secondary ABCD surveys?

The Primary ABCD Survey:

Airway: Open the airway.
Breathing: Provide positive-pressure ventilation.
Circulation: Give chest compressions; give cycles of **30 compressions** and **two breaths** until the defibrillator arrives.
Defibrillation: Assess for and shock ventricular fibrillation/pulseless ventricular tachycardia (V-fib/pulseless VT). Give one shock and resume cardiopulmonary resuscitation (CPR) immediately for five cycles.

The Secondary ABCD Survey:

Airway: Place advanced airway device as soon as possible.
Breathing: Confirm advanced airway device placement by physical exam and confirmation device, secure the airway device, and confirm effective oxygen and ventilation.

Circulation: Establish an intravenous (IV) access, identify the rhythm, and administer drugs appropriate for the rhythm and condition.

Differential diagnosis: Search for and treat identified reversible causes.

2. How is the diagnosis of cardiac arrest established?

By definition, the patient is in full cardiac arrest if he or she:

- Is not responsive
- Is not breathing
- Has no pulse

3. What are the three mechanisms of cardiac arrest?

1. V-fib/pulseless VT
2. Pulseless electrical activity
3. Asystole

    V-fib is most commonly present during the first minute following the onset of cardiac arrest.

4. Which types of chest pain suggest cardiac ischemia?

- Uncomfortable squeezing pressure, fullness, or pain in the center of the chest lasting longer than 15 min
- Pain that radiates to the shoulder, neck, arm, and jaws
- Pain between the shoulder blades
- Chest discomfort with light-headedness, fainting, sweating, and nausea
- A feeling of distress, anxiety, or impending doom

5. What is the recommended initial management for a stable adult patient with chest pain that is suggestive of ischemia?

1. Call for help.
2. Perform immediate assessment including:
    - Vital signs and SaO_2 monitoring
    - IV access and electrocardiogram (ECG)
    - Targeted history and physical exam
    - Initial serum cardiac marker levels, electrolytes, and coagulation studies
    - Portable chest x-ray
3. Immediate general treatment:
    - Oxygen at 4 L/min
    - Aspirin (160-325 mg)
    - Nitroglycerin (sublingual or spray)
    - Morphine (IV) if pain is not relieved by nitroglycerin
    - Memory aid: "MONA" greets all patients (**M**orphine, **O**xygen, **N**itroglycerin, **A**spirin).

6. What is the initial assessment of a 12-lead ECG in patients with cardiac ischemia?

- ST-segment elevation or new-onset left bundle branch block (LBBB) strongly suggests a myocardial injury. New LBBB is caused by occlusion of the left anterior descending (LAD) branch of the left coronary artery. LAD occlusion causes a loss of large amount of myocardium.
- ST-segment depression or T-wave inversion (ischemia)
- Nondiagnostic or normal ECG

7. What is the relationship between 12-lead EGC findings and coronary artery disease?

ECG relationship:

- Anterior myocardium injury or infarct: leads V3 and V4
- Septal myocardium injury or infarct: leads V1 and V2

- Lateral myocardium injury or infarct: leads I, aVL, V5, and V6
- Inferior myocardium injury or infarct: leads II, III, and aVF
    Coronary artery branches relationship:
- LAD artery occlusion: leads V1 through V6
- Circumflex artery occlusion: leads I, aVL, possibly V5, and V6
- Right coronary artery occlusion: leads II, III, aVF

8. What actions should be taken for patients with acute myocardial injury?
1. Start adjunctive treatments:
    - IV beta blockers
    - IV nitroglycerin
    - IV heparin
    - ACE inhibitors
2. Select a reperfusion therapy: The key to reperfusion therapy is to begin as early as possible (up to or at least 12 hr after onset of symptoms).
    - Angiography
    - Angioplasty with or without stent
    - Cardiothoracic surgery backup
    - Fibrinolytic therapy if no contraindications and patient is younger than age 75
3. Assess clinical status for patients with an onset of symptoms more than 12 hr:
    - Unstable patients: Perform cardiac catheterization and possible revascularization with angioplasty or coronary artery bypass graft (CABG) for unstable patients.
    - Stable patients: Admit to cardiac care unit, start adjunctive treatment, order serial cardiac markers and serial ECG.

9. What actions should be taken for patients with acute myocardial ischemia?
1. Adjunctive treatment:
    - Heparin
    - Aspirin 160-325 mg/day
    - Glycoprotein IIb/IIIa receptor inhibitors
    - Nitroglycerin IV
    - Beta blockers
2. Assess clinical status:
    - Unstable patients: Perform cardiac catheterization and possible revascularization with angioplasty or CABG for unstable patients.
    - Stable patients: Admit to cardiac care unit, start adjunctive treatment, order serial cardiac markers and serial ECG.

10. What is the most common arrhythmia following electrical shock?
The most common arrhythmia caused by electrocution is **V-fib;** hence cardiac arrest is the primary cause of death from electrical shock. Other rhythms that may occur following electrical shock are VT progressing to V-fib and asystole.

Electrical shock is the cause of more than 1000 deaths/year in the United States. It results in injuries ranging from unpleasant sensation to instant cardiac death. Exposure to high-tension current (>1000 V) is more likely to produce serious injury. However, death can result from exposure to relatively low voltage (100 V) household currents. Alternating current (AC) is more dangerous than direct current (DC). AC produces muscle tetany, which may prevent the victim from releasing the electrical source and thus prolong the contact.

11. What is V-fib?
V-fib is a cardiac dysrhythmia that occurs when multiple areas within the ventricles display unsynchronized depolarization and repolarization. As a result, the ventricles do not contract as a unit. Instead, the ventricles appear to quiver, or fibrillate, as multiple areas of the ventricle are contracting and relaxing in a disorganized fashion. The net result is no cardiac output and no pulse.

12. **How are V-fib/pulseless VT treated initially according to the American Heart Association (AHA) recommendations?**

1. The initial treatment for V-fib is always **defibrillation.**
2. Begin with the universal algorithm:
   - Assess the airway, breathing, and circulation (ABCs).
   - Ascertain that the patient is in cardiac arrest.
   - Begin CPR with cycles of 30 compressions and two breaths until defibrillator is attached, and confirm V-fib.
3. Give one shock:
   - Manual biphasic: device specific (120-200 J)
   - AED: device specific
   - Monophasic: 360 J
4. If V-fib persists:
   - Resume CPR immediately, intubate, and establish IV access.
   - Administer epinephrine 1 mg IV/IO (intraosseous) and repeat every 3-5 min, or you may administer one dose of vasopressin 40 U IV/IO to replace the first or second dose of epinephrine.
5. Give five cycles of CPR.
6. Give one shock if the rhythm is shockable.
7. Resum CPR immediately after the shock.
8. Consider antiarrhythmic medications.

13. **What medications are used in the treatment of refractory V-fib/pulseless VT?**

Amiodarone is a complex agent with multiple effects on sodium, potassium, and calcium channels. Amiodarone possesses both alpha- and beta-adrenergic blocking properties. 300 mg IV push for cardiac arrest from V-fib/VT that persists after multiple shocks. If V-fib/pulseless VT recurs, then administer a second dose of 150 mg IV. Maximum cumulative dose: 2.2 g over 24 hr.

Lidocaine is generally accepted as the initial antifibrillatory agent in the treatment of V-fib/pulseless VT at a recommended dose of 1-1.5 mg/kg (about 50-150 mg for an average adult patient). The bolus of lidocaine may be repeated in 3-5 min up to a total dose of 3 mg/kg.

Magnesium sulfate is given in a dose of 1-2 g IV push for patients with known low or suspected low serum magnesium, such as patients with alcoholism or other conditions associated with malnutrition or hypomagnesemic states. Also use magnesium sulfate for patients with a *torsades de pointes* pattern of V-fib or VT.

Procainamide is given up to 50 mg/min (maximum total 17mg/kg) for patients with V-fib/pulseless VT who respond to shocks with intermittent return of a pulse or a non–V-fib rhythm, but then recurs.

14. **What is tachycardia?**

Tachycardia means that there is a rapid heart rate. The normal adult heart rate is considered by most to be between 60 and 100 beats/min. Thus a heart rate of >100 beats/min can be classified as tachycardia. Not all patients with a heart rate of 100 beats/min or more will require treatment. The following cardiac rhythms are considered tachyarrhythmias:

1. Atrial flutter (A-flutter)/atrial fibrillation (A-fib)
2. Narrow-complex tachycardia:
   - Junctional tachycardia
   - Paroxysmal supraventricular tachycardia (PSVT)
   - Multifocal or ectopic atrial tachycardia
3. Wide-complex tachycardia:
   - SVT with aberrant conduction
   - Stable polymorphic VT (with and without normal baseline QT interval)
   - Stable monomorphic VT
   - *Torsades de pointes*

A patient with tachycardia or tachyarrhythmia needs treatment when there are signs and symptoms associated with the rapid heart rate. The following signs and symptoms indicate that the patient is already or is becoming hemodynamically unstable:

    Symptoms: shortness of breath, chest pain, dyspnea on exertion, and altered mental status

    Signs: pulmonary edema, rales, rhonchi, hypotension, orthostasis, jugular vein distention, peripheral edema, ischemic ECG changes

    Ventricular rate > 150 beats/min

15. Which tachyarrhythmias are supraventricular?

If the QRS complex is narrow, then the tachyarrhythmia is **supraventricular.** This means the arrhythmia is originating at or above the level of the atrioventricular (AV) node:

- Sinus tachycardia
- A-fib
- A-flutter
- PSVT

If the QRS complex is wide, then the tachycardia is of **ventricular** origin:

- Wide-complex tachycardia of uncertain type
- VT

16. How is the decision made to cardiovert a patient with tachycardia?

According to the AHA algorithm for tachycardia:

- Assess the patient using the primary and secondary ABCD surveys.
- Assess the patient's vital signs and heart rate if above 150 beats/min.
- Take a focused history.
- Conduct a focused physical exam.
- Perform a 12-lead ECG.

    Determine if the patient is hemodynamically stable:

- If there are no serious signs or symptoms of hemodynamic instability, treatment begins with diagnosis of the specific tachyarrhythmia and specific treatment for the particular tachyarrhythmia.
- If the patient presents with serious signs and symptoms related to the tachycardia, then assess the ventricular rate. If the rate is above 150 beats/min, then consider a brief trial of medications based on specific arrhythmia, or proceed to **cardioversion:**

    Have available: oxygen saturation monitor, suction device, IV line, and intubation equipment. Premedicate whenever possible (e.g., fentanyl, midazolam, or morphine).

    Synchronized cardioversion: VT, PSVT, A-fib, and A-flutter with 100 J, 200 J, 300 J, 360 J monophasic energy (Two exceptions are A-flutter, which often responds to lower energy levels such as 50 J, and the polymorphic VT, which often requires higher energy levels.)

    Synchronized cardioversion is not performed when tachycardia is a reflection of another underlying condition—for example, tachycardia that develops in response to severe hypotension, myocardial infarction (MI), or pulmonary edema.

17. What is the pathophysiology of PSVT?

PSVT is a distinct clinical syndrome characterized by repeated episodes of tachycardia with abrupt onset lasting a few seconds to many hours. PSVT is due to a reentry mechanism involving the AV node alone or automatic focus.

18. What are the types of narrow-complex tachycardia?

- PSVT: caused by a reentry circuit mechanism
- Ectopic or multifocal atrial tachycardia: caused by an automatic focus
- Junctional tachycardia: caused by automatic focus that originates within or near the AV node

    Reentry tachycardia responds well to antiarrhythmic medications and electrical cardioversion.

    Automatic focus tachycardias do not respond to electrical cardioversion and should be treated with medications that suppress the ectopic foci.

19. **According to AHA protocol, what is the treatment of supraventricular, narrow complex tachycardia with reentry (PSVT) in a stable patient?**
1. Consider vagal maneuver (carotid body massage or Valsalva)
2. Treatment with adenosine:
   - Begin with 6 mg IV push given rapidly over 1-3 sec followed by a normal saline bolus of 20 mL; elevate extremity. A second and a third dose can be given if needed.
   - Second dose of 12 mg
   - Third dose of 12 mg
3. AV nodal blockade:
   - Beta blocker
   - Calcium channel blocker
   - Digoxin
   - DC cardioversion
4. Consider antiarrhythmics:
   - Procainamide
   - Amiodarone
   - Sotalol (Oral form only in the United States; the IV form is not approved for use in the United States.)

20. **What are the signs and symptoms of A-fib and A-flutter?**

A-fib may result from multiple areas of reentry within the atria or from multiple ectopic foci. A-fib may be associated with sick sinus syndrome, hypoxia, increased atrial pressure, and pericarditis. Because there is no uniform atrial depolarization, no P-wave will be seen on ECG. Hypotension may result from A-fib.

A-flutter is the result of reentry circuit within the atria. A-flutter rarely occurs in the absence of organic disease. It is seen in association with mitral or tricuspid valvular disease, acute cor pulmonale, and coronary artery disease. Signs and symptoms include hypotension, ischemic pain, and severe congestive heart failure.

21. **How are A-fib and A-flutter treated?**

According to the AHA, the protocol for treatment of A-fib and A-flutter is:
1. Rule out precipitating causes for A-fib and A-flutter:
   - Heart failure
   - Acute MI
   - Hyperthyroidism
   - Hypoxia
   - Pulmonary embolism
   - Substance abuse
   - Hypokalemia
   - Hypomagnesemia
2. Control the rate:
   - Preserved heart function: diltiazem (or another calcium channel blocker) or metoprolol (or another beta blocker), flecainide, propafenone, procainamide, amiodarone, or digoxin
   - Impaired heart function: diltiazem, digoxin, or amiodarone
   - Patients with Wolff-Parkinson-White (WPW) syndrome: Avoid adenosine, calcium channel blockers, beta blockers, and digoxin to control the rate. Convert the rhythm (electrical cardioversion if drug therapy is unsuccessful) or if the duration is 48 hr or less.
   - Preserved heart function: DC cardioversion, amiodarone, ibutilide, flecainide, propafenone, procainamide
   - Impaired heart function: DC cardioversion, amiodarone.
3. Convert the rhythm if the duration is > 48 hr:
4. Urgent cardioversion: begins with IV heparin, followed by transesophageal echocardiogram to exclude atrial clot. Then cardiovert within 24 hr and give anticoagulation for 4 weeks.
5. Delayed cardioversion: anticoagulation for 3 weeks, then cardiovert and anticoagulate for 4 more weeks.

22. What are the types of wide-complex tachycardias and their AHA treatment recommendations?

1. Unknown type:
   - Attempt to identify and distinguish between VT and SVT with aberrant conduction due to the different treatment option for SVT that might compromise a patient with VT.
   - Always assume that any wide-complex tachycardia is VT until proven otherwise, because there is little danger in treating a wide-complex SVT as if it were VT.
   - **Treatment:** DC cardioversion, procainamide, or amiodarone for preserved cardiac function. Treat with DC cardioversion or amiodarone for impaired cardiac function.
2. Monomorphic VT:
   - QRS complexes appear identical in shape.
   - **Treatment:** procainamide, amiodarone, lidocaine, or sotalol with normal cardiac function. Lidocaine or amiodarone should be given to patients with impaired cardiac function.
3. Polymorphic VT:
   - QRS complexes are subdivided into normal baseline QT and prolonged baseline QT interval.
   - Associated with metabolic derangement such as electrolyte abnormalities or drug toxicities.
   - **Treatment:** search for the metabolic derangement. Use DC cardioversion, procainamide, amiodarone, or beta blockers.
   - *Torsades de pointes* is an example of this VT with unique rhythm strip. The drug of choice for *torsades* associated with hypomagnesemia is magnesium sulfate.

23. What is WPW syndrome? Which drugs can be harmful in the treatment of A-fib or A-flutter associated with WPW syndrome?

If there is an extra conduction pathway, the electrical signal may arrive at the ventricles too soon. This condition is called Wolff-Parkinson-White (WPW) syndrome. It is in a category of electrical abnormalities called "preexcitation syndromes."

It is recognized by certain changes on the ECG, which is a graphical record of the heart's electrical activity. The ECG will show that an extra pathway or shortcut exists from the atria to the ventricles.

Many people with WPW syndrome who have symptoms or episodes of tachycardia (rapid heart rhythm) may have dizziness, chest palpitations, fainting or, rarely, cardiac arrest. Other people with WPW syndrome never have tachycardia or other symptoms. About 80% of people with symptoms first have them between the ages of 11 and 50.

Drugs that selectively block the AV node without also blocking coexisting accessory conduction pathways (e.g., adenosine, calcium channel blockers, beta blockers, and digoxin) are contraindicated when preexcitation syndromes are present. These medications can increase conduction through the accessory pathway and paradoxically increase the heart rate. For patients with A-fib or A-flutter, this poses severe risks and is associated with a very high incidence of clinical deterioration.

24. What is bradycardia?

The term *bradycardia* simply means that the heart rate is slow. Normal adult heart rate is considered by most to be 60-100 beats/min. According to this definition, every patient with a heart rate <60 beats/min is bradycardic. Not all patients with a heart rate <60 beats/min will need treatment. Autonomic influence or intrinsic disease affecting the cardiac conduction system most often causes bradycardia.

A patient may have a relative bradycardia. An example is the patient with severe hypotension but with a heart rate of 70 beats/min; the heart rate of 70 in a hypotensive patient may not sustain the cardiac output.

25. What are the principal bradyarrhythmias?
- Sinus bradycardia

- A-fib with slow ventricular response
- AV block:
  First-degree heart block
  Second-degree heart block, types I and II
  Third-degree heart block
- Relative bradycardia
  Other rhythms that may also be considered bradyarrhythmias are:
- Pulseless electrical activity
- Asystole

26. When does sinus bradycardia need treatment?

A patient with a slow heart rate needs treatment only if there are serious signs or symptoms associated with the slow heart rate that indicate the patient is already or is becoming hemodynamically unstable. These signs and symptoms include:

Signs: hypotension, congestive heart failure, pulmonary congestion, and acute MI
Symptoms: chest pain, shortness of breath, and decrease level of consciousness

27. How is a patient with a bradyarrhythmia initially managed according to AHA protocol?

1. Supportive actions:

- Assess ABCs
- Oxygen, IV, monitors, and pulse oximetry
- 12-lead ECG
- Chest x-ray
- Brief history and targeted physical exam

2. Determine if bradycardia is hemodynamically significant.

- Monitor patient.
- Be prepared to begin transcutaneous pacing (TCP) on standby.
  If the patient is hemodynamically unstable:
- Atropine, 0.5-1.0 mg IV
- TCP
- Dopamine infusion, 5-20 μg/kg/min
- Epinephrine infusion, 2-10 μg/min
- Isoproterenol infusion, 2-10 μg/min

28. What is meant by the term *heart block?*

Heart block is used interchangeably with the correct term, *atrioventricular (AV) block.* AV block describes a delay or interruption in conduction between the atria and the ventricles, which may be caused by one or more of the following:

- Lesion in the conduction pathway
- Prolonged refractory period along the conduction pathway
- Supraventricular heart rates that surpass the refractory period of the AV node

29. What is first-degree heart block?

First-degree heart block is the prolonged delay in conduction at the AV node or the bundle of His. The diagnosis of first-degree heart block is based on the PR interval. First-degree heart block exists when the PR interval is longer than 0.2 sec.

30. According to AHA protocol, how is first-degree heart block treated?

First-degree heart block requires no treatment unless there are associated symptoms.

31. What is second-degree heart block?

In second-degree heart block, not every atrial impulse is able to pass through the AV node into the ventricles. The atrial impulses that are conducted to the ventricle will stimulate ventricular contraction. Therefore the ratio of P to QRS will be > 1:1.

Type I second-degree heart block (Wenckebach):

- Occurs at the level of the AV node
- Is usually due to increased parasympathetic tone or drug effects

- Is characterized by progressive elongation of the PR interval
- Conduction velocity through AV node gradually decreases until impulse is blocked, resulting in skipped ventricular beat.
    Type II second-degree heart block:
- Occurs below the level of the AV node, uncommonly at the bundle of His
- Is usually due to lesion along pathway
- Has a PR interval that does not lengthen before skipped ventricular beat
- May have more than one skipped ventricular beat in a row
- Has a poorer prognosis than type I second-degree heart block
- Is more likely to progress to complete heart block than type I

32. According to AHA protocol, how is type I second-degree heart block treated?

Type I second-degree heart block rarely requires treatment unless symptoms associated with bradycardia develop. Treatment should be directed at addressing the underlying cause of the block, such as:

- Decreased parasympathetic tone
- Digitalis toxicity
- Propranolol toxicity/overdose
- Verapamil toxicity/overdose

    If serious symptoms occur, then the following treatment is recommended:

- Atropine, 0.5-1.0 mg
- TCP
- Dopamine infusion beginning with 5 μg/kg/min
- Epinephrine infusion, 1-2 μg/min
- Fluid challenge if appropriate

33. According to AHA protocol, how is type II second-degree heart block treated?

Type II second-degree heart block requires no treatment unless symptoms associated with bradycardia develop. If serious symptoms develop, then the following treatment is recommended:

- Atropine, 0.5-1.0 mg
- TCP
- Dopamine beginning with 5 μg/kg/min
- Epinephrine infusion, 1-2 μg/min
- Fluid challenge if appropriate

34. What is third-degree heart block?

Third-degree heart block occurs when no atrial impulses are transmitted to the ventricles. The atrial rate will be equal to or greater than the ventricular rate. If block occurs at the AV node, a junctional pacemaker may initiate ventricular depolarizations at a regular rate of 40-60 beats/min. If the block is infranodal, usually both bundle branches are blocked and there is significant disease of the conduction pathway.

35. According to AHA protocol, how is third-degree heart block treated?

Third-degree heart block is treated only if there are signs and symptoms that the patient is or is becoming hemodynamically unstable. Recommended treatment for third-degree heart block is:

- Atropine, 0.5-1.0 mg
- TCP
- Dopamine infusion beginning with 5 μg/kg/min
- Epinephrine infusion, 1-2 μg/min
- Fluid challenge if appropriate

36. What is pulseless electrical activity (PEA)?

This term is used to describe a group of diverse ECG rhythms that manifest electrical activity but are similar in that the patient will be without a pulse. Therefore the PEA is a nonperfusing rhythm.

    The types of rhythms included in the PEA group are:

- **EMD:** organized ECG rhythm present, no pulse
- **Pseudo-EMD:** as above, but with some meaningful cardiac contraction
- **Idioventricular, ventricular escape:** wide QRS, no atrial activity, and no pulse
- **Bradyasystolic:** profound bradycardia with periods of asystole, no pulse
    PEA is almost always a secondary disorder resulting from some underlying condition.

37. What are the causes of PEA?

The underlying causes of PEA can be remembered easily using the mnemonic five *H*'s and five *T*'s:

Five causes that start with "**H**":

Hypovolemia

Hypoxia

Hydrogen ion (acidosis)

Hyperkalemia/hypokalemia

Hypothermia

Five causes that start with "**T**":

Table (ABCDs)—*a*ntidepressants, *b*eta blockers, *c*alcium channel blocker, *d*igitalis

Tamponade (cardiac)

Tension pneumothorax

Thrombosis (coronary)

Thrombosis (pulmonary)

Alternatively, the causes of PEA can be divided into three basic categories:

1. Inadequate ventilation:
   - Intubation of right mainstem bronchus
   - Tension pneumothorax
   - Bilateral pneumothorax
2. Inadequate circulation:
   - Pericardial effusion with tamponade
   - Myocardial rupture
   - Ruptured aortic aneurysm
   - Massive pulmonary embolus
   - Hypovolemia
3. Metabolic disorder:
   - Electrolyte disturbances (hyperkalemia or hypokalemia, hypomagnesemia)
   - Persistent severe acidosis (diabetic ketoacidosis or lactic acidosis)
   - Tricyclic overdose
   - Hypothermia

38. According to AHA protocol, how is PEA treated?

1. Continue CPR.
2. Intubate/establish IV access.
3. Assess blood flow using Doppler.
4. Consider and treat underlying causes.
5. Epinephrine, 1 mg IV/IO. Repeat every 3-5 min, or you may give one dose of vasopressin 40 U IV/IO to replace the first or second dose of epinephrine.
6. Atropine, 1 mg IV push if pulse is present and absolute bradycardia is < 60 beats/min. Repeat every 3-5 min (up to three doses).

39. What is asystole?

The term *asystole* indicates the absence of ventricular activity. The patient will be without pulse. ECG will show characteristic flat-line tracing without P-waves and QRS complexes. The underlying causes of asystole can be remembered using the mnemonic *PHD:*

Preexisting acidosis

Hypoxia, hyperkalemia, hypokalemia, hypothermia

Drug overdose

40. How is a flat-line rhythm verified to be asystole?

- The patient will be pulseless.
- The patient will be unresponsive.

- The monitoring leads are correctly hooked up.
- There will be flat-line recording in more than one lead.

41. What four conditions other than asystole can lead to a flat-line tracing on ECG?

1. Fine V-fib
2. Loose electrode leads
3. No power
4. Signal gain is turned down

42. What four conditions are pulseless?

There are four conditions in which the patient will present without a pulse and are therefore considered nonperfusing conditions:

1. V-fib
2. Pulseless VT
3. PEA:
   - Electromechanical dissociation
   - Pseudo-EMD (pulse will be very faint and evident only by Doppler)
   - Ventricular escape rhythms
   - Postdefibrillation idioventricular rhythms
4. Asystole

43. According to AHA protocol, what is the treatment for asystole?

The treatment sequence for asystole is virtually the same algorithm for PEA:

1. Continue CPR.
2. Intubate/establish IV access.
3. Confirm asystole.
4. Consider and treat underlying causes.
5. TCP only if started early.
6. Epinephrine, 1 mg IV/IO. Repeat every 3-5 min, or you may give one dose of vasopressin 40 U IV/IO to replace the first or second dose of epinephrine.
7. Atropine, 1 mg IV/IO. Repeat every 3-5 min (up to three doses).

44. What is shock?

The term *shock* denotes a clinical syndrome in which there is inadequate cellular perfusion and inadequate oxygen delivery for the metabolic demands of the tissues. Types of shock include:

- Cardiogenic shock
- Hypovolemic shock
- Septic shock
- Neurogenic shock
- Flow disruption shock
- Anaphylactic shock

In general, shock is characterized by:

- Increased vascular resistance
- Cool mottled skin
- Oliguria
- Tachycardia
- Adrenergic response
- Diaphoresis
- Anxiety
- Vomiting
- Diarrhea
- Myocardial ischemia
- Mental status changes

45. What is the pathophysiology of acute cardiogenic pulmonary edema?

Acute cardiogenic pulmonary edema results from an increase in pulmonary venous pressure that leads to engorgement of the pulmonary vasculature. Lung compliance will decrease, and small airway resistance will increase. Lymphatic flow increases, presumably to maintain the pulmonary extravascular liquid volume. The net result is dyspnea and hypoxia, followed by shock.

46. What drugs are useful in the treatment of acute cardiogenic pulmonary edema?

- Norepinephrine
- Furosemide

- Dopamine
- Dobutamine
- Nitroglycerin
- Nitroprusside

- Amrinone
- Aminophylline
- Thrombolytic agents
- Digoxin

47. When is synchronized cardioversion used?
- Tachycardia
- PSVT
- A-fib
- A-flutter

48. What are the signs and symptoms of cardiac tamponade?
- Persistent tachycardia with falling blood pressure
- Pulsus paradoxus
- Pulsatile neck veins
- Enlarging heart shadow on chest x-ray

49. What are the signs and symptoms of hypovolemic shock?
- Cardiac output will be low due to inadequate left ventricular filling.
- Hypotension may lead to changes in the ECG.

50. How is hypovolemic shock treated?
- Volume loss can be diagnosed through history and clinical evaluation.
- Replace volume with crystalloid or colloid solution when the hematocrit is normal.
- With active bleeding, hemostasis must be achieved first. If the hematocrit is dangerously low, transfusion of whole blood or packed red blood cells is indicated.

51. What are the four life-threatening conditions that may mimic acute MI and lead to cardiovascular collapse?
- Massive pulmonary embolism
- Hypovolemic and septic shock
- Cardiac tamponade
- Aortic dissection

52. What drugs can be administered through the endotracheal tube?
L-E-A-N (**L**idocaine, **A**tropine, **E**pinephrine, **N**arcan). Administer all tracheal medications at 2-2.5 times the recommended IV dosage, diluted in 10 mL of normal saline or distilled water. Tracheal absorption is greater with the distilled water as the diluent than with normal saline, but distilled water has a greater adverse effect on PaO_2.

53. How is sudden cardiac death defined?[*]
Sudden V-fib or PEA. Acute coronary ischemia and preexisting cardiac disease are the most common causes. V-fib is becoming less common.

54. Is there an immediate need for an airway?[*]
No. Defibrillation and chest compression should be initiated first. Waiting for intubation to be completed before initiation of these interventions is one of the most common mistakes in advanced life support. Children, in whom primary respiratory arrest is more common, are an exception. Restoration of ventilation in children often reveals that pulselessness was severe shock, not cardiac arrest.

55. Is the central line the best access to the circulation?[*]
Yes. Large volumes of fluid can be delivered to the venous system more quickly, however,

---

[*]Reprinted from Paradis NA, Harken AH: Cardiopulmonary resuscitation. In Harken AH, Moore EE (eds): *Abernathy's Surgical Secrets*, 5th ed. Philadelphia, 2005, Mosby.

via large-bore peripheral venous catheters. A 14-gauge, 5-cm catheter (peripheral) can deliver twice the flow of a 16-gauge, 20-cm catheter (central). Central line placement may be associated with significant complications, including pneumothorax, air embolus, and arterial puncture. In hypovolemic patients, in whom central veins are collapsed and peripheral veins are constricted, venous cannulation can be difficult.

56. Does a central line offer therapeutic and diagnostic advantages?[*]
Yes. A central line permits bolus administration of drugs to the right side of the heart. Identification of a high central venous pressure may indicate the need to treat reversible causes of PEA, such as cardiac tamponade or tension pneumothorax.

57. Which is preferred—colloid or crystalloid resuscitation fluid?[*]
Colloid advocates claim that the big molecules remain in the intravascular space and are more effective in elevating blood volume. Crystalloid advocates state that capillaries leak albumin, especially in the shock state. Resuscitation with crystalloid is clearly safe. Given its availability, low cost, and safety, crystalloid (lactated Ringer's solution) is the choice for initial fluid resuscitation. When true cardiac arrest has occurred, however, volume is of little importance.

58. In a patient exhibiting asystole, bradycardia, PEA, or fine fibrillation, what is your primary goal?[*]
Adequate vital organ perfusion, especially to the coronary arteries. Done properly, CPR may cause PEA to progress to stable hemodynamics or V-fib to become "coarse enough" for successful countershock.

59. What are the drugs commonly used during resuscitation? What are their appropriate dosages?[*]
Oxygen: To reverse hypoxia, always provide 100% oxygen initially.
Epinephrine: alpha- and beta-adrenergic agonist. IV dose is 5-10 mL of 1:10,000 solution. Because of the short duration of action, a repeat dose may be necessary after 5 min. Epinephrine is inactivated by alkali; do not mix with bicarbonate solutions. Although it enhances myocardial performance, epinephrine greatly increases myocardial oxygen demand. Ventilate!
Vasopressin: antidiuretic hormone. A first-line pressor during cardiac arrest. Administer one time as a bolus of 40 U.
Amiodarone: first-line, broad-spectrum antidysrhythmic possibly useful in treating V-fib/VT cardiac arrest and atrial arrhythmias. It is active at cardiac sodium, potassium, and calcium channels and has alpha- and beta-adrenergic blocking properties. In cardiac arrest, it is administered as a 300-mg rapid IV infusion. Amiodarone may cause hypotension and bradycardia; a pressor drug, such as epinephrine or dopamine, should be readily available or already administered.
Atropine: parasympatholytic (vagolytic) agent that increases the discharge rate of the sinus node. Atropine is useful in treating sinus bradycardia associated with hemodynamic compromise. An IV dose of 0.5 mg is repeated at 5-min intervals until a desirable rate is achieved (at least 60 beats/min). Increased heart rate increases myocardial oxygen demand; atropine should be used only if the bradycardia causes hemodynamic compromise (heart rate < 60 beats/min).
Dopamine: catecholamine precursor of norepinephrine active at dopaminergic receptors. Stimulates the heart and vasoconstricts (high dose) the periphery. Use as a vasopressor to treat hypotension secondary to bradycardia or decreased peripheral vasomotor tone. Dosage should be adjusted based on clinical end points starting at 2-5 µg/kg/min up to 20 µg/kg/min. The principal toxicity, seen with prolonged dosages >10 µg/kg/min, is splanchnic and systemic vasoconstriction with resultant injury.
Dobutamine: synthetic catecholamine that is a cardiac beta-receptor agonist used to treat cardiogenic shock. It increases cardiac contractility. Reflex peripheral vasodilation may

require combination with a pressor drug, such as dopamine. Dosage should be adjusted based on clinical end points starting at 5 μg/kg/min up to 20 μg/kg/min.

Sodium bicarbonate ($NaHCO_3$): no longer commonly used in cardiac arrest; in shock, it is used to reverse acidosis (hypoxia-induced anaerobic metabolism leads to acid accumulation). The initial dose is 1 mEq/kg. One ampule (50 mL) contains 50 mEq of sodium bicarbonate. Bicarbonate combines with hydrogen ions to form CO_2 and water; adequate ventilation is required for bicarbonate therapy to be fully effective. Overzealous use of bicarbonate may result in hypernatremia/hyperosmolality (each HCO_3^- is accompanied by a sodium ion).

Magnesium: effective in treating drug-induced *torsades de pointes* or VT. Administer 1-2 g IV over 3-5 min. May cause hypotension.

Calcium chloride or gluconate: positive inotropic agent. Calcium ions bind to troponin (the cardiomyocyte-specific calcium regulatory protein used to diagnose an acute myocardial infarction), which enhances the formation of cross-bridges between muscle contractile filaments with resultant fiber shortening. Dose is calcium chloride (or gluconate), 500 mg IV push. Do not mix with bicarbonate because it will precipitate.

Lidocaine: local anesthetic that suppresses ventricular arrhythmias (automatic and reentrant). An IV bolus of 1 mg/kg is followed by IV infusion at 2-4 mg/min. An additional IV bolus can be given at 10 min after initial dose if arrhythmias persist. Amiodarone is accepted as a preferred agent for treatment of arrhythmias.

Adenosine: a naturally occurring vasodilating hormone that is synthesized by vascular endothelial cells and dramatically slows AV nodal conduction. It is useful in the therapy of supraventricular tachyarrhythmias. Dose is 6 mg or 12 mg injected in a rapid IV bolus (which may be repeated several times). The half-life of IV adenosine is only 12 sec. Measurable systemic hypotension occurs in <2% of patients because adenosine is metabolized before it reaches the systemic vessels.

Verapamil: slow-channel calcium blocker used to block the AV node and to treat PSVT that causes hemodynamic compromise. Dose is 0.1 mg/kg. Dilute drug with 10 mL of saline, and infuse 1 mL/min until the SVT either breaks or blocks. Repeat dose after 30 min if not effective. The drug reduces systemic vascular resistance and may cause hypotension.

60. What measures should be considered postresuscitation to improve the chances of a good outcome?*

Lab and clinical data support use of mild hypothermia (34° C for 24 hr) in patients who remain comatose after resuscitation from cardiac arrest. Hypotension or causes of increased cerebral oxygen use (e.g., as seizures or fever) should be treated aggressively.

BIBLIOGRAPHY

1. Cohn E, Gilroy-Doohan M: Flip and See ECG, 2nd ed. Philadelphia, 2002, Saunders.
2. Cummins RO (ed): Advanced Cardiac Life Support. Dallas, 2004, American Heart Association.
3. Dubin D: Rapid interpretation of EKGs, 6th ed. Tampa, Fla, 2000, Cover Publishing Company.
4. Grauer K, Cavallaro D: Arrhythmia Interpretation: ACLS Preparation and Clinical Approach. St Louis, 1997, Mosby.
5. Kudenchuk PJ, Cobb LA, Copass MK et al: Amiodarone for resuscitation after out-of-hospital cardiac arrest due to ventricular fibrillation. N Engl J Med 341:871-878, 1999.
6. Lindner KH, Dirks B, Strohmenger HU et al: Randomised comparison of epinephrine and vasopressin in patients with out-of-hospital ventricular fibrillation. Lancet 349:535-537, 1997.
7. Mild therapeutic hypothermia to improve the neurologic outcome after cardiac arrest. N Engl J Med 346:549-556, 2002.
8. Paradis NA, Harken AH: Cardiopulmonary resuscitation. In Harken AH, Moore EE (eds): Abernathy's Surgical Secrets, 5th ed. Philadelphia, 2005, Mosby.
9. Thaler MS: The Only EKG Book You'll Ever Need. Philadelphia, 1997, Lippincott-Raven.

14. ADVANCED TRAUMA LIFE SUPPORT

Edward Kozlovsky, DMD, and Shahid R. Aziz, DMD, MD, FACS

1. **What is the appropriate systematic approach to be used in the rapid assessment of the injuries and treatment to be provided to the seriously injured patient?**

   Primary and secondary surveys are used for rapid, systematic, and thorough evaluation of the injured patient.

   Primary survey:
   - Airway and cervical spine protection
   - Breathing
   - Circulation with control of external hemorrhage
   - Disability: brief neurologic evaluation
   - Exposure/environment: Completely undress the patient, but prevent hypothermia.

   Secondary survey (physical exam and history):
   - Head and skull
   - Maxillofacial and intraoral
   - Neck
   - Chest
   - Abdomen (including back)
   - Perineum/rectum/vagina
   - Musculoskeletal
   - Neurologic exam

2. **What are the indications for definitive airway placement in the trauma patient?**
   - Unconscious patient
   - Severe maxillofacial trauma
   - Risk for aspiration (bleeding/vomiting)
   - Risk for obstruction (neck hematoma, laryngeal/tracheal injury, stridor)

3. **What are the benefits of endotracheal intubation?**

   Endotracheal intubation provides:
   - A definitive airway
   - A supplemental oxygen delivery port
   - A way to support ventilation
   - A means of providing pulmonary care
   - Prevention against aspiration

4. **Which initial radiographic studies should be obtained for a blunt trauma patient?**

   Cervical spine, anteroposterior chest, and anteroposterior pelvis radiographs should be obtained via portable means in the resuscitation area.

5. **What are the approximate Pao_2 vs. O_2 hemoglobin saturation levels for Pao_2 of 90 mm Hg, Pao_2 of 60 mm Hg, Pao_2 of 30 mm Hg, and Pao_2 of 27 mm Hg (Table 14-1)?**

Table 14-1	O_2 Saturation Levels and Corresponding Pao_2 Levels
Pao_2 LEVELS	O_2 HEMOGLOBIN SATURATION LEVELS
90 mm Hg	100%
60 mm Hg	90%
30 mm Hg	60%
27 mm Hg	50%

6.　**What is the initial fluid of choice in resuscitation, and why?**
　　Lactated Ringer's solution is the first choice in the fluid resuscitation of the injured patient. It is an isotonic electrolyte solution that provides transient intravascular expansion. It also stabilizes vascular volume by replacing accompanying fluid losses into the interstitial and intercellular spaces.

7.　**What determines the maximum rate of fluid administration through a catheter?**
　　The rate is determined by the internal diameter of the catheter and inversely by its length. The size of the vessel into which the catheter is placed has no effect on flow rate.

8.　**What is the optimal urinary output for adult and pediatric trauma patients?**
　　In an adult patient, urinary output should be at least 0.5 mL/kg/hr; in a pediatric patient older than age 1, it should be 1 mL/kg/hr.

9.　**What is the definition of *shock*?**
　　Shock is defined as an abnormality of the circulatory system that results in inadequate organ perfusion and tissue oxygenation.

10.　**What are the most common forms of shock encountered in trauma patients?**
　　Most injured patients in shock are hypovolemic, but they may suffer from neurogenic, cardiogenic, or septic shock.

11.　**What is the most common cause of shock in the injured patient?**
　　Hemorrhage.

12.　**What is the earliest measurable circulatory sign of shock?**
　　Tachycardia. The release of endogenous catecholamines increases peripheral vascular resistance. This increases diastolic blood pressure and reduces pulse pressure but does not increase organ and tissue perfusion.

13.　**What is cardiogenic shock?**
　　Cardiogenic shock occurs when the blood flow decreases due to an intrinsic defect in cardiac function—either the heart muscle or the heart valves. A classic example is an acute myocardial infarction resulting in ischemic damage to the heart muscle impeding cardiac contractility. The decreased contractility causes a decrease in stroke volume, resulting in decreased cardiac output and blood pressure; high left ventricular filling pressures (backward failure); increased systemic vascular resistance (from vasoconstriction, which is a sympathetic compensatory response to the low blood pressure); and increased heart rate (sympathetic compensatory response to the low blood pressure). Other features of cardiogenic shock, such as cool extremities, decreased urine output, and sweating, may also be explained by the sympathetic compensatory response.

14.　**What is neurogenic shock?**
　　Neurogenic shock is caused by the sudden loss of the descending sympathetic nervous system control of the smooth muscle in vessel walls. This can result from severe central nervous system (CNS) (brain and spinal cord) damage. With the loss of background sympathetic stimulation, the visceral and lower extremity vessels suddenly relax, resulting in a sudden decrease in peripheral vascular resistance and decrease in blood pressure. Loss of sympathetic stimulation of the heart will decrease the patient's ability to become tachycardic and may even cause bradycardia. Central venous pressure (CVP) monitoring is recommended to avoid fluid overload and congestive failure during fluid resuscitation. Atropine and vasopressors are used in the treatment of neurogenic shock to maintain blood pressure and organ perfusion.

15. What is the normal blood volume of an adult and a pediatric patient?

The normal blood volume of an adult is approximately 7% of body weight. The blood volume of obese adults is estimated based on their ideal body weight. The blood volume of a child is calculated as 8%-9% of body weight (80-90 mL/kg).

16. What are the four classes of hemorrhage?

Hemorrhage is defined as an acute loss of circulating blood volume.

- **Class I hemorrhage**—in which up to 15% of total blood volume is lost. Except for minimal tachycardia, no other sign may be apparent.
- **Class II hemorrhage**—in which 15%-30% of blood volume lost. Evidence of tachycardia and tachypnea and a decrease in pulse pressure will be noted. This decrease in pulse pressure is the result of elevation of the diastolic pressure, which is a natural response as a result of increased peripheral resistance brought on by catecholamine circulation. In Class II hemorrhage, early CNS changes take place, leading to anxiety and, at times, minimal confusion. The urinary output becomes significantly less.
- **Class III hemorrhage**—in which 30%-40% of blood volume (almost 3 L in an adult) is lost. All the typical signs and symptoms of shock are obvious.
- **Class IV hemorrhage**—in which more than 40% of blood volume is lost. The patient is cold and pale with significant loss of blood pressure, narrowed pulse pressure, negligible urine output, and depressed mental status.

17. What is a tension pneumothorax?

Tension pneumothorax develops when air enters the pleural space, but a flap-valve mechanism prevents its escape. Intrapleural pressure rises, causing total lung collapse and a shift of the mediastinum to the opposite side, with resulting impairment of venous return and a fall in cardiac output.

18. How is tension pneumothorax diagnosed and treated?

Tension pneumothorax is a true surgical emergency that requires immediate diagnosis and treatment. Diagnosis of tension pneumothorax should be made based on the clinical evaluation. Symptoms such as acute respiratory distress, subcutaneous emphysema, absent breath sounds, hyperresonance to percussion, and tracheal shift support the diagnosis. Tension pneumothorax requires immediate thoracic decompression and is managed initially by rapidly inserting a needle into the second intercostal space along the midclavicular line of the affected hemithorax. Insertion of a chest tube into the fifth intercostal space, usually at the nipple level, just anterior to the midaxillary line, is required for the definitive treatment of tension pneumothorax.

19. What is focused assessment sonography (FAST) and its indications?

FAST is a rapid bedside ultrasound exam performed to identify intraperitoneal hemorrhage or pericardial tamponade. FAST examines four areas for free fluid: perihepatic and hepatorenal space, perisplenic, pelvis, pericardium. FAST assessment is indicated in trauma patients who have a history of abdominal trauma, are hypotensive, or are unable to provide a reliable history because of impaired consciousness resulting from head injury or drugs. FAST is an adjunct to the ATLS (Advanced Trauma Life Support) primary survey and therefore follows the performance of the ABCs (*a*irway, *b*reathing, and *c*irculation).

20. What is diagnostic peritoneal lavage (DPL) and its indications?

DPL involves passing a small catheter into the peritoneal cavity, usually at the umbilicus or just inferior to it (3-4 cm). If blood can be aspirated through this catheter, this is referred to as a diagnostic positive aspiration (DPA). If no blood can be aspirated, a liter of warm crystalloid solution is run into the peritoneal cavity and then allowed to drain out by gravity after sitting for 5-10 min. This lavage fluid is then sent to the lab for analysis of red blood cell (RBC) count, white blood cell (WBC) count, and any bowel contents (fecal or food matter). A rule of thumb for a positive DPL is the inability to read newsprint through the lavage fluid. Further surgical intervention is required if lab results of the submitted specimen indicate the presence of 100,000 RBCs/mm^3 or more, and >WBCs/mm^3. DPL is used as an alternative to the FAST scan to identify intraperitoneal hemorrhage in blunt abdominal trauma. The role of DPL in the hemodynamically normal patient with penetrating abdominal injury is to identify hollow viscus injury (stomach, small bowel, colon) or diaphragmatic injury. The primary disadvantages of DPL are that it is invasive, does not evaluate the retroperitoneum, and has a significant false-positive rate.

21. What are the recommended tests for the hemodynamically abnormal and normal patient with blunt abdominal trauma?

The hemodynamically abnormal patient with blunt abdominal injuries should be rapidly assessed for intraabdominal bleeding or contamination from the gastrointestinal tract by performing DPL or FAST. The hemodynamically normal patient without peritonitis should be evaluated by contrast-enhanced CT.

22. What is the difference between epidural and subdural hematomas?

Epidural hematomas occur in 0.5% of all brain-injured patients. These hematomas are located outside the dura but within the skull and are typically biconvex or lenticular in shape. Epidural hematomas are usually the result of a tear of the middle meningeal artery and are most often located in the temporal or temporoparietal region. Although the majority are of arterial origin, they also may result from a tear of a major venous sinus.

Subdural hematomas occur in approximately 30% of severe brain injuries. They result from tearing of small surface vessels of the cerebral cortex and commonly cover the entire surface of the hemisphere. An acute subdural hematoma usually results in much more severe brain damage than an epidural hematoma.

23. What are the symptoms and signs of an epidural hematoma?
- Loss of conscious state followed by an intervening lucid interval
- Secondary depression of consciousness
- Development of hemiparesis on the contralateral side
- A fixed and dilated pupil on the ipsilateral side of the impact area

24. What is the Glasgow Coma Scale?

The Glasgow Coma Scale (GCS) provides a quantitative measure of a patient's level of consciousness. The GCS comprises the sum of scores for three areas of assessment: (1) eye opening; (2) verbal response; (3) best motor response. The maximum GCS score is 15, and the minimum is 3.

Eye Opening Response
- Spontaneous—open with blinking at baseline: **4 points**
- To verbal stimuli, command, speech: **3 points**
- To pain only (not applied to face): **2 points**
- No response: **1 point**

Verbal Response
- Oriented: **5 points**
- Confused conversation, but able to answer questions: **4 points**
- Inappropriate words: **3 points**
- Incomprehensible speech: **2 points**
- No response: **1 point**

Motor Response
- Obeys commands for movement: **6 points**

- Purposeful movement to painful stimulus: **5 points**
- Withdraws in response to pain: **4 points**
- Flexion in response to pain (decorticate posturing): **3 points**
- Extension in response to pain (decerebrate posturing): **2 points**
- No response: **1 point**

25. How is GCS used to classify the severity of brain injury?
- Severe head injury (coma)—GCS score of 8 or less
- Moderate head injury—GCS score of 9-13
- Mild head injury—GCS score of 14-15

26. What is spinal shock?
    Loss of reflexes and flaccidity, seen after spinal cord injury. Owing to shock, the injured cord may appear completely functionless, although all areas are not necessarily destroyed.

27. What are the clinically assessable spinal cord tracts?
The corticospinal tract—located in the posterolateral segment of the cord; controls motor power on the ipsilateral side of the body. It is tested by involuntary response to painful stimuli or voluntary muscle contractions.
The spinothalamic tract—located in the anterolateral part of the cord; carries temperature and pain sensations from the contralateral side of the body. It is tested by gentle touch or pinprick.
The posterior columns—transmit proprioception, vibration, and light touch sensation from the ipsilateral side. They are tested by location sense in the toes and fingers or by using a tuning fork to test for vibration sense.

28. What are the classifications of spinal cord injuries?
    Spinal cord injuries are classified based on:
1. Level
2. Severity of neurologic deficit
3. Spinal cord syndrome
4. Morphology

29. What are the most common spinal cord syndromes?
Central cord syndrome—identified by greater loss of motor function in the upper extremities than the lower extremities, with varying sensory loss
Anterior cord syndrome—identified by paraplegia with loss of temperature and pain sensation

30. What are three proper ways for assessment of the trauma patient's extremities?
1. **Primary survey**—identification of life-threatening injury
2. **Secondary survey**—identification of limb-threatening injuries
3. **Continuous reevaluation**—systematic review to decrease the chances of missing any other musculoskeletal injury

31. What is compartment syndrome, and how it is treated?
    Compartment syndrome is an extremity-threatening and life-threatening condition observed when perfusion pressure falls below tissue pressure in a closed anatomic space. This is often secondary to a crush injury of the affected extremity. Owing to the high intracompartmental pressure, blood flow through the capillaries stops, causing cessation of oxygen delivery to the extremity's soft tissue (Fig. 14-1). Hypoxic injury causes cells to release vasoactive substances (e.g., histamine, serotonin) that increase endothelial permeability. This allows capillaries to continue fluid loss, which increases tissue pressure. Nerve conduction slows; tissue pH falls as a result of anaerobic metabolism, creating damage to surrounding tissue; and muscle tissue suffers necrosis, releasing myoglobinemia. The end result is loss of the extremity, which can be life

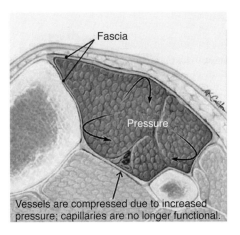

Fig. 14-1 Compartment syndrome in the anterior compartment. (From Flandry F: Compartment Syndrome: Swelling Out of Control. The Hughston Health Alert, vol 17, No. 2, Spring 2005. Copyright Hughston Sports Medicine Foundation, Inc., Columbus, Ga.)

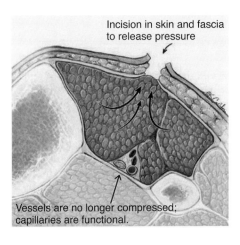

Fig. 14-2 Fasciotomy procedure. (From Flandry F: Compartment Syndrome: Swelling Out of Control. The Hughston Health Alert vol 17, No. 2, Spring 2005. Copyright Hughston Sports Medicine Foundation, Inc., Columbus, Ga.)

threatening. If intracompartmental pressures rises to >30 mm Hg, intervention is required. Fasciotomy is the only proven method for the treatment of compartment syndrome (Fig. 14-2).

32. What are the different degrees of thermal burns?
First-degree burn—identified by erythema with absence of blisters
Second-degree burn (partial-thickness burn)—identified by a mottled or erythematous appearance with swelling and blister formation. The surface may be wet and weeping; it is painful and hypersensitive.
Third-degree burn (full-thickness burn)—identified by skin that appears dark, translucent, leathery, mottled. The surface does not blanch with pressure. The skin is dry, painless, and red.

It is important to ascertain the depth of a burn to properly plan for wound care and predict cosmetic and functional outcome.

33. What is the most common cause of cardiac arrest in the pediatric patient?
Hypoxia is the most common cause of cardiac arrest in the pediatric patient. Before cardiac arrest, hypoventilation causes a respiratory acidosis, which is the most common acid-base abnormality during resuscitation of the pediatric trauma patient.

BIBLIOGRAPHY

1. Abubaker O, Benson K (eds): Oral and Maxillofacial Surgery Secrets. Philadelphia, 2001, Hanley & Belfus.
2. Advanced Trauma Life Support Student Course Manual, 7th ed. Chicago, 2004, American College of Surgeons.
3. Bickell WH, Wall MJ Jr, Pepe PE et al: Immediate versus delayed fluid resuscitation for hypotensive patients with penetrating torso injuries. N Engl J Med 331:1105-1109, 1994.
4. Burris D, Rhee P, Kaufmann C et al: Controlled resuscitation for uncontrolled hemorrhagic shock. J Trauma 46:216-223, 1999.
5. Mattox KL, Feliciano DV, Moore EE (eds): Trauma, 4th ed. New York, 2000, McGraw-Hill.
6. Pezzella AT, Silva WE, Lancey RA: Cardiothoracic trauma. Curr Probl Surg 35:649-650, 1998.
7. Root HD: Abdominal trauma and diagnostic peritoneal lavage revisited. Am J Surg 159:363-364, 1990.

15. TRACHEOSTOMY AND CRICOTHYROTOMY

Timothy S. Bartholomew, DDS, and A. Omar Abubaker, DMD, PhD

1. What are the different methods of achieving and securing an airway in an emergency?

Simple maneuvers for airway management include head tilt and chin lift or jaw thrust in the noninjured patient. Other adjunctive methods of airway management include the use of oral and nasal airways. The definitive method for airway control is by oral and nasal intubation. However, there may be situations in which this is difficult, impossible, or contraindicated, such as in severe panfacial trauma, massive upper airway bleeding, spasm of facial muscles, and laryngeal stenosis or deformities of the oronasopharynx. In such instances, if nonsurgical airway is unsuccessful, cricothyrotomy, whether by needle or surgical technique, may be the quickest, easiest, safest, and most effective way to obtain a patent airway.

2. What is the advantage of cricothyrotomy?

Cricothyrotomy should be viewed as the method of choice in procuring a patent airway in patients with acute airway obstruction. Cricothyrotomy has the following advantages over the standard tracheostomy, which makes it a very versatile procedure:

- It is faster.
- It is technically easier to perform with minimal instrumentation inside and outside an operating room setting.
- The incidence of operative and postoperative complications is low.
- It is safer to perform in patients with definite or suspected cervical spine injury or pharyngeal pathology.

3. When should cricothyrotomy be replaced with tracheostomy?

Unless the plan is to discontinue the access altogether, cricothyrotomy should be converted to tracheostomy within a maximum of 5-7 days.

4. What anatomy is pertinent to cricothyrotomy?

The thyroid cartilage consists of two quadrilateral-shaped laminae of hyaline cartilage that fuse anteriorly. The anterosuperior edge of the thyroid cartilage, the laryngeal prominence, is known as the Adam's apple. The angle at which these laminae converge is more acute in men than women and therefore is more easily located in men. The thyroid prominence is the most important landmark in the neck when performing a cricothyrotomy. The next cartilaginous ring below the larynx (and the only complete ring) is the cricoid cartilage. It helps to maintain the laryngeal lumen and forms the inferior border of the cricothyroid membrane. This membrane, another important landmark, is a dense fibroelastic membrane located between the thyroid cartilage superiorly and the cricoid cartilage inferiorly and bounded laterally by the cricothyroid muscles. It is approximately 22-30 mm wide, 9-10 mm high, and 13 mm inferior to the vocal cords. This membrane can be identified by palpating a notch (a slight indentation or dip) in the skin inferior to the laryngeal prominence in an adult. Although the right and left cricothyroid arteries (branches of the right and left superior thyroid arteries, respectively) traverse the superior part of the cricothyroid membrane, these vessels are not of clinical significance or the cause of problems when performing a cricothyrotomy.

The tissue layers involved in cricothyrotomy include the subcutaneous tissue, cervical fascia, cricothyroid membrane, and tracheal mucosa. The distance from skin to tracheal lumen is only 10 mm in most adult patients. In contrast to the main body of the trachea, the posterior wall at this level of the upper airway is rigidly separated from the esophagus by the tall posterior cricoid cartilage shield, making esophageal perforation unlikely during cricothyrotomy. The highly vascular thyroid gland lies over the trachea at the level of the second and third tracheal rings. If the tracheal rings or the thyroid gland is encountered when performing a cricothyrotomy, the incision is too low in the neck and must be redirected more superiorly.

5. What is the cricothyrotomy technique?

If there are no known or suspected cervical spine injuries, the patient's head may be hyperextended. Identify and palpate the notch or dip in the neck below the laryngeal prominence. Once the pertinent landmarks are identified, the right-handed surgeon then stabilizes the thyroid cartilage between the thumb and middle finger of his left hand and identifies the cricothyroid space with his left index finger. If local anesthetic is used, it should also be injected into the tracheal lumen to diminish the cough reflex during tube placement. A 3-4-cm transverse or vertical skin incision is made. A vertical incision is preferred in an emergency situation because if the skin incision is too high or too low, it may be extended easily, saving time and avoiding a second incision. A short, horizontal stab incision (about 1 cm long) is made with a No. 11 blade in the lower part of the cricothyroid membrane (nearer the cricoid ring) to avoid the cricothyroid arteries. Mayo scissors are spread horizontally in the incision to widen the space. Alternatively, the handle of the scalpel may be inserted and twisted 90 degrees. Next, the opening is enlarged with Trousseau dilators or a curved hemostat. After stabilization of the larynx, the tracheostomy tube is inserted, the dilator or hemostat is removed, and the cuff of the tracheostomy tube is inflated (Fig. 15-1).

6. When is a tracheostomy the preferred emergency surgical airway?

In pediatric patients younger than ages 10-12. The small 3-mm-wide cricothyroid membrane and poorly defined anatomic landmarks make cricothyrotomy all but impossible in children.

7. What are the indications for a tracheostomy?

- Airway obstruction, such as from trauma, foreign bodies, irritants, anomalies, vasomotor incidents, laryngeal dysfunction, tumors, and obstructive sleep apnea syndrome
- For control of mucous secretion retention caused by inability to cough or expectorate, as in comatose and trauma patients
- Mechanical respiratory support, as in acute or chronic respiratory or central nervous system (CNS) diseases, multiple trauma patients
- Elective, such as for major head and neck procedures

8. What are the surface anatomy landmarks for tracheostomy?

The most important anatomic landmarks for the tracheostomy procedure are the thyroid notch, cricoid ring, sternal notch, and innominate artery, which is above the sternal notch in

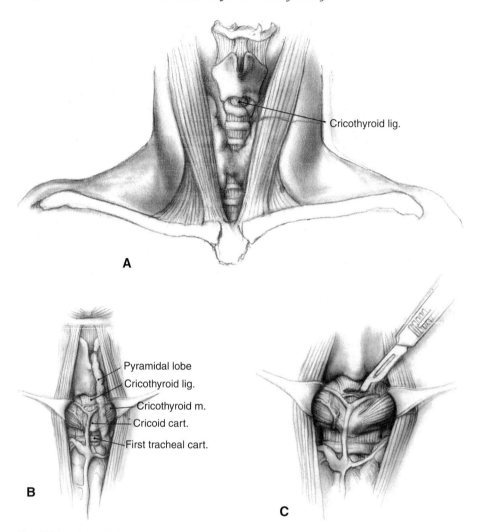

Fig. 15-1   **A** and **B**, Surface anatomy and landmarks for cricothyroidotomy. **C,** A horizontal stab incision is made through the ligament. (From Morris WM: Cricothyroidotomy. In Loré JM, Medina JE [eds]: An Atlas of Head and Neck Surgery, 4th ed. Philadelphia, 2005, Saunders.)

approximately 25% of patients. The location for skin incision (approximately 4-6 cm long) for tracheostomy should be about 2 cm below the cricoid ring or midway between this ring and the sternal notch.

9.   From skin to the trachea, what are the layers encountered during dissection for a tracheostomy?

- Skin
- Subcutaneous connective tissue
- Platysma
- Investing fascia
- Linea alba of the infrahyoid muscles
- Thyroid isthmus
- Pretracheal fascia
- Tracheal rings

10. What are the important principles in tracheostomy?
- Hyperextension of the neck, except in patients with suspected cervical spine injuries, facilitates the procedure.
- Always suture the flange of the tracheostomy tube to the skin.
- Never suture the skin incision tightly around the tube; leave the wound open to allow air to leak out.
- Upon decannulation, place tape across the stoma; do not suture the stoma closed.
- The cricoid cartilage and first tracheal ring must not be injured.
- The incision must not extend below the fourth ring (usually at rings 2 and 3).

11. What is the technique for performing a tracheostomy?
A 4- to 6-cm incision is carried through skin, subcutaneous tissue, and platysma. Flaps are retracted superiorly, and a vertical incision is made in the fascia overlying the strap muscles. After the cricoid cartilage is identified, the thyroid isthmus may be retracted superiorly or divided and tied off. This exposes the second, third, and fourth tracheal rings. Using a hypodermic needle and a syringe, aspirate air from the trachea and inject 1-2 mL of local anesthetic to minimize coughing when entering the trachea. Make a 1-cm horizontal incision into the trachea above and below the ring of choice. This ring is cut so that a small rectangular window into the trachea is made. Place sutures in each side of the trachea to facilitate locating the tracheal stoma should the tube become dislodged. Insert the tracheostomy tube into the opening, taking care not to tear the cuff and not to insert the tube in the space anterior or lateral to the trachea. Once the tube is in place, inflate the cuff and check the chest for breath sounds. Leave the skin edges around the tube open or only partially closed with nonresorbable sutures, leaving a small space to minimize the danger of air escape into the subcutaneous tissue. Suture the tube to the skin, and secure it with a tape tied in a square knot around the neck (Fig. 15-2).

12. What major vessels may be encountered during tracheostomy?
The anterior jugular vein and the jugular venous arch are found in the suprasternal space of Burns. The infrahyoid vein and artery and thyroid artery all lie in the space between the pretracheal and infrahyoid fascia.

13. Which tracheal rings are covered by the thyroid isthmus?
The second through fourth rings.

14. What are the advantages of an inverted-U entrance incision into the trachea?
This incision prevents the cannula from being inserted anterior to the trachea. In addition, the patient can breath more easily through the stoma if the cannula is lost, and changing the cannula is easier.

15. What instrument is used to assist with insertion of the tracheostomy tube?
The Trousseau dilator.

16. Why are high-volume, low-pressure tracheostomy tube cuffs preferable?
High-volume, low-pressure tracheostomy tube cuffs prevent occlusion of submucosal capillaries of the tracheostomy and therefore decrease the risk of tracheal stenosis (submucosal capillaries are occluded at pressures >25 cm H_2O).

17. What are the possible intraoperative complications associated with tracheostomy?
Hemorrhage. The anterior jugular system and its anastomoses, thyroid isthmus, high aortic arch (in children and the elderly) may be elevated into the surgical field by neck hyperextension, thyroid veins and arteries, left innominate or brachiocephalic veins, or erosion of the tracheostomy tube through the anterior tracheal wall.

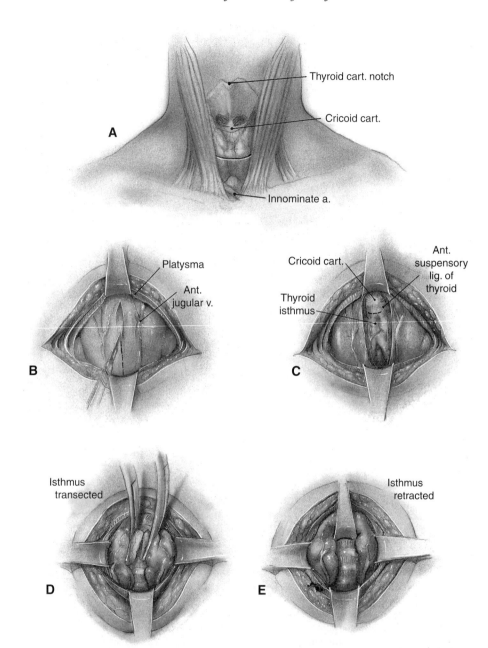

Fig. 15-2 **A,** Surface anatomy landmarks for tracheostomy. **B,** After skin and platysma incisions are completed, a vertical incision is made in the fascia at midline between the strap muscles. **C,** The cricoid cartilage and thyroid isthmus exposed. **D-F,** The thyroid isthmus transected, retracted, and secured with ligature.

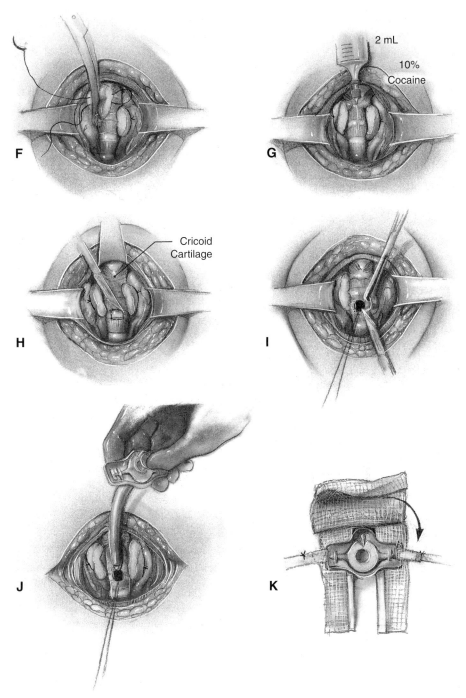

Fig. 15-2, cont'd **G,** Using a smaller gauge needle, air is aspirated into the syringe, and 2% lidocaine (Xylocaine) is injected into the lumen of the trachea. **H** and **I,** A window is cut into the second, third, or fourth ring of the trachea. Alternatively, the ring is left pedicle inferiorly and sutured to the skin. **J** and **K,** The tracheostomy tube is inserted into the trachea and secured in place. (From Loré JM: The trachea and mediastinum. In Loré JM, Medina JE [eds]: An Atlas of Head and Neck Surgery, 4th ed. Philadelphia, 2005, Saunders.)

Subcutaneous emphysema. This can result from a wound that has been closed too tightly around the tracheostomy tube or sutures that are placed after decannulation.

Recurrent laryngeal nerve injury. The laryngeal nerve innervates the trachea, esophagus, and all the intrinsic muscles of the larynx except the cricothyroid. Damage to this nerve produces vocal cord paralysis.

Pneumothorax or pneumomediastinum. These are more common in pediatrics, in which the lung apex extends farther into the lower neck. It can also result from false passage of a tracheostomy tube between the anterior tracheal surface and the mediastinal tissues.

18. What are the possible postoperative complications associated with tracheostomy?

Atelectasis. This is caused if blood or foreign material is aspirated into the tube or if the tracheostomy tube is directed into one mainstem bronchus, resulting in collapse of the opposite lung.

Tracheoesophageal fistula. This rarely occurs in an orderly tracheostomy. It may accompany emergency stab-type tracheotomy or if an ill-fitting tracheostomy tube rubs against the posterior tracheal wall.

Subglottic edema and tracheal stenosis. These are preventable by entering the trachea below the second tracheal ring. The most common symptom is increasing stridor.

Pneumonia

Difficult decannulation

Persistent fistula after decannulation. Vertical incisions heal more rapidly than horizontal ones. This may require operative closure with resection of the tracheotomy tract.

Tracheo-innominate fistula. Minor bleeding from tracheostomy tube may herald this. Overinflating the tracheostomy cuff or endotracheal tube while attempting to compress the innominate artery anteriorly against the sternum with a finger inserted through the tracheostomy wound usually treats such bleeding. This is usually associated with an anomalous, superiorly placed artery crossing the trachea or use of a tracheal ring below the four rings.

19. What are the steps involved in the decannulation of the tracheotomy?

Once the problem that required tracheostomy has been resolved, the process of removing the tracheostomy tube should begin. The initial step in this process is to change to a smaller size tube. Then, a capping trial can be attempted: The cuff is deflated for progressively longer periods of time until the patient can tolerate this with good oxygenation and phonation. If the patient tolerates this, remove the tube altogether. Reapproximate the wound edges and place additional pressure dressing. Instruct the patient to apply pressure on the dressing when talking and coughing for the first 3-5 days. Change the pressure dressing as needed. Occasionally, rigid endoscopy may be done to assess the patency of the aerodigestive tract.

20. What is the postoperative care for a tracheostomy?

Once the tracheostomy procedure is completed, diligent postoperative care and observation are essential to prevent postoperative complication associated with this procedure. Both the surgeons and the nursing staff should supply this care, including:

- Performing a chest x-ray in the recovery room to check tube position
- Changing the tube on the third or fourth postoperative day
- Using humidified air to keep the tracheal mucosa moist
- Frequently suctioning the tracheostomy tube, because the tracheotomy reduces the efficiency of coughing and initially there are more secretions from the trachea
- Performing routine wound care and changing the tracheostomy tube

BIBLIOGRAPHY

1. Bradley PJ: Management of airway and tracheostomy. In Hibbert J (ed): Otolaryngology: Laryngology and Head and Neck Surgery, 6th ed. Bath, England, 1997, Butterworth-Heinemann.
2. Braun RF, Cutilli BJ: Cricothyrotomy. In Braun RF, Cutilli BJ (eds): Manual of Emergency Medical Treatment for the Dental Team. Baltimore, 1999, Williams & Wilkins.
3. Demas PN, Sotereanos GC: The use of tracheotomy in oral and maxillofacial surgery. J Oral Maxillofac Surg 46:483-486, 1988.
4. Feinberg SE, Peterson LJ: Use of cricothyrotomy in oral and maxillofacial surgery. J Oral Maxillofac Surg 45:873-878, 1987.
5. Lewis RJ: Tracheostomy. Indications, timing, and complications. Clinic Chest Med 13:137-149, 1992.
6. Loré JM: Emergency procedures. In Loré JM, Medina JE (eds): An Atlas of Head and Neck Surgery, 4th ed. Philadelphia, 2005, Saunders.
7. Montgomery WW: Surgery of the Upper Respiratory System, 2nd ed. Philadelphia, 1989, Lea & Febiger.
8. Parsons DS, Smith WC: Difficult tracheostomy decannulation. In Gates GA (ed): Current Therapy in Otolaryngology—Head and Neck Surgery, 6th ed. St Louis, 1998, Mosby.
9. Weissler MC: Tracheostomy and intubation. In Bailey BJ (ed): Head and Neck Surgery—Otolaryngology. Philadelphia, 1993, J.B. Lippincott.

16. MALIGNANT HYPERTHERMIA

Kathy A. Banks, DMD

1. What is malignant hyperthermia (MH)?

A hypermetabolic state involving skeletal muscle that is precipitated by certain anesthetic agents in genetically susceptible individuals.

2. Which patients are at risk of developing MH?

Patients at risk of developing MH include those with:

- A diagnosis of MH (see question 6)
- A first-degree relative with a diagnosis of MH
- An elevated resting creatine kinase (CK) and family with suspected MH tendency
- Central core disease
- Musculoskeletal disease associated with MH (see question 5)

3. How is MH inherited?

MH is an autosomal-dominant disease that is thought to be caused by a defect on chromosome 19. Chromosome 7q and chromosome 17 also have been implicated. It also has been postulated that MH and central core disease may be allelic and thus can be co-inherited.

4. What is the incidence of MH?

Less than 0.5% of all patients who are exposed to anesthetic agents.

5. With which muscle diseases has MH been associated?

- Dystrophinopathy
- Phosphorylase deficiency
- Minicore disease
- Myotonia
- King-Denborough and Barnes myopathies

6. How are susceptible patients diagnosed?

The diagnosis of MH in susceptible patients is made by the muscle contracture test. Muscle fibers from MH-positive patients produce an exaggerated response to electrical stimulation when exposed to halothane and caffeine. When a muscle contracture test is not possible, muscle biopsy may be performed. Characteristic findings on muscle biopsy include variable muscle fiber size, increased number of internalized nuclei, and the presence of "moth-eaten" fibers. These findings are nonspecific and cannot be used alone to establish diagnosis. Patients with MH also may have elevated baseline CK levels.

7. Which anesthetic drugs are known to trigger MH?

Inhalation anesthetics:
- Halothane
- Enflurane
- Isoflurane
- Desflurane
- Sevoflurane

Depolarizing neuromuscular blockade agents:
- Succinylcholine
- Decamethonium
- Suxamethonium

8. Which other drugs are suspected of causing MH?
- Ketamine
- Catecholamines
- Phenothiazines
- Monoamine oxidase (MAO) inhibitors

9. What are the five major clinical characteristics of MH?
1. Acidosis
2. Rigidity
3. Fever
4. Hypermetabolism
5. Myoglobinuria

10. What are the three early presenting signs and symptoms of MH during an anesthetic procedure?
1. Early masseter contracture following administration of succinylcholine
2. An unexplained rise in end-tidal CO_2 following induction of anesthesia
3. An unexplained tachycardia following induction of anesthesia

11. What are the other clinical findings in MH?
- Cyanosis and skin mottling
- Hypertension
- Tachypnea
- Elevated CK and potassium
- Cardiac dysrhythmias
- Cardiac arrest

12. What is the pathogenesis of MH?

Abnormal calcium channels of the sarcoplasmic reticulum impair the ability to sequester calcium, which leads to decreased control of cytosolic calcium levels. The defect causes a calcium-induced calcium release (positive feedback) that is abnormal in skeletal muscle. Exposure to certain "MH-triggering" anesthetics causes a sudden, prolonged release of calcium. This excessive release of calcium leads to excessive muscle contraction and oxygen consumption, elevated temperature, and depletion of high-energy phosphate compounds. Energy exhaustion limits calcium reuptake by the sarcoplasmic reticulum, ultimately leading to cell lysis. Glycogenolysis and leakage of organic acids into the blood result in acidosis. The hypermetabolic state manifests as muscle rigidity, acidosis, hypercarbia, hypertension, and tachypnea. Potassium and myoglobin released from the lysed cells cause hyperkalemia and myoglobinuria.

Hyperkalemia, hypercarbia, and acidosis lead to cardiac dysrhythmia or arrest. Myoglobinuria leads to renal failure. Proteins released from lysed myocytes such as CK can be measured.

13. What are the effects of myoglobinuria associated with MH on the kidneys?
Rhabdomyolysis results in release of excessive amounts of heme protein myoglobin in the urine. The urine becomes cola colored. Acute tubular obstruction with myoglobin and free chelatable iron leads to necrosis and renal failure.

14. What is the initial management of an acute attack of MH in the adult patient?
1. Discontinue the anesthetic agent.
2. Hyperventilate with 100% oxygen.
3. Administer dantrolene sodium intravenously until heart rate and end-tidal CO_2 decrease.
4. Begin infusion of iced intravenous (IV) fluids (avoid lactated Ringer's).
5. Cool patient with iced saline lavage of stomach, bladder, and rectum; cooling blankets; and ice packs.
6. Draw blood for serum electrolytes, arterial blood gases, prothrombin time (PT), partial thromboplastin time (PTT), and myoglobin studies.
7. Monitor vital signs, electrocardiogram (ECG), end-tidal CO_2, blood gases, temperature, and urine output.
8. Treat metabolic acidosis with sodium bicarbonate.
9. Treat arrhythmias with antiarrhythmic drugs (avoid calcium channel blockers).
10. Treat hyperkalemia with glucose and insulin.
11. Maintain urinary output of greater than 2 mL/kg/hr with hydration and diuretics (furosemide or mannitol).

15. How is cardiac arrest managed in children during an acute MH attack?
Treat hyperkalemia first.

16. What is the postoperative management of a patient who has experienced an acute attack of MH?
- Continuous monitoring in the intensive care unit (ICU) setting for a minimum of 24 hr
- Follow-up measurements of blood gases, potassium, calcium, and urine myoglobin
- Administration of IV dantrolene sodium

17. What is dantrolene sodium, and how does it work?
Dantrolene sodium is a hydantoin-derivative muscle relaxant that exerts its muscle-relaxant effect by interfering with excitation-contraction coupling in the muscle fiber. Dantrolene sodium is used in the treatment of MH because it blocks calcium release from the sarcoplasmic reticulum calcium channels.

18. What is the recommended dose of dantrolene sodium for treatment of MH?
- 2-3 mg/kg IV every 5 min up to a total dose of 10 mg/kg
- 1 mg/kg IV every 6 hr for 24-48 hr in recovery
- Then oral dantrolene for an additional 24 hr

19. What is the mortality rate associated with MH?
The mortality rate is greater than 40% when dantrolene is not administered. The mortality rate approaches 0% with the administration of dantrolene and appropriate treatment.

20. How can MH be prevented?
- Those at risk for MH should not be given triggering agents.
- Identify patients at risk for development of MH in the preoperative phase.

21. How do you manage a known or suspected MH patient?

When a known or suspected MH patient is about to undergo a procedure that requires the use of an anesthetic agent, a series of steps can be taken to prevent the occurrence of MH:

1. Preoperative preparations
   - Ensure that the anesthetic vaporizers on the anesthesia machine are disabled by removing, draining, or taping in the "off" position.
   - Flow 10 L/min O_2 through the circuit via the ventilator for at least 20 min. If the fresh gas hose is replaced, 10 min is adequate. During this time, a disposable, unused breathing bag should be attached to the Y-piece of the circle system, and the ventilator should be set to inflate the bag periodically.
   - Use a new or disposable breathing circuit.
   - Place a cooling blanket on the table.
   - Dantrolene prophylaxis should be considered on an individual basis but is not recommended for most MH-susceptible patients. When used, dosage is 2.5 mg/kg IV starting immediately before anesthesia. Dantrolene can worsen muscle weakness in patients with muscle disease and should be used with caution. For most procedures, even those requiring general anesthesia, dantrolene prophylaxis may be omitted.

2. Intraoperative considerations
   - Consider an alternative anesthetic technique, such as spinal, epidural, regional, or local anesthesia. Local anesthetics do not trigger MH; thus any type of regional anesthesia is safe for MH-susceptible patients.
   - Safe general anesthesia agents include benzodiazepines, opioids, barbiturates, propofol, ketamine, nitrous oxide, and etomidate. Pancuronium, atracurium, vecuronium, doxacurium, or curare may be used for relaxation. Neostigmine and atropine are used for reversal without problems.
   - Avoid using unsafe drugs and MH triggers such as halothane, enflurane, isoflurane, desflurane, sevoflurane, ether, methoxyflurane, cyclopropane, and succinylcholine.
   - Use adequate monitoring techniques to check blood pressure, central temperature, ECG, pulse oximeter, and capnograph. Monitoring the respiratory rate and volume is strongly recommended if a general anesthetic is used. Use an arterial line, central venous pressure, or other invasive monitor when appropriate for the surgical procedure and underlying medical condition.

22. What conditions mimic MH?
- Endocrine disorders (thyrotoxicosis, anticholinergic syndrome)
- Sepsis
- Drug use (amphetamines, cocaine)

23. What is molecular genetic testing for MH?
- A DNA sample may be obtained from a person's blood and evaluated for one of the genetic changes that predispose for MH.
- If a person is known to be MH susceptible and has a DNA change known to be causative for MH, then his or her relatives may be diagnosed as MH susceptible through a DNA test and will not have to undergo a muscle biopsy test.
- If the DNA test in an MH-susceptible person is negative for mutations, this does not mean the patient is at risk for MH.
- The muscle contracture test is still the gold standard for testing for MH.

24. Is there a hotline or website to obtain more information on MH?

Yes. The telephone hotline is in operation 24 hours a day, 7 days a week to help in the management of ongoing MH. Within the United States, the number is (800) MH-HYPER.

Outside the United States, call (800) 644-9737 or (315) 464-7079. In addition, information can be faxed free of charge by calling (800) 440-9990. The URL is http://www.mhaus.org.

BIBLIOGRAPHY

1. Bertorini TE: Myoglobinuria, malignant hyperthermia, neuroleptic malignant syndrome and serotonin syndrome. Neurol Clin 15:649-671, 1977.
2. Carr AS, Lerman J, Cunliffe M et al: Incidence of malignant hyperthermia reactions in 2214 patients undergoing muscle biopsy. Can J Anesth 42:281-286, 1995.
3. Gronert GA, Mott J, Lee J: Aetiology of malignant hyperthermia. Br J Anaesth 60:253-267, 1988.
4. Malignant Hyperthermia Association of the United States, http://www.mhaus.org
5. Malignant Hyperthermia Association of the United States: Preventing Malignant Hyperthermia: An Anesthesia Protocol [brochure]. Sherburne, NY, 1999, MHAUS.
6. Murphy F: Hazards of anesthesia. In Longnecker DE, Murphy FL (eds): Dripps/Eckenhoff/Vandam: Introduction to Anesthesia, 9th ed. Philadelphia, 1997, Saunders.

Part V
Management Considerations

17. CARDIOVASCULAR DISEASES

A. Omar Abubaker, DMD, PhD, and James A. Giglio, DDS, MEd

ISCHEMIC HEART DISEASE, MYOCARDIAL INFARCTION, AND VALVULAR HEART DISEASE

1.   What are the known risk factors for the development of ischemic heart disease (IHD)?
Age, male gender, positive family history, hypertension, smoking, hypercholesterolemia, and diabetes mellitus. Sedentary lifestyle and obesity are often associated factors.

2.   What are the determinants of myocardial oxygen supply and demand?
Oxygen (O_2) supply to the myocardium is determined by oxygen content and coronary blood flow. Oxygen content can be calculated by the following equation:

$$O_2 \text{ content} = [1.39 \text{ mL } O_2/\text{g of hemoglobin} \times \text{hemoglobin (g/dL)} \times \% \text{ saturation}] + [0.003 \times \text{Pao}_2]$$

Coronary blood flow occurs mainly during diastole, especially to the ventricular endocardium. Coronary perfusion pressure is determined by the difference between diastolic blood pressure and left ventricular end-diastolic pressure (LVEDP). Anemia, hypoxemia, tachycardia, diastolic hypotension, hypocapnia (coronary vasoconstriction), coronary occlusion (IHD), vasospasm, increased LVEDP, and hypertrophied myocardium all may adversely affect myocardial O_2 supply.
Myocardial O_2 demand is determined by heart rate, contractility, and wall tension. Increases in heart rate increase myocardial work and decrease the relative time spent in diastole (decreased supply). Contractility increases in response to sympathetic stimulation, which increases O_2 demand. Wall tension is the product of intraventricular pressure and radius. Increased ventricular volume (preload) and increased blood pressure (BP) (afterload) both increase wall tension and O_2 demand.

3.   What is the pathophysiology of myocardial ischemia?
Ischemia occurs when coronary blood flow is inadequate to meet the needs of the myocardium. Atherosclerotic lesions that occlude 50%-75% of the vessel lumen are considered hemodynamically significant. Nonstenotic causes of ischemia include aortic valve disease, left ventricular hypertrophy, ostial occlusion, coronary embolism, coronary arteritis, and vasospasm.
The right coronary artery system is dominant in 80%-90% of people and supplies the sinoatrial node, atrioventricular node, and right ventricle. Right-sided coronary artery disease often manifests as heart block and dysrhythmias. The left main coronary artery gives rise to the circumflex artery and left anterior descending artery, which supply the majority of the interventricular septum and left ventricular wall. Significant stenosis of the left main coronary artery (left main disease) or the proximal circumflex and left anterior descending arteries (left main equivalent) may cause severely depressed myocardial function during ischemia.

4. What is the pathogenesis of a perioperative myocardial infarction?

A myocardial infarction (MI) is usually caused by platelet aggregation, vasoconstriction, and thrombus formation at the site of an atheromatous plaque in a coronary artery. Sudden increases in myocardial O_2 demand (tachycardia, hypertension) or decreases in O_2 supply (hypotension, hypoxemia, anemia) can precipitate MI in patients with IHD. Complications of MI include dysrhythmias, hypotension, congestive heart failure (CHF), acute mitral regurgitation, pericarditis, ventricular thrombus formation, ventricular rupture, and death.

5. What clinical factors increase the risk of a perioperative MI following noncardiac surgery?

IHD (prior MI or angina) and CHF are historically the strongest predictors of an increased risk for perioperative MI. Other risk factors include valvular heart disease (particularly aortic stenosis), arrhythmias caused by underlying heart disease, advanced age, type of surgical procedure, and poor general medical status. Hypertension alone does not place a patient at increased risk for perioperative MI, but these patients are at increased risk for IHD, CHF, and stroke.

6. How can cardiac function be evaluated on history and physical exam?

If a patient's exercise capacity is excellent even in the presence of IHD, then chances are good that the patient will be able to tolerate the stresses of surgery. Poor exercise tolerance in the absence of pulmonary or other systemic disease indicates an inadequate cardiac reserve. All patients should be questioned about their ability to perform daily activities, such as cleaning, yard work, shopping, and golfing, for example. The ability to climb two to three flights of stairs without significant symptoms (angina, dyspnea, syncope) is usually an indication of adequate cardiac reserve. Signs and symptoms of CHF including dyspnea, orthopnea, paroxysmal nocturnal dyspnea, peripheral edema, jugular venous distention, a third heart sound, rales, and hepatomegaly must be recognized preoperatively.

7. What is the significance of a history of angina pectoris?

Angina is a symptom of myocardial ischemia, and nearly all patients with angina have coronary artery disease. Stable angina is defined as no change in the onset, severity, and duration of chest pain for at least 60 days. Syncope, shortness of breath, or dizziness that accompanies angina may indicate severe myocardial dysfunction resulting from ischemia. Patients with unstable angina are at high risk for developing an MI and should be referred for medical evaluation immediately. Patients with diabetes mellitus and hypertension have a much higher incidence of silent ischemia. Perioperatively, most ischemic episodes are silent (as determined by ambulatory and postoperative electrocardiogram [ECG]) but probably significant in the final outcome of surgery.

8. Should all cardiac medications be continued throughout the perioperative period?

Patients with a history of IHD are usually taking medications intended to decrease myocardial oxygen demand by decreasing the heart rate, preload, or contractile state (beta blockers, calcium channel antagonists, nitrates) and to increase the oxygen supply by causing coronary vasodilation (nitrates). These drugs are generally continued throughout the perioperative period. Abrupt withdrawal of beta blockers can cause rebound increases in heart rate and BP. Calcium channel blockers can exaggerate the myocardial depressant effects of inhaled anesthetics but should be continued perioperatively.

9. What ECG findings support the diagnosis of IHD?

The resting 12-lead ECG remains a low-cost, effective screening tool in the detection of IHD. It should be evaluated for the presence of ST-segment depression or elevation, T-wave inversion, old MI as demonstrated by Q waves, disturbances in conduction and rhythm, and left ventricular hypertrophy. Ischemic changes in leads II, III, and aVF suggest right coronary artery disease, leads I and aVL monitor circumflex artery distribution, and leads V3-V5 look at the distribution of the left anterior descending artery. Poor progression of anterior forces suggests significant left ventricular dysfunction, possibly related to IHD.

10. **What tests performed by medical consultants can help further evaluate patients with known or suspected IHD?**

Exercise ECG is a noninvasive test that attempts to produce ischemic changes on ECG (ST depression = 1 mm from baseline) or symptoms by having the patient exercise to maximum capacity. Information obtained relates to the thresholds of heart rate and BP that can be tolerated. Maximal heart rates and BP response, as well as symptoms, guide interpretation of results.

Exercise thallium scintigraphy increases the sensitivity and specificity of the exercise ECG. The isotope thallium is almost completely taken up from the coronary circulation by the myocardium and can then be visualized radiographically. Poorly perfused areas that later refill with contrast delineate areas of myocardium at risk for ischemia. Fixed perfusion defects indicate infarcted myocardium.

Dipyridamole thallium imaging is useful in patients who are unable to exercise. This testing is frequently required in patients with peripheral vascular disease who are at high risk for IHD and limited by claudication. Dipyridamole is a potent coronary vasodilator that causes differential flow between normal and diseased coronary arteries detectable by thallium imaging.

Echocardiography can be used to evaluate left ventricular and valvular function and to measure ejection fraction. Stress echocardiography (dobutamine echo) can be used to evaluate new or worsened regional wall motion abnormalities in the pharmacologically stressed heart. Areas of wall motion abnormality are considered at risk for ischemia.

Coronary angiography is the gold standard for defining the coronary anatomy. Valvular and ventricular function can be evaluated and measurements of hemodynamic indices taken. Because angiography is invasive, it is reserved for patients who require further evaluation based on previous tests or who have a high probability of severe coronary disease.

11. **Based on the initial evaluation, which patients should be referred for further testing?**

Patients at risk for IHD but with good exercise tolerance may not require further work-up, especially if they are undergoing procedures with a low to moderate risk of perioperative MI. Patients with decreased exercise tolerance for unclear reasons or with unreliable histories should be evaluated with dipyridamole thallium testing.

Patients with documented IHD (prior MI or chronic stable angina) with good exercise tolerance can sometimes proceed with low-risk surgery without further evaluation. Patients with known IHD and poor exercise tolerance should be referred for dipyridamole thallium testing or coronary angiography before all but the most minor surgical procedures.

12. **Which surgical procedures carry the highest risk of perioperative MI?**

In general, major abdominal, thoracic, and emergency surgeries carry the highest risk of perioperative MI. The highest-risk noncardiac procedure is aortic aneurysm repair. These patients have a high incidence of IHD, and cross-clamping of the aorta during surgery and postoperative complications can place great stress on the heart.

13. **How long should a patient with a recent MI wait before undergoing elective noncardiac surgery?**

The risk of reinfarction during surgery after a prior MI has traditionally depended on the time interval between the MI and the procedure. The highest risk of reinfarction is between 0 and 3 months post-MI; lower risk is from 3-6 months; and a baseline risk level is reached after 6 months (approximately 5% in most studies).

14. **What if surgery cannot safely be delayed for 6 months?**

The patient's functional status after rehabilitation from an MI is probably more important than the absolute time interval. Patients with ongoing symptoms may be candidates for coronary revascularization before their noncardiac procedure. Patients who quickly return to good functional status after an MI can be considered for necessary noncardiac surgery between 6 weeks and 3 months without undue added risk.

15. How is premedication useful in the setting of IHD and surgery?

Patient anxiety can lead to catecholamine secretion and increased oxygen demand. In this regard, the goal of premedication is to produce sedation and amnesia without causing deleterious myocardial depression, hypotension, or hypoxemia. Morphine, scopolamine, and benzodiazepines, alone or in combination, are popular choices to achieve these goals. All premedicated patients should receive supplemental oxygen. Patients who use sublingual nitroglycerin should have access to their medication. Transdermal nitroglycerin can be applied in the perioperative period as well.

16. What are the hemodynamic goals of induction and maintenance of general anesthesia in patients with IHD?

The anesthesiologist's goal must be to maintain the balance between myocardial O_2 supply and demand throughout the perioperative period. During induction, wide swings in heart rate and BP should be avoided. Ketamine should be avoided because of the resultant tachycardia and hypertension. Prolonged laryngoscopy should be avoided, and the anesthesiologist may wish to blunt the stimulation of laryngoscopy and intubation by the addition of opiates, beta blockers, or laryngotracheal or intravenous lidocaine.

Maintenance drugs are chosen with knowledge of the patient's ventricular function. In patients with good left ventricular function, the cardiac depressant and vasodilatory effects of inhaled anesthetics may reduce myocardial O_2 demand. A narcotic-based technique may be chosen to avoid undue myocardial depression in patients with poor left ventricular function. Muscle relaxants with minimal cardiovascular effects are usually preferred.

BP and heart rate should be maintained near baseline values. This can be accomplished by blunting sympathetic stimulation with adequate analgesia and aggressively treating hypertension (anesthetics, nitroglycerin, nitroprusside, beta blockers), hypotension (fluids, sympathomimetics, inotropic drugs), and tachycardia (fluids, anesthetics, beta blockers).

17. What monitors are useful for detecting ischemia intraoperatively?

The V5 precordial lead is the most sensitive single ECG lead for detecting ischemia and should be monitored routinely in patients at risk for IHD. Lead II can detect ischemia of the right coronary artery distribution and is the most useful lead for monitoring P waves and cardiac rhythm.

Transesophageal echocardiography can provide continuous intraoperative monitoring of left ventricular function. Detection of regional wall motion abnormalities with this technique is the most sensitive for myocardial ischemia.

The pulmonary artery occlusion (wedge) pressure gives an indirect measurement of left ventricular volume and is a useful guide for optimizing intravascular fluid therapy. Sudden increases in the wedge pressure may indicate acute left ventricular dysfunction resulting from ischemia. The routine use of pulmonary artery catheters in patients with IHD has not been shown to improve outcome. However, close hemodynamic monitoring (including pulmonary artery catheter data) may be beneficial, depending on the patient's condition and the nature of the surgical procedure.

18. What is the basic pathophysiology of valvular heart disease?

Mitral and aortic stenosis cause pressure overload of the left ventricle, which produces hypertrophy with a cardiac chamber of normal size. Mitral and aortic regurgitation causes volume overload, which leads to hypertrophy with a dilated chamber. The net effect of left-sided valvular lesions is an impedance to forward flow of blood into the systemic circulation. Although right-sided valvular lesions occur, left-sided lesions are more common and usually more hemodynamically significant. This chapter deals only with left-sided lesions.

19. What are common findings of the history and physical exam in patients with valvular heart disease?

A history of rheumatic fever, intravenous drug abuse, or heart murmur should alert the examiner to the possibility of valvular heart disease. Exercise tolerance is frequently decreased. Patients may exhibit signs and symptoms of CHF, including dyspnea, orthopnea, fatigue, pulmonary rales, jugular venous congestion, hepatic congestion, and dependent edema. Compensatory increases in sympathetic nervous system tone manifest as resting tachycardia, anxiety, and diaphoresis. Angina may occur in patients with hypertrophied left ventricle, even in the absence of coronary artery disease. Atrial fibrillation frequently accompanies diseases of the mitral valve.

20. Which tests are useful in the evaluation of valvular heart disease?

The **EGC** should be examined for evidence of ischemia, arrhythmias, atrial enlargement, and ventricular hypertrophy. The **chest radiograph** may show enlargement of cardiac chambers, suggest pulmonary hypertension, or reveal pulmonary edema and pleural effusions. **Cardiac catheterization** is the gold standard in the evaluation of such patients and determines pressures in various heart chambers, as well as pressure gradients across valves. **Cardiac angiography** allows visualization of the coronary arteries and heart chambers.

21. How is echocardiography helpful?

Doppler echocardiography characterizes ventricular function and valve function. It can be used to measure the valve orifice area and transvalvular pressure gradients, which are measures of the severity of valvular dysfunction. The function of prosthetic valves is also measured echocardiographically.

22. Which invasive monitors aid the anesthesiologist in the perioperative period?

An arterial catheter provides beat-to-beat BP measurement and continuous access to the bloodstream for sampling. Pulmonary artery catheters enable the anesthetist to measure cardiac output and provide central access for the infusion of vasoactive drugs. The pulmonary capillary wedge pressure is an index of left ventricular filling and is useful for guiding intravenous fluid therapy. Transesophageal echocardiography can be used intraoperatively to evaluate left ventricular volume and function, to detect ischemia (segmental wall motion abnormalities), and intracardiac air, and to examine valve function before and after repair.

23. What is a pressure-volume loop?

A pressure-volume loop plots left ventricular pressure against volume through one complete cardiac cycle. Each valvular lesion has a unique profile that suggests compensatory physiologic changes by the left ventricle.

24. What is the pathophysiology of aortic stenosis?

Aortic stenosis is a fixed outlet obstruction to left ventricular ejection. Concentric hypertrophy (thickened ventricular wall with normal chamber size) develops in response to the increased intraventricular systolic pressure and increased wall tension necessary to maintain forward flow. Ventricular compliance decreases, and end-diastolic pressures increase. Contractility and ejection fraction are usually maintained until late in the disease process. Atrial contraction may account for up to 40% of ventricular filling (normally 20%). Aortic stenosis is usually secondary to calcification of a congenital bicuspid valve or rheumatic heart disease. Patients often present with angina, dyspnea, syncope, or sudden death. Angina occurs in the absence of coronary artery disease because the thickened myocardium is susceptible to ischemia (increased oxygen demand)

and elevated end-diastolic pressure reduces coronary perfusion pressure (decreased oxygen supply).

25. What is the pathophysiology of aortic insufficiency?

Chronic aortic insufficiency is usually rheumatic in origin. Acute aortic insufficiency may be secondary to trauma, endocarditis, or dissection of a thoracic aortic aneurysm. The left ventricle experiences volume overload, because part of the stroke volume regurgitates across the incompetent aortic valve in diastole. Eccentric hypertrophy (dilated and thickened chamber) develops. A dilated orifice, slower heart rate (relatively more time spent in diastole), and increased systemic vascular resistance increase the amount of regurgitant flow. Compliance and stroke volume may be significantly increased in chronic aortic insufficiency, whereas contractility gradually diminishes. Ideally, such patients should have valve replacement surgery before the onset of irreversible myocardial damage. In acute aortic insufficiency, the left ventricle is subjected to rapid, massive volume overload with elevated end-diastolic pressures and displays poor contractility. Hypotension and pulmonary edema may necessitate emergent valvular replacement.

26. What is the pathophysiology of mitral stenosis?

Mitral stenosis is usually secondary to rheumatic disease. Critical stenosis of the valve occurs 10-20 years after the initial infection. As the orifice of the valve narrows, the left atrium experiences pressure overload. In contrast to other valvular lesions, the left ventricle shows relative volume underload resulting from the obstruction of forward blood flow from the atrium. The elevated atrial pressure may be transmitted to the pulmonary circuit and thus may lead to pulmonary hypertension and right-sided heart failure. The overdistended atrium is susceptible to fibrillation with resultant loss of atrial systole, leading to reduced ventricular filling and cardiac output. Symptoms (fatigue, dyspnea on exertion, hemoptysis) may be worsened when increased cardiac output is needed, as with pregnancy, illness, anemia, and exercise. Blood stasis in the left atrium is a risk for thrombus formation and systemic embolization.

27. What is the pathophysiology of mitral regurgitation?

Chronic mitral regurgitation is usually due to rheumatic heart disease, ischemia, or mitral valve prolapse. Acute mitral regurgitation may occur in the setting of myocardial ischemia and infarction with papillary muscle dysfunction or chordae tendineae rupture. In chronic mitral regurgitation, the left ventricle and atrium show volume overload, which leads to eccentric hypertrophy. Left ventricular systolic pressures decrease as part of the stroke volume escapes through the incompetent valve into the left atrium, leading to elevated left atrial pressure, pulmonary hypertension, and eventually right-sided heart failure. As in aortic insufficiency, regurgitant flow depends on valve orifice size, time available for regurgitant flow, and transvalvular pressure gradient. The valve orifice increases in size as the left ventricle increases in size. In acute mitral regurgitation, the pulmonary circuit and right side of the heart are subjected to sudden increases in pressure and volume in the absence of compensatory ventricular dilatation, which may precipitate acute pulmonary hypertension, pulmonary edema, and right-sided heart failure.

PERIOPERATIVE CONSIDERATIONS IN VALVULAR HEART DISEASE

28. What are the surgical risks for patients with valvular heart disease?

Patients with valvular heart disease present varying degrees of surgical risk, depending on the nature and severity of the valvular disease. The risk is generally one of three types:
1. Hemodynamic risks
2. Risks associated with **medications** taken for this disease
3. Risk of bacterial endocarditis

29. Is the following statement true or false? Patients with valvular stenosis are at greater surgical risk than those with valvular regurgitation.

True. Among patients with valvular heart disease, valvular stenosis poses higher risks intraoperatively than valvular regurgitation, although careful fluid management is important in both entities. Such management prevents increases in afterload and possibly pulmonary edema. In addition, patients with valvular stenosis are poorly tolerant of tachyarrhythmias, and care should be taken to avoid them.

30. What is the perioperative management of medications for valvular heart disease?

Patients with valvular heart disease, especially with mechanical valves, and patients with mitral stenosis often receive anticoagulation therapy to render the prothrombin time at 1.3-1.5 times control, or an international normalized ratio (INR) of 2-3. When oral surgical procedures are to be performed on these patients, the risk of thromboembolism has to be weighed against the risks of postoperative hemorrhage. A decision should be made, in consultation with the patient's cardiologist, on stopping such medications.

In general, if the risk of thromboembolism is moderate, Coumadin can be stopped for 72 hr preoperatively and resumed the same or following day postoperatively. If the patient is at high risk for thromboembolic phenomena, then heparin can be started intravenously after Coumadin has been discontinued; heparin is discontinued 6 hr before surgery. Once hemostasis of the surgical site is assured, heparin and Coumadin can be resumed postoperatively, but close monitoring for evidence of hemorrhage is continued.

31. Which cardiac conditions require preoperative antibiotic prophylaxis for prevention of bacterial endocarditis (Box 17-1)?

Box 17-1 *Stratification of Cardiac Conditions for Risk of Endocarditis*	
ENDOCARDITIS PROPHYLAXIS RECOMMENDED	ENDOCARDITIS PROPHYLAXIS NOT RECOMMENDED
High Risk	**Negligible Risk**
Prosthetic heart valves	Isolated secundum atrial septal defect
Prior bacterial endocarditis	Surgical repair of atrial septal defect,
Complex cyanotic congenital heart disease	ventricular septal defect, or patent ductus
Surgically constructed systemic pulmonary	arteriosus (without residua beyond 6 months)
shunts or conduits	Prior coronary artery bypass graft
	Mitral valve prolapse without regurgitation
Moderate Risk	Physiologic, functional, or innocent heart
Most other congenital cardiac	murmurs
malformations	Previous Kawasaki disease without valvular
Acquired valvular dysfunction	dysfunction
Hypertrophic cardiomyopathy	Previous rheumatic fever without valvular
Mitral valve prolapse with regurgitations	dysfunction
and/or thickened leaflets	Cardiac pacemakers and implanted
	defibrillators

Adapted from Dajani AS, Taubert KA, Wilson W et al: Prevention of bacterial endocarditis. Recommendations by the American Heart Association. JAMA 277:1794-1801, 1997.

32. **Which dental and oral surgical procedures require preoperative antibiotic prophylaxis for prevention of bacterial endocarditis (Box 17-2)?**

Box 17-2 *Dental Procedures and Endocarditis Prophylaxis*	
RECOMMENDED IN HIGH- AND MODERATE-RISK CARDIAC CONDITIONS	ENDOCARDITIS PROPHYLAXIS NOT RECOMMENDED
Exodontia	Restorative dentistry
Periodontal procedures	Nonintraligamentary local anesthetic injections
Incision and drainage of abscesses	Postoperative suture removal
Dental implant placement and uncovering	Placement of removable orthodontic or prosthodontic appliances
Reimplantation of avulsed teeth	Taking oral impressions
Endodontic therapy or apical surgery	Shedding (naturally) of primary teeth
Placement of intermaxillary fixation	
Reduction of contaminated maxillofacial fractures	
Osteotomies	
Subgingival placement of antibiotic fibers or strips	
Intraligamentary local anesthetic injections	
Prophylactic dental or implant cleaning	
Intraoral biopsies	

Adapted from Dajani AS, Taubert KA, Wilson W et al: Prevention of bacterial endocarditis. Recommendations by the American Heart Association. JAMA 277:1794-1801, 1997.

33. **What are the different antibiotic prophylactic regimens for dental and oral surgical procedures (Table 17-1)?**

Table 17-1 *Antibiotic Prophylactic Regimens for Dental and Oral Surgical Procedures*

	ANTIBIOTIC	REGIMEN[*]
Standard prophylaxis	Amoxicillin	Adults: 2 g PO; children: 50 mg/kg PO 1 hr before procedure
Unable to take oral medications	Ampicillin	Adults: 2 g IM or IV; children: 50 mg/kg IM or IV within 30 min of procedure
Penicillin allergy	Clindamycin or	Adults: 600 mg PO; children: 20 mg/kg PO 1 hr before procedure
	+ cephalexin or cefadroxil	Adults: 2 g PO; children: 50 mg/kg PO 1 hr before procedure
	Azithromycin or clarithromycin	Adults: 500 mg PO; children: 15 mg/kg PO 1 hr before procedure

Table 17-1   *Antibiotic Prophylactic Regimens for Dental and Oral Surgical*
Procedures—cont'd

	ANTIBIOTIC	REGIMEN*
Penicillin allergy and unable to take oral medications	Clindamycin or + cefazolin	Adults: 600 mg IM or IV; children: 20 mg/kg IM or IV within 30 min of procedure Adults: 1 g IM or IV; children: 25 mg/kg IM or IV within 30 min of surgery

Adapted from Dajani AS, Taubert KA, Wilson W et al: Prevention of bacterial endocarditis. Recommendations by the American Heart Association. JAMA 277:1794-1801, 1997.
Note: Do not use cephalosporins in individuals with immediate-type hypersensitivity reaction to penicillin.
IM, Intramuscularly; *IV,* intravenously; *PO,* orally.
*Total children's dose should not exceed adult dose.

HYPERTENSION

34. What is hypertension?

Hypertension is a sustained, elevated arterial blood pressure resulting from increased peripheral vascular resistance. An adult patient with a BP reading above 140/90 mm Hg is generally considered to be hypertensive.

35. What are the general categories of hypertension, based on the presentation and level of need for treatment?

Hypertension clinically presents in one of four generally recognized settings: hypertensive emergencies, hypertensive urgencies, mild uncomplicated hypertension, and transient hypertensive episodes.

36. What is the difference between hypertensive emergency and hypertensive urgency? How are these conditions managed?

A hypertensive *emergency* is an increased BP **with end-organ damage or dysfunction.** The brain, heart, or kidneys may be affected. BP can be as high as systolic >210 mm Hg and diastolic >120 mm Hg. Treatments for a hypertensive emergency should be rapid and aggressive, attempting to lower the BP within 60 min in a controlled fashion.

Hypertensive *urgency* is an elevation of BP to a potentially harmful level **without end-organ dysfunction.** Hypertensive urgency should be treated over a longer period (1-2 days).

37. What is the difference between primary and secondary hypertension?

Primary or essential hypertension is a sustained, elevated BP of unknown etiology. **Secondary** hypertension is an elevated BP that results from an identifiable cause, such as renal artery stenosis; chronic renal parenchymal disease; aldosteronism/Cushing's syndrome; acromegaly; hypercalcemia; coarctation of the aorta; pheochromocytoma; or oral contraceptives.

38. During the perioperative period, when are the highest mean arterial pressure (MAP) readings typically recorded?

The highest MAP is typically observed in response to laryngoscopy and intubation. A single dose of a beta-adrenergic blocker 90 min before induction in a patient with hypertension has been shown to reduce intraoperative BP, myocardial ischemia, and postoperative morbidity.

39. How is hypertension classified?

There are different systems for classifying hypertension. For example, hypertension can be classified as high normal, mild, moderate, or severe based on the diastolic pressure alone (85-89, 90-104, 105-114, and >115, respectively). However, hypertension typically is classified based on both the systolic and diastolic pressures into four stages. BP readings below these stages are considered either normal (< 130 for systolic and < 85 for diastolic), or high normal (130-139 for systolic and 85-89 for diastolic). The four stages of hypertension are:

- **Stage I (mild):** 140-159 systolic and 90-99 diastolic
- **Stage II (moderate):** 160-179 systolic and 100-119 diastolic
- **Stage III (severe):** 180-209 systolic and 110-119 diastolic
- **Stage IV (very severe):** >210 systolic and >120 diastolic

40. What behavior modifications can help treat hypertension?

Patients with hypertension are encouraged to modify their lifestyle. Weight loss (10 lb or more in overweight people), limitation of alcohol intake to <1 oz /day for men and 0.5 oz for women, and aerobic physical activity for 30-45 min three to five times/week are recommended. Patients are also encouraged to maintain adequate intake of potassium, calcium, and magnesium; reduce sodium, fat, and cholesterol; and quit smoking. All these measures have been shown to lower BP (Table 17-2).

Table 17-2   *Classification of Adult Blood Pressure and Treatment Modifications*

CATEGORY	SYSTOLIC (mm Hg)	DIASTOLIC (mm Hg)	TREATMENT
Normal	<130	<85	No modification
High normal	130-139	85-89	No modification
Hypertension			
Stage I	140-159	90-99	No modification, medical referral, inform patient
Stage II	160-179	100-109	Selective care,* medical referral
Stage III	180-209	110-119	Emergent nonstressful procedures† Immediate medical referral or consultation
Stage IV	≥210	≥120	Emergent nonstressful procedures† Immediate medical referral

*Selective care may include but is not limited to atraumatic removal of teeth, biopsies, etc.
†Emergent nonstressful procedures may include but are not limited to procedures that alleviate pain, infection, or masticatory dysfunction. These procedures should have limited physiologic and psychological effects (e.g., incision and drainage of an abscess). In all cases the medical benefit of the procedure should outweigh the risk of complications secondary to the patient's hypertensive state.

41. What pharmacologic therapy exists for hypertension?

Drug therapy for hypertension is based on the individual's needs and condition. For example, initial drug therapy for uncomplicated hypertension consists of diuretics and beta blockers. **Beta blockers** also may be prescribed for patients with hypertension after experiencing an MI. **Diuretics** can be used when there is concomitant CHF. **Calcium channel blockers** are recommended for older patients with IHD. **Angiotensin-converting enzyme (ACE) inhibitors** benefit hypertensive patients who have diabetes and proteinuria.

Note: Nonsteroidal antiinflammatory drugs (NSAIDs) may reduce the efficacy of ACE inhibitors, diuretics, and beta blockers. However, the reduction appears to be more likely in the NSAID class, dose, and duration not commonly prescribed for oral and maxillofacial surgery procedures. In addition, calcium channel blockers may cause gingival hyperplasia similar to the hyperplasia associated with Dilantin used to treat epilepsy.

42. Is it safe to administer local anesthesia with epinephrine to a hypertensive patient?

Cartridges of local anesthetic as used in dentistry contain epinephrine concentrations of 1:50,000 (0.02 mg/mL), 1:100,000 (0.01 mg/mL), or 1:200,000 (0.005 mg/mL). One cartridge contains 1.8 mL solution of local anesthetic and epinephrine; therefore one cartridge with an epinephrine concentration of 1:100,000 contains 1.8 mL × 0.01 mg/mL or 0.018 mg of epinephrine. According to American Dental Association/American Heart Association guidelines, a patient with cardiovascular disease can receive up to 0.04 mg of epinephrine, or up to two cartridges of agent.

If, however, the patient has poorly controlled hypertension or an otherwise significant medical risk, then the use of epinephrine becomes a clinical judgment of risk vs. benefit and is performed on a case-by-case basis. These patients are medical risks, not only concerning epinephrine, but also because of their overall poor medical status.

43. What is the Goldman Cardiac Risk Index? Which factors are most important in assigning risk?

The Goldman Cardiac Risk Index was established based on the study of more than 1000 patients undergoing noncardiac surgery who were evaluated preoperatively. The evaluation examined certain variables obtained from the history, physical exam, ECG, and general status (pulmonary, kidney, or liver disease) and factored in the type of operation to determine the risk factors that predispose a patient to a cardiac event.

The cardiac risk index is based on a point system, and patients are assigned to four different cardiac risk index classes (Tables 17-3 and 17-4). According to this study, the presence of an S_3

Table 17-3 *Points Awarded for Cardiac Risk Factors*

RISK FACTOR	POINTS
Third heart sound or jugular venous distention	11
Recent myocardial infarction	10
Rhythm other than sinus or premature atrial contractions on last ECG	7
>5 premature ventricular contractions/min at any time	7
Intraperitoneal, intrathoracic, or aortic operation	3
Age > 70 years	5
Important aortic stenosis	3
Emergent operation	4
Poor general medical condition	3
$\quad$ Po_2 < 60 or Pco_2 > 50 mm Hg	
$\quad$ K^+ < 30 mEq/L	
$\quad$ HCO_3^- < 20 mEq/L	
$\quad$ Creatinine > 3 mg/dL or BUN > 50 mg/dL	
$\quad$ Chronic liver disease	

Adapted from Goldman L: Multifactorial index of cardiac risk in noncardiac procedures. N Engl J Med 297:945-950, 1977.
BUN, Blood urea nitrogen; *ECG,* electrocardiogram.

Table 17-4 *Goldman Cardiac Risk Index*

CLASS	POINT TOTAL	NO OR ONLY MINOR COMPLICATION (n = 943) (%)	LIFE-THREATENING COMPLICATIONS* (n = 39) (%)	CARDIAC DEATHS (n = 19) (%)
I (n = 537)	0-5	532 (99)	4 (0.7)	1 (0.2)
II (n = 316)	6-12	295 (93)	16 (5)	5 (2)
III (n = 130)	13-25	112 (86)	15 (11)	3 (2)
IV (n = 18)	>26	4 (22)	4 (22)	10 (56)

Adapted from Goldman L: Multifactorial index of cardiac risk in noncardiac procedures. N Engl J Med 297:945-950, 1977.
*Documented intraoperative or postoperative myocardial infarction, pulmonary edema, or ventricular tachycardia.

heart sound, indicating heart failure or MI within the last 6 months, poses the greatest risk for a significant perioperative event.

44. What are the different sympathetic nervous system receptors relative to hypertension and antihypertensive agents?
These receptors are classified into two major categories: **alpha and beta receptors.** Each of these is further divided into two subdivisions: alpha 1 and alpha 2, and beta 1 and beta 2 receptors.
- Alpha 1 site stimulation causes constriction of vascular smooth muscles and thus increases peripheral vascular resistance.
- Alpha 2 stimulation inhibits the release of norepinephrine (the negative feedback to sympathetic neurons).
- Beta 1 stimulation increases heart rate and the strength of cardiac contraction.
- Beta 2 stimulation causes dilatation of smooth muscles of the blood vessels and airway, relaxation of uterine smooth muscle, and a variety of endocrine effects, including secretion of renin.

45. Is the following statement true or false? There are six different categories of oral antihypertensive agents.
False. Antihypertensive agents are generally classified into three major categories based on their mechanisms of action: diuretics, sympatholytics, and vasodilators (Table 17-5).

Table 17-5 *Categories and Classes of Oral Antihypertensive Agents*

CATEGORY	CLASS	SUBCLASS	AGENT
Diuretics	Thiazide type		Chlorothiazide, chlorthalidone, hydrochlorothiazide, indapamide, metolazone
	Potassium-sparing		Spironolactone, triamterene, amiloride
	Loop		Bumetanide, ethacrynic acid, furosemide, torsemide

Table 17-5 *Categories and Classes of Oral Antihypertensive Agents—cont'd*

CATEGORY	CLASS	SUBCLASS	AGENT
Sympatholytics	Adrenergic-receptor blockers	Beta	Acebutolol, atenolol, betaxolol, bisoprolol, carteolol, metoprolol, nadolol, penbutolol, pindolol, propranolol, timolol
		Alpha: alpha 1	Doxazosin, prazosin, terazosin
		alpha 1 + alpha 2	Phenoxybenzamine
		Alpha and beta	Labetalol
	Central alpha 2 agonists		Clonidine, guanabenz, guanfacine, methyldopa
	Postganglionic blockers		Bethanidine, guanadrel, guanethidine, reserpine
Vasodilators	Calcium channel blockers	Benzothiazepine Phenylalkylamines Dihydropyridines	Diltiazem, verapamil, amlodipine, felodipine, isradipine, nicardipine, nifedipine
	ACE inhibitors		Benazepril, captopril, enalapril, fosinopril, lisinopril, quinapril, ramipril
	Direct vasodilators		Hydralazine, minoxidil

Adapted from Dym H: The hypertensive patient. Therapeutic modalities. Oral Maxillofac Clin North Am 10: 349-362, 1998.

46. **What are the doses, mechanisms of action, and possible complications of commonly used antihypertensive agents (Table 17-6)?**

Table 17-6 *Doses, Mechanisms of Action, and Possible Complications of Antihypertensive Drugs*

AGENT AND DOSE	MECHANISM OF ACTION	POSSIBLE COMPLICATIONS
Diuretics		
Thiazide 25-50 mg/day	Increases urinary excretion of Na and water by inhibiting Na reabsorption in cortical diluting tubule in nephron; exact mechanism of anti-hypertension is unknown; may be partially from direct arteriolar vasodilation	Hypokalemia, dehydration, hyperglycemia, hyperuricemia, decreased lithium clearance
Loop diuretics 40-240 mg/day	Inhibits Na and chloride reabsorption in proximal ascending loop of Henle; also has renal and peripheral vasodilatory effects	Hypokalemia, dehydration, hypochloremic alkalosis

Continued

Table 17-6 *Doses, Mechanisms of Action, and Possible Complications of Antihypertensive Drugs—cont'd*

AGENT AND DOSE	MECHANISM OF ACTION	POSSIBLE COMPLICATIONS
Spironolactone 50-100 mg/day	Potassium-sparing; competitively inhibits aldosterone effects on distal renal tubules (increases Na and water excretion); also may block aldosterone effect on vascular smooth muscle	Hyperkalemia, gynecomastia, dehydration
Central Antiadrenergics		
Alpha-methyldopa PO 500-2000 mg/day IV 250-500 mg over 30-60 min q6h	Metabolite (alpha-methylnorepinephrine) stimulates inhibitory alpha-adrenergic receptors and inhibits sympathetic nervous system outflow, thus decreasing total peripheral resistance	Sedation, hepatic dysfunction, lupuslike symptoms, rebound hypertension, positive Coombs' test
Clonidine PO 0.1-2.4 mg/day topical transdermal patch q7d	Stimulates inhibitory alpha 2 receptors and inhibits sympathetic outflow	Sedation, xerostomia, rebound HTN, 50% decrease in minimal alveolar concentrations of volatile anesthetic
Peripheral Antiadrenergics		
Prazosin (Minipress) 2-20 mg/day	Selective and competitive postsynaptic alpha-receptor blockade leads to arterioles and vasodilation	Alters test results for pheochromocytoma, false-positive test results for ANA, increased liver function tests
Terazosin (Hytrin) 1-5 mg/PO/day	Selectively inhibits alpha receptors in vascular smooth muscles; dilates both arteriolar and venules	Decreases hematocrit, hemoglobin, albumin, leukocytes, and total protein
Guanethidine (Ismelin) 100-300 mg/day	Peripherally inhibits alpha receptors and release of NE; depletes stores of NE in adrenergic nerve endings	Peripherally inhibits alpha receptors and release of NE; depletes stores of NE in adrenergic nerve endings
Labetalol 100-400 mg PO twice daily 10-80 mg IV q10min	Competitive antagonist at beta- and alpha-adrenergic receptors	Contraindicated in asthmatic, second- or third-degree AV block, CHF, or "brittle" diabetes

Adapted from Dym H: The hypertensive patient. Therapeutic modalities. Oral Maxillofac Clin North Am 10: 349-362, 1998.

Table 17-6 *Doses, Mechanisms of Action, and Possible Complications of Antihypertensive Drugs—cont'd*

AGENT AND DOSE	MECHANISM OF ACTION	POSSIBLE COMPLICATIONS
Vasodilators		
Hydralazine 10-50 mg PO four times/day 5-10 mg IV q20min	Direct relaxing effect on vascular smooth muscle (arterioles) veins	Lupuslike syndrome in 1%-20% of patients on long-term therapy, decreases DBP > SBP, increases heart rate
Minoxidil 5-10 mg/day PO		Fluid retention, pericardial effusion, and hypertrichosis
ACE Inhibitors		
Benazepril (Lotensin) 10-40 mg/day PO	Competes with ACE, prevents pulmonary conversion of angiotensin I to angiotensin II (a potent vasoconstrictor); decreases peripheral arterial resistance; leads to decreased aldosterone secretion, thereby reducing Na and water retention	10% get rash with fever and joint pain, proteinuria, neutropenia, and cough
Captopril (Capoten) 6.25-150 mg PO three times/day		
Enalapril (Vasotec) 5-40 mg/day PO 1.25 mg/IV q6h		
Lisinopril (Zestril) 10-40 mg/day PO		
Calcium Channel Blockers		
Diltiazem (Cardizem) 30-90 mg PO four times/day 0.25 mg/kg IV over 2 min 5-15 mg/hr IV drip	Blocks calcium movement across cell membranes, causing arterial vasodilation; nifedipine is the most potent peripheral and coronary artery vasodilator of calcium channel blockers; diltiazem has less negative inotropic effects than verapamil and has some selective coronary vasodilatory effects	CHF, nodal changes, edema, headaches, hyperkalemia, flushing, tachycardia (with nifedipine only)
Isradipine (DynaCirc) 2.5-5 mg PO twice daily		
Nifedipine (Procardia) 10-30 mg PO three times/day		
Verapamil (Calan, Isoptin) 0.075-0.3 mg/kg IV over 2 min 80-120 PO three times/day		

ACE, Angiotensin-converting enzyme; *ANA,* antinuclear antibody; *AV,* atrioventricular; *CHF,* congestive heart failure; *DBP,* diastolic blood pressure; *HTN,* hypertension; *IV,* intravenously; *Na,* sodium; *NE,* norepinephrine; *PO,* orally; *q6h,* every 6 hr; *q7d,* every 7 days; *q10min,* every 10 min; *q20min,* every 20 min; *SBP,* systolic blood pressure.

47. What are the commonly used *parenteral* agents used for treatment of hypertensive emergencies (Table 17-7)?

Table 17-7 *Parenteral Drugs Used for Treatment of Hypertensive Emergencies*

DRUG	DOSAGE	ONSET OF ACTION	ADVERSE EFFECTS
Vasodilators			
Nitroprusside (Nipride, Nitropress)	0.25-10 µg/kg/min as IV infusion	Instantaneous	Nausea, vomiting, muscle twitching, sweating, thiocyanate, intoxication
Nitroglycerin	5-100 g/min as IV infusion	2-5 min	Tachycardia, flushing, headache, vomiting, methemoglobinemia
Diazoxide (Hyperstat)	50-100 mg IV bolus repeated or 15-30 mg/min by IV infusion	2-4 min	Nausea, hypotension, flushing, tachycardia, chest pain
Hydralazine (Apresoline)	10-20 mg IV bolus	10-20 min	Tachycardia, flushing, headache, vomiting, aggravation of angina
Enalapril (Vasotec IV)	1.25-5 mg IV bolus q6h	15 min	Precipitous fall in blood pressure in high renin states; response variable
Nicardipine	5-10 mg/hr as IV infusion	10 min	Tachycardia, headache, flushing, local phlebitis
Adrenergic Inhibitors			
Phentolamine (Regitine)	5-15 mg IV bolus	1-2 min	Tachycardia, flushing
Trimethaphan (Arfonad)	0.5-5 mg/min as IV infusion	1-5 min	Paresis of bowel and bladder, orthostatic hypotension, blurred vision, dry mouth
Esmolol (Brevibloc)	500 µg/kg/min for first 4 min, then 150-300 µg/kg/min as IV infusion	1-2 min	Hypotension
Propranolol (Inderal)	1-10 mg load; 3 mg/hr	1-2 min	Beta-blocker side effect, e.g., bronchospasm, decreased cardiac output
Labetalol (Normodyne, Trandate)	10-80 mg IV bolus q10min 0.5-2 mg/min IV as infusion	5-10 min	Vomiting, scalp tingling, burning in throat, postural hypotension, dizziness, nausea

Adapted from Dym H: The hypertensive patient. Therapeutic modalities. Oral Maxillofac Clin North Am 10: 349-362, 1998.

IV, Intravenous; *q6h,* every 6 hr; *q10min,* every 10 min.

48. What are the commonly used *oral* drugs for treatment of hypertensive *urgencies* (Table 17-8)?

Table 17-8 *Oral Drugs Used for Hypertensive Urgencies*				
DRUG	CLASS	DOSAGE	ONSET	DURATION
Nifedipine (Procardia)	Calcium entry blocker	5-10 mg sublingual	5-15 min	3-5 hr
Clonidine (Catapres)	Central sympatholytic	0.2 mg initially, then 0.1 mg/hr up to 0.7 mg total	0.5-2 hr	6-8 hr

Adapted from Dym H: The hypertensive patient. Therapeutic modalities. Oral Maxillofac Clin North Am 10:349-362, 1998.

CONGESTIVE HEART FAILURE

49. What is congestive heart failure?

Congestive heart failure (CHF) results from impaired pumping ability by the heart. A ventricular ejection fraction below 50% is indicative of CHF. Causes of CHF include MI, IHD, poorly controlled hypertension, structural heart defects, and cardiomyopathy.

50. What are the potential effects of long-term hypertension on end organs?

Chronically elevated BP often leads to serious consequences for the heart, central nervous system, and kidneys. Persistent hypertension may lead to left ventricular hypertrophy; angina pectoris with the potential for MI; CHF; and cardiomyopathy. Neurologic complications of hypertension include retinal damage with focal spasm; narrowing of arterioles or papilledema, or both; cerebral infarction or hemorrhage; cerebral vascular microaneurysms (Charcot-Bouchard aneurysms); hypertensive encephalopathy; and stroke. Renal complications include renal insufficiency and renal failure.

51. What are the clinical signs and symptoms of CHF?

Fatigue and dyspnea on exertion are often the primary symptoms of CHF. Patients may also report ankle edema and 2- to 3-pillow orthopnea. Palpitation, nocturia, cough, nausea, and vomiting are associated findings. Physical findings include gallop rhythm (S_3 or S_4), murmurs, and jugular venous distention. Pulmonary exam may reveal rales over the lung bases and decreased breath sounds. Cyanosis is often present in severe CHF.

52. What are the different classifications of heart failure?

There are different methods of classification of heart failure, such as left-sided vs. right-sided, high output vs. low output, backward vs. forward, acute vs. chronic, and compensated vs. decompensated.

53. What are the causes of heart failure?

Cardiac	Noncardiac
Ischemia	Hypertension
• Cardiomyopathy	Pulmonary embolus
• Toxic	High-output states
• Metabolic	Thyrotoxicosis
• Infectious, inflammatory	

- Infiltrative
- Genetic
- Idiopathic

Valvular heart diseases
- Aortic stenosis, regurgitation
- Mitral stenosis, regurgitation

Restrictive disease
- Pericardial
- Myocardial

Congenital disease

Electrical abnormalities
- Tachydysrhythmias
- Ventricular dyssynergy

54. What are the major physiologic alterations in patients with heart failure?

- Loss of artery compliance
- Arteriolar narrowing
- Vascular smooth muscle hypertrophy
- Enhanced vasoconstrictor activity secondary to elevated sympathetic nervous system activity
- Activation of the renin-angiotensin system resulting in sodium and water retention
- Increased levels of argentine vasopressin and endothelin
- Possible decrease in the local release of endothelium-derived relaxing factor (nitric oxide)

55. Which lab studies are useful in evaluating the patient with CHF?

Chest x-ray, ECG, echocardiogram, and radionuclear ventriculography are all useful in the evaluation of patients with heart failure. **Chest x-ray** may show cardiomegaly or evidence of pulmonary vascular congestion, including perihilar engorgement of the pulmonary veins, cephalization of the pulmonary vascular markings, or pleural effusions. The **ECG** in these patients is often nonspecific, although 70%-90% of patients demonstrate ventricular or supraventricular dysrhythmias. **Echocardiography** is used to demonstrate chamber size, wall motion, valvular function, and left ventricular wall thickness. **Radionuclear ventriculography** is helpful in providing an assessment of left ventricular ejection fraction.

56. How is the severity of heart failure classified?

The status of patients with CHF is typically classified on the basis of symptoms, impairment of lifestyle, or severity of cardiac dysfunction. The New York Heart Association uses four categories that describe the symptomatic limitations of the patient with heart failure. These classifications are:

Class I—Ordinary physical activity does not cause symptoms.
Class II—Ordinary physical activity causes symptoms.
Class III—Less than ordinary activity results in symptoms.
Class IV—Symptoms occur at rest.

57. What are the principles of management for CHF?

The mnemonic MOIST 'N DAMP is helpful in listing the methods generally used in combination for the management of CHF:

- **M**orphine
- **O**xygen
- **I**notropes (digitalis)
- **S**it-'em-up
- **T**ourniquets

- **N**itrates

- Diuretics
- ACE inhibitors and afterload reduction (aminophylline)
- Mechanical ventilator
- Phlebotomy

58. What are the different classes of drugs used in the treatment of heart failure?

Drugs used in the treatment of CHF typically fall into one of five categories: diuretics, ACE inhibitors, calcium channel blockers, digitalis, and beta blockers.

Diuretics are used when patients with CHF exhibit signs or symptoms of circulatory congestion. *Thiazide* diuretics are often used for mild fluid retention. *Loop* diuretics, such as furosemide, may be substituted when thiazides fail to produce an adequate response. Addition of a second diuretic, such as metolazone, may induce an effective diuresis in patients resistant to loop diuretics alone.

ACE inhibitors are effective therapy for patients who can tolerate them. They improve left ventricular function and exercise tolerance and may prolong life. Hypotension and azotemia are the major side effects. A dry cough is fairly common but rarely necessitates discontinuation of therapy. A combination of the vasodilators hydralazine and isosorbide dinitrate also has been shown to be effective in improving exercise tolerance and life span.

Calcium channel blockers may produce favorable hemodynamic responses, but negative inotropic effects. These agents are used in patients with concurrent myocardial ischemia.

Digitalis is effective in patients with underlying arterial fibrillation or a dilated left ventricle with poor systolic function.

Beta blockers may produce favorable long-term effects in patients with IHD.

59. What are the signs and symptoms of digitalis toxicity?

Patients with digitalis toxicity may present with any of the following signs and symptoms: anorexia, nausea, vomiting, abdominal pain, confusion, paresthesias, amblyopia, and scotomata. ECG findings are usually nonspecific and include atrial or ventricular dysrhythmias, such as premature ventricular contractions, bigeminy, trigeminy, ventricular tachycardia, delayed atrioventricular node conduction, and complete heart block. Older patients and patients with hypothyroidism, decreased renal function, hypokalemia, hypercalcemia, and/or hypomagnesemia are more predisposed to digitalis toxicity.

60. What are the important elements of postoperative care for patients with CHF?

The peak evidence of postoperative MI occurs about 72 hr postoperatively; therefore closely monitor the patient's cardiac status during this period. Improve pulmonary function with incentive spirometry, pulmonary toilet, and bronchodilators when appropriate. Observation of renal function and urine output is also important in these patients, because postoperative renal failure has ominous implications. Pain must be well controlled to minimize physiologic stress.

Other possible postoperative complications to avoid include gastrointestinal ischemia, bleeding, stroke, graft infection, distal arterial thrombosis, and pulmonary embolism.

BIBLIOGRAPHY

1. Dajani AS, Taubert KA, Wilson W et al: Prevention of bacterial endocarditis. Recommendations by the American Heart Association. JAMA 277:1794-1801, 1997.
2. Dym H: The hypertensive patient. Therapeutic modalities. Oral Maxillofac Surg Clin North Am 10:349-362, 1998.
3. Eagle KA, Coley CM, Nussbaum SR et al: Combining clinical and thallium data optimizes preoperative assessment of cardiac risk before major vascular surgery. Ann Intern Med 110:859-866, 1989.
4. Glick M: New guidelines for prevention, detection, evaluation, and treatment of high blood pressure. J Am Dent Assoc 129:1588-1594, 1998.
5. Goldman L, Caldera DL, Nussbaum SR et al: Multifactorial index of cardiac risk in patients in noncardiac surgical procedures. N Engl J Med 297:945-950, 1977.

6. McCabe JC, Roser SM: Evaluation and management of the cardiac patient for surgery. Oral Maxillofac Surg Clin North Am 10:429-443, 1998.
7. Muzyka BC, Glick M: The hypertensive dental patient. J Am Dent Assoc 128:1109-1120, 1997.
8. Seres T: Congestive heart failure. In Duke J (ed): Anesthesia Secrets, 3rd ed. Philadelphia, 2006, Mosby.

18. RESPIRATORY DISORDERS

Robert E. Doriot, DDS, and Kenneth J. Benson, DDS

1.   What is the normal adult oxyhemoglobin dissociation curve for blood at 37%, pH of 7.4, Pco₂ of 40 mm Hg (Fig. 18-1)?

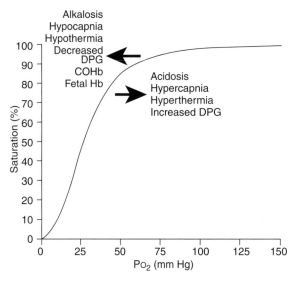

Fig. 18-1   Normal oxyhemoglobin dissociation curve. *DPG*, Diphosphoglycerate; *COHb*, Carboxyhemoglobin; *Hb*, hemoglobin. (From Hess D: Arterial blood gases. In Parsons PE, Heffner JE [eds]: Pulmonary/Respiratory Therapy Secrets, 3rd ed. Philadelphia, 2006, Mosby.)

2.   Which way would this curve shift if the pH was more acidic?
To the right.

3.   What are the general rules concerning the dissociation curve shifts?
• A low pH or a high Pco₂ shifts the curve to the right.
• A high pH or a low Pco₂ shifts the curve to the left.
• Elevated body temperature shifts the curve to the right.
• Lower body temperature shifts the curve to left.

4.   How does the interpretation of the curve change when the curve shifts to the left?
With a shift to the left, a lower Po₂ is required to bind a given amount of oxygen (O₂). The lower the oxygen half-saturation pressure (P-50), the higher the affinity of hemoglobin for O₂; the higher the P-50, the lower the affinity of hemoglobin for O₂. If the curve is shifted to the right, the P-50 increases, and if the curve is shifted to the left, the P-50 decreases.

5. Which way does carbon monoxide move the curve?
Small amounts of carbon monoxide in blood increase the affinity of remaining oxygen for hemoglobin and, therefore, cause a leftward shift of the curve.

6. What is 2,3-diphosphoglycerate (2,3-DPG)?
2,3-DPG is produced by erythrocytes and normally is present in fairly high concentrations in red blood cells (RBCs).

7. When is 2,3-DPG produced?
2,3-DPG is produced mainly during chronic hypoxic conditions. An increase in 2,3-DPG shifts the curve to the right and allows more O_2 to be released from hemoglobin at a particular O_2 level.

8. How does decreased 2,3-DPG affect the dissociation curve?
With a decrease in 2,3-DPG, the curve will shift to the left, indicating an increased affinity for O_2 by hemoglobin. Hemoglobin does not release O_2 in the tissues except at a very low Po_2.

9. How does 2,3-DPG affect blood supply in blood banks?
Blood stored for as little as 1 week will have depleted 2,3-DPG unless steps are taken to restore normal levels of 2,3-DPG.

10. How does the aging process affect $PaCO_2$?
$PaCO_2$ and alveolar ventilation are unchanged by the aging process.

11. How does the aging process affect Pao_2?
Pao_2 decreases with age. This decrease can be calculated according to the following formula:

$$Pao_2 = 100.1 - (0.323 \times \text{age in years})$$

Thus the Pao_2 of a 30-year-old would be calculated as $100.1 - (0.323 \times 30) = 90.41$.

12. How is the forced expiratory volume in 1 sec (FEV1) changed with age?
FEV_1 declines linearly with age increase.

13. What are the most significant changes of pulmonary function associated with aging?
- Loss of lung elasticity, which leads to increased mean alveolar diameter and volume and reduced FEV_1
- Decreased power of the respiratory musculature
- Increased rigidity of rib cage
  All these changes start becoming apparent in the third decade of life.

14. What does PEEP mean?
*P*ositive *e*nd-*e*xpiratory *p*ressure during mechanical ventilation. PEEP aids in preventing alveolar and small airway collapse and may help recruit lung units that were previously collapsed.

15. What are the beneficial effects of PEEP?
- Increased functional residual capacity
- Increased compliance
- Increased Pao_2
- Increased ventilation-perfusion (V/Q) ratio (when initially low)
- Decreased pulmonary shunt

16. What is the effect of PEEP on cardiac output?

Because of increased intrathoracic pressure and decreased venous return when using PEEP, cardiac output may be decreased as a result.

17. What are the normal blood gas values?

pH 7.40 ± 0.05 units

(H^+) 40 ± 5 mEq/L

Pco_2 40 ± 5 mm Hg

As a rule, each 0.1 increment of pH corresponds to 12 mm Hg of Pco_2, which equals a base change of 6 mEq/L.

- Golden rule No. 1: A pH of 0.08 = $PaCO_2$ of 10 mm Hg.
- Golden rule No. 2: A pH of 0.15 = base change of 10 mEq/L.

18. What are acidosis and alkalosis?

Acidosis is the metabolic state when only excessive quantities of metabolic acids are produced or when the buffering systems or renal function are abnormal. **Alkalosis** occurs when there is excessive ingestion of a base (e.g., bicarbonate) or a loss of excess acid (e.g., hypovolemia, vomiting).

19. How is the diagnosis of respiratory acidosis made?

Respiratory acidosis is usually evident from the clinical exam, especially if respiration is obviously depressed. Analysis of arterial blood gases (ABGs) will confirm the diagnosis: arterial pH will be < 7.35, and Pco_2 will be > 45 mm Hg.

20. What are some causes of respiratory acidosis?

Any disease or condition that may affect the respiratory function can cause respiratory acidosis, including:

- Chronic obstructive pulmonary disease (COPD)
- Pulmonary edema
- Cardiac arrest
- Pneumonia
- Chest wall or airway injury
- Drug effects
- Central nervous system (CNS) depression
- Extreme obesity (e.g., pickwickian syndrome)

21. How is the diagnosis of respiratory alkalosis made?

Clinically, respiratory alkalosis usually manifests as hyperventilation. However, depending on its severity and acuteness, hyperventilation may not be evident, but an analysis of arterial blood gases will demonstrate an arterial pH of >7.45 and a Pco_2 of <35 mm Hg.

22. What are some causes of respiratory alkalosis?

- Hyperventilation
- CNS injury
- Fever
- Pulmonary embolus
- Excessive mechanical ventilation

23. With what is bronchial carcinoma most often associated?

Up to 50% of cases of carcinoma of the hypopharynx and upper part of the esophagus are associated with Plummer-Vinson syndrome.

24. Where is the respiratory center?

The respiratory center is a widely dispersed group of neurons located bilaterally in the reticular substance of the medulla oblongata and pons.

25. What influences the respiratory center?

Excess CO_2 and hydrogen ions (H^+) affect respiration mainly by direct excitatory effects on the respiratory center itself. Oxygen does *not* have a significant direct effect on the respiratory center. O_2 acts almost entirely peripherally on the carotid and aortic bodies.

26. How does metastatic bronchiogenic carcinoma usually reach the mandible?

The mandible is affected by metastatic tumors much more often than the maxilla is. Studies have shown that 82%-85% of metastatic tumors involve the mandible. The molar area is predominantly involved because it contains a rich deposit of hematopoietic tissue. Also, because the mode of spread is usually hematogenous, tumor cells tend to be deposited in the vascular medullary tissue.

27. What is the normal rate of breathing?

The respiratory rate (RR) is 10-20 breaths/min in normal adults and 44 breaths/min in infants. An RR >20/min is considered tachypnea, and an RR <10/min is bradypnea.

28. What is Cheyne-Stokes breathing?

Periods of hyperpnea (deep breathing) alternating with periods of apnea. Children and the elderly normally show this pattern in sleep. In normal adults, causes of this pattern of breathing include heart failure, uremia, drug-induced respiratory depression, and brain damage.

29. What causes stridor?

Stridor, an airway emergency that demands immediate attention, is caused by partial obstruction of the airway at the level of larynx or trachea.

30. What is the definition of acute respiratory failure?

Respiratory failure is an inadequate exchange of O_2 and CO_2 secondary to failure of the ventilatory apparatus or gas exchange system. It results in hypoventilation and therefore hypercapnia and hypoxemia.

31. How is the diagnosis of respiratory failure made?

Respiratory failure is primarily based on arterial blood gases: hemoglobin saturation of <92% (which corresponds to a PaO_2 of <60 mm Hg, a $PaCO_2$ of >50 mm Hg, and a pH of <7.35 [respiratory acidosis]).

32. How is respiratory failure treated?

Secure and maintain a patent airway in order to deliver appropriate O_2 therapy using mechanical or supportive ventilation. The airway may be in the form of oral and nasal endotracheal intubation, tracheostomy, or cricothyrotomy.

33. What are the indications for elective intubation and mechanical ventilation?

The indications for intubation and mechanical ventilation are based on clinical and lab values. These include:

- Respiratory rate >30-40 breaths/min
- Negative inspiratory pressure <25 cm H_2O
- Vital capacity <10-15 mL/kg or a $PaCO_2$ >50 mm Hg with a pH <7.3

34. What are the guidelines for withdrawing mechanical ventilatory support (weaning parameters)?

Mechanical ventilation can be withdrawn if one or more of the following parameters is met:

- PaO_2 >60 mm Hg with an FiO_2 <0.4
- $PaCO_2$ (35-45) acceptable with normal pH
- Tidal volume >4-5 mL/kg
- Vital capacity >10-15 mL/kg
- Minute ventilation <10 L/min
- Respiratory rate <25 breaths/min
- Negative inspiratory pressure >20 cm H_2O

35. What is pleural effusion?

Pleural effusion occurs when fluid accumulates in the pleural space (i.e., volume overload, infection) and the air-filled lung separates from the chest wall.

36. What is atelectasis?

Atelectasis occurs when mucus or a foreign object obstructs airflow in a mainstem bronchus causing collapse of the affected lung tissue into an airless state. It typically occurs 36 hr postoperatively and presents with mild dyspnea.

37. How is postoperative atelectasis managed?

Treatment of postoperative atelectasis is aimed at expansion of the lung, and, for most patients, incentive spirometry is adequate. However, in patients with severe atelectasis, endotracheal suction and even bronchoscopy may be warranted.

38. What are the signs of pneumothorax?

Pneumothorax occurs when air leaks into the pleural space, causing the lung to recoil from the chest wall. The signs of intraoperative pneumothorax include unexplained hypotension, ventilatory hypoxia with bulging diaphragm, jugular venous distention, tympanic thorax, and trachea deviated to one side. In an awake patient, a pneumothorax typically presents with dyspnea, chest pain, absence of breath sounds on the affected side, and evidence of pneumothorax on chest x-ray. Tracheal deviation may be present.

39. What is the appropriate treatment of pneumothorax?

Pneumothorax is definitively treated with placement of a thoracostomy tube connected to closed suction of 20 cm H_2O. However, if tension pneumothorax is suspected, immediate needle decompression through the second intercostal space in the midclavicular line using a 14-gauge needle should be performed.

40. What is the mechanism of asthma?

Asthma is a chronic disorder characterized by inflammation and increased responsiveness of the tracheobronchial tree to diverse stimuli resulting in a varying degree of airway obstruction.

41. What is the clinical presentation of acute asthma?

Patients present with dyspnea or tachypnea, wheezing, hypoxemia, and, occasionally, hypercapnia.

42. What is the appropriate management of an acute asthma attack?

An acute asthmatic attack is best treated by administration of supplemental O_2 with inhaled beta-adrenergic agonistic (albuterol, 3.0 mL [2.5 mg], in 2 mL of normal saline every 4-6 hr, in a nebulizer). If the patient is resistant to beta agonists, theophylline should be considered. Therapy also may include parenteral steroids, such as methylprednisolone (50-250 mg over 4-6 hr). In a severe asthmatic attack that is unresponsive to the above, administer 0.3 mg of 1:1000 epinephrine subcutaneously.

43. What drugs interfere (interact) with aminophylline?

The most commonly cited drug is erythromycin, which increases serum levels of aminophylline. Cimetidine also increases serum levels of aminophylline.

44. Why do chronic emphysema patients have a barrel-chest appearance?

In patients with emphysema, the distal air spaces become enlarged, and the lungs become hyperinflated.

45. What is adult respiratory distress syndrome (ARDS)?
ARDS is a C5a-induced neutrophil aggregation in the lung. This aggregation is one of the major mechanisms of pathology of ARDS. The damaged capillaries leak protein-rich fluid into the interstitium, which leads to changes in pulmonary function.

46. What causes ARDS?
ARDS usually results from an injury to the alveolar-capillary membrane. It also can be caused by an existing underlying disease, such as systemic sepsis, fat embolism, head injury, aspiration, pancreatitis, or inhalation injury. Patients typically show severe dyspnea and hypoxemia refractory to supplemental O_2 with diffuse pulmonary infiltrates on chest radiograph.

47. What is the appropriate management of ARDS?
Management of ARDS includes immediate transfer to an intensive care unit and placement of a pulmonary artery catheter with mechanical ventilation to maintain the pulse oximetry (SpO_2) >90%, which corresponds to Po_2 >60 mm Hg. In addition, the pulmonary capillary pressure should be kept in the range of 12-15 mm Hg, and the cardiac index should be maintained above 3 L/min/m^2. Treatment of ARDS is generally supportive to achieve O_2 saturation of 90% while minimizing barotrauma and oxygen toxicity.

48. What are the features of ARDS?
- History of major insult
- Increased respiratory distress
- Diffuse infiltration on chest x ray
- Hypoxemia (PaO_2 <60 mm Hg with FiO_2 >0.6)
- Respiratory alkalosis
- Normal pulmonary capillary wedge pressure (PCWP)
- Decreased pulmonary compliance
- Increased shunt function
- Increased dead space and ventilation

49. What is the appropriate management of aspiration of gastric contents?
Treatment of aspiration is generally supportive and should include administration of O_2, endotracheal intubation, and antibiotics. The patient should not be given anything orally (NPO), and may require total parenteral nutrition or enteral feedings. These patients generally will present with acute dyspnea and fever 2-3 hr after the event, secondary to chemical pneumonitis. Note that the chest radiograph in these patients may be normal initially but eventually will demonstrate diffuse interstitial infiltrates.

50. What are the possible complications of aspiration?
ARDS, pneumonia, and lung disease.

51. What are the signs and symptoms of pulmonary embolus (PE)?

Symptoms of PE	Signs of PE
Dyspnea	Tachypnea
Chest pain	Tachycardia
Cough	Possible syncope
Possible hemoptysis	

52. How is PE diagnosed?
PE should be considered in any postoperative patient with unexplained dyspnea, hypoxia, or tachypnea. Immediate SpO_2, electrocardiogram (ECG), and chest x-ray should be obtained.

Desaturation will be evident, and nonspecific ST or T wave changes will be noted. Spiral computed tomography (CT) scans are helpful in diagnosis.

53. What is the appropriate management of postoperative PE?
Treatment should include the administration of O_2 to correct hypoxemia and intravenous fluids to maintain blood pressure. In addition, intravenous or subcutaneous heparin should be initiated immediately with a target partial thromboplastin time (PTT) of 1.5-2.4 times the control. Warfarin therapy should be started while the patient is on heparin until the patient's therapeutic prothrombin time (PT) is reached (within 5-7 days). The treatment is continued for 2-3 months. Finally, placement of an inferior vena cava (IVC) filter should be considered. Embolectomy may also be considered.

BIBLIOGRAPHY

1. Barash P, Cullen B, Stoelting R et al (eds): Clinical Anesthesia, 2nd ed. Philadelphia, 1996, Lippincott-Raven.
2. Bates B, Bickley L, Hoekelman R: The thorax and lungs. In Bates B (ed): A Guide to Physical Examination and History Taking, 6th ed. Philadelphia, 1995, J.B. Lippincott.
3. Kollef M, Goodenberger D: Critical care and medical emergencies. In Ewald G, McKenzie C (eds): The Washington Manual of Medical Therapeutics. Boston, 1995, Little, Brown.
4. Miller R, Stoelting R: Acid-base and blood gas analysis. In Miller R (ed): Basics of Anesthesia, 3rd ed. New York, 1994, Churchill Livingstone.
5. Pettit TW, Cobb JP: Critical care. In Doherty GM, Wells SA, Baumann DS et al (eds): The Washington Manual of Surgery. Boston, 1997, Little, Brown.
6. Roser SM: Management of the medically compromised patient. In Kwon P, Laskin D (eds): Clinician's Manual of Oral and Maxillofacial Surgery, 2nd ed. Chicago, 1997, Quintessence.

19. HEMATOLOGY

James A. Giglio, DDS, MEd, and Robert E. Doriot, DDS

1. Which blood clotting factors are dependent on vitamin K for their synthesis?
Factors II, VII, IX, and X.

2. Which blood test is used to monitor the effect of warfarin?
Prothrombin time (PT) test.

3. What is the international normalized ratio (INR)?
The INR is a calculated value developed to normalize the reporting of PT.

$$INR = \left(\frac{\text{patient protime}}{\text{mean of the normal range}} \right)^{ISI}$$

The ISI is the International Sensitivity Index value assigned by the manufacturer to each lot of thromboplastin calibrated to the World Health Organization reference material. The INR standardizes reporting of anticoagulation activity and monitors patients on stabilized oral anticoagulant therapy only. The therapeutic INR range is 2.0-3.0 for most clinical situations. Patients with mechanical prosthetic heart valves are maintained at 2.5-3.5.

4.   What are the three phases of hemostasis?
Vascular, platelet, and coagulation phases.

5.   What effect can long-term antibiotic therapy have on hemostasis?
Long-term antibiotic therapy can suppress the normal flora in the gastrointestinal tract that are necessary for the synthesis of vitamin K. Clotting factors II, VII, IX, and X require vitamin K for their synthesis.

6.   What disease is a factor IX deficiency?
Hemophilia B or Christmas disease.

7.   If warfarin (Coumadin) is to be discontinued before oral surgery, how soon should this occur before the planned procedure?
Although dose dependent, in general, the duration of action for warfarin is 3-5 days with an onset in 12-24 hr. The half-life is 1.5-2.5 days. Warfarin should be discontinued at least 3 days before the procedure, and a PT test should be done within 24 hr of the surgery.

8.   How does administering vitamin K affect warfarin?
Vitamin K reverses the action of warfarin. Once vitamin K is administered, the patient may be resistant to further anticoagulation with warfarin for a few days. In addition, certain patients may have an underlying thrombotic tendency that puts them at risk for thrombosis and embolic complications should the effects of the anticoagulant be stopped abruptly. Therefore administering vitamin K or abruptly stopping warfarin medication can be harmful to some patients.

9.   How does heparin affect blood clotting?
Heparin is a naturally occurring conjugated polysaccharide formed by many cells including mast cells located in connective tissue, especially in the lung. Heparin calcium is commercially prepared from porcine intestinal connective tissue, whereas the sodium form is prepared from either porcine intestinal connective tissue or bovine lung. Heparin affects the intrinsic and common pathways of blood coagulation. It prevents the formation of prothrombin activator and inhibits the action of thrombin on fibrinogen. Heparin increases the normal clotting time (4-6 min) to 6-30 min. Its duration of action is 3-4 hr.

10.   How can the effects of heparin be reversed?
Protamine sulfate is used to reverse the effects of heparin. Protamine, which itself is an anticoagulant, must be administered with caution. When protamine is given with heparin, the anticoagulant effect of both drugs is lost. Careful control of the protamine dosing is necessary to prevent bleeding from an overdose. Too rapid administration of protamine can result in hypertensive and anaphylactoid reactions.

11.   How does aspirin affect blood coagulation?
Aspirin (acetylsalicylic acid [ASA]) and other nonsteroidal antiinflammatory drugs (NSAIDs) affect the platelet phase of coagulation. These drugs alter cyclooxygenase activity within platelets. Cyclooxygenase controls the release of the adhesive proteins from platelets that are necessary for them to aggregate and "stick together" in response to trauma. Inhibition of cyclooxygenase activity by either aspirin or another NSAID will cause the development of an ineffective platelet plug, resulting in prolonged bleeding. This side effect of ASA has led to its accepted controlled use as a prophylactic measure against coronary and cerebral vessel thrombosis.

12. What are the components of the extrinsic, intrinsic, and common pathways of the coagulation cascade?

The components of the intrinsic pathway are factors VIII, IX, XI, and XII. The components of the extrinsic pathways include tissue factors and factor VII. The common pathway involves factors X and XIII, prothrombin, thrombin, fibrinogen, and fibrin.

13. What factors are measured by PT and which ones are measured by partial thromboplastin time (PTT)?

PT measures factors II, VII, IX, X, and fibrinogen. PTT measures the integrity of the intrinsic pathways before the activation of factor X and the activity of factors I, II, V, VIII, IX, X, XI, and XII, and fibrinogen.

14. What are the indications for transfusion of fresh frozen plasma (FFP)?

Fresh frozen platelets are used for replacement of deficiencies of factors II, V, VII, IX, and XI when specific component therapy is not available or desirable. In an average-size adult, each unit of FFP increases the level of all clotting factors by 2%-3%, and most bleeding can be controlled by transfusion of FFP at a dose of 10 mL/kg of body weight.

15. What is anemia?

A decrease in the oxygen-carrying capacity of the blood. General symptoms include weakness, fatigue, palpitations, tingling, and numbness of the fingers and toes, a burning tongue, bone pain, and shortness of breath. Clinical signs of anemia include pallor, spooning and brittle nails, and a smooth, red tongue caused by loss of filiform papillae.

16. What causes iron deficiency anemia?

Iron deficiency anemia is caused by low serum ferritin and blood loss. A diagnosis of iron deficiency anemia is based on a low hemoglobin, a low white blood cell (WBC) count and microcytic, hypochromic erythrocytes. Iron supplement and correction of any underlying cause of blood loss is the treatment for this anemia. Plummer-Vinson syndrome is a clinical triad of esophageal webbing, dysphagia, and oral symptoms of glossitis and xerostomia in a patient with iron deficiency anemia.

17. What is pernicious anemia?

Red blood cells (RBCs) require vitamin B_{12} and folic acid for their maturation and development. Vitamin B_{12} requires intrinsic factor, which is secreted by the parietal cells in the stomach, for its absorption. Pernicious anemia will develop if there is a deficiency of intrinsic factor, folic acid, or vitamin B_{12}.

18. What causes sickle cell anemia?

Sickle cell anemia is caused by a defect in the beta chain of hemoglobin causing the RBCs to become sickle shaped when exposed to low oxygen tension or increased pH. The inherent defect causing sickle cell anemia is the substitution of valine for glutamic acid on the beta chain of the hemoglobin molecule.

19. What is the perioperative management of a patient with sickle cell disease?

Perioperative management of a sickle cell anemia patient involves avoiding all possible precipitating factors, which include hypoxia, dehydration, stress, and infection. This can be done with intravenous (IV) fluids, sedation, oxygen supplementation, and all measures that prevent infection, including antibiotic coverage. In patients with severe sickle cell disease who are undergoing major surgical procedures, exchange transfusions may be used to dilute the defective RBCs by 50%, keeping the hematocrit under 35%. Treatment of sickle cell crisis involves maintenance of hydration, administration of oxygen, and analgesics.

20. What is the result of a deficiency of glucose-6 phosphate dehydrogenase (G-6-PD)?

RBC glucose is metabolized by either the glycolytic or the hexose monophosphate shunt pathways. Reduced nicotinamide adenine dinucleotide phosphate (NADPH) formed by the hexose monophosphate shunt is necessary to rid the cell of oxidants. G-6-PD is a necessary enzyme for the hexose monophosphate shunt pathway to function properly. A deficiency of G-6-PD results in accumulation of cell oxidants and ultimately hemolysis of RBCs. ASA medications should not be prescribed to patients with G-6-PD deficiency because they can cause hemolysis.

21. What is the normal WBC count?

Between 4500 and 11,000/mm^3. An increase in WBCs is termed *leukocytosis*, and a decrease is *leukopenia*.

22. What are the forms of leukemia?

Leukemia can be either acute or chronic. There are two types of acute leukemia: acute lymphocytic and acute myelogenous leukemia. Chronic leukemia is classified as chronic lymphocytic or chronic myelogenous leukemia.

23. Which form of leukemia is most often associated with the Philadelphia chromosome?

Chronic myelogenous leukemia. This marker can be found in the metaphase and is associated with a poor prognosis.

24. What is the primary difference between Hodgkin's disease and non-Hodgkin's lymphoma?

Both diseases are lymphoproliferative diseases. Hodgkin's disease usually begins as a single tumor focus, whereas non-Hodgkin's lymphoma is usually multifocal.

25. What is Plummer-Vinson syndrome?

Plummer-Vinson syndrome occurs with iron deficiency anemia and is a predisposing factor to oral carcinoma. It is found primarily in women in the fourth and fifth decades of life. Clinical signs include cracking at the lip commissure; lemon-tinted pallor; smooth, red, painful tongue with atrophy of the filiform; and, later, fungiform papillae. A characteristic esophageal webbing or stricture is also identified. Iron deficiency anemia responds well to iron replacement therapy.

26. What is von Willebrand's disease? How is it managed in a patient who is about to undergo surgery?

Von Willebrand's disease is an inherited disorder in which von Willebrand's factor, required for platelet adhesion, is either deficient or defective. Management of von Willebrand's disease depends on the severity of the disease, because bleeding is variable from patient to patient. In mild cases, one of the following routes can be followed: preoperative administration of 50-100 g/kg of IV aminocaproic acid (Amicar); oral Amicar 3 hr after surgery, and then every 6 hr for 7 days; or IV infusion of 0.3 mg/kg of desmopressin (DDAVP) diluted in 50 mL of normal saline over 15-30 min, which will produce maximum levels of factor VIIIc in 90-120 min and will last for 6 hr. A high-concentration intranasal form of desmopressin shows a response similar to the IV preparation. In severe cases, a transfusion of cryoprecipitate (20 bags) is warranted to achieve factor VIIIc and factor VIIIvw levels of 1 U/mL immediately before surgery. In addition, Amicar should be initiated 12-24 hr preoperatively and continued for 12 days.

27. How would you differentiate hemophilia A and B?

Hemophilia A is an X-linked recessive disorder in which factor VIII is deficient, whereas the affected serine protease in type B is factor IX. Initially, the two coagulation disorders will appear similar, with elevated PTT and normal PT and bleeding time, but they are managed differently.

28. What are some other causes of bleeding disorders?

Liver disease, anticoagulant therapy, aspirin therapy, disseminated intravascular coagulation (DIC), vitamin K deficiency, malabsorption syndrome, thrombocytopenia, polycythemia vera, iron deficiency, vitamin B_{12} deficiency, and thalassemia major can also cause bleeding disorders.

29. What is DIC?

Disseminated intravascular coagulation is the consequence of intravascular activation of both the coagulation and fibrinolytic systems. DIC varies greatly in its clinical presentation because it can show up as either bleeding or thrombosis. Generally, treatment involves correction of the underlying process, which can be neoplasm, infection, liver disease, snake bites, spider bites, obstetric complications, trauma, shock, extensive burns, connective tissue diseases, or acute leukemia (for more on DIC, see Chapter 4).

30. How should a patient with hemophilia A who is about to undergo a surgical procedure be managed?

Patients with hemophilia A are managed according to the severity of their disorder and anticipated blood loss. Patients with severe hemophilia should receive replacement of factor VIII with factor VIII concentrate. The minimal level of factor VIII required for hemostasis is 30%, and the half-life of factor VIII in the circulation is 10 hr. A loading dose of 30 U/kg immediately before surgery is followed by continuous infusion of 3 U/kg for 5 days and then a single dose of 30 U/kg for an additional 5 days. Patients with less severe disease can be managed with cryoprecipitate or DDAVP, 0.3 mg/kg every 24 hr, and/or Amicar, 4 g by mouth every 4 hr for 5-7 days.

31. What is the replacement therapy for hemophilia B?

Replacement therapy for hemophilia type B is similar to that for factor VIII deficiency, but the dosing interval differs because the half-life of factor IX is 24 hr. Factor IX concentrate should be given every 18-24 hr.

32. What is low-molecular-weight heparin, and how is it used in oral and maxillofacial surgery?

Standard unfractionated heparin (UFH) is formed from a heterogenous combination of sulfated mucopolysaccharides. Its anticoagulant activity is unpredictable, so it must be carefully monitored with the PTT test. Low-molecular-weight heparin (LMWH—fractionated heparin) is formed from depolymerization of heparin into lower-molecular-weight particles. Because LMWH has increased bioavailability compared with UFH, it can be given as a fixed dose and without the need for monitoring with the PTT test.

It is useful in oral and maxillofacial surgery for patients who cannot stop oral anticoagulation therapy. Patients stop warfarin therapy, and the INR is allowed to normalize while the LMWH is administered to maintain anticoagulation therapy. When the INR returns to an acceptable level, the surgery can be performed and scheduled for early in the day. The LMWH is withheld the day of surgery and resumed in the evening. Warfarin can be resumed the following day, and the LMWH is continued until the INR returns to the desired therapeutic range.

33. What is tranexamic acid, and how is it used?

Tranexamic acid is an antifibrinolytic agent that is used to promote stability of a formed blood clot. The final phase in the common pathway to blood clot formation is the activation of fibrinogen to fibrin in the presence of thrombin. Fibrin forms the basis for the blood clot. Fibrinolysis or clot breakdown begins in the presence of plasmin that is formed from activated plasminogen. Tranexamic acid inhibits the activation of plasminogen, thereby promoting stability of the blood clot.

34. How is tranexamic acid used to control postoperative bleeding following removal of teeth?

Because of its antifibrinolytic properties, tranexamic acid can be used effectively as a topical agent and mouthrinse to promote clot stability in patients receiving warfarin anticoagulation therapy. The anticoagulation therapy does not have to be altered or stopped. A compounding pharmacy first prepares a 4.8% tranexamic acid solution. Immediately after surgery, sutures are placed and the patient is asked to bite firmly on a 2 -× 2-inch gauze pack first soaked in the prescription solution. The process is repeated until bleeding stops. The patient then rinses for 2 min, four times/day, for 4-5 days.

BIBLIOGRAPHY

1. Beirne O, Koehler J: Surgical management of patients on warfarin sodium. J Oral Maxillofac Surg 54:1115-1118, 1996.
2. Herman W, Konzelman J, Sutley S: Current perspectives on dental patients receiving Coumadin anticoagulant therapy. J Am Dent Assoc 128:327-335, 1997.
3. Lew D: Blood and blood products. In Kwon PH, Laskin DM (eds): Clinician's Manual of Oral and Maxillofacial Surgery, 2nd ed. Carol Stream, Ill, 1997, Quintessence.
4. Little J, Falace D, Miller C et al: Dental Management of the Medically Compromised Patient, 6th ed. St Louis, 2002, Mosby.
5. Todd DW, Roman A: Outpatient use of low-molecular-weight heparin in an anticoagulated patient requiring oral surgery: case report. J Oral Maxillofac Surg 59:1090-1092, 2001.

20. LIVER DISEASES

Mark A. Oghalai, DDS

1. What are common risk factors for developing liver disease?

- Intravenous drug abuse
- Cocaine use
- Contact with blood
- Blood transfusion before 1989
- Alcohol abuse
- Multiple sexual contacts
- Diabetes
- Family history of liver disease
- Intake of certain medications and food supplements

2. Which liver function tests are useful for assessing hepatocellular damage?

Alanine aminotransferase (ALT) and aspartate aminotransferase (AST). These enzymes are released from damaged hepatocytes. ALT is a more sensitive indicator of liver damage because it is found only in hepatic cells, whereas AST is also found in heart, skeletal muscle, pancreas, kidney, and red blood cells. Increased bilirubin, decreased albumin, decreased cholesterol, and abnormal prothrombin time (PT) are other lab abnormalities found in liver disease.

3. How is drug metabolism affected by liver cirrhosis?

Fibrosis leads to decreases in blood flow from the hepatic artery to the most distal areas of the liver. These areas are concentrated with the cytochrome P450 system, which is important in metabolizing many drugs. Prolonged plasma half-life of these drugs is a consequence of cirrhosis.

4. What are the signs of liver failure?
- Jaundice
- Portal hypertension (dilated chest; abdominal or rectal veins; liver and spleen enlargement)
- Hepatic encephalopathy
- Asterixis
- Palmar erythema
- Testicular atrophy
- Ascites
- Dupuytren's contracture
- Gynecomastia
- Spider telangiectasia

5. What lab test is used to assess hepatic dysfunction secondary to biliary obstruction?
Alkaline phosphatase (ALP). ALP is present in bile duct cells; even slight degrees of bile duct obstruction result in large increases in plasma concentration.

6. How is drug protein binding affected by liver disease?
Decreased albumin production by the liver results in a decreased number of protein-binding sites. The amount of unbound, pharmacologically active drug is, in turn, increased.

7. What is the effect of inhaled anesthetics on hepatic blood flow?
A 20%-30% decrease in hepatic blood flow results from decreased perfusion pressure.

8. What is the effect of positive pressure ventilation on hepatic blood flow?
Decreased hepatic blood flow secondary to increased central venous pressure decreases hepatic perfusion pressure.

9. What class of drugs can cause spasm of the choledochoduodenal sphincter?
Opioids.

10. Which inhaled anesthetic is best for maintaining hepatic blood flow and hepatocyte oxygenation?
Isoflurane.

11. Which muscle relaxant is the best choice to use in a patient with liver dysfunction?
Cis-atracurium, because it is eliminated by Hofmann elimination and therefore is independent of liver function.

12. How does liver dysfunction affect metabolism of procaine?
The liver is responsible for the production of pseudocholinesterase, which metabolizes procaine (and other ester anesthetics). Decreased production can result in prolonged half-life of these drugs.

13. What mechanism is responsible for metabolism of amide anesthetics?
Hepatic microsomal enzymes have the major role in metabolism of amide local anesthetics. A decrease in liver function can therefore prolong the plasma half-life of amide anesthetics.

14. What is the most accurate test for evaluation of liver disease?

The liver biopsy. It can detect cirrhosis, fibrosis, fat deposition, iron overload, and inflammatory processes, as well as determine the prognosis.

15. How can liver disease affect the bleeding time?

The bleeding time may be increased in patients with portal hypertension by splenic sequestration of platelets leading to thrombocytopenia.

16. Which clotting factors does the liver produce?

Factors II, V, VII, IX, and X. These factors are vitamin K–dependent clotting factors.

17. What lab values will be affected by a deficiency in the factors produced by the liver?

PT and partial thromboplastin time (PTT).

18. What is the treatment for bleeding diathesis from liver disease?

Fresh frozen plasma (FFP). If the patient is thrombocytopenic, he or she may need platelet transfusion as well. Vitamin K–dependent clotting factors alone are not sufficient because they do not include factor V, which is also produced in the liver.

19. What is Gilbert's syndrome?

Gilbert's syndrome, the most common cause of idiopathic hyperbilirubinemia, is an autosomal dominant trait with variable penetrance. Decreased bilirubin uptake by hepatocytes results in increased plasma concentration of unconjugated bilirubin.

20. What are the most common drugs used in the dental office that are metabolized primarily by the liver?

Local anesthetics, including articaine (Septocaine), lidocaine (Xylocaine), mepivacaine (Carbocaine), prilocaine (Citanest), and bupivacaine (Marcaine), are metabolized by the liver. Analgesics that are metabolized in the liver include aspirin, acetaminophen (Tylenol), codeine, meperidine (Demerol), and ibuprofen (Motrin). Commonly used sedation drugs that are metabolized in the liver include diazepam (Valium) and midazolam (Versed). Valium is metabolized into the active metabolites desmethyldiazepam and oxazepam, thereby prolonging its effects on the central nervous system. Antibiotics that are metabolized in the liver include ampicillin, penicillin, clindamycin, erythromycin, and tetracycline. Erythromycin inhibits substrates CYP1A2 and 3A4, thereby increasing plasma concentrations of many other drugs. Because of this, close scrutiny of other medicines a person may be taking is required when prescribing erythromycin.

21. What are the different types of viral hepatitis?

To date, five distinct types of hepatitis have been designated according to the etiologic viruses: types A, B, C, D (delta), and E. Each of these viruses belongs to a different family of virus with distinct antigenic properties.

22. What are the differences among the various viral hepatitides?

Hepatitis A virus (HAV) is a 28-nm RNA virus whose mode of transmission is primarily fecal-oral. The diagnostic marker for hepatitis A is anti-HAV. Infected patients are treated with immune globulin and will develop lifetime immunity to HAV. A vaccine is available for HAV.

Hepatitis B virus (HBV) is a 42-nm DNA virus whose mode of transmission is predominately parenteral or through sexual contact. Diagnostic markers for HBV include immunoglobulin M (IgM) anti-HBc (acute), HBsAg (acute/chronic/infective), HBeAg (infectious), anti-HBs (recovery/immunity), and anti-HBcIg (ongoing or past infection). Infected patients are treated with hepatitis B immunoglobulin and will develop lifetime immunity. A vaccine is available for HBV.

Hepatitis C virus (HCV) is a 38-50–nm RNA virus whose mode of transmission is predominantly parenteral. Diagnostic markers include anti-HCV (recovery/immunity) and HCV RNA (infectivity). Effectiveness of treatment modalities for infected patients has not yet been established. Immunity following infection is weak and ineffective, and no vaccine currently exists.

Hepatitis D virus (HDV) is a viral infection that occurs only in patients with preexisting HBV. This co-infection often causes marked decline in hepatic function and may cause fulminate hepatic failure. HDV is usually transmitted by needles in drug users.

Hepatitis E virus (HEV) is a 32-nm RNA virus whose mode of transmission is predominately fecal-oral. The diagnostic marker used is anti-HEV (recovery). No treatment is currently used for infected patients. Infected patients will develop lifetime immunity, but no vaccine is currently available for HEV.

23. What are the orofacial features of patients with chronic alcoholism?

- Poor oral hygiene
- Jaundice of the oral mucosa
- Glossitis
- Parotid gland enlargement
- Angular cheilosis
- Impaired healing
- Candidiasis
- Bruxism
- Petechiae
- Xerostomia

24. What precautions should be taken before oral and maxillofacial surgery in a patient with viral hepatitis?

The patient's liver function status should be determined by means of liver function enzymes (AST, ALT, ALP). Drug choice and dosage should be determined with these lab values in mind. The patient's bleeding tendency should also be assessed by PT, PTT, international normalized ratio (INR), and bleeding time. For patients undergoing major surgical procedures, if the PT or PTT is more than $1^1/_2$ times > control values or if the INR is ≥ 3.0, transfusion of FFP should be considered. This supplies the patient with factors II, VII, IX, X, XI, XII, and XIII and heat-labile factors V and VII. In patients with a platelet count of <50,000/mm^3, platelet administration to a level above 50,000 mm^3 is indicated. Universal precautions should also be taken to prevent hepatitis exposure to the surgeon and assistants.

25. What is the preoperative therapy for patients with liver disease?

Preoperative maximization of liver function in patients with liver disease should include evaluating and optimizing the nutritional status and correcting electrolyte and coagulation abnormalities. The patient should stop alcohol intake and increase protein intake. If the patient has active hepatitis, all elective surgeries should be postponed until the hepatitis has resolved completely. Defects in coagulation should be corrected with FFP. If the patient is taking steroids, intravenous corticosteroids should be given. Finally, preoperative or operative sedation should be done to a degree that is compatible with the patient's decreased ability to metabolize drugs by the liver, especially benzodiazepines, barbiturates, and other sedatives.

26. What are the intraoperative considerations in patients with liver disease?

It is important to maintain adequate liver perfusion during surgery by maintaining adequate blood pressure. This can be done by infusing saline, FFP, and platelets if there is thrombocytopenia. If the patient swallowed blood, the stomach should be evacuated to prevent protein loading and false-positive blood in the stool. If the patient is taking corticosteroids, supplemental steroids should be given.

27. What are the surgical considerations in post–liver transplant patient?

During the first 3 months of the postoperative period, and in patients with chronic rejection of the graft, only emergency oral surgical procedures should be rendered. Such procedures should be performed only after consultation with the patient's transplant service, and whenever possible, antibiotic prophylaxis should be given to prevent bacterial endarteritis. After the first 3 months, the patient is usually on immunosuppressants. If the patient has a stable functional graft, good liver function is established. However, there is still the risk of acquired infection including influenza, fungal infections, and posttransplant viral infections. In these patients, prevention and treatment of any possible infection is important, and consideration must be given to the patient's immunosuppressant doses, supplementation of steroids (if necessary), and use of effective infection control measures.

BIBLIOGRAPHY

1. Cerulli MA: Management of the patient with liver diseases. Oral Maxillofac Surg Clin North Am 10:465-470, 1998.
2. Douglas LR, Douglas JB, Sieck JO et al: Oral management of the patient with end-stage liver disease and the liver transplant patient. Oral Surg Oral Med Oral Pathol Oral Radiol Endod 86:55-64, 1998.
3. Duke J: Renal function and anesthesia. In Duke J (ed): Anesthesia Secrets, 3rd ed. Philadelphia, 2006, Mosby.
4. Little JW, Falace DA: Liver disease. In Little JW, Falace DA (eds): Dental Management of the Medically Compromised Patient, 6th ed. St Louis, 2002, Mosby.
5. Stoelting RK, Dierdorf SF: Diseases of the liver and biliary tract. In Stoelting RK, Dierdorf SF (eds): Anesthesia and Co-Existing Disease, 3rd ed. London, 1993, Churchill Livingstone.
6. Stoelting RK, Miller RD: Liver and biliary tract disease. In Stoelting RK, Miller RD (eds): Basics of Anesthesia, 3rd ed. New York, 1994, Churchill Livingstone.
7. Ziccardi VB, Abubaker AO, Sotereanos GC et al: Maxillofacial considerations in orthotopic liver transplant patient. Oral Surg Oral Med Oral Pathol 71:21-26, 1991.

21. RENAL DISEASES

Mark A. Oghalai, DDS

1. What are five main functions of the kidney?
1. Elimination of metabolic waste
2. Maintenance of fluid balance
3. Maintenance of electrolyte balance
4. Maintenance of acid and base balance
5. Endocrine and metabolic functions, including erythropoietin secretion and vitamin D conversion

2. Which compound is used as a sensitive, indirect measurement of glomerular filtration rate (GFR)?
Creatinine is used because it is filtered by the glomeruli but minimally secreted or reabsorbed.

3. What is renal failure?
Renal failure is defined as impairment in renal function, as measured by the GFR. It is classified as either acute or chronic.

4. What is acute renal failure (ARF)?
This syndrome is characterized by sudden decline in renal function, resulting in retention

of nitrogenous waste with corresponding elevations of serum creatinine and blood urea nitrogen (BUN). It is usually reversible if treated early.

5.   What are the major classes of ARF?
- **Prerenal.** This class is the most common type and is associated with insufficient renal perfusion. Examples include hypovolemia, impaired cardiac function, and sepsis.
- **Renal.** Glomerular diseases, acute tubular necrosis, and acute interstitial nephritis fall under this classification.
- **Postrenal.** This type of renal failure includes bilateral urethral obstruction and bladder neck obstruction.

6.   What is chronic renal failure (CRF)?
CRF is an irreversible, advanced, and progressive renal insufficiency.

7.   What are the major causes of CRF?
- Diabetic nephropathy
- Hypertension

8.   What are the clinical manifestations of CRF and end-stage renal disease (ESRD)?
The clinical manifestations of CRF and ESRD depend on the stage of the disease and include:
- Fluid and electrolyte disturbances
- Hypertension and pericarditis
- Uremia and uremic osteodystrophy
- Tiredness and insomnia
- Peripheral neuropathy
- Anemia and thrombocytopenia
- Nausea and vomiting
- Pruritus and hyperpigmentation

9.   What are the main treatment options for ESRD?
- Peritoneal dialysis
- Hemodialysis
- Renal transplant

10. What endocrine abnormality is often associated with CRF?
Secondary hyperparathyroidism. As the kidneys lose their ability to convert vitamin D, intestinal absorption of calcium decreases, causing hyperparathyroidism.

11. What are the oral manifestations of renal disease?
Patients with renal disease or CRF often demonstrate orofacial signs and symptoms that are not necessarily specific for ESRD but are related to the systemic manifestations of the disease. The most common of these manifestations are:
- Enamel hypoplasia and staining of teeth
- Halitosis and metallic taste
- Stomatitis and xerostomia secondary to fluid intake restriction
- Gingival bleeding, ecchymosis, petechiae, and pale and inflamed gingiva
- Osteolytic bone defects in the mandible, mandibular condyles, and maxilla; loss of lamina dura; and decreased trabeculation of bone
- Skeletal facial deformities secondary to altered growth
- Accelerated dental calculus accumulation

12. What are the lab findings in patients with CRF?
- Elevated BUN and creatinine resulting from decreased glomerular filtration
- Metabolic acidosis secondary to impaired tubular function, causing an accumulation of ammonia

- Multiple electrolyte abnormalities, including hyperkalemia, hypocalcemia, and hypermagnesemia
- Anemia from decreased renal production of erythropoietin

13. How does renal disease affect the pharmacodynamics of administered drugs?

The effects of drugs may be potentiated by increased volume of distribution, decreased protein binding, and decreased glomerular filtration and renal tubular secretion. Renal failure may modify drug bioavailability, distribution, pharmacologic action, or elimination when the kidney excretes the drug or its metabolites. For the ESRD patient, most drugs are administered in an initial loading dose to provide therapeutic blood concentrations. Sustained effects are controlled by dosage adjustments and time-interval alterations and are based on serum drug levels.

14. How do nonsteroidal antiinflammatory drugs (NSAIDs) affect renal function?

NSAIDs inhibit prostaglandin synthesis and therefore decrease prostaglandin-associated intrinsic renal vasodilatation.

15. What classes of drugs should be avoided in patients with renal disease?
- Nephrotoxic drugs, including NSAIDs, aminoglycosides, and intravenous (IV) dyes
- Drugs that are converted to toxic metabolites, including meperidine and propoxyphene
- Drugs that contain excessive electrolytes, including penicillin G and magnesium citrate

16. What analgesics should be avoided in patients with renal disease?
- Aspirin
- Acetaminophen
- NSAIDs
- Meperidine (accumulation of meperidine can result in seizures)
- Morphine (dose decreased secondary to accumulation of morphine-6-glucuronide)

17. What antibiotics should be avoided in patients with renal disease?
- Cephalosporins
- Erythromycin
- Tetracycline
- Aminoglycosides

18. In severe renal dysfunction patients, are metabolic end products from local anesthetics contraindicated?

No. Local anesthetics are metabolized in the liver and plasma, then excreted. Therefore anesthetics can accumulate and not be a factor in patients with renal disease.

19. What effect might general anesthetics have on renal blood flow and GFR?

General anesthetics that can cause myocardial depression also can cause decreased renal blood flow and a GFR that is proportional to the depth of anesthesia. Methoxyflurane is no longer in use because of fluoride-induced nephrotoxicity. Halothane, enflurane, and isoflurane produce much lower fluoride levels and are safer to use with regard to nephrotoxicity. Therefore it is important to choose the type of agent and the appropriate level of anesthesia in renal failure patients to minimize further injury and likelihood of renal failure.

20. Which metabolites from halogenated general anesthetics can lead to nephrotoxic renal failure?

Inorganic fluoride from the metabolism of methoxyflurane. Sevoflurane also increases inorganic fluoride, and its use is controversial in patients with renal disease.

21. Which halogenated general anesthetics do not significantly increase plasma inorganic fluoride concentrations?

Isoflurane, halothane, and desflurane.

22. At what time before and after surgery should dialysis be performed?

One day before surgery and 1-2 days after surgery to correct potassium and fluid balance while minimizing bleeding complications.

23. What lab tests should be performed for renal failure patients before surgery?

CRF patients should have bleeding time, prothrombin time (PT), partial thromboplastin time (PTT), platelet count, complete blood cell count (CBC), and serum potassium and protein levels. Bleeding time is the most sensitive test for a bleeding tendency in CRF patients. If the bleeding time is elevated, the patient should receive vigorous dialysis and, if necessary, deamino-D-arginine vasopressin (DDAVP) intravenously or nasally, at a dose of 0.3 µg/kg, 30 min before surgery. Hyperkalemia also can be corrected with preoperative dialysis. If surgery is emergent and dialysis cannot be performed preoperatively, hyperkalemia should be treated aggressively to decrease the arrhythmogenic effect of hyperkalemia. This can be done by IV infusion of calcium chloride, glucose, and insulin to drive extracellular potassium into cells.

24. What is the cause of CRF-induced anemia?

Decreased erythropoietin production from the kidneys.

25. What is the treatment for CRF-induced anemia before surgery?

Anemia in CRF patients should be treated with administration of recombinant human erythropoietin until the patient's hematocrit is raised to at least 30%-33%.

26. What is the difference between peritoneal dialysis and hemodialysis?

In peritoneal dialysis, a hypertonic solution is placed into the peritoneal cavity and removed a short time later. During the removal process, dissolved solutes such as urea are drawn out. Peritoneal dialysis does not require anticoagulation and is less expensive than hemodialysis. However, peritoneal dialysis requires more frequent sessions than hemodialysis, is less effective, and has a higher incidence of complications such as infection, hypoglycemia, and protein loss. The most common use for peritoneal dialysis is the treatment of patients with ARF.

Hemodialysis is the most commonly used method of dialysis for CRF and is performed at 2- to 3-day intervals. Surgical placement of a permanent arteriovenous (AV) fistula for large-bore cannulation is required; the patient's blood is filtered through a dialysis machine and returned to the patient via the AV fistula. Administering heparin prevents clotting. Patients receiving hemodialysis are at risk for contracting hepatitis B, hepatitis C, and HIV because of multiple blood exposures. In addition, these patients are at risk for infection of their AV shunts, which predisposes them to septic emboli, septicemia, infective endarteritis, and infective endocarditis.

27. What steps should be taken before oral surgical procedures in ESRD patients?

- Review lab values to detect possible bleeding diathesis (bleeding time, platelet count, PT, PTT).
- Monitor blood pressure.
- Avoid nephrotoxic drugs such as acyclovir, aspirin, NSAIDs, and high-dose acetaminophen.
- Decrease dosage of drugs metabolized by the kidney.
- Aggressively manage orofacial infections.
- Ensure that patients receiving hemodialysis do not undergo surgery for at least 4 hr after hemodialysis to avoid heparin-induced bleeding.

28. What presurgical adjustments need to be made in drug dosing or interval in patients with CRF (Table 21-1)?

Table 21-1 *Presurgical Drug Adjustments Made in Chronic Renal Failure Patients*

DRUG	PRESURGERY ADJUSTMENT
Aspirin	Increase interval between doses and avoid drug completely if glomerular filtration rate is low
Acetaminophen	Increase interval between doses and avoid drug completely in cases of severe failure
Penicillin V, cephalexin, tetracycline	Increase interval between doses in severe failure
Ketoconazole	Reduce dose
Lidocaine, codeine, erythromycin, clindamycin, metronidazole	No adjustment necessary

29. What medical considerations should be given to patients receiving dialysis before oral surgical procedures?

No adjustments are required for patients receiving peritoneal dialysis, but there are several concerns for patients receiving hemodialysis. Surgically created bacteremia can cause infection of the AV fistula. Because graft endothelialization takes up to 3-6 months after placement, standard American Heart Association antibiotic prophylaxis is strongly recommended for the first 6 months after fistula placement and may be beneficial for all graft patients undergoing oral surgery. The arm that contains the AV shunt should not be used for blood pressure recording because the shunt could collapse. Likewise, IV administration of medications should be avoided in the arm because clot formation could jeopardize the shunt. The quality of the AV thrill should be assessed initially and then periodically during surgery. During long surgeries, the use of a circulating heating pack over the arm is advocated.

Patients should be screened for bleeding tendencies because hemodialysis destroys platelets. Surgery should be delayed for at least 4 hr after hemodialysis to prevent heparin-induced bleeding. Patients should be screened periodically for hepatitis B, hepatitis C, and HIV. Universal precautions should be followed by the surgical team when treating any patient undergoing hemodialysis. The positioning of the access site must be observed during surgery to avoid pressure on the site.

30. How are bleeding problems prevented and managed in patients with renal failure?

Bleeding encountered in patients with renal failure is best managed initially with local hemostatic procedures, such as good surgical technique, primary wound closure whenever possible, hemostatic agents and topical thrombin, and electrocautery. Preoperative IV (0.3 µg/kg) or intranasal (3.0 µg/kg) DDAVP temporarily corrects the increase in bleeding time in uremic patients for up to 4 hr. It also may be useful as a therapeutic modality in acute postsurgical hemorrhage. Cryoprecipitate has a peak effect in 4-12 hr and duration of 24-36 hr but generally is reserved for acute bleeding that is not easily managed. Conjugated estrogen, which has a duration of up to 30 days and peak effects in approximately 2-5 days, also may be used.

BIBLIOGRAPHY

1. Bennett WM, Muther RS, Parker RA et al: Drug therapy in renal failure: dosing guidelines for adults. Part I: antimicrobial agents, analgesics. Ann Intern Med 93:62-89, 1980.
2. Carl W, Wood RH: The dental patient with chronic renal failure. Quintessence Int 7:9-15, 1976.
3. Duke J: Renal function and anesthesia. In Duke J (ed): Anesthesia Secrets, 3rd ed. Philadelphia, 2006, Mosby.

4. Little JW, Falace DA: Chronic renal failure and dialysis. In Little JW, Falace DA (eds): Dental Management of the Medically Compromised Patient, 6th ed. St Louis, 2002, Mosby.
5. Silverstein KE, Adams MC, Fonseca RJ: Evaluation and management of the renal failure and dialysis patient. Oral Maxillofac Surg Clin North Am 10:417-427, 1998.
6. Stoelting RK, Dierdorf SF: Renal disease. In Stoelting RK, Dierdorf SF (eds): Anesthesia and Co-Existing Disease, 3rd ed. London, 1993, Churchill Livingstone.
7. Stoelting RK, Miller RD: Renal disease. In Stoelting RK, Miller RD (eds): Basics of Anesthesia, 3rd ed. Philadelphia, 1994, Churchill Livingstone.
8. Swell SB: Dental care for patients with renal failure and renal transplants. J Am Dent Assoc 104:171-177, 1982.
9. Westbrook DS: Dental management in patients receiving hemodialysis and kidney transplants. J Am Dental Assoc 96:464-468, 1978.
10. Ziccardi VB, Saini J, Demas PN et al: Management of the oral and maxillofacial surgery patient with end-stage renal disease. J Oral Maxillofac Surg 50:1207-1212, 1992.

22. ENDOCRINE DISEASES

Maria J. Iuorno, MD, MS

1. What is calcitonin?

Calcitonin, a 32-amino acid polypeptide, is a hormone produced by the parafollicular cells or C cells of the thyroid gland.

2. What are the signs and symptoms associated with adrenal insufficiency?

Chronic Signs and Symptoms	Associated Mineralocorticoid Deficiency Symptoms
Anorexia	Acute (adrenal crises) mental status changes
Bronzing of the skin	Confusion
Dehydration	Hyperkalemia
Dizziness	Hyponatremia
Fatigue	Hypotension
Hypertension	Lethargy
Hypoglycemia	
Nausea	
Vomiting	
Weakness	
Weight loss	

3. Where is aldosterone produced?

Aldosterone, a mineralocorticoid, is produced within the zona glomerulosa of the adrenal cortex.

4. What influence does aldosterone have on sodium (Na) and potassium (K)?

Major influence is on Na balance by increasing renal tubular reabsorption of Na in distal tubular segment (mostly collecting tubules). The net result is Na resorption and K excretion.

5. Which hormone is also known as vasopressin?

Antidiuretic hormone (ADH).

6. **Where is ADH produced and released?**
    Posterior pituitary.

7. **What effect will an increased release of ADH have on urine concentration?**
    Because ADH affects the renal collecting tubule's permeability, water will be reabsorbed, resulting in a more concentrated urine.

8. **What causes ADH release?**
    ADH is released in response to changes in the serum osmolality detected by the hypothalamus. Osmolality that decreases to about 295 mOsm/kg initiates release.

9. **Where are angiotensin I and II produced?**
    In the kidney.

10. **How does angiotensin II cause an increase in blood pressure?**
    Angiotensin II actively increases vascular tone, stimulates catecholamine release, and increases Na reabsorption (at the distal tubule). It also stimulates release of aldosterone from zona glomerulosa of the adrenal cortex.

11. **What are the diagnostic criteria for differentiating among acute tubular necrosis, prerenal azotemia, and postrenal obstruction (Table 22-1)?**

Table 22-1   *Differing Diagnostic Criteria for Acute Tubular Necrosis, Prerenal Azotemia, and Postrenal Obstruction*

	PRERENAL AZOTEMIA (OBSTRUCTION)	ATN (TUBULAR INJURY)	POSTRENAL OBSTRUCTION
Urine osmolality	>500	<350	Varies
U/P osmolality	>1.25	<1.1	Varies
U/P urea	>8	<3	Varies
U/P creatinine	>40	<20	<20
Urine Na	<20	>40	>40
FENa	<1	>3	>3

ATN, Acute tubular necrosis; *U/P*, urea/plasma ratio; *Na*, sodium; *FENa*, fractional excretion of sodium.

12. **What is azotemia?**
    Nitrogen retention resulting from factors other than primary renal disease.

13. **What is the syndrome of inappropriate secretion of ADH (SIADH)?**
    SIADH is the nonphysiologic secretion of ADH from sites other than the pituitary gland. It is the most common cause of hospital-acquired hyponatremia. Several conditions can cause SIADH:
    - Some tumors, such as oat cell lung carcinoma (small cell), secrete biologically active ADH.
    - Central nervous system (CNS) disorders, such as meningitis and encephalitis, may affect osmoreceptors that regulate pituitary ADH secretion.
    - Pulmonary infections cause decreased serum Na concentration by an unknown mechanism.
    - Pharmacologic agents such as clofibrate, cyclophosphamide, and the oral hypoglycemic

chlorpropamide enhance secretion of ADH or duplicate the kidney's response to ADH.
• Mechanical ventilation, narcotics, hypercarbia, and pain may trigger ADH.

14. How is SIADH diagnosed?

Clinical exam may reveal weakness, lethargy, seizure, confusion, and coma.

Lab findings usually show persistent hyponatremia, serum hyposmolarity > plasma, and an inappropriately concentrated urine and abnormally high Na. Dehydration must be ruled out before diagnosis of SIADH can be made.

15. What is the treatment for SIADH?

Treatment for SIADH depends on the symptoms. Mild to moderate symptoms are treated with fluid restriction (500-1000 mL/24 hr). Severe water intoxication (symptomatically severe hyponatremia) requires hypertonic saline (3%, 200 mL) in addition to free water restriction. Water restriction is effective in most cases of chronic SIADH. Demeclocycline, which inhibits ADH action at the renal tubular cell, can also be used.

16. What is diabetes insipidus (DI)?

DI is a disease of ADH deficiency. It is less common than SIADH and occurs primarily after head trauma, cranial surgery, anoxic encephalopathy, metastatic neoplasms to the pituitary (e.g., breast cancer), and granulomatous destruction (e.g., sarcoid) of the posterior pituitary. Drugs that inhibit ADH release (phenytoin and ethanol) can stimulate a mild form of DI. Idiopathic central DI causes polyuria, polydipsia, and astounding urine volumes (5-10 L/day).

17. How is DI diagnosed?

DI is characterized by dilute urine with increased serum osmolality. The diagnosis is made by fluid restriction for 6-10 hr. A patient with an intact neurohypophyseal axis will increase urine osmolality up to 500-1400 mEq/L while keeping serum osmolality < 295 mEq/L. A patient with full-blown DI cannot protect his or her serum osmolality. As a result, levels of serum osmolality >320 with a urine osmolality <200 may be seen. When this patient is given parenteral ADH, the urine osmolality rises significantly.

18. How is central DI treated?

Treatment for central DI depends on etiology. DI due to trauma or surgery is often transient and self-limited. DDAVP (1-deamino-8-D-arginine vasopressin), an ADH analogue with an antidiuretic pressor activity ratio of 2000:1, is the treatment of choice for DI from other etiologies. Duration of action is 6-20 hr when taken intranasally or subcutaneously. It requires once- or twice-daily dosing.

19. What is nephrogenic DI, and how does it differ from central DI?

In nephrogenic DI, the renal distal tubular cells are unable to respond to ADH. Causes of nephrogenic DI include lithium use and pregnancy. Nephrogenic DI is differentiated from central DI by evidence that ADH administration will not increase urine osmolality. Nephrogenic DI should be treated with thiazide diuretics and strict salt restriction. Psychogenic polydipsia (compulsive water drinking) may mimic DI.

20. What is the result of resection of the parathyroid gland?

Hypoparathyroidism is characterized by decreased excretion of calcium. Blood chemistry shows low serum calcium and high serum phosphorus. If calcium falls to 7-8 mg/dL, neuromuscular symptoms will develop. If serum levels fall to 5-6 mg/dL, tetany and the characteristic carpopedal spasms are apparent. Chronic calcinosis sometimes precedes idiopathic hypoparathyroidism, possibly inducing an immune response.

21. What are the three types of multiple endocrine neoplasia syndrome (MENS) (Table 22-2)?

Table 22-2	*Three Types of Multiple Endocrine Neoplasia Syndrome (MENS)*
TYPE	CHARACTERISTICS
MENS I	Hyperplasia of pituitary, parathyroid, adrenal cortex, pancreatic islet cells, and peptic ulcer
MENS II MENS IIa MENS IIb	Parathyroid tumor: adenoma, pheochromocytoma, and medullary carcinoma of thyroid
MENS III	Mucocutaneous neuroma, pheochromocytoma, and medullary carcinoma of thyroid and a marfanoid appearance

22. What are MENS IIa and MENS IIb associated with?

MENS IIa is associated with hyperparathyroidism, and MENS IIb is associated with marfanoid habitus and hyperplastic joints.

23. How is adrenal crisis recognized? How is it treated?

Adrenal crisis is characterized by acute-onset fatigue, mental status changes, and hypotension. Electrolyte abnormalities are also present in the form of hyponatremia, hyperkalemia, and nonanion gap acidosis. Appropriate therapy includes 0.9% normal saline infusion and corticosteroid replacement with hydrocortisone, 100 mg intravenously (IV) every 6-8 hr. If an adrenocorticotropic hormone (ACTH; cosyntropin) stimulation test is needed, dexamethasone (2-4 mg every 8 hr) should be used for replacement instead; this drug, unlike hydrocortisone, is not measured as serum cortisol in the blood. Mineralocorticoid replacement with Florinef is not indicated in the acute management of adrenal crisis.

24. How do you test for primary adrenal insufficiency?

The gold standard test for primary adrenal failure is the ACTH (cosyntropin) stimulation test. Cosyntropin (Cortrosyn) is an ACTH analogue that stimulates the adrenal gland and its ACTH receptor. The test is performed by drawing a serum cortisol between 7:00 AM and 8:00 AM, administering cosyntropin (125 mg intramusculary [IM] or IV), and drawing the serum cortisol again at 30 min and 60 min after cosyntropin administration. The serum cortisol level should rise to >20 μg/dL if there is adequate adrenal function.

25. How long can high-dose exogenous corticosteroids produce potential significant adrenal insufficiency?

Exogenous steroids in excess of 10-20 mg of prednisone daily can produce significant endogenous adrenal axis suppression after 2 weeks in chronic therapy for such conditions as asthma, chronic obstructive pulmonary disease (COPD), and rheumatoid arthritis. Preoperatively, these patients should be treated with high-dose (100 mg of hydrocortisone) stress-level steroids for at least 24 hr before surgery and every 8 hr thereafter to avoid adrenal crisis.

26. What are some clinical signs and symptoms of anterior pituitary tumors?

The many functional types of anterior pituitary tumors are based on the predominant pituitary hormone that the tumor secretes. These tumors also produce functional deficiencies of the anterior pituitary. Common tumors are shown in Table 22-3.

Table 22-3   Clinical Signs of Anterior Pituitary Tumors

HORMONE-ASSOCIATED TUMORS	SIGNS AND SYMPTOMS
Prolactin	Amenorrhea or galactorrhea in women
Nonsecreting chromophobe adenoma	Often none, unless large
Luteinizing hormone and follicle-stimulating hormone secretory (gonadotropin-secretory) tumor	Impotence in men
Asymptomatic, TSH-secreting, ACTH-secreting tumors	Cushing's disease
Growth hormone–secreting tumors	Acromegaly

TSH, Thyroid-stimulating hormone; *ACTH,* adrenocorticotropic hormone.

Typical signs, such as impotence, amenorrhea, headaches, bitemporal hemianopia, and visual field disturbance worsen as the tumor increases in size.

27. What are the preferred medical agents used to treat hypertension in hyper-aldosteronism?

The usual agents are K^+-sparing diuretics. Hyperaldosteronism is characterized by K-wasting hypertension. Spironolactone is the drug of choice because it is a direct aldosterone antagonist at the level of the kidneys. Aldactone is an alternative.

28. What are the characteristic electrolyte abnormalities of hyperaldosteronism?

Hyperaldosteronism is usually characterized by extreme hypokalemia (<3.1) and possible signs of insufficiency, such as increased serum creatinine and blood urea nitrogen (BUN). The hypokalemia may be exacerbated by the use of loop diuretics, such as furosemide and thiazide drugs.

29. What is appropriate therapy for the treatment for symptomatic hypercalcemia?

Symptomatic hypercalcemia can be life threatening and needs to be treated on an emergency basis. Usually, therapy includes aggressive IV hydration with normal saline (not lactated Ringer's solution, which contains calcium). After 6-12 hr of hydration, furosemide (Lasix) therapy may be initiated to help with aggressive diuresis of calcium. IV pamidronate, a bisphosphonate, may be given (60 mg IV over 4-6 hr) to help sequester serum calcium back into bony sites. A one-time dose will deliver adequate therapy for up to 2 weeks.

30. What is the proper management of a palpable solitary nodule within the thyroid gland?

An isolated palpable nodule needs to be evaluated for thyroid cancer. Thyroid cancer is usually occult and slow growing, which permits time for evaluation. Masses > 1 cm are more suspicious for malignancy. Palpable nodules may be evaluated first by fine-needle aspiration biopsy. The results of the biopsy can be read quickly by a pathologist; if the preliminary results come back consistent with malignancy, the patient should be referred for surgery. If the results are benign, the nodule may be checked every 6 months to evaluate for a size increase. Lesions that are undetermined can undergo thyroid iodine I^{123} scanning. "Cold" nodules with low uptake are suspicious for malignancy and should be referred to surgery. Also, at the initial visit, a thyroid-stimulating hormone (TSH) test may be drawn. If TSH is low or suppressed, the patient should be referred for thyroid scan to rule out a benign "hot" nodule.

31. What lab thyroid function test and findings characterize sick euthyroid syndrome?

Sick euthyroid syndrome is a euthyroid condition common in the critically ill patient. It is due to excessive conversion of thyroxine (T_4) to reverse triiodothyronine (rT_3) instead of its more potent isomer, T_3, and possibly hypothalamic suppression of TSH. These patients are clinically euthyroid. Lab findings include a normal to low TSH, low to normal T_4, and low free T_4 index. Direct free T_4 by equilibrium dialysis, however, is normal. Reverse T_3 is high, and T_3 is low.

32. Does empiric therapy benefit critically ill patients with euthyroid sick syndrome?

Studies of critically ill patients 24-72 hr after coronary artery bypass grafting failed to demonstrate that patient survival and morbidity improved after therapy with exogenous T_3 (Cytomel).

33. What common postoperative complication is associated with subclinical hypothyroidism?

Significant respiratory suppression with inability to wean from a respirator can be seen in patients who have even mild untreated hypothyroidism that is otherwise asymptomatic. Thyroid function tests alone may be needed to make this diagnosis. Preoperative TSH is the best screening test. This test would be elevated even in mild hypothyroidism.

34. What is the most common cardiac arrhythmia present in the elderly with hyperthyroidism?

Hyperthyroidism in the elderly may be of the **clinical** form or the **apathetic** form. In the latter, patients rarely present with classic signs and symptoms, such as anxiety, sweating, weight loss, or palpitations. Rather, they may present with depressed mood or somnolence, cognitive impairment, or poor appetite. A TSH that is suppressed is the most sensitive indicator of hyperthyroidism. Even patients who are elderly and symptomatic are at significantly increased risk for cardiac arrhythmia—most commonly atrial fibrillation.

35. What are the contraindications to the use of metformin (Glucophage) in type 2 diabetes?

Metformin therapy is strictly contraindicated in alcoholics, patients with significant renal insufficiency or failure (serum creatinine >1.5 in men and >1.4 for women), and patients with liver disease. These conditions considerably increase the risk of the fatal side effect, lactic acidosis. Patients who are older than age 70 and those with cardiac ejection fractions <50% also are not candidates for metformin therapy. Patients about to receive iodine contrast for cardiac catheterization or who are to undergo major surgery should stop metformin therapy 48-72 hr before the procedure.

BIBLIOGRAPHY

1. Arnaud CN: The calcitropic hormones and metabolic bone disease. In Greenspan FS, Baxter JD (eds): Basic and Clinical Endocrinology, 4th ed. Stamford, Conn, 1994, Appleton & Lange.
2. Deftos LJ, Catherwood BD: Syndromes involving multiple endocrine glands. In Greenspan FS, Baxter JD (eds): Basic and Clinical Endocrinology, 4th ed. Stamford, Conn, 1994, Appleton & Lange.
3. Favus JJ (ed): Primer on the Metabolic Bone Diseases and Disorders of Mineral Metabolism, 3rd ed. New York, 1996, Lippincott-Raven.
4. Greenspan FS: The thyroid gland. In Greenspan FS, Baxter JD (eds): Basic and Clinical Endocrinology, 4th ed. Stamford, Conn, 1994, Appleton & Lange.
5. Halpern LR, Chase DC: Perioperative management of patients with endocrine dysfunction: physiology, presurgical, and postsurgical treatment protocols. Oral Maxillofac Surg Clin North Am 10:491, 1998.
6. Karam JH, Forsham PH: Diabetes mellitus. In Greenspan FS, Baxter JD (eds): Basic and Clinical Endocrinology, 4th ed. Stamford, Conn, 1994, Appleton & Lange.
7. McDermott MT (ed): Endocrine Secrets, 4th ed. Philadelphia, 2005, Hanley & Belfus.

8. Orth DN, Kovacs WJ: Adrenal cortex. In Wilson JD, Daniel F, Kronenberg HM et al (eds): Williams Textbook of Endocrinology, 9th ed. Philadelphia, 1998, Wilson & Foster.
9. Reeves FG, Bichel CB, Andreoli TE: Posterior pituitary and water metabolism. In Wilson JD, Daniel F, Kronenberg HM et al (eds): Williams Textbook of Endocrinology, 9th ed. Philadelphia, 1998, Wilson & Foster.

23. THE DIABETIC PATIENT

Bradley A. Gregory, DMD

1. What is diabetes?

Diabetes is a chronic disorder of carbohydrates, fat, and protein metabolism whereby a defective or deficient insulin secretory response leads to impaired glucose use. Diabetes creates a physiologic predisposition for developing generalized microvascular, macrovascular, and neuropathic complications.

2. How is glucose normally metabolized?

Blood glucose level is normally maintained between 60 and 130 mg/dL. Excess glucose is converted to glycogen, which is stored mostly in liver and muscle. Triglycerides (omega-3 fatty acids attached to glycerol) are used during periods of energy deprivation through lipolysis, and various amino acids can be converted to glucose in the liver through gluconeogenesis.

3. How does insulin facilitate uptake of glucose into cells?

Insulin is released in a rapid surge during the first 10-30 min after a meal. This is followed by a second phase of a slower, sustained release of insulin. Insulin receptors in the cell membrane have alpha and beta subunits. Insulin binds to subunit alpha, which causes the aforementioned change in subunit beta. Subunit beta promotes the activity of the enzyme tyrosine kinase. Tyrosine kinase is essential because it phosphorylates intracellular insulin receptors that bring glucose into the cell.

4. From where is insulin secreted?

Insulin is secreted from the beta cells of the endocrine pancreas.

5. How does insulin lower the plasma glucose?

Insulin promotes glucose uptake into most tissues *except* brain, kidney tubules, intestinal mucosa, and red blood cells. Insulin promotes glycogenesis, the formation of glycogen from glucose. At the same time, it will inhibit glycogenolysis. Insulin also inhibits gluconeogenesis, especially in the liver and kidneys.

6. How does insulin lower blood levels of amino acids?

Insulin promotes the uptake of amino acids into muscles. This facilitates protein synthesis. At the same time, insulin inhibits proteolysis.

7. What is the effect of insulin on free fatty acids (FFAs)?

Insulin lowers the blood levels of FFAs by promoting their uptake into adipose tissue. In addition, insulin promotes the formation of triglycerides (lipogenesis). Also, insulin inhibits hormone-sensitive lipase, which is the enzyme necessary for the breakdown of triglycerides into FFAs.

8. From where is glucagon secreted?

Glucagon is secreted from alpha cells of the endocrine pancreas. It is also found in the gastrointestinal mucosa.

9. What metabolic effects does glucagon regulate?

The metabolic effects exerted on liver, muscle, and adipose tissue are opposite those of insulin. Glucagon mobilizes stored energy by promoting glycogenolysis (especially at the liver), gluconeogenesis, and lipolysis by activating hormone-sensitive lipase. Other effects of glucagon include stimulating the secretion of insulin by increasing plasma glucose and stimulating the secretion of growth hormone.

10. How is cortisol secreted and regulated?

Corticotropin-releasing hormone (CRH) is released from the hypothalamus. CRH stimulates the release of adrenocorticotropic hormone (ACTH) from the anterior pituitary. ACTH stimulates cortisol release from the zona fasciculata of the adrenal glands, causing negative feedback to CRH and ACTH.

11. What metabolic role does cortisol play in glucose metabolism?

Cortisol protects plasma glucose and stores glucose as glycogen by promoting the breakdown of protein from muscle, stimulating hepatic gluconeogenesis and glycogenesis, and facilitating lipolysis by growth hormone and epinephrine. Cortisol also has an antiinsulin effect on muscle and adipose tissue.

12. How does epinephrine exert its metabolic controls?

Effects are mediated through beta receptors located on the exterior of cells. The inhibition of insulin secretion at the beta cells of the pancreas is through alpha receptors. Epinephrine stimulates gluconeogenesis at the liver through alpha receptors.

13. What is the role of epinephrine in glucose regulation?

The overall goal of epinephrine is to protect plasma glucose. In the muscle and liver, it promotes glycogenolysis. Epinephrine promotes gluconeogenesis as well. In addition, it will inhibit insulin release and stimulate glucagon release through alpha receptors in the pancreas. In the bloodstream, it will inhibit glucose uptake. Finally, epinephrine stimulates hormone-sensitive lipase to facilitate lipolysis in muscle and adipose tissue.

14. What is the role of growth hormone in glucose regulation?

Growth hormone is secreted by stimuli such as exercise-induced hypoglycemia, fasting, and stress from trauma, fever, and surgery. Growth hormone release is inhibited by glucose and FFAs. Growth hormone increases plasma glucose, mobilizes FFAs and protein stores by promoting lipolysis, increases glycogenolysis, and inhibits glucose uptake by muscle and adipose tissue.

15. What are the four different types of diabetes mellitus?

1. **Type 1 diabetes.** This form is usually associated with young people. These patients require insulin to maintain glucose homeostasis secondary to beta cell destruction in the pancreas.
2. **Type 2 diabetes.** These patients' cells have lost their sensitivity to insulin secondary to environmental and genetic factors. Therefore their muscle and adipose cells cannot transport glucose.
3. **Gestational diabetes.** This usually develops secondary to pregnancy. Up to 40% of women with gestational diabetes will develop type 2 diabetes within 10 years of developing gestational diabetes.
4. **Secondary diabetes.** This is related to a specific cause, such as removal of the pancreas.

16. What is the pathogenesis of type 1 diabetes?
- A **genetic susceptibility** predisposes some people to autoimmunity against beta cells of the pancreas.
- **Autoimmunity** develops spontaneously or, more commonly, is stimulated by an environmental agent.
- **Environmental injury** can damage beta cells, which are then recognized as foreign by the immune defenses.

17. What is the pathogenesis of type 2 diabetes?
- Genetics play a significant, but not well understood, part.
- Type 2 diabetes is a combination of insulin resistance and an insulin secretory defect.
- Environmental factors play a very important role. This includes obesity, which will not cause diabetes but can unmask it. Also in this group are inactivity, pregnancy, and stress. Stress releases cortisol and catecholamines, which oppose insulin and raise the blood sugar level.

18. What metabolic abnormalities are associated with type 1 diabetes?
   Abnormalities are classified into those of carbohydrate, protein, and lipid metabolism.
- Type 1 patients generally have a combination of glucose underutilization and excessive glucose production resembling the fasting state. Glucose is unable to get into certain tissues, which causes the renal threshold to be surpassed, resulting in polyuria. Polyuria leads to dehydration, which triggers polydipsia. In addition, because cells are not getting nourishment, patients experience polyphagia.
- These patients break down protein from muscle to make glucose. Proteins are required for antibody production, white blood cell production, and healing of wounds. Deficiency of these proteins leads to susceptibility of infections and poor wound healing.
- Insulin deficiency leads to lipolysis of triglycerides into FFAs, which yields acetyl coenzyme A (CoA). Ultimately, ketone bodies are formed, which can lead to metabolic acidosis.

19. What metabolic abnormalities are associated with type 2 diabetes?
   The metabolic abnormalities are classified as insulin resistance, loss of sensitivity of cells to insulin, and a decrease in insulin secretion. Insulin is unable to get into cells because either a postreceptor defect prevents uptake or there is a problem of insulin binding to target cells in the liver, muscle, and adipose tissue. In addition, type 2 diabetics may have a gradual decrease in basal levels of insulin secretion because the pancreas loses sensitivity to glucose level changes.

20. Which acute complication is most often associated with type 1 diabetes?
   Diabetic ketoacidosis (DKA) almost exclusively occurs in type 1 diabetics. DKA is the result of severe insulin deficiency coupled with an absolute or relative increase of glucagon.
   Patients with DKA usually have blood glucose levels >250 mg/dL, ketones in the urine and serum, pH <7.2, and plasma bicarbonate <15 mEq/L. Clinical manifestations include nausea and vomiting to compensate for the metabolic acidosis and Kussmaul respirations to reduce carbon dioxide levels in blood. The goals of treatment are to correct dehydration by starting 0.9% normal saline intravenously, using regular insulin, reversing the acidosis, and treating the potassium deficiency.

21. What is the acute complication most associated with type 2 diabetes?
   Hyperosmolar nonketotic coma usually occurs in patients who are age 65 or older. The symptoms may go unrecognized for weeks. These patients have enough insulin to prevent a ketotic state, but they are severely hyperglycemic (usually >600 mg/dL). Left untreated, they

become severely dehydrated and progress into a comatose state. The treatment includes increased insulin and slow fluid replacement to prevent cerebral edema because of the sorbitol accumulation in the brain.

22. What tissues do not require insulin for glucose transport?
- Nervous tissue
- Lens of the eye
- Kidney tubules
- Brain
- Blood vessels

23. What pathophysiologic mechanisms cause major chronic complications of diabetes?
- Neuropathy
- Macroangiopathy
- Microangiopathy
- Retinopathy
- Nephropathy

24. What biochemical pathways are suspected of contributing to diabetic complications?
The suspected pathways are enzymatic glycosylation and the buildup of sorbitol. *Enzymatic glycosylation* is the process by which glucose attaches to proteins throughout the body at a rate proportional to the plasma glucose concentration. The proteins glycosylated include serum albumin, collagen, basic myelin protein, and low-density lipoproteins (LDLs). The function of the proteins is altered.

Hyperglycemia leads to buildup of glucose in tissues that do not require insulin for uptake. Excess glucose is metabolized to sorbitol, which creates an osmotic gradient favoring water diffusing into the cell.

25. What is the enzyme that is responsible for the breakdown of glucose into sorbitol?
Aldose reductase.

26. How do advanced glycosylation end-products (AGEs) contribute to diabetic complications?
AGEs are the result of enzymatic glycosylation. They get incorporated into the collagen that comprises the basement membranes of capillaries located in the eye, kidney, nerves, and skin. This results in thickening of basement membranes and a reduction in production of relaxing factors by the endothelium, causing vasoconstriction and, ultimately, hypertension. In addition, AGEs irreversibly attach to collagen walls in larger vessels. This impedes the normal efflux of LDLs entering the vessel wall and promotes cholesterol deposition.

27. How does sorbitol accumulation lead to diabetic complications?
Cells of the tissues that do not require insulin for glucose transport (see question 22) become hypertonic. In Schwann's cells, the hypertonicity causes loss of feeling in extremities and a decrease in sensation. In the lens of the eye, water accumulation leads to cataracts, macular edema, and glaucoma. Damage to endothelial cells leads to thickening of basement membranes, resulting in microangiopathies of the retina, arterioles of the kidneys, and small vessels of the skin.

28. What is the importance of nonenzymatic glycosylation of hemoglobin?
The degree of nonenzymatic glycosylation is dependent on the amount of plasma glucose levels. Therefore high levels result in more glycosylation of hemoglobin. The normal hemoglobin A1c is 4%-6%. In diabetics, levels may reach 16%-20%. Because the lifespan of a red blood cell is about 120 days and the glycosylation occurs continuously over that span, hemoglobin A1c concentrations provide an index of the average blood glucose over the preceding 60-90 days.

29. How does glycosylation of platelets affect microvascular disease?
Glycosylation of platelets increases platelet adhesiveness. This allows platelets to produce excessive thromboxane, which makes the platelets hypercoagulable. This hypercoagulable state predisposes a diabetic to microvascular disease.

30. What are the criteria for the diagnosis of diabetes mellitus?
The diagnosis is made based on one or more of the following criteria:
- Signs and symptoms plus a random plasma glucose concentration ≥200 mg/dL
- A fasting plasma glucose ≥126 mg/dL at least two times
- Oral glucose tolerance test with a 2-hr postload glucose concentration ≥200 mg/dL and a time 0 serum glucose level >126 mg/dL

31. What test is accepted by the American Diabetes Association for diagnosing diabetes?
The fasting plasma glucose test is a diagnostic marker for diabetes. The patient fasts overnight for at least 8 hr, and the test is performed the next morning. This test is performed only on nonpregnant adults who are not taking any medications or have any other metabolic conditions that would lead to abnormal results. A normal fasting plasma glucose is usually 65-110 mg/dL.

32. What is the oral glucose tolerance test, and how is it performed?
This test measures a person's ability to handle a glucose load over a period of time. The patient fasts overnight. In the morning, the fasting blood glucose is determined. The patient then ingests a 75-g glucose load. In children and nonpregnant adults, the blood glucose is tested every 30 min for 2 hr. The test is considered normal if the fasting blood glucose is < 110 mg/dL and the 2-hr postload blood glucose is < 140 mg/dL.

33. What are the different categories of hypoglycemia?
Categories of hypoglycemia can be broken down depending on the level of plasma glucose and associated signs and symptoms (Table 23-1).

Table 23-1 *Categories of Hypoglycemia*		
	PLASMA GLUCOSE LEVEL	SIGNS/SYMPTOMS
Mild	60-70 mg/dL	Tachycardia, palpitations, pallor, shakiness, irritability
Moderate	50-60 mg/dL	Impaired central nervous system function: confusion, inability to concentrate, slurred speech, blurred vision
Severe	≤ 40-50 mg/dL	Loss of consciousness, difficulty awakening, seizures

34. How do you treat mild to moderate hypoglycemia?
Initially, treat with 10-15 g of carbohydrates. Give the patient 1/2 cup of orange juice or a *regular* soda, 3-5 hard candies, 1 cup of milk, 3 glucose tablets, *or* 2 tbsp of raisins. Evaluate plasma glucose levels as soon as possible. If symptoms do not improve in 15 min, treat with an additional 10-15 g of a carbohydrate source.

35. How do you treat severe hypoglycemia?

If a glucagon kit is available, the patient should be given an injection of glucagon. The adult dose is 1 mg; children younger than age 5 years, 0.5 mg; and infants younger than 1 year, 0.25 mg. If no kit is available and the patient can swallow without risk of aspiration, 15-50 g of a carbohydrate source can be given on the inside of the cheek. Sources include glucose gel, 1-4 tsp of honey (except in infants), syrup, *or* jelly. When the patient is more alert, follow with a liquid such as orange juice.

36. What is the best route to administer agents to stimulate insulin release?

Oral glucose and amino acids have a greater stimulatory effect on insulin than intravenously administered solutions because of stimulation of intestinal hormones by ingested substances. These hormones include gastric inhibitory peptide, cholecystokinin (CCK), glucagon, and gastrin. All are stimulators of insulin secretion.

37. What are the different insulin preparations (Table 23-2)?

Table 23-2	*Insulin Preparations*			
	TYPE OF INSULIN	ONSET	PEAK	DURATION
Short-acting	Regular	0.5-1 hr	2-4 hr	5-7 hr
Intermediate-acting	Isophane (NPH)	1-2 hr	6-14 hr	18-24 hr
	Lente	1-2 hr	6-14 hr	18-24 hr
Long-acting	Ultralente	6 hr	18-26 hr	36+ hr

38. How do you manage the postsurgical patient with diabetes that is controlled by diet only?

If plasma glucose levels exceed and remain above 250 mg/dL as a consequence of surgical stress or infection, sliding-scale insulin therapy should be instituted.

39. How do you manage a surgical patient who controls diabetes with oral hypoglycemic agents?

Use of oral agents other than chlorpropamide should be stopped on the day of the procedure. Chlorpropamide, which has a longer half-life than other oral hypoglycemics, should be discontinued the day before surgery. These patients often require insulin perioperatively during major surgical procedures. Postoperatively, follow the same regimen adhered to for diabetes controlled by diet.

40. What is the management of a patient with insulin-controlled diabetes who is undergoing major surgery?

Most diabetic patients who receive insulin use a combination of intermediate-acting (NPH) and regular insulin. In these patients, total insulin dosage is usually given in the morning or divided between morning and afternoon. Usually, two thirds of the total dose is NPH, and one third is regular insulin. Management of these patients in the perioperative period includes:

- Half of the normal daily insulin is given as NPH in the morning. An intravenous (IV) line is placed and lactated Ringer's solution started. A preoperative blood sugar is obtained.
- During surgery, plasma glucose, serum electrolytes, and arterial blood gases (ABGs) should be monitored. Additional regular insulin is provided as needed by titrating an insulin infusion of 5-10 U/hr either subcutaneously or in the IV fluids.

- Postoperatively, blood glucose is checked every 4-6 hr. Regular insulin should be administered to maintain plasma glucose between 150 and 200 mg/dL.
- Once the patient has resumed oral intake, NPH insulin is started. The patient's plasma glucose is monitored, and the insulin dosage is adjusted with regular insulin as needed.

41. How do you manage a patient with insulin-controlled diabetes who is undergoing ambulatory surgery?

Half the daily NPH insulin dose is given on the morning of surgery, and the regular insulin is withheld if the patient is expected to be able to resume oral intake shortly after surgery. The remaining half of NPH is given in the afternoon, but not too late in the afternoon. If given too late in the afternoon, the peak effect of the NPH will occur while the patient is sleeping.

42. What oral hypoglycemic is categorized as a biguanide?

Metformin (Glucophage) reduces hepatic glucose production and enhances glucose utilization by muscle. It is normally used by type 2 diabetics.

43. What is the pharmacology of the sulfonylureas?

These type 2 diabetic agents acutely increase insulin secretion from the beta cells and potentiate insulin action on several extrahepatic tissues. Long-term sulfonylureas increase peripheral utilization of glucose, suppress hepatic gluconeogenesis, and possibly increase the sensitivity or number of peripheral insulin receptors.

44. What drugs make up the sulfonylureas (Table 23-3)?

Table 23-3	*Sulfonylureas*		
DRUG	BRAND NAME	DOSE	DURATION
Tolbutamide	Orinase	2 g	6-12 hr
Tolazamide	Tolinase	250 mg	10-18 hr
Glipizide	Glucotrol	10-15 mg	12 hr
Glyburide	Micronase	5-10 mg	16 hr
Acetohexamide	Dymelor	1 g	8-12 hr
Chlorpropamide	Diabinese	250 mg	1-3 days

45. What are the contraindications to the use of metformin in type 2 diabetes?

Metformin therapy is strictly contraindicated in alcoholics, patients with significant renal insufficiency or failure (serum creatinine >1.5 and >1.4 for women), and patients with liver disease. These conditions considerably increase the risk of lactic acidosis, a fatal side effect. Patients who are older than age 70 and those with cardiac ejection fractions <79% also are not candidates for metformin therapy. Patients who are about to receive iodine contrast dye, such as before cardiac catheterization, or who are to undergo major surgery should discontinue metformin 48-72 hr before the procedure.

46. What is the pharmacology of the meglitinides?

These type 2 diabetic agents quickly stimulate insulin release by the beta cells of the pancreas to reduce postprandial hyperglycemia. These drugs are taken before each of three meals.

47. What drugs make up the meglitinides (Table 23-4)?

Table 23-4 *Meglitinides*

DRUG	TRADE NAME	DOSE	ONSET OF ACTION	DURATION
Repaglinide	Prandin	0.5 mg-2 mg bid	15-60 min	4-6 hr
Mitiglinide	Starlix	120 mg bid 1-30 min before meals	20 min	4 hr

bid, Twice a day.

48. What is the pharmacology of the thiazolidinediones?

These type 2 diabetic drugs lower blood glucose by improving the target cell response to insulin in muscle and fat. At the same time, they do not increase pancreatic secretion of insulin. The thiazolidinediones are taken once or twice a day with food. These drugs can be used by themselves or in combination with sulfonylureas, metformin, or insulin. However, thiazolidinediones can have a rare but serious effect on liver function requiring regular liver function tests. This could affect the length of time that the amide local anesthetics are in circulation.

49. What drugs make up the thiazolidinediones (Table 23-5)?

Table 23-5 *Thiazolidinediones*

DRUG	TRADE NAME	DOSE	ONSET OF ACTION	DURATION
Rosiglitazone	Avandia	4-8 mg qd or bid	Delayed	12 weeks
Pioglitazone	Actos	14-45 mg qd	Delayed	Several weeks
Troglitazone	Rezulin	Not available	Not available	Not available

qd, Daily; *bid,* twice a day.

50. What is the pharmacology of the alpha-glucosidase inhibitors?

These type 2 diabetic agents help the body to lower blood glucose levels by competitively inhibiting pancreatic alpha-amylase and intestinal brush border alpha-glucoside resulting in delayed breakdown of ingested complex carbohydrates therefore slowing the absorption of glucose. These drugs should be taken with the first bite of a meal. The alpha-glucosidase inhibitors can be used alone or in combination with a sulfonylurea metformin, or insulin.

51. What drugs make up the alpha-glucosidase inhibitors?

Acarbose (Precase) and miglitol (Glyset). These drugs have < 2% absorption as active drug because they work in the gastrointestinal tract. The metabolism is exclusively via the gastrointestinal tract.

52. What is the oral combination drug Avandamet?

Avandamet is a combination of metformin and Avandia that is used to treat type 2 diabetics who are not adequately controlled with metformin alone. The dosage is determined by starting Avandia 4 mg/day and adding it to the current metformin dose. If the patient is already taking Avandia, then add metformin so that the patient is getting a l000 mg/day.

53. What is the oral combination drug Metaglip?

Metaglip is the combination of glipizide (Glucotrol) and metformin. This drug can be used as initial therapy for management of type 2 diabetes when hyperglycemia cannot be controlled with diet and exercise, or as second-line treatment when neither drug by itself controls hyperglycemia. Dosages are expressed as glipizide/metformin components. When used as initial therapy, 1.25 mg/250 mg is taken daily or twice daily with meals. As second-line therapy, 2.5 mg/500 mg or 5 mg/500 mg is given twice daily with meals.

54. What is the oral combination drug Glucovance?

Glucovance is the combination of glyburide and metformin. It can be used for initial management of type 2 diabetes, or as second-line therapy when a sulfonylurea or metformin alone cannot control hyperglycemia. In addition, Glucovance with a thiazolidinedione may be required to achieve adequate control.

55. What is the dosage of Glucovance?

Glucovance dosages are expressed as glyburide/metformin components. When used as initial therapy, 1.25 mg/250 mg is taken with a meal once daily. Patients with an HgA_{1c} >9% or fasting plasma glucose >200 mg/dL are started at 1.25 mg/250 mg twice daily. The maximum dose is not to exceed 10 mg/2000 mg. For those patients previously treated with a sulfonylurea or metformin alone, the initial dose is 2.5 mg/500 mg or 5 mg/500 mg twice a day.

56. What is pramlintide?

Its brand name is Symlin, and it is a synthetic form of the hormone amylin which is produced in the beta cells of the pancreas. It is an injectable drug that has been recently approved by the FDA. Pramlintide has been approved for type 1 diabetics who are not achieving their A_{1c} goal levels, and for type 2 diabetics using insulin and unable to achieve their A_{1c} goals. It has been shown to modestly improve HgA_{1c} levels, as well as promote modest weight loss without causing increased hypoglycemia.

57. What is exenatide?

Exenatide (Byetta) is a synthetic version of exendin-4, a hormone first isolated from the saliva of the Gila monster. It is an injectable drug approved by the FDA for the treatment of type 2 diabetics who have not been able to achieve their target HgA_{1c} levels using metformin, a sulfonylurea, or combination drug. Exenalide works to lower blood glucose levels by increasing insulin secretion. As with pramlintide, Exenalide is injected with meals, and patients using it have experienced improved HgA_{1c} levels and modest weight loss.

58. How do insulin pumps work?

Insulin pumps deliver short-acting insulin 24 hr a day through a catheter placed subcutaneously. Insulin doses are separated into basal rates, boluses, and doses to correct glucose levels.

59. What is a basal rate and a bolus?

A basal rate is a constant rate of insulin delivered over 24 hr, keeping blood glucose levels in range between meals and overnight. The rate of insulin can be programmed to deliver different amounts of insulin at different times of the day and night. A bolus amount of insulin is used to cover the carbohydrate in each meal or snack. There are buttons on the insulin pump that will deliver the bolus if the meal is larger than planned, and a larger bolus of insulin can be programmed to cover it.

60. What is the physiologic effect of a decrease in plasma glucose?
A decrease protects plasma glucose levels. Therefore there would be increased production of glucagon, epinephrine, growth hormone, and cortisol to increase plasma glucose.

61. What are the lab findings in type 2 diabetes?
- High plasma glucose
- Glucose in the urine
- High urine volume

62. What is the response of insulin and glucagon to dietary protein?
An increase in both hormones.

63. Which hormones are considered ketogenic? Why?
Epinephrine, glucocorticoids, glucagon, and growth hormone because they promote lipolysis.

64. What is the response by insulin to parasympathetic stimulation?
Insulin release will be increased.

65. How will epinephrine released from the adrenal medulla affect plasma glucose?
Epinephrine decreases glycogen synthesis in the liver. In addition, its release is increased in response to hypoglycemia.

66. Where is the major site of action for glucagon?
The breakdown of hepatic glycogen to glucose.

67. What hormones antagonize the action of insulin on blood sugar?
- Growth hormone
- Cortisol
- Glucagon
- Epinephrine

68. What are the effects of infection and surgical stress on blood sugar in diabetic patients?
Surgical stress can be related to trauma to the tissues during the procedure, pain that the patient experiences after the procedure, and anxiety before and after the surgery. Infections cause stress on tissues and can cause trauma to tissues. Stress leads to surges of epinephrine. As discussed earlier, epinephrine will antagonize insulin and cause an increase in plasma glucose. In addition, stress from surgery and infections may override negative feedback mechanisms to result in cortisol surge. Cortisol will contribute to the effects of epinephrine on glucose.

69. What are the most common types of infections in diabetics, and why?
Diabetic patients have enhanced susceptibility to infections of the skin, tuberculosis, pneumonia, and pyelonephritis. Together, these infections cause the death of about 5% of diabetics. In addition, diabetics are very susceptible to fungal infections. The susceptibility to infections is a combination of impaired leukocyte function, inability to make antibodies against the bacteria, and vascular insufficiency.

BIBLIOGRAPHY

1. Cada DJ, Covington TR, Hebel SK (eds): Drug Facts and Comparisons. St Louis, 1998, Wolters Kluwer.
2. Kumar V, Abbas A, Fausto N: Robbins & Cotran Pathologic Basis of Disease, 7th ed. Philadelphia, 2005, Saunders.
3. Roser M: Management of the medically compromised patient. In Kwon PH, Laskin DM (eds): Clinician's Manual of Oral and Maxillofacial Surgery. Carol Stream, Ill, 1997, Quintessence.
4. Steil CF: Diabetes: an overview. In: CVS Pharmacy Pharmaceutical Care Module—Diabetes. Woonsocket, RI, 1998, CVS Pharmacy.

24. THE IMMUNOCOMPROMISED SURGICAL PATIENT

A. Omar Abubaker, DMD, PhD, and Noah Sandler, DMD, MD

1. **What are the types of immunodeficiency?**
   Immunodeficiency can be either **primary** or **acquired** (secondary). Primary immunodeficiency is usually caused by a defect in a specific aspect of the immune system, such as a specific immunoglobulin. Acquired immunodeficiency can be secondary to disease or iatrogenic causes, such as the result of chemotherapy, and may involve more than one aspect of the immune system.

2. **What are the common causes of immunosuppression and immunodeficiency?**
   Immunodeficiency can be caused by any of several factors, including:
   - Acquired/congenital immunodeficiency
   - Advanced age
   - Burns
   - Diabetes
   - Iatrogenic causes (such as posttransplant drug immunosuppression)
   - Malignancy
   - Malnutrition
   - Organ failure
   - Radiation
   - Surgery
   - Trauma

3. **What are the different classes of systemic immunity?**
   Systemic immunity can be classified into an **antigen-specific** or **nonspecific immunity**. Antigen-specific can be either humoral or cell-mediated immunity. Parts of the nonspecific immunity system are the phagocytes and complement cascade.

4. **What is the effect of deficiency in cell-mediated immunity, and what are the appropriate methods of testing for such deficiency?**
   Deficiencies in cell-mediated immunity predispose the patient to infection from gram-negative organisms, mycobacteria, viruses, *Pneumocystis carinii*, and *Toxoplasma*. The best test for cell-mediated immunity is delayed-type hypersensitivity (DTH) skin testing, in which patients' reactions to intradermal injections of *Candida*, tuberculin, *Trichophyton*, and other antigens are observed. Direct measurement of T-cell function by the use of monoclonal antibodies is, however, a more specific test. The ratio of helper T cells (CD4) to suppressor T cells (CD8) (normally 1.8:2.2) is often used as a measure of this immune-type function.

5. **How is deficiency in humoral immunity manifested, and what are the appropriate methods of testing for humoral immunity?**
   Deficiency in humoral immunity predisposes patients to infection from pyogenic bacteria, hepatitis viruses, *Cytomegalovirus*, parasites, and *P. carinii*. Measuring serum immunoglobulin levels tests humoral immunity. Testing for the presence of antibodies to previous vaccination or infections can also indicate the status of the patient's humoral immunity. Other tests for humoral immunity, such as circulating B-cell count and in vitro B-cell testing, can also be performed.

6. **What infections are caused by deficiency in polymorphonuclear neutrophils (PMNs)?**
   Deficiencies of neutrophilic leukocytes predispose patients to infections from staphylococci, *Serratia*, *Escherichia coli*, *Pseudomonas*, *Proteus*, *Enterobacter*, *Salmonella*, *Candida*, and

208

Aspergillus. Neutrophil absolute count and most functions of polymorphonuclear leukocytes can be tested.

7. What is the effect of deficiency in complement, and how can complement functions be tested?

Deficiency in complement predisposes patients to infections from *Neisseria* and viruses. The status of complement cascade can be measured by the $C'H_{50}$ (50% hemolyzing dose of complement) assay and by individual assay or C3 and C4 levels.

8. What are the possible complications of immunosuppressive drugs in transplant patients?

Although newer immunosuppressive medications have reduced the amount and severity of acute transplant rejection, these new regimens are not without consequences. An increased risk of infection is seen in these patients secondary to decreased host resistance, with an increased risk for graft rejection in patients with severe infection. Infection is also the leading cause of death in transplant patients. Therefore any transplant patients with active infections should be treated aggressively. Another risk for transplant patients is the increased incidence of de novo cancer. There may be a 100-fold increased incidence of cancer in the transplant patient. The most prevalent neoplasms are lymphoma and squamous cell carcinoma of the lips and skin. The incidence of tumors such as non-Hodgkin's lymphoma is approximately 2%, and this risk increases with the duration of immunosuppressive therapy. Most of these lesions occur in the head and neck, gastrointestinal tract, and transplanted allograft. These lesions are seen primarily with the use of cyclosporine and tacrolimus and are believed to be related to the inhibition of Epstein-Barr virus (EBV) cytotoxic T cells. Transplant patients on immunosuppressive therapy therefore should be examined carefully for lip and skin lesions, nonhealing ulcers, and lymphadenopathy, and questionable lesions should undergo biopsy.

9. What are the most common types of orofacial infection seen in immunocompromised patients?

T-cell deficiency is commonly found in posttransplant patients on immunosuppressive therapy, in AIDS patients, in some patients with certain forms of carcinoma, and in patients receiving treatment for cancer. Viral and fungal infections are more common in these patients. Viral infections are most often produced by the Herpesviridae family (i.e., herpes simplex, varicella zoster virus, and cytomegalovirus). The clinical presentation of these infections is typically an acute, vesiculobullous lesion with a lack of inflammatory response in leukopenic patients. If not treated aggressively with antiviral agents, such as acyclovir or ganciclovir, these infections can lead to significant local and possible systemic morbidity.

Among fungal infections, *Candida albicans* is the most common fungal pathogen, but others such as *Aspergillus* and *Cryptococcus* are commonly encountered. The more aggressive fungi show an invasive behavior that often involves deeper tissues. Patients should be monitored carefully for signs of local tissue trauma that may predispose them to viral or fungal colonization.

10. What are the characteristics of bacterial oral infections in immunocompromised patients?

Oral infections in immunocompromised patients typically occur with significant local symptoms and may spread to involve adjacent or distant anatomic sites. These infections tend to progress more rapidly and may produce systemic symptoms or local osteomyelitis. Infections may be caused by gram-negative enteric flora secondary to colonization of these organisms in the oral cavity. These bacteria are often resistant to penicillin and cephalosporins. Broad-spectrum antibiotic prophylaxis should be used empirically before definitive identification of the causative microorganism in immunocompromised patients with evidence of infection.

11. What are the general principles of the preoperative evaluation of immuno-compromised patients?

Immunosuppression is not in itself a contraindication to well-planned surgery. The general approach to the care of these patients when they are to undergo surgery is to increase host resistance to infection and to maximize wound healing. The patient's immune status should be evaluated by means of a history, physical exam, and lab studies. The history should include questions about the patient's underlying disease, previous infections, use of medications and other therapy, previous anesthesia, and trauma. The physical exam should also determine the patient's nutritional status and include a search for signs of existing infection and lymphadenopathy.

High-risk patients should have elective procedures scheduled at the beginning of the day. The possibility of reducing the dosages of immunosuppressive drugs must be weighed against the effect this might have on the reason why the patient is being treated with these agents. Other considerations include the removal of any infected foreign bodies; assessment of the need of invasive devices; restoration of cardiac and renal function, including tissue perfusion; correction of nutritional deficiencies, if present; assessment of the patient's need for vaccinations; and the administration of prophylactic antibiotics. Also, regardless of the etiology, hemostasis should be achieved with pressure, packing, or suturing, and if the platelet count is below $50,000/mm^3$, platelet transfusion should be considered. In the case of dental extractions, alveolectomy and primary closure are recommended. If platelet counts are $< 40,000/mm^3$, platelets should be transfused 30 min before surgery to achieve platelet levels of more than $40,000/mm^3$. One unit (pack) of platelets typically raises the platelet count by $10,000/mm^3$. Although correcting the patient's immunodeficiency is usually difficult or impossible, defects in B-cell function may be partially treated by administering immunoglobulin.

12. What preoperative lab studies should be included in evaluation of immuno-compromised patients?
- Chest radiograph
- Urinalysis
- Serum albumin determination
- Liver and kidney function tests
- Culture of material from any infected sites

Because some of these patients may present with neutropenia as well as thrombocytopenia, other tests include:
- Complete blood count with platelet count
- Prothrombin time (PT)
- Partial thromboplastin time (PTT)

Specific testing of the patient's T cells, B cells, PMNs, and complement should be checked before surgery.

13. What are the effects of chemotherapeutic and immunosuppressant drugs on the immune system?

The effects of these drugs vary from agent to agent. For example, chemotherapeutic agents depress the number and activity of the neutrophilic leukocytes. The nadir of white cell counts varies with the agents used but generally occurs 10-20 days after administration. The patient is susceptible to infection when the absolute neutrophil count (ANC) falls below $1500/mm^3$. The susceptibility increases significantly when the count falls below $500/mm^3$. Corticosteroids, on the other hand, decrease the leukocyte response to inflamed tissue and depress T-cell function. Wound healing is slowed, and the ability to localize infection is reduced. Cyclosporine has almost no effect on the local inflammatory reaction but causes the initiation of interleukin-2 production and the suppression of T-helper and cytotoxic cells. Antilymphocyte antibodies appear to work by lysing target cells. With all these agents, increased dosage is associated with increased predisposition to infection. These patients should receive prophylactic antibiotics before most surgical procedures.

14. When should prophylactic antibiotics be used in chemotherapy patient?

Prophylactic antibiotics should be considered if the granulocyte count is $< 2000/mm^3$. Surgery generally should be performed at least 3 days before chemotherapy is initiated in cancer patients because granulocyte levels may fall below $500/mm^3$ 1 week after the initiation of many types of chemotherapeutic agents. When surgery needs to be performed during severe neutropenia (granulocyte counts $<500/mm^3$), it is recommended that the procedure be performed in a hospital setting with broad-spectrum antibiotic prophylaxis administered during the perioperative period.

15. What type of virus is HIV, and what is its cell target?

Human immunodeficiency viruses (HIVs) are a group of retroviruses that can be acquired by the transmission of body fluids, including transfusions, and through the infection of infants by infected mothers. The specific target of the virus is the CD4 T-cell lymphocytes. The virus multiplies in the cell and eventually destroys it. Cell-mediated immunity is thereby severely affected.

16. What are the general categories of HIV-infected patients?

- Asymptomatic patients with evidence of HIV infection demonstrated by the presence of HIV antibodies in the serum or in the secretions of these patients
- Patients with AIDS-related complex (ARC), manifested by presence of symptoms including lymphadenopathy, unexplained fever, weight loss, and hematologic and neurologic abnormalities
- Patients with AIDS as defined by the Centers for Disease Control and Prevention (CDC) (i.e., HIV infection and CD4 lymphocyte count <200)

17. What are the lab tests to determine the status of the HIV patient?

Diagnosis of HIV infection is made by detection of antibodies to HIV. Antibodies to HIV are determined by the enzyme-linked immunosorbent assay (ELISA) method or by the Western blot method; both tests require the patient's consent in many states.

The status of patient with HIV infection and potential risk of surgery is evaluated by assessing the viral load (as determined by the HIV RNA), and the CD4+ lymphocyte count. Information regarding the overall physical status of the patient and the patient's symptomatic and physical manifestation of HIV-related diseases are also helpful in assessing the HIV patient risk for surgery.

Viral load measurements give an indication of the amount of current viral activity and have been shown to correlate with disease progression. Studies have demonstrated that viral loads of more than 30,000-50,000 HIV RNA copies/mL of plasma correlate with a poor prognosis, whereas viral loads of < 5000 copies/mL correlate with better short-term prognosis.

The CD4+ lymphocyte gives an indication of the degree of immunologic destruction. Lab findings in patients with AIDS include low lymphocyte counts and depressed CD4 T cells, with the CD4-to-CD8 ratio of 1:0 or less (normally 1.8:2.2).

18. What are the clinical manifestations of AIDS?

Signs and Symptoms	Opportunistic Infections
Lymphadenopathy	*P. carinii* (pulmonary)
Weight loss	Toxoplasmosis (cerebral)
Diarrhea	Cryptosporidiosis (diarrhea)
Thrombocytopenia	Candidiasis (esophageal)
Anemia	*Cryptococcus* (meningitis)

Leukopenia
Neurologic Abnormalities
Dementia
Encephalopathy
Central nervous system toxoplasmosis
Lymphoma

Herpes
Varicella viruses (skin)
Histoplasmosis
Tuberculosis
Neoplasms
Kaposi's sarcoma
Lymphoma

19. What are the principles of drug therapy of AIDS patients?

The major goal of therapy of patients with AIDS is treatment of the opportunistic infections, including antiviral therapy. Prophylaxis is essential for all persons with symptomatic HIV disease, AIDS, or CD4+ counts <200/µL. Survival has also been prolonged in HIV-positive patients by prophylaxis against opportunistic infections such as *P. carinii* pneumonia (PCP), the mycobacterium avium complex (MAC), and other fungal infections. PCP prophylaxis commonly is with trimethoprim-sulfamethoxazole, although dapsone-trimethoprim or clindamycin-primaquine may be used alternately. Prophylaxis for MAC usually consists of a macrolide antibiotic, clarithromycin, or azithromycin and is recommended when the CD4+ cell count falls below 75 or 50/µL. Prophylaxis against *Candida* or other fungal diseases is currently not recommended, although many immunocompromised patients may be taking an antifungal medication, such as fluconazole or another azole, when they have manifestations of fungal infection. Current antiretroviral therapies have been shown to reduce viral counts and slow disease progression, and they can be effective in raising the CD4+ lymphocyte counts considerably. The most effective antiretroviral treatment strategies are multiple drug therapies that combine nucleoside analogue drugs with protease inhibitors and, when patients are able to tolerate these regimens, triple drug therapy with two nucleoside analogue drugs plus a protease inhibitor.

20. What are the considerations in the surgical treatment of an HIV-infected person?

Patients with early HIV infection and with no immunologic impairment generally tolerate elective oral surgical procedures well, and recent studies have demonstrated no increased incidence in infection, bleeding, or dry socket in extractions. In fact, routine prophylactic antibiotics are not indicated for these patients and may even further predispose them to candidiasis or drug reactions. In contrast, patients with AIDS and ARC are not good surgical candidates because of their hematologic abnormalities and predisposition to AIDS infection. Patients with mandibular fractures who have AIDS infection have an increased incidence of postoperative infections compared with asymptomatic HIV-positive patients. Accordingly, it is recommended that patients with AIDS (as defined by CD4+ count of < 200 cells/µL or history of AIDS-defining illness such as lymphoma, tuberculosis, or *P. carinii*) should not undergo elective surgery. When urgent and emergency surgery is necessary, these patients should receive broad-spectrum prophylactic antibiotics before undergoing any surgical procedure, and proper attention to the prevention of wound infection must be given to prevent transmission of the virus to personnel caring for the patient.

21. What are the potential drug interactions in HIV-infected patients?

See Table 24-1.

22. What is the management of health care workers exposed to HIV-infected blood or body fluids?

The rate of seroconversion of health care workers exposed to HIV-infected blood or body fluid has been reported to be 0.42%. The management of occupational exposures of contaminated or suspected contaminated fluids is controversial. Currently, the CDC recommends that, after informed consent is obtained, the patient should be tested for HIV. If the patient is HIV positive,

Table 24-1   Potential Interactions of Drugs Used by HIV-Infected Patients

DRUG	DRUG USED TO TREAT HIV	MECHANISM OF INTERACTION	EFFECT	RECOMMENDATION
Benzodiazepines	Ritonavir, indinavir (protease inhibitors)	Inhibition of hepatic metabolism	↑ Concentration of benzodiazepines	Adjust benzodiazepines dosage, use alternate agent, or monitor closely for toxicity
Cisapride	Azole antifungals, clarithromycin, ritonavir, indinavir	Inhibition of hepatic metabolism	Cardiotoxic effects (including fatal arrhythmias)	Avoid concomitant use
Clarithromycin	Ritonavir, indinavir	Inhibition of hepatic metabolism	↑ Concentration of clarithromycin	Dosage reduction not required for patients with normal renal function
Didanosine (nucleoside analogue)	Oral ganciclovir	Unknown	↑ Didanosine	Monitor for didanosine toxicity; dosage reduction may be required
Ganciclovir	Zidovudine (thymidine analogue)	Pharmacodynamic interaction	Enhanced bone marrow toxicity	May require decreased dose of zidovudine or concomitant G-CSF
Ketoconazole	Saquinavir (protease inhibitor)	Inhibition of hepatic metabolism	↑ Saquinavir concentration	Under investigation to maximize saquinavir exposure

Adapted from Sandler NA, Braun TW: Current surgical management of the immunocompromised patient. Oral Maxillofac Surg Clin North Am 10:445-455, 1998.
G-CSF, Granulocyte colony-stimulating factor.

Continued

Table 24-1   *Potential Interactions of Drugs Used by HIV-Infected Patients—cont'd*

DRUG	DRUG USED TO TREAT HIV	MECHANISM OF INTERACTION	EFFECT	RECOMMENDATION
Metronidazole	Ritonavir (liquid only)	Alcohol in liquid formulation	Disulfiram-like reaction	Monitor for toxicity; change form of ritonavir
Opiate analgesics (especially meperidine, propoxyphene, fentanyl)	Ritonavir	Inhibition of hepatic metabolism	↑ Opiate concentration	Use alternate pain medication; monitor for toxicity
Terfenadine, astemizole (H₁ antihistamines)	Azole antifungals, clarithromycin, ritonavir	Inhibition of hepatic metabolism	Accumulation of cardiotoxic unmetabolized antihistamine	Avoid concomitant use

the exposed health care worker should undergo HIV testing immediately and then at 6 weeks, 12 weeks, and 6 months. Initiation of zidovudine prophylaxis after exposure remains controversial because of its yet unproven efficacy.

23. What is the mechanism of action of immunosuppressive agents used in transplant patients?

Several new immunosuppressive agents are available for clinical use or are undergoing clinical trials in this country. These new drugs suppress the immune system at sites complementary to traditional immunosuppressive medications (Fig. 24-1). Many transplant patients currently are on two or more of these drugs in an attempt to prevent rejection. This may predispose the patient to overimmunosuppression or potential drug interactions.

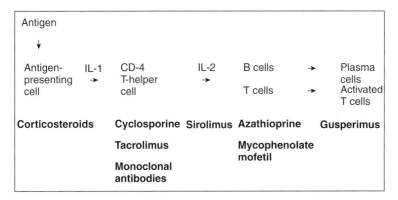

Fig. 24-1   Sites of action of immunosuppressive drugs used in transplant patients. *IL,* Interleukin. (Modified from Sandler NA, Braun TW: Current surgical management of the immunocompromised patient. Oral Maxillofac Surg Clin North Am 10:445-455, 1998.)

24. What are the side effects of immunosuppressive drugs in transplant patients?

See Table 24-2.

25. What are the oral manifestations of cyclosporine use?

Cyclosporine is associated with gingival hyperplasia in the dental papillae of the anterior teeth, which typically occurs after 3-6 months of immunosuppressant therapy. Studies suggest that approximately 30% of patients medicated with cyclosporine alone experience significant gingival changes. Calcium channel blocking agents that may be prescribed to counter the hypertension caused by cyclosporine may also induce gingival hyperplasia with an additive effect to that of cyclosporine. When the two drugs are used simultaneously, they can result in a nearly 40% incidence of gingival hyperplasia. Other significant risk factors that influence gingival overgrowth include age and sex (with younger men having an increased susceptibility), duration of therapy, serum creatinine levels, and the HLA-B37 haplotype. Decreases in the dosage of the drug or discontinuing the drug early may result in reversal of this side effect. However, surgical intervention that consists of gingivectomy and tissue recontouring is often necessary to improve aesthetics and function.

26. What are the different drug interactions of cyclosporine/tacrolimus?

See Table 24-3.

Table 24-2   *Side Effects of Immunosuppressive Drugs Used in Transplant Patients*

MEDICATION	POTENTIAL SIDE EFFECTS
Corticosteroids	Cushing's syndrome, adrenal insufficiency
Azathioprine	Myelodepression (leukopenia, thrombocytopenia)
Cyclosporine	Nephrotoxicity, neurotoxicity, hypertension, hepatotoxicity
Tacrolimus	Nephrotoxicity, neurotoxicity, diabetogenic effects
Mycophenolate mofetil	Myelodepression (leukopenia, anemia), gastrointestinal (diarrhea, emesis)
Sirolimus	Myelodepression (leukopenia, thrombocytopenia), potential nephrotoxicity
Gusperimus	Myelodepression (leukopenia, anemia, thrombocytopenia)
Monoclonal antibodies	Central nervous system (seizure, encephalopathy, psychosis)*

Adapted from Sandler NA, Braun TW: Current surgical management of the immunocompromised patient. Oral Maxillofac Surg Clin North Am 10:445-455, 1998.
*Increased risk of encephalopathy and psychosis reported with indomethacin use.

Table 24-3   *Drug Interactions of Cyclosporine and Tacrolimus*

DRUG	CLASS	MECHANISM
Increased Cyclosporine		
Metoclopramide	Prokinetic	↑ Cyclosporine absorption
Cisapride	Prokinetic	↑ Cyclosporine absorption
Erythromycin	Macrolide antibiotic	Mechanism unclear
Increased Cyclosporin/Tacrolimus		
Clotrimazole	Imidazole	Inhibit cytochrome P450
Fluconazole	Antifungal	Inhibit cytochrome P450
Corticosterone	Corticosteroid	Inhibit cytochrome P450
Dexamethasone	Corticosteroid	Inhibit cytochrome P450
Bromocriptine	Dopamine agonist	Inhibit cytochrome P450
Cyclosporine/tacrolimus	Immunosuppressant	Inhibit cytochrome P450
Ergotamine	Alpha blocker	Inhibit cytochrome P450
Nifedipine	Ca channel blocker	Inhibit cytochrome P450
Diltiazem	Ca channel blocker	Inhibit cytochrome P450
Verapamil	Ca channel blocker	Inhibit cytochrome P450
Cimetidine	H_2 blocker	Inhibit cytochrome P450
Omeprazole	H/K ATPase blocker	Inhibit cytochrome P450

Adapted from Sandler NA, Braun TW: Current surgical management of the immunocompromised patient. Oral Maxillofac Surg Clin North Am 10:445-455, 1998.
ATPase, Adenosine triphosphatase.

Table 24-3 *Drug Interactions of Cyclosporine and Tacrolimus—cont'd*		
DRUG	CLASS	MECHANISM
Increased Tacrolimus		
Danazol	Androgen	↑ Renal impairment
Grapefruit juice		Inhibit intestinal cytochrome P450
Decreased Cyclosporine/Tacrolimus		
Rifampin	Antibiotic	↑ Cytochrome P450 activity
Phenytoin	Anticonvulsant	↑ Cytochrome P450 activity
Phenobarbital	Anticonvulsant	↑ Cytochrome P450 activity
Decreased Cyclosporine		
Sulfadimidine	Antibiotic	↑ Cytochrome P450 activity
Trimethoprim	Antibiotic	↑ Cytochrome P450 activity
Decreased Tacrolimus		
Carbamazepine	Anticonvulsant	↑ Cytochrome P450 activity
Primidone	Anticonvulsant	↑ Cytochrome P450 activity

27. What is tacrolimus, and what are its major side effects?

Tacrolimus (FK-506) is a macrolide immunosuppressant isolated from *Streptomyces tsukubaensis* in 1984. This drug is 50-100 times more potent than cyclosporine. Initially used during episodes of severe graft rejection, it is now used for baseline immunosuppression.

The principal adverse effects associated with tacrolimus are similar to those of cyclosporine and include nephrotoxicity and neurotoxicity. In addition, diabetogenic effects are seen. The mechanism by which tacrolimus causes nephrotoxicity is related to an alteration of prostaglandin metabolism, by inducing vasoconstriction, and reduction in renal blood flow and a resultant decreased glomerular filtration rate. With the addition of a nonsteroidal antiinflammatory drug (NSAID), the renal blood flow can become even more impaired. Therefore the routine prescription of NSAIDs to patients on tacrolimus should be avoided. Drugs that may induce nephrotoxicity and contribute to renal impairment, such as aminoglycosides, trimethoprim-sulfamethoxazole, amphotericin B, and acyclovir, also should be avoided in patients who are taking tacrolimus.

28. Does tacrolimus interact with any drugs that are routinely used in oral and maxillofacial surgery patients?

Yes. Tacrolimus is eliminated in the liver by cytochrome P450 isoenzymes and therefore may show a rise in concentration with the concomitant use of macrolide antibiotics, such as erythromycin or clarithromycin, azole antifungal agents, or corticosteroids. Also, the antihistamines terfenadine (Seldane) and astemizole (Hismanal) have been associated with cardiac arrhythmias after coadministration with tacrolimus or cyclosporine. Concurrent use of NSAIDs or nephrotoxic antibiotics and tacrolimus also increases the potential for nephrotoxicity.

29. What are the oral manifestations of graft-vs.-host disease in the transplant patient?

Graft-vs.-host disease results from the action of T cells in the transplanted organ against histocompatibility antigens of the host tissue. The oral cavity can be affected, along with the liver, skin, and gastrointestinal tract. More than 80% of patients with graft-vs.-host disease have oral lesions, which in many cases may be the first symptom. The clinical presentation of oral graft-vs.-host disease resembles that of other collagen vascular diseases, such as systemic lupus erythematosus or lichen planus. The oral mucosa may show erythema, ulceration, white striations, atrophy, or a pseudomembranous covering. Symptoms may range from mild discomfort to burning and severe pain and salivary dysfunction. Graft-vs.-host disease is treated by augmenting immunosuppressive therapy. Careful monitoring of the patient for signs of overimmunosuppression should also be performed during this period.

30. What are the perioperative considerations of postsplenectomy patients?

Postsplenectomy patients have the potential to develop overwhelming sepsis with shock and disseminated intravascular coagulation (DIC). The most common organisms causing such infections are *Pneumococcus, Meningococcus,* and *Haemophilus*. Therefore before splenectomy, patients should receive vaccination with pneumococcal polysaccharide. Prophylactic antibiotics should be given before surgical procedures in contaminated sites, such as the oral cavity. Early aggressive treatment of infections in these patients is recommended.

BIBLIOGRAPHY

 1. Carpenter CC, Fischl MA, Hammer SM et al: Antiretroviral therapy for HIV infection in 1996: recommendations of an international panel. International AIDS Society-USA. JAMA 276:146-164, 1996.
 2. Centers for Disease Control and Prevention: USPHA/IDSA guidelines for the prevention of opportunistic infections in persons infected with human immunodeficiency virus: a summary. MMWR Morb Mortal Wkly Rep 44:1-34, 1995.
 3. Deeks SG, Smith M, Holodniy M et al: HIV-1 protease inhibitors: a review for clinicians. JAMA 277:145-153, 1997.
 4. Dodson TB, Parrott DH, Nguyen T et al: HIV status and the risk of postoperative complications. J Oral Maxillofac Surg 49(suppl 1):81-82, 1991.
 5. Grant D, Wall W, Duff J et al: Adverse effects of cyclosporine therapy following liver transplantation. Transplant Proc 19:3463-3465, 1987.
 6. Ho M, Dummer JS: Risk factors and approach to infections in transplant recipients. In Mandell GL, Douglas RG, Bennett JE (eds): Principles and Practices of Infectious Diseases, 4th ed. New York, 1995, Churchill Livingstone.
 7. Lockhart PB, Sonis ST: Relationship of oral complications to peripheral blood leukocyte and platelet counts in patients receiving cancer chemotherapy. Oral Surg Oral Med Oral Pathol 48:21-28, 1979.
 8. Martinez-Gimeno C, Acero-Sanz J, Martin-Sastra R et al: Maxillofacial trauma: influence of HIV infection. J Craniomaxillofac Surg 20:297-302, 1992.
 9. Matsuda H, Iwasaki K, Shiriga T et al: Interactions of FK506 (tacrolimus) with clinically important drugs. Res Commun Mol Pathol Pharmacol 91:57-64, 1996.
10. Maxymiw WG, Wood RE: The role of dentistry in patients undergoing bone marrow transplantation. Br Dent J 167:229-234, 1989.
11. Mignat C: Clinically significant drug interactions with new immunosuppressive agents. Drug Safety 16:267-278, 1997.
12. Pernu HE, Pernu LM, Huttunen K et al: Gingival overgrowth among renal transplant recipients and uremic patients. Nephrol Dial Transplant 8:1254-1258, 1993.
13. Peterson DE, Sonis ST: Oral complications of cancer chemotherapy: present status and future studies. Cancer Treat Rep 66:1251-1256, 1982.
14. Portery SR, Scully C, Luker J: Complications of dental surgery in persons with HIV disease. Oral Surg Oral Med Oral Pathol 75:165-167, 1993.

15. Reichart PA, Gelderblom HR, Becker J et al: AIDS and the oral cavity. The HIV-infection virology, etiology, origin, immunology, precautions and clinical observation in 110 patients. Int J Oral Maxillofac Surg 16:129-153, 1987.
16. Robinson PG, Cooper H, Hatt J: Healing after dental extractions in men with HIV infections. Oral Surg Oral Med Oral Pathol 74:426-430, 1992.
17. Roser SM: Management of the medically compromised patient. In Kwon PH, Laskin DM (eds): Clinician Manual of Oral and Maxillofacial Surgery, 2nd ed. Chicago, 1996, Quintessence.
18. Samaranayake LP: Oral mycoses in HIV infection. Oral Surg Oral Med Oral Pathol 73:171-180, 1992.
19. Schmidt B, Kearns G, Parrott D et al: Infection following treatment of mandibular fractures in human immunodeficiency virus in seropositive patients. J Oral Maxillofac Surg 53:1134-1139, 1995.
20. Thomason JM, Seymour RA, Rice N: Determinants of gingival overgrowth severity in organ transplant patients. An examination of the role of HLA phenotype. J Clin Periodontol 23:628-634, 1996.
21. Thomason JM, Seymour RA, Rice N: The prevalence and severity of cyclosporine and nifedipine-induced gingival overgrowth. J Clin Periodontol 20:37-40, 1993.
22. Wysocki GP, Gretzinger HA, Laupacis A et al: Fibrous hyperplasia of the gingiva: a side effect of cyclosporine A therapy. Oral Surg Oral Med Oral Pathol 55:274-278, 1983.
23. Yee J, Christou NV: Perioperative care of the immunocompromised patient. World J Surg 17:207-214, 1993.

25. THE JOINT REPLACEMENT PATIENT

Kathy A. Banks, DMD

1.   What are the two most common causes of prosthetic joint infections?

The majority of prosthetic joint infections are the result of **wound contamination** occurring during placement of the prosthesis. Signs and symptoms of infection may occur immediately after joint placement or may arise weeks to months later. A smaller proportion of prosthetic joint infections are attributed to **hematogenous spread** of bacteria from distant sites of infection.

2.   What major change in the surgical technique of prosthetic joint replacement is responsible for the low rate of postoperative infection?

Prophylactic antibiotic therapy is the single most important change in surgical technique and is mostly responsible for the low incidence (about 1%) of postoperative infections involving prosthetic joints. Prophylactic antibiotic therapy significantly decreases the risk of both early and late infections caused by wound contamination at the time of joint prosthesis placement. Antibiotic-impregnated cement used in the retention of the prosthesis and improvements in aseptic technique are contributing factors.

3.   What bacteria most commonly are cultured from infected prosthetic joints?

Staphylococcus aureus and *Staphylococcus epidermidis,* because the majority of infections involving prosthetic joints are caused by staphylococcal contamination during the placement of the prosthesis.

4.   Which bacteria have been identified in cases of infected prosthetic joints arising by hematogenous spread of infection to the prosthesis from oral sites of infection?

Streptococcus viridans and *Streptococcus sanguis.*

5. **Which medical conditions place patients with prosthetic joints at high risk for developing hematogenous infection of the prosthetic joint?**
- Active rheumatoid arthritis
- Systemic lupus erythematosus
- Severe type 1 insulin-dependent diabetes mellitus
- Steroid therapy
- Hemophilia
- Immunosuppressive disease
- First 2 years after joint placement

6. **What conditions seem to predispose a prosthetic joint to development of infection?**
- Loose prosthesis
- First 2 years after joint placement
- Second or third prosthesis in place
- Previous infection involving the joint
- Acute skin infections

7. **Late infections involving prosthetic joints are associated with acute infections of which major organ systems?**
- Oral cavity
- Skin
- Respiratory system
- Urogenital
- Gastrointestinal

8. **Which bacteria most commonly cause infected prosthetic joints in the "high risk" group of patients?**
    S. aureus and *S. epidermidis*. The origin of the bacteria causing the joint infection is not different in this group.

9. **What criteria are used to establish a diagnosis of hematogenous infection in prosthetic joint replacement?**
    The same strain of bacteria must be cultured from the following three sites:
    1. Infected joint
    2. Primary focus of infection
    3. Blood

10. **What are the treatment options for a patient with an infected prosthetic joint?**
- Remove the joint prosthesis.
- Salvage the prosthesis with surgical debridement and antibiotic therapy.
- Salvage the prosthesis with aspiration of pus and antibiotic therapy.

11. **When can transient oral bacteremias occur?**
- During mastication
- During tooth brushing and flossing, and dental prophylaxis
- Sporadically in patients with moderate to severe periodontal disease
- Sporadically in patients with moderate to severe odontogenic infections
- During invasive dental and otolaryngology procedures

12. **Which bacteria have been associated with transient oral bacteremias?**
    S. viridans and *S. sanguis*.

13. **Which dental procedures have the highest incidence of bacteremia?**
- Dental extractions
- All periodontal procedures
- Endodontic instrumentation
- Initial placement of orthodontic bands
- Intraligamentary injections of local anesthesia
- Dental prophylaxis of teeth or implants where bleeding is expected

14. Which dental procedures have the lowest incidence of bacteremia?
- Restorative dentistry:
  - With or without retraction cord
  - Placement of post and core buildup
  - Placement of rubber dam
  - Placement of removable appliances
- Injections of local anesthetic (except intraligamentary injections)
- Suture removal
- Taking oral impressions
- Fluoride treatments
- Taking oral radiographs
- Orthodontic bracket placement and adjustment

15. What are the risks of antibiotic therapy?
- Gastrointestinal upset
- Cross reactions with other drugs
- Emergence of resistant bacterium
- Allergic reactions
- Anaphylaxis
- Hearing loss
- Death

16. What steps can be taken to minimize transient oral bacteremia in the prosthetic joint replacement patient?
- Elimination of active dental and periodontal disease before the joint replacement surgery
- Oral rinsing with chlorhexidine solution before dental, periodontal, and dental extraction procedures
- Aggressive treatment of acute dental and oral infections with antibiotics, surgery, and culture and sensitivity testing

17. What are the current recommendations of the American Dental Association and the American Academy of Orthopedic Surgeons regarding the use of antibiotic prophylaxis for routine dental procedures in patients with prosthetic joint replacements?
- Antibiotic prophylaxis is not indicated for dental patients with pins, plates, or screws, nor is it routinely indicated for most dental patients with total joint replacements.
- Empiric prophylactic antibiotic therapy should be considered for patients who are considered to be at high risk for developing hematogenous prosthetic joint infection.
- The dentist is encouraged to consult with the orthopedic surgeon regarding the decision of whether to treat with antibiotic prophylaxis.

18. What are the current antibiotic prophylaxis guidelines recommended by the American Dental Association for dental patients with prosthetic joint replacements?
See Table 25-1.

Table 25-1   *American Dental Association Antibiotic Prophylaxis Guidelines for Patients with Prosthetic Joint Replacements*

PATIENT STATUS	ANTIBIOTIC	DOSE	ADMINISTRATION
Able to take oral penicillin	Cephalexin *or*	2 g	PO 1 hr before dental procedure
	Cephradine *or*	2 g	
	Amoxicillin	2 g	
Unable to take oral medications	Cefazolin *or*	1 g	IM or IV 1 hr before dental procedure
	Ampicillin	2 g	
Allergic to penicillin	Clindamycin	600 mg	1 hr before dental procedure
Allergic to penicillin and unable to take oral medications	Clindamycin	600 mg	IV 1 hr before dental procedure

PO, Orally; *IM,* intramuscularly; *IV,* intravenously.

BIBLIOGRAPHY

1. Ainscow DA, Denham RA: The risk of haematogenous infection in total joint replacements. J Bone Joint Surg 66(B):580-582, 1984.
2. Bartzokas C, Johnson R, Jane M et al: Relation between mouth and haematogenous infection in total joint replacements. BMJ 309:506-508, 1994.
3. Burton DS, Schurman DJ: Salvage of infected total joint replacements. Arch Surg 112:574-578, 1977.
4. Cozen L: Infection after knee replacement surgery. Orthopedics 1:222-223, 1978.
5. Little JW: Patients with prosthetic joints: are they at risk when receiving invasive dental procedures? Spec Care Dentist 17:153-160, 1997.
6. Wahl M: Myths of dental-induced prosthetic joint infections. Clin Infect Dis 20:1420-1425, 1995.

26. THE PREGNANT ORAL AND MAXILLOFACIAL SURGERY PATIENT

Terrence R. Nedbalski, DDS, and Brenda Price, MD

1. **What is the normal human gestation time?**
Pregnancy lasts approximately 275 days, or ≈ 40 weeks divided into trimesters.

2. **A 22-week pregnant women is in which trimester?**
She is in her second trimester. The trimester system is:
- First trimester (0-14 weeks)
- Second trimester (14-27 weeks)
- Third trimester (28-40 weeks)

3. **What are the development milestones for a normally developing fetus?**
- 24 weeks : low end of fetal survival
- 34 weeks: lung maturation; fetal survival increases exponentially. Mortality is equal to 37 weeks; however, there is a much higher morbidity. Common fetal complications include feeding and temperature control issues, as well as an increased risk of neonatal jaundice.
- 37 weeks: Fetal mortality same as at 40 weeks; therefore this is considered a term pregnancy.
- 39 weeks: Fetal morbidity is so low as to permit elective delivery.

4. **When does organogenesis take place?**
   Weeks 3-14.
- Weeks 1-2: embryo implantations—all or no response to embryo insult
- Weeks 3-14: organogenesis—extremely sensitive to exogenous insults
- Weeks 14–27: fetus less sensitive to exogenous insult. Fetal heart sound can be heard for first time.
- Weeks 28-40: Fetus becomes sensitive to transplacental carcinogens.

5. **When is the safest time to perform surgery on a pregnant patient?**
   In the second trimester.

6. **Why are the first and third trimesters a less optimal time to perform oral and maxillofacial surgery (OMFS) on the pregnant patient?**
   During the first trimester, the fetus is the most vulnerable in terms of organogenesis and response to exogenous insult. During the third trimester, there is the risk of inducing a preterm delivery and all its sequelae.

7. **What is the OB/GYN "point of view" in timing the treatment of the gravid OMFS patient?**
   Let the fetus "incubate" until the patient approaches the most probable or achievable milestone weighed against the mother's health needs. In regard to treatment of the pregnant patient, tread lightly in the first trimester. Get all urgent care out of the way in the second trimester in the hopes of avoiding having to induce in the early part of the third trimester owing to high morbidity. In the third trimester, get as far down the developmental line as you can, constantly weighing benefit to the mother vs. risk to the fetus.

8. **What are the FDA categories for pregnant and lactating patients?**
   A: Controlled studies in humans have failed to demonstrate a risk to the fetus, and the possibility of fetal harm seems remote.
   B: Animal studies have not indicated fetal risk, and there are no human studies; or animal studies have shown a risk, but controlled human studies have not.
   C: Animal studies have shown a risk, but there are no controlled human studies; or no studies are available in humans or animals.
   D: Evidence of human fetal risk exists, but in certain situations, the drug may be used despite its risk.
   X: Evidence of fetal abnormalities or fetal risk based on human experience exists. The risk outweighs any possible benefit for use during pregnancy.

9. **What are the FDA drug classes for antibiotics commonly used in OMFS?**
   Class B: Penicillin, erythromycin, clindamycin, cephalosporins, metronidazole
   Class D: Tetracycline, quinolones

10. **What are the FDA drug classes for analgesics?**
    Class B:

- Acetaminophen
- Ibuprofen (*can* be given in first 32 weeks; past that, theoretical risk of premature closure of the patent ductus arteriosus [PDA]. This is true of all nonsteroidal antiinflammatory drugs [NSAIDs])
- Oxycodone
- Morphine
- Fentanyl
- Meperidine
- Hydrocodone
  There is concern for fetal dependence with any opioid, as well as respiratory depression in the newborn recently exposed to opioids.
  Class C:
- Codeine: associated with first trimester malformations; can use in second or third trimester
- Aspirin: associated with late-term intrauterine growth restriction

11. What are the FDA drug classes for common sedatives used in OMFS?
Both benzodiazepines and barbiturates pose a risk for fetal craniofacial anomalies and are FDA Class D drugs.

12. What are the FDA drug classes for common local anesthetics used in OMFS?

Category B	Category C
Lidocaine	Articaine
Prilocaine	Bupivacaine
Etidocaine	Mepivacaine

13. What difficulties would you encounter when attempting to intubate a pregnant patient?
During pregnancy, there is significant increased friability of the upper respiratory tract mucosa. This friability leads to bleeding and blood obscuring the airway during endotracheal intubation, especially nasal endotracheal intubation. Also, the standard signs predicting difficulty of intubation in a nonpregnant patient (short thyromental distance, large neck circumference, etc.) may not be present, and therefore ease of intubation may be misleading.

14. What is the incidence of failed intubation in the pregnant patient vs. the nonpregnant patient?
The incidence of failed intubations overall is 1:2230. The incidence of failed intubations in gravid patients is 1:280.

15. What happens to cardiac output during pregnancy?
Cardiac output increases 30%-50% during pregnancy. There is a 20%-30% increase in heart rate and a 20%-50% increase in stroke volume. Cardiac output increases during the fist trimester, plateaus during the second, and shows minimal increases in the third trimester.

16. What happens to blood volume during pregnancy?
Blood volume increases 25%-52% and red blood cell mass increases 20% by late pregnancy. This is a protective mechanism against volume depletion during peripartum or postpartum hemorrhage. The average blood loss from a normal vaginal delivery is 500 mL. The average blood loss from a cesarean delivery is 1000 mL. To naturally help prevent the chance of thrombotic events, pregnant women experience a maternal hemodilution, with an optimal hematocrit (Hct) value of 30%-38%.

17. What are the changes in respiration system?
A lowered O_2 reserve, with increased O_2 consumption. The diaphragm is displaced superiorly, leading to a 15%-20% change in functional residual capacity. The pregnant patient

needs extensive preoxygenation before induction (treated similarly to obese patients during induction).

18. What changes occur in the clotting cascade in pregnancy?
Thrombin-mediated fibrin generation increases, which, paired with increased hematocrit, leads to hypercoagulability.

19. Which clotting factors are altered during pregnancy?
Factors XI and XII are increased during pregnancy.

20. What are the elements of Virchow's triad?
A hypercoagulable state, venous stasis, and endothelial wall damage.

21. How does the pregnant patient fulfill *all* the elements of Virchow's triad?
Increased Hct along with increased fibrin generation causes a hypercoagulable state; pressure on the inferior vena cava and iliac vein by the uterus causes venous stasis; stasis, in turn, causes endothelial wall damage, which predisposes to venous thrombus.

22. What is the incidence of thrombotic events in a postoperative pregnant patient?
All the above lead to a **fivefold** increase in thrombotic events.

23. What are the changes you would notice on an arterial blood gas test in a pregnant patient?
Hyperventilation increases by 42% during pregnancy. Increased renal bicarbonate excretion, along with postural changes, leads to a moderate level of baseline hypoxemia. The gravid patient is expected to have a mild respiratory alkalosis (pH 7.40-7.46), which is important in determining ventilatory patterns under general anesthesia.

24. What level of x-ray radiation to a fetus will cause teratogenicity?
Analysis of human data shows that fetuses of < 16 weeks who had an acute exposure of 0.5 Gy had a higher risk of growth restriction, microcephaly, and mental retardation. During the fetal period, the fetus becomes less sensitive to radiation but retains central nervous system sensitivity that may lead to growth restriction at term. Diagnostic radiographs that deliver < 0.05 to 0.1 Gy are not believed to be teratogenic. Virtually all plain film and computed tomography (CT) scan irradiation delivers < 0.01 Gy to the fetus.

25. What type of radiographic studies delivers the greatest amount of radiation?
The greatest exposure to the fetus is during abdominal and pelvic irradiation.

26. What is the incidence of a teratogenic malformation from two periapical radiographs on a properly shielded pregnant patient in her first trimester?
Nine in 1 billion. Background radiation in the United States is 0.0008 cGy daily. The exposure to two periapical films is 700 times < the average background radiation in 1 day.

27. What are common radiation dosages for radiographic studies performed in OMFS?
(1 cGy = 0.01 Gy = 1 rad; 0.001 rad = 1 mrad)
- Full dental series < 0.01 mrad
- Skull < 0.01 mrad
- Cervical spine < 0.01 mrad
- Chest < 0.06 mrad
- CT scan (head) 0.1- 0.3 mrad

28. How should a pregnant patient be positioned for surgery?
During the second and third trimesters, a decrease in blood pressure can occur while the patient is in a supine position. This is attributed to a decreased venous return to the heart from the

compression of the inferior vena cava by the gravid uterus. This also can compress the descending aorta and common iliac arteries, both of which will lead to a potential decrease in CO by 14%. Not all pregnant patients are susceptible, but a decrease in uteroplacental perfusion can still occur. Position the patient in the *left lateral decubitus position* by placing the patient in a 5%-15% tilt during surgery.

29. Is N_2O contraindicated in pregnant patients?

Potential teratogenic effects of N_2O are related to its ability to inactivate methionine synthase. It is responsible for converting homocysteine and methyltetrahydrofolate to methionine and tetrahydrofolate, which are needed for synthesis of DNA. Folate supplementation preoperatively has been recommended. N_2O is used heavily in European obstetrics.

Rowland, Baird, and Shore et al. looked at dental assistants who showed a higher level of spontaneous abortion when they were exposed to *nonscavanged* N_2O for > 3 hours/week.

Axelson, Ahlborg, and Bodin et al. showed that midwives who worked at night had a higher correlation of spontaneous abortion from heavy work and night hours than from exposure to N_2O.

30. What FDA classification is N_2O for pregnant patients?

Not rated.

31. What is the risk of using NSAIDs during pregnancy?

The PDA, which joins the fetal aorta to the pulmonary artery, begins to close at birth. After 32 weeks, its remaining open is dependent on fetal prostaglandins. Inhibiting these prostaglandins at this point may result in fetal death secondary to compromised fetal circulation.

32. What is the incidence of closure of the PDA following oral NSAID use?

There had never been a documented case of PDA closure following oral NSAID use. It is avoided for its theoretical and medicolegal ramifications.

BIBLIOGRAPHY

1. Axelsson G, Ahlborg G Jr, Bodin L: Shift work, nitrous oxide exposure, and spontaneous abortion among Swedish midwives. Occup Environ Med 53:374-378, 1996.
2. Briggs F: Drugs in Pregnancy and Lactation: A Reference Guide to Fetal and Neonatal Risk, 3rd ed. Baltimore, 1990, Williams & Wilkins.
3. Cunningham FG, Gant NF, Leveno KJ et al: Williams Obstetrics, 21st ed. New York, 2001, McGraw-Hill.
4. Little JW, Falace DA: Dental Management of the Medically Compromised Patient. St Louis, 1993, Mosby.
5. Pradel C: The pregnant oral and maxillofacial surgery patient. Oral Maxillofac Surg Clin North Am 10:471-489, 1998.
6. Rowland AS, Baird DD, Shore DL et al: Nitrous oxide and spontaneous abortion in female dental assistants. Am J Epidemiol 141:531-538, 1995.
7. Turner M, Aziz S: Management of the pregnant oral and maxillofacial surgery patient. J Oral Maxillofac Surg 60:1479-1488, 2002.

Part VI
Management of the Oral and Maxillofacial Surgery Patient

27. APPLIED OROFACIAL ANATOMY

A. Omar Abubaker, DMD, PhD, and Kenneth J. Benson, DDS

1. **What are the sources for the blood and nerve supply to the sternocleidomastoid muscle (SCM)?**

   The blood supply to the SCM is provided from two sources. The superior thyroid artery supplies the middle third of the muscle, whereas the occipital artery branches supply the remainder of the muscle. The nerve supply is from the spinal accessory (cranial nerve [CN] XI) and from C2 and C3.

2. **What are the sources of the blood and nerve supply to the temporomandibular joint (TMJ)?**

   The major arterial supply to the TMJ is derived from the superficial temporal artery and from the maxillary artery posteriorly, and from smaller masseteric, posterior deep temporal, and lateral pterygoid arteries anteriorly. The venous drainage is through a diffuse plexus around the capsule and rich venous channels that drain the retrodiscal tissue.

   The nerve supply is from the auriculotemporal nerve, which provides the principal sensory innervation to the TMJ. The nerve gives off two or three branches, which enter the capsule inferiorly, medially, and laterally. The masseteric nerve also innervates the capsule from the frontal and medial sides of the joint. The posterior deep temporal nerve supplies the TMJ laterally and anteriorly.

3. **How many origins and insertions does each masticatory muscle have?**

   For each muscle of mastication, there are two insertions and two origins.

4. **What is the function of the lateral pterygoid muscle?**

   The lateral pterygoid muscle is triangular in shape and runs in a slightly inferior and posterior horizontal direction. The muscle has superior and inferior heads. The **superior head** arises from the infratemporal surface of the greater wing of the sphenoid and inserts into the articular capsule and disc. The function of the superior head is to stabilize the condyle and disc during closing movement.

   The **inferior head** originates from the lateral surface of the lateral pterygoid plate and inserts into the pterygoid fovea of the neck of the condyle. The inferior head aids in translation of the condyle over the articular eminence during opening of the mouth.

5. **Which muscles make up the pterygomandibular raphe?**

   The buccinator muscle anteriorly and the superior constrictor of the pharynx posteriorly make up the pterygomandibular raphe.

6.   What embryologic structures form the external nose?

The **maxillary processes,** which originate from the dorsal ends of the first (mandibular) arch and the lateral nasal processes, grow toward the midline to merge with the downward-growing frontonasal process to form the external nose. The **frontonasal process** then continues to elongate, forming the median nasal process and fetal philtrum. The lateral nasal processes form the lateral portion of the adult nose (i.e., lower lateral cartilage and lobule). The **olfactory placode,** an ectodermal thickening, invaginates as a pit between the medial portion of the frontonasal process and the lateral nasal process. The olfactory placode finally comes to rest high in the nose as the analogue of the olfactory epithelium.

7.   What nasal bones and cartilages make up the external nasal skeleton?

Several bones and cartilages make up the external nose and give it its characteristic pyramidal shape (Fig. 27-1). The nasal bones articulate with the nasal part of the frontal bone superiorly and the nasal process of the maxilla laterally. The nasal bones are attached at their inferior aspect to the upper lateral cartilages. The upper lateral cartilages in turn attach their inferior portion to the lower lateral cartilages and, medially, to the cartilaginous septum.

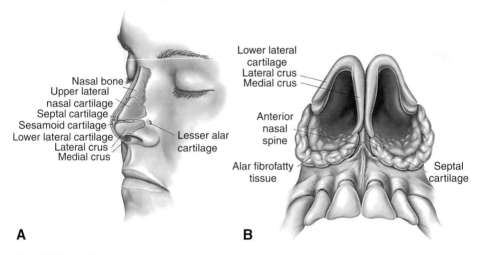

Fig. 27-1   A, Normal anatomy and underlying soft tissues of the nose. **B,** Normal position of the nasal septum and nasal spine. (From Bertz JE: Nasal injuries. In Fonseca RJ [ed]: Oral and Maxillofacial Surgery, 3rd vol. Philadelphia, 2000, Saunders.)

Small rudimentary cartilages known as *sesamoid cartilages,* or *alar cartilages,* give additional support to the lateral nasal ala, where the lower lateral cartilage extends to meet the cheek. The fibrofatty tissue of the lower lateral cartilage, which contains the sesamoid cartilages, is known as the *lobule.*

The nasal septum is made up of quadrangle cartilage that continues with the lateral nasal cartilage toward the bridge of the nose, forming the cartilaginous portion of the septum. Posteriorly and above, the septal cartilage with the perpendicular plate of the ethmoid and the inferior edge of the septum fits into a groove on the vomer and the nasal crest.

8.   What is the vascular supply to the nose?

Branches from both the external and internal carotid arteries supply the nose. The external nose is supplied by the dorsal nasal of the ophthalmic artery superiorly, and the septal and lateral nasal of the angular artery inferiorly. The lower part of the dorsum of the nose is supplied by the external nasal, from the anterior ethmoidal artery.

The external carotid artery via the terminal branches of the internal maxillary artery, namely the sphenopalatine and greater palatine arteries, supplies the posterior inferior part of the internal nose. Branches from the anterior and posterior ethmoid arteries of the ophthalmic artery supply the anterior inferior nasal cavity, which is a branch of the internal carotid artery. Venous drainage of the nose corresponds to the arterial nomenclature and occurs through the sphenopalatine, ophthalmic, and anterior facial veins.

9. How is the sensory nerve supply to the nose mapped?

- Olfactory fibers are located in the superior portion of the internal nose and serve the sensory function of smell.
- The sensory innervation of the skin of the root of the nose is derived from the supratrochlear and infratrochlear branches of the ophthalmic nerve.
- Branches of the infraorbital nerve supply the skin on the lower half of the nose's side.
- Nasociliary branches of the ophthalmic nerve supply the skin over the lower dorsum of the nose down to the tip.
- The trigeminal nerve supplies general sensory innervation to the anterior internal nose through the anterior ethmoidal, external, and internal nasal branches.
- The lateral posterior superior, pharyngeal, and lateral posterior inferior branches of the maxillary nerve supply the posterior portion.
- The terminal branches of the infraorbital nerve supply the lining of the nasal vestibule.
- The internal nasal (anterior ethmoidal) and medial posterior superior branches supply the septum anterior and posterior portions, respectively.

10. How is the motor nerve supply to the nose mapped?

- The autonomic nerve supply of the nose controls the secretory function of the mucous glands.
- The preganglionic sympathetic innervation originates from the hypothalamus, passes through the thoracolumbar region of the spinal cord, and synapses in the superior cervical ganglion in the neck.
- Postganglionic sympathetic fibers then pass through the sphenopalatine ganglion to reach the nasal glands along the posterior nasal nerves.
- The parasympathetic nerve supply to the nose originates in the superior salvatory nucleus of the midbrain to reach the sphenopalatine ganglion through the greater petrosal nerve.
- The postganglionic fibers are carried out along the vidian nerve to finally reach the nose via the posterior nasal nerve.
- The motor nerve supply to all the muscles of the external nose is by way of the facial nerve.

11. What are the most common vessels involved with anterior epistaxis?

Kiesselbach's plexus of septum arterioles is the source of 90% of nosebleeds. Four anastomosed arteries make up this plexus: the sphenopalatine, anterior ethmoidal, greater palatine, and superior labial arteries. The nasopalatine branch of the descending palatine artery anastomoses with septal branches of the sphenopalatine artery, the anterior ethmoidal artery, and superior lateral branches of the superior labial branch of the facial artery. Traumatic nasal bleeding can be caused by laceration of the nasal mucosa, and any of the nasal vessels can be the source of the bleeding (Fig. 27-2).

12. How does lymphatic drainage of the nose occur?

The lymphatics of the nose arise from the superficial portion of the mucous membrane and travel posteriorly to the retropharyngeal lymph nodes. Anteriorly, the lymphatics drain into the submandibular lymph nodes or the upper deep cervical nodes.

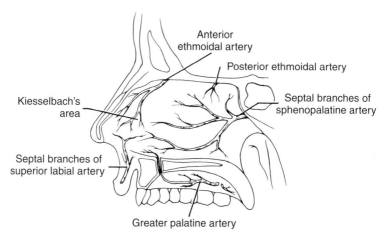

Anterior
ethmoidal artery

Posterior ethmoidal artery

Kiesselbach's
area

Septal branches of
sphenopalatine artery

Septal branches of
superior labial artery

Greater palatine artery

Fig. 27-2   Vessels that make up Kiesselbach's plexus. (From Abelson RI: Epistaxis. In Paparella MM, Shumrick DA, Gluckman JL et al [eds]: Otolaryngology, 3rd ed. Philadelphia, 1991, Saunders.)

13. Where do the paranasal sinuses drain?
   The sphenoid sinus drains into the sphenoethmoidal recess. The posterior ethmoid sinus drains into the superior nasal meatus, and the nasolacrimal duct drains into the inferior nasal meatus. All other sinuses (maxillary, frontal, and anterior and middle ethmoidal) drain into the middle nasal meatus.

14. What are Arnold's and Jacobson's nerves? Which organ do they supply?
   Both nerves provide sensory innervation to the ear. Arnold's nerve is a branch of the vagus nerve (CN X) and supplies the concha and auditory canal. Jacobson's nerve is a branch of the glossopharyngeal nerve (CN IX) and supplies the concha, canal, and middle ear.

15. What other nerves supply the ear?
   The auriculotemporal nerve (CN V3) supplies the root helix, crus, tragus, and canal, whereas the auricular branch off the facial nerve (CN VII) supplies the concha and canal. Thus, in all, four cranial nerves (V, VII, IX, and X) provide sensory innervation for the ear.

16. What is the sensory innervation to the larynx?
   The **vagus nerve** innervates the larynx via two laryngeal branches, the *internal laryngeal* and the *recurrent laryngeal*. The internal laryngeal branch provides sensory innervation to the mucous membrane above the vocal fold, whereas the recurrent laryngeal nerve provides sensory innervation to the mucous membrane below the vocal fold.
   Motor function of the laryngeal muscles and vocal cords also is provided by the laryngeal branches of the vagus nerve (fibers of CN XI traveling with CN X). The *external laryngeal* branch innervates the cricothyroid muscle, and the recurrent laryngeal branch innervates all other intrinsic muscles.

17. What is the interval between open eyelids called?
   The palpebral fissure (rima).

18. What is the average height of the inferior and superior tarsi?
   The superior tarsus is 8-12 mm; the inferior tarsus is 5-7 mm.

19. What is the autonomic innervation to the lacrimal gland?

Preganglionic parasympathetic fibers originate at the superior salivatory nucleus and are carried along the facial nerve to reach the sphenopalatine ganglion by the greater petrosal nerve. The postganglionic parasympathetic fibers travel through the zygomatic nerve to reach the lacrimal gland along the lacrimal nerve. Postganglionic sympathetic fibers from the superior cervical sympathetic ganglion travel through the deep petrosal nerve to reach the lacrimal gland in the same fashion as the parasympathetic fibers.

20. What are the components of the lacrimal drainage system?

Approximately 12 small ducts under the outer corner of the upper eyelid drain tears onto the conjunctiva. From the superior and inferior puncta at the upper and lower eyelids at the medial canthus, the **lacrimal canaliculi** travel first vertically, then medially and downward (of the superior canaliculi), and finally upward and medially (of the inferior canaliculi) to converge at the **lacrimal sac.** The canaliculi length is approximately 8 mm. Often the canaliculi converge before the lacrimal sac and create a small dilation called the **sinus of Maier.** The lacrimal sac is 12 mm long and is found in the anterior aspect of the medial orbital wall. The **lacrimal crest** is covered by periosteum. The medial palpebral ligament lies anterior and superior to the sac. The lacrimal sac empties into the nasolacrimal duct, which drains into the inferior nasal meatus of the nose.

21. What is the relationship of the nasolacrimal duct to the nasal cavity and maxillary sinus?

The nasolacrimal duct lies within the thin, bony wall between the maxillary sinus and the nasal cavity. The duct ends at the inferior nasal meatus through the valve of Hasner. The position of the nasolacrimal duct beneath the inferior turbinate is 11-14 mm posterior to the piriform aperture and 11-17 mm above the nasal floor (Fig. 27-3).

22. Which bones form the orbital cavity?

- Lacrimal
- Ethmoid
- Palatine
- Frontal

- Sphenoid
- Zygomatic
- Maxillary

23. What is Whitnall's orbital tubercle?

Whitnall's orbital tubercle is a bony protuberance present at the lateral orbital wall approximately 5 mm behind the lateral orbital rim. The tubercle is the area for attachment of the lateral horn of the levator aponeurosis, lateral palpebral ligament, and lateral check ligament. The attachment of these structures is in that order, from anterior to posterior.

24. Which orbital voluntary muscle does *not* originate at the orbital apex?

The inferior oblique muscle arises from the medial portion of the floor of the orbit just posterior to the orbital rim. The muscle then passes laterally and inserts on the posterolateral sclera.

25. What is the anatomy, nerve supply, and function of the extraocular muscles?

See Table 27-1.

26. What are the distance limits from the lateral, inferior, superior, and medial orbital rims for safe posterior dissection?

Although the distance from the orbital rim to the orbital apex is 4-4.5 cm, subperiosteal dissection along the orbital walls can be safely extended only up to 25 mm posteriorly from the inferior orbital rim and 25 mm from the lateral orbital rim. From the anterior lacrimal crest, dissection can be extended 25 mm posteriorly with minimal danger to the posterior orbital

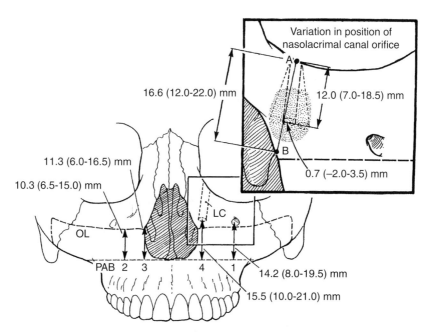

Fig. 27-3 The relationship of the nasolacrimal duct to the nasal floor and turbinates. Heights (means and ranges) are from the piriform aperture base *(PAB)* to the infraorbital foramen *(1)*, the simulated osteotomy *(2)*, the anterior attachment of the inferior turbinate *(3)*, and the inferior orifice of the nasolacrimal canal *(4)*. The inset illustrates the variation in position of the nasolacrimal canal orifice relative to the x line drawn between the lacrimal fossa *(A)* and the anterior attachment of the inferior turbinate *(B)*. *LC,* Nasolacrimal canal; *OL,* simulated high-level Le Fort I osteotomy. (Modified from You-ZH, Bell WH, Finn RA: Location of the nasolacrimal canal in relation to the high Le Forte I osteotomy. J Oral Maxillofac Surg 50:1075-1080, 1992.)

Table 27-1 *Anatomy, Nerve Supply, and Function of the Extraocular Muscles*

MUSCLE	ORIGIN	INSERTION	NERVE SUPPLY	FUNCTION
Levator palpebrae superioris	Lesser wing of sphenoid	Anterior surface and upper border of superior tarsal plate		
• Voluntary portion			Oculomotor nerve	Raises upper eyelid
• Involuntary portion			Sympathetic nerves	
Superior rectus	Common tendinous ring	Sclera 6 mm behind corneal margin	Oculomotor nerve	Raises and medially rotates cornea
Inferior rectus	Common tendinous ring	Sclera 6 mm behind corneal margin	Oculomotor nerve	Depresses cornea, medially rotates cornea

Table 27-1 *Anatomy, Nerve Supply, and Function of the Extraocular Muscles—cont'd*

MUSCLE	ORIGIN	INSERTION	NERVE SUPPLY	FUNCTION
Lateral rectus	Common tendinous ring	Sclera 6 mm behind corneal margin	Abducent nerve	Moves cornea laterally
Medial rectus	Common tendinous ring	Sclera 6 mm behind corneal margin	Oculomotor nerve	Moves cornea medially
Superior oblique	Body of sphenoid	By way of pulley and attached to sclera behind coronal equator of eyeball; line of pull of tendon passes medial to vertical axis	Trochlear nerve	Moves cornea downward and laterally
Inferior oblique	Anterior part of floor of orbit	Attached to sclera behind coronal equat or; line of pull of tendon passes medial to vertical axis	Oculomotor nerve	Moves cornea upward and laterally

Adapted from Snell RS: Clinical Anatomy for Medical Students, 5th ed. Boston, 1996, Little, Brown.

contents. From the superior orbital rim, dissection can be extended 30 mm. However, because most traumatic forces tend to displace all or part of these rims posteriorly, this displacement should be considered when carrying out posterior dissection in the orbit (Fig. 27-4).

27. What occurs during the autonomic nerve supply to the pupil?

Postganglionic sympathetic fibers have their cell bodies in the superior cervical ganglion. These nerves reach the dilator pupil muscles via the **short and long ciliary nerves.** Preganglionic parasympathetic fibers have their cell bodies in the Edinger-Westphal nucleus in the brain and travel to the ciliary ganglion in the orbit via the oculomotor nerve. The short ciliary nerves from the ciliary ganglion to the sphincter pupillary muscles carry the postganglionic fibers. Parasympathetic fibers contribute to pupillary constriction; the sympathetic supply activates pupillary dilator muscles.

28. What are the sebaceous and sweat glands of the eyelids called?

The sebaceous glands of the eyelid are called the *glands of Zeis.* The sweat glands of the eyelid are called the *glands of Moll.*

29. What are crocodile tears?

This condition results after injury to the fibers of the facial nerve carrying parasympathetic secretory fibers that normally innervate the salivary gland. The injury causes the fibers to heal in contact with fibers supplying the lacrimal gland, leading to "crying" when the patient eats.

30. What are the contents of the carotid sheath?

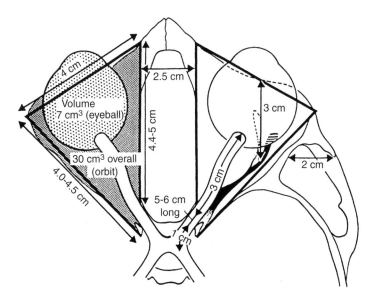

Fig. 27-4 Major orbital dimensions and relationships. (Modified from Ochs M, Buckley M: Anatomy of the orbit. Oral Maxillofac Surg Clin 5:420, 1993.)

The carotid sheath contains the carotid artery, the jugular vein, and the vagus nerve. Within the carotid sheath, the vagus nerve (CN X) lies posterior to the common carotid artery and internal jugular vein.

31. How many branches does the external carotid artery give off? What are they?

The external carotid artery branches from the common carotid artery at the level of the upper border of the thyroid cartilage to be the principal artery supplying the anterior aspect of the neck, face, scalp, oral and nasal cavities, bones of the skull, and dura mater. Note that the orbit and its contents are the only structures that are not supplied by the external carotid. There are eight branches (order of appearance from inferior to superior): (1) the superior thyroid, (2) the ascending pharyngeal, (3) the lingual, (4) the facial, (5) the occipital, (6) the posterior auricular, (7) the internal maxillary, and (8) the superficial temporal.

32. What is the course of the facial artery in the submandibular triangle?

The facial artery passes from behind and medial to the submandibular gland, up and over the gland, to emerge from the submandibular space laterally. It then proceeds into the face at the level of the anterior border of the masseter muscle. Thus the facial artery may or may not be encountered in the incision and removal of the gland, and therefore may not require removal, but would have to be located during dissection by pinpointing the two lymph nodes, which overlie it at the level of the inferior border of the mandible.

Superior and deep to these lymph nodes is the marginal mandibular branch of the facial nerve. Posterior to the nodes is the facial vein. Because the vein is lateral to the gland, it is often necessary to ligate and cut this vessel during the dissection to remove the gland.

33. What is the relationship of the lingual nerve to Wharton's duct?

The submandibular gland, or Wharton's duct, is about 5 cm in length, and its lumen is 2-4 mm in diameter. It runs anteriorly above the mylohyoid muscle and on the lateral surface of the hyoglossus and genioglossus muscles. At first, the duct lies below the lingual nerve. Then, as the lingual nerve descends, it crosses lateral to the duct. As the duct and lingual nerve pass below the sublingual gland, the lingual nerve passes below the duct and crosses it medially. As the nerve continues toward the genioglossus, the duct continues anteriorly and medially. The duct loops from below upward beneath the lingual nerve at the level of the third molar and then crosses above the lingual nerve at about the level of the second molar. Thus the nerve loops almost completely around the duct (Fig. 27-5).

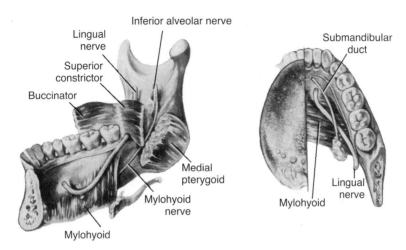

Fig. 27-5   The course and relationships of the submandibular gland duct. (From Sinnatamby CS: Last's Anatomy: Regional and Applied, 10th ed. Edinburgh, 1999, Churchill Livingstone.)

34. What are the relationships and the course of the hypoglossal nerves in the submandibular triangle?

The hypoglossal nerve emerges from the hypoglossal canal and passes laterally between the internal jugular vein and the internal and external carotid arteries. It then descends steeply and crosses the stylohyoid and posterior belly of the digastric muscles on their medial surfaces. The hypoglossal nerve courses forward and upward on the lateral surface of the hyoglossus muscle and is accompanied by branches of the sublingual vein entering the oral cavity at the posterior border of the mylohyoid muscle, slightly above the digastric tendon. Here, beneath the tongue, the nerve curves forward and upward on the lateral surface of the genioglossus muscle, splitting into several branches that go into the substance of the tongue. These branches supply all extrinsic and intrinsic muscles of the tongue except the palatoglossus, which is supplied by CN XI via CN X.

35. What are the boundaries and significance of Lesser's triangle?

The triangle is made up by the angle between the tendon of the digastric muscle inferiorly, the hypoglossal nerve superiorly, and the posterior border of the mylohyoid muscle. The hyoglossal and mylohyoid muscles form the floor of this triangle. This triangle is useful in localization and ligation of the artery that lies at the inner surface (beneath) of the hyoglossus muscle deep to the floor of the triangle.

36. What is the superficial musculoaponeurotic system (SMAS)?

The SMAS is a layer of tissue that includes the platysma, risorius, triangularis, and auricularis muscles. Some authors also include the frontalis and the other muscles of facial expression in this tissue layer. The SMAS is connected to the dermis by a dense network of fibrous septae. These septae allow for movement of the overlying skin when the muscles in this tissue layer contract, giving rise to changes in facial expression. The skin can be dissected from the underlying SMAS by transection of these connecting fibrous septa, such as during rhytidectomy. The significance of the SMAS is related to its relationship to the nerves in the face: facial motor nerves deep to it, and sensory nerves more superficial to it (Fig. 27-6).

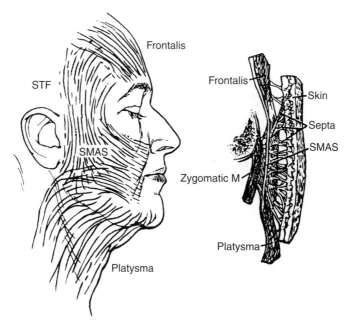

Fig. 27-6   Anatomy of the superficial musculoaponeurotic system *(SMAS)*. *STF,* Superficial temporal fascia. (From Rees TD, Aston SJ, Thorne CHM: Blepharoplasty and fascioplasty. In McCarthy JG [ed]: Plastic Surgery. Philadelphia, 1990, Saunders.)

37. What are the layers of the scalp?

The scalp is made up of five tissue layers, the first three of which are intimately bound together and move as one unit called the *scalp proper*. The layers are:

• **Skin**
• **Connective tissue layer**
• **Aponeurosis**
• **Loose areolar tissue occupying the subgaleal space**
• **Periosteum or pericranium**

The aponeurosis is the tendinous sheet that connects the frontalis muscles to the occipitalis posteriorly and auricularis muscles and superficial temporal fascia laterally. Because the aponeurosis layer is the most distinct layer and covers the cranium like a helmet, it is also called the *galea*, which is Latin for "helmet."

38. How does blood supply and nerve supply to the scalp occur?

The scalp has a rich network of nerve and blood supply. Both the sensory nerves and the arteries of the scalp run in a radial fashion anterior to posterior, posterior to anterior, and laterally to the midline from both sides. All these vessels and nerves meet at the vertex of the cranium, providing an even richer network of nerves and vessels in this region.

The **sensory nerves** supplying the cranium are a pair of supratrochlear and supraorbital nerves anteriorly (V1); the greater and third occipital nerves posteriorly (from the cervical); and the zygomaticotemporal (V2), auriculotemporal (V3), and lesser occipital nerves (C2-C3) laterally. The arterial supply consists of the supratrochlear and supraorbital arteries anteriorly (from the internal carotid); the occipital artery posteriorly; and the zygomaticotemporal, superficial temporal, and posterior auricular laterally (all from the external carotid) (Fig. 27-7).

The **motor nerves** to the muscles of the scalp (frontalis, occipitalis, and auricularis muscles) are supplied by the temporal and posterior auricular branches of the facial nerve.

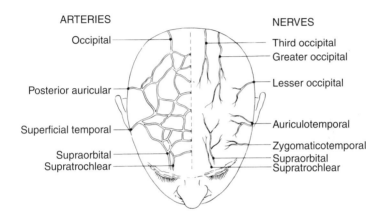

ARTERIES
- Occipital
- Posterior auricular
- Superficial temporal
- Supraorbital
- Supratrochlear

NERVES
- Third occipital
- Greater occipital
- Lesser occipital
- Auriculotemporal
- Zygomaticotemporal
- Supraorbital
- Supratrochlear

Fig. 27-7   Nerve and blood supply of the scalp. (From Welch TB, Boyne PJ: The management of traumatic scalp injuries: report of cases. J Oral Maxillofacial Surg 49:1007-1014, 1991.)

39. What is the extension of the galea of the scalp into the temporal region?
The musculoaponeurotic layer covering the cranium is made of fascia (galea) in some locations and of muscles (frontalis, occipitals, and auricularis) in others. When this layer reaches the temporal region it is called the *superficial temporal fascia* or the *temporoparietal fascia*.

40. What is the extension of the temporoparietal fascia in the face?
The temporoparietal fascia in the temporal region of the face is confluent with the SMAS. This system consists of muscles of facial expression in some locations, and in other locations where there are no muscles, it consists of a dense fascial layer.

41. What are the other fascial layers of the temporal region?
In the temporal region, the temporalis fascia (the deep temporal fascia) becomes the extension of the pericranium, forming the periosteum covering the skull. In the preauricular region, roughly 2 cm superior to the zygomatic arch, the temporalis fascia splits into two layers (or leaflets): superficial and deep. These fascial layers form a pocket that contains the temporal fat pad. The two layers attach to the zygomatic arch and fuse with its periosteum (Fig. 27-8).

42. What is the extension of the temporalis fascia below the level of the zygomatic arch?
The temporalis fascia extends below the zygomatic arch to invest muscles of mastication and adjacent structures, namely the masseter muscle and parotid gland. This layer is called *parotideomasseteric fascia*.

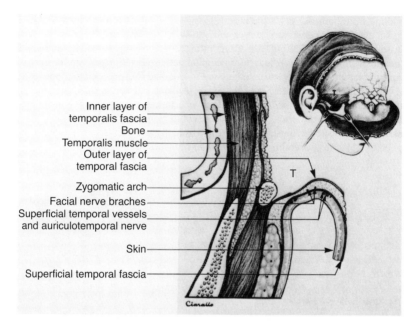

Inner layer of
temporalis fascia
Bone
Temporalis muscle
Outer layer of
temporal fascia

Zygomatic arch
Facial nerve braches
Superficial temporal vessels
and auriculotemporal nerve

Skin

Superficial temporal fascia

Fig. 27-8   Cross-section showing the level of dissection of the coronal flap in the temporal region. (From Bell WH: Modern Practice in Orthognathic and Reconstructive Surgery, 2nd vol. Philadelphia, 1992, Saunders.)

43. What are the extensions of the SMAS and parotideomasseteric fascia in the neck?

In the neck, the extension of the SMAS is the superficial cervical fascia, which is similar to the SMAS in containing the muscle of facial expression of the neck, the *platysma*. This layer is loose in most areas, but is bound firmly to the underlying structures in a few places. The continuation of the parotideomasseteric fascia in the neck is the deep cervical fascia. This fascia also varies in thickness and splits in various sites to enclose the muscles of the neck, the submandibular gland, and the thyroid glands.

44. What is the blood supply to the temporalis muscle and the temporalis fascia?

The muscle is supplied primarily by the anterior and posterior deep temporal arteries (branches of the internal maxillary artery) and to a lesser extent by the superficial temporal artery.

The middle temporal artery, a branch of the superficial temporal artery, is the main supply to the fascia.

45. What is the blood supply to the temporal fat pad?

The blood supply to the temporal pad fat is from the middle temporal artery, which is a branch of the superficial temporal artery.

46. What is the function and foramina of the 12 cranial nerves?

See Table 27-2.

47. At what distance from the stylomastoid foramen does the facial nerve bifurcate?

The nerve bifurcates into two main trunks (the zygomatico facial and the mandibular cervical) at variable distances after the nerve exits the skull, but on the average this distance is 1.3 cm.

Table 27-2   *Cranial Nerve Components, Function, and Foramen of Exit from the Cranium*

NERVE	COMPONENTS	FUNCTION	SKULL OPENING
I. Olfactory	Sensory	Smell	Opening in cribriform plate of ethmoid
II. Optic	Sensory	Vision	Optic canal
III. Oculomotor	Motor	Lifts upper eyelid, turns eyeball upward, downward, and medially; constricts pupil; accommodates eye	Superior orbital fissure
IV. Trochlear	Motor	Assists in turning eyeball downward and laterally	Superior orbital fissure
V. Trigeminal			
• Ophthalmic division	Sensory	Cornea, skin of forehead, scalp, eyelids, and nose; also mucous membrane of paranasal sinuses and nasal cavity	Superior orbital fissure
• Maxillary division	Sensory	Skin of face over maxilla and the upper lip; teeth of upper jaw; mucous membrane of nose, the maxillary air sinus, and palate	Foramen rotundum
• Mandibular division	Motor	Muscles of mastication, mylohyoid, anterior belly of digastric, tensor veli palatini, and tensor tympani	Foramen ovale
	Sensory	Skin of cheek, skin over mandible, lower lip, and side of head; teeth of lower jaw and temporomandibular joint; mucous membrane of mouth and anterior two thirds of tongue	
VI. Abducent	Motor	Lateral rectus muscle; turns eyeball laterally	Superior orbital fissure
VII. Facial	Motor	Muscles of face, the cheek, and scalp; stapedius muscle of middle ear; stylohyoid; and posterior belly of digastric	Internal acoustic meatus, facial canal, stylomastoid foramen
	Sensory	Taste from anterior two thirds of tongue; floor of mouth and palate	
	Secretomotor parasympathetic	Submandibular and sublingual salivary glands, the lacrimal gland, and glands of nose and palate	

Continued

Table 27-2 *Cranial Nerve Components, Function, and Foramen of Exit from the Cranium—cont'd*

NERVE	COMPONENTS	FUNCTION	SKULL OPENING
VIII. Vestibulocochlear			
• Vestibular	Sensory	Position and movement of head	Internal acoustic meatus
• Cochlear	Sensory	Hearing	
IX. Glossopharyngeal	Motor	Stylopharyngeus muscle: assists swallowing	
	Secretomotor parasym-pathetic	Parotid salivary gland	Jugular foramen
	Sensory	General sensation and taste from posterior third of tongue and pharynx; carotid sinus and carotid body	
X. Vagus	Motor	Constrictor muscles of pharynx and intrinsic muscles of larynx; involuntary muscle of trachea and bronchi, heart, alimentary tract from pharynx to splenic flexure of colon; liver and pancreas	Jugular foramen
	Sensory	Taste from epiglottis and vallecula and afferent fibers from structures named above	
XI. Accessory			
• Cranial root	Motor	Muscles of soft palate, pharynx, and larynx	Jugular foramen
• Spinal root	Motor	Sternocleidomastoid and trapezius muscles	
XII. Hypoglossal	Motor	Muscles of tongue controlling its shape and movement (except palatoglossus)	Hypoglossal canal

Adapted from Snell RS: Clinical Anatomy for Medical Students, 5th ed. Boston, 1996, Little, Brown.

48. At what distance from the external auditory canal does the facial nerve bifurcate?
The point of bifurcation of the facial nerve is located 1.5-2.8 cm inferior to the lowest concavity of the bony external auditory canal.

49. What is the "danger zone" for the frontal branch of the facial nerve as it crosses the zygomatic arch?
The frontal branch of the facial nerve crosses superficial to the zygomatic arch in an area that lies 0.8-3.5 cm anterior to the anterior concavity of the bony external auditory

canal (an average of 2 cm anterior to the canal). A danger zone for injuring the frontal branch of the facial nerve during surgical procedures in the temporal and preauricular regions is located between two parallel lines drawn in the temporal region. The anterior line is drawn from the inferior attachment of the earlobe to the most lateral extension of the eyebrow. The posterior line is drawn from a midpoint on the tragus of the ear to the most superior forehead crease of the forehead, or at least 2 cm from the first line or 2 cm above the supraorbital regions.

50. What is the "danger zone" for the marginal mandibular branch of the facial nerve?

The mandibular branch of the facial nerve courses in an area where incisions to approach the mandible and mandibular condyle are commonly placed. Accordingly, this area is considered a danger zone for injury to this branch. The zone is located between the inferior border of the mandible and a line in the retromandibular and submandibular region. This line extends from anterior to posterior and is 2 cm (1 thumb-breadth) behind the gonion and posterior border of the ascending ramus, 2 cm below the gonion, extending forward 2 cm below the inferior border of the mandible as far anteriorly to the level of the second premolar tooth. The anterior border of the zone is located at the intersection of two lines: a horizontal line 2 cm below and parallel to the inferior border of the body of the mandible, and another along the long axis of the lower second premolar.

51. How can the main trunk of the facial nerve be located during a parotidectomy?

As the facial nerve trunk travels from the stylomastoid foramen to the parotid gland, it passes anterior to the posterior belly of the digastric muscle, lateral to the styloid process and the external carotid artery, and posterior to the facial vein. Start a parotidectomy by mobilizing the tail of the parotid superiorly and retracting the anterior border of the sternocleidomastoid laterally, to identify the posterior belly of the digastric muscle. Follow this muscle superiorly toward its insertion at the mastoid tip. After bluntly separating the parotid from its attachment to the cartilage of the external auditory canal, the **tragal pointer** (outer surface of the external auditory cartilage) comes into view. The facial nerve trunk lies approximately 1 cm deep and slightly anteroinferior to the tragal pointer.

52. What are the branches of the facial nerve?

The facial nerve trunk has six major branches: temporal, zygomatic, buccal, mandibular, cervical, and auricular. The auricular branch comes off before the facial nerve turns into the parotid body, and innervates the superior auricular, posterior auricular, and occipitalis muscles, as well as provides sensation to the area behind the earlobe. Within the parotid, the facial nerve divides into two main branches, the temporofacial and cervicofacial, which further divide into the temporal, zygomatic, buccal, mandibular, and cervical branches. The stylohyoid and posterior digastric are other minor branches of the nerve.

53. What is the relationship of the facial nerve to the parotideomasseteric fascia?

As the facial nerve branches leave the parotid gland, the parotideomasseteric fascia covers them. The SMAS is located superficial to this layer.

54. How do the facial muscles of expression receive their innervation?

All facial muscles except the mentalis, levator angularis superioris, and buccinator receive their innervation along their deep surfaces. However, because these three muscles are located deep within the facial soft tissue and lie deep to the plane of the facial nerve, they receive their innervation along their superficial surfaces. All other facial muscles of expression are located superficial to the plane of the facial nerve and thus receive their innervation along their deep or posterior surfaces. For example, the platysma, orbicularis oculi, and zygomaticus major and minor are situated superficial to the level of the facial nerve.

55. What is the relationship of the frontal branch of the facial nerve to the SMAS and temporoparietal fascia?

Inferior to the zygomatic arch, the frontal branch of the facial nerve travels deep to the SMAS. As it crosses over the zygomatic arch it becomes very superficial. At this point it is sandwiched between the periosteum (extension of the temporal fascia) and the temporoparietal fascia (extension of the SMAS). Superior to the zygomatic arch, the frontal branch of the facial nerve travels within or on the undersurface of the temporoparietal fascia, but superficial to the outer layer of the temporal fascia.

56. How do the frontal and mandibular branches of the facial nerve differ from other facial branches?

Crossover communication between the frontal branch and adjacent branches and between the mandibular branch and adjacent branches is only about 15%. Crossover among the other branches is approximately 70%. Injury to either the frontal or mandibular branches leads to more marked deficit compared with the results of injury to the other branches.

57. What is the relationship of the frontal and mandibular branch courses of the facial nerve?

The frontal branch of the facial nerve crosses the zygomatic arch deep to the SMAS and in the temporal region deep to the temporoparietal fascia (superficial temporal fascia). The nerve usually lies within 2 cm from the lateral border of the eyebrow and enters the frontalis muscle from its deep surface.

The mandibular branch courses within 2 cm of the inferior border of the mandible, posterior to the facial artery. The mandibular branch is at risk during an anterior dissection because in this area, it becomes more superficial. It lies deep to the platysma and superficial to the facial artery.

58. How do you evaluate the five branches of the facial nerve during a physical exam?

Test each of the five branches of the nerve in the following manner:
- Cervical—contract the platysma muscles
- Marginal mandibular—whistle or pucker the lips
- Buccal—smile or show teeth
- Zygomatic—squeeze eyes shut tightly
- Temporal—raise eyebrows

59. What are the most common causes of facial nerve paralysis?

Facial nerve paralysis, which may be unilateral or bilateral, can be a manifestation of any of several disease processes. These diseases can be idiopathic, neoplastic, traumatic, infectious, or congenital. The paralysis can also result from a systemic/metabolic process (Box 27-1).

60. What is the retromandibular approach?

This approach is useful for procedures involving ramus and areas on or near the condylar neck/head. The incision begins 0.5 cm below the earlobe and continues 3.0-3.5 cm inferiorly, approximately 2 cm posterior to the ramus. In some patients, this may limit the direct proximity of the skin incision to the mandible, which is one of the main advantages of this technique. Accordingly, some surgeons recommend placement of the incision more anteriorly at the posterior ramus, just below the earlobe. The deeper dissection of this approach is carried out bluntly through the parotid gland in an anteromedial direction (in the anticipated direction of the facial nerve) toward the posterior border of the mandible. The facial nerve, if identified, is avoided and deeper dissection is continued until the pterygomasseteric sling is identified and incised. The submasseteric dissection is continued to expose the ramus and condyle as needed.

Box 27-1	*Causes of Facial Nerve Paralysis*

Idiopathic
Bell's palsy
Recurrent facial palsy
Melkersson-Rosenthal syndrome

Neoplasia
Cholesteatoma
Facial neuroma
Glomus jugulare or tympanicum
Carcinoma (primary or metastatic)
Schwannoma of lower cranial nerves
Meningioma
Histiocytosis
Rhabdomyosarcoma
Leukemia

Trauma
Temporal bone fractures[*]
Birth trauma
Facial contusions/lacerations
Penetrating wounds to face and temporal bone
Iatrogenic injury

Infection
Herpes zoster oticus (Ramsay-Hunt syndrome)
Otitis media with effusion
Acute suppurative otitis media
Coalescent mastoiditis
Chronic otitis media
Malignant otitis externa (*Pseudomonas* osteomyelitis)
Tuberculosis
Lyme disease[*]
AIDS
Infectious mononucleosis

Congenital
Compression injury
Moebius syndrome[*]
Lower lip paralysis

Metabolic and Systemic
Pregnancy
Diabetes mellitus
Sarcoidosis[*]
Guillain-Barré syndrome[*]
Autoimmune disorders

Modified from Coker NJ: Acute paralysis of the facial nerve. In Bailey BJ: Head and Neck Surgery—Otolaryngology. Philadelphia, 1993, J.B. Lippincott.
*May present as bilateral facial paralysis.

61. Where should the skin incision be placed during a submandibular approach to avoid the mandibular branch of the facial nerve?

The submandibular approach is often referred to as the Risdon approach. It may be used to access the mandibular angle, ramus, condyle, inferior border of the mandibular body, and submandibular gland. The exact location of the skin incision differs, mostly due to the disagreement over the course of the marginal mandibular branch of the facial nerve.

Dingman and Grabb showed, in 192 patients, that this branch is below the inferior border of the mandible, posterior to where the nerve crosses the facial artery. Anterior to that point, the facial nerve is above the inferior border in 100% of patients. In another study, Ziarah and Atkinson found that in 53% of patients the marginal mandible of the facial nerve is below the inferior border of the mandible, posterior to the facial vessels, and in 6% this nerve continues to be below the inferior border anterior to the facial vessels.

Based on these findings, and to err well on the safe side, the recommended placement of the submandibular incision is **1.5-2.0 cm (a thumb-breadth) below the inferior border of the mandible.**

62. In a patient with a 3-cm vertical laceration of the anterior border of the masseter muscle, what findings are likely?

In such an injury there is a likelihood for paralysis of the frontalis, orbicularis oculi, nasalis muscles, and orbicularis oris. The paralysis of these muscles is due to severance of the frontal, zygomatic, and buccal branches of the facial nerve, respectively. The parotid duct and the parotid gland may also be involved.

63. What are the structures involved in resection of the mandible from midramus to the mental foramen?

Composite resection of the body of the mandible usually involves removal of bone, muscles, glands, lymph nodes, and vessels. The muscles involved are the masseter, medial pterygoid, platysma, mylohyoid, buccinator, depressor anguli oris, depressor labii inferioris, superior pharyngeal constrictor, and a small portion of the temporalis. The submandibular gland, sublingual glands, and the submandibular lymph nodes surrounding superficial and deep cervical nodes also are removed, depending on the extent of the resection. The facial artery, anterior facial vein, and marginal mandibular branch of the facial nerve also are occasionally removed.

64. What is the anatomy of taste sensory function?

Taste sensory function from the anterior part of the tongue is carried along the chorda tympani of the trigeminal nerve through the submandibular ganglion to reach the facial nerve. From the posterior or pharyngeal part of the tongue, taste sensation is carried along the glossopharyngeal nerve, through the pterygopalatine ganglion, to the major petrosal nerve, and then the facial nerve. From the palatal region, the sensation is carried via the palatine nerves, which also pass through the pterygopalatine ganglion to ultimately reach the facial nerve.

Along with the facial nerve, taste fibers reach the tractus solitarius, which is concerned with visceral function, including taste. Some textbooks state that taste fibers from the posterior part of the tongue reach the tractus solitarius directly by the glossopharyngeal nerve.

65. What is the anatomy of the zygoma?

The zygoma is a pyramidal bone of the midface. Its anterior convexity gives prominence to the malar eminence of the cheek, and its posterior concavity contributes to the shape of the temporal fossa. The zygoma forms the superolateral and superoanterior portions of the maxillary sinus. It articulates with the frontal, temporal, maxillary, and sphenoid bones. Superolaterally, the frontal process of the zygoma articulates with the zygomatic process of the frontal bone and forms the lateral orbital wall along with its intraorbital articulation with the sphenoid bone. The temporal process of the zygoma articulates posterolaterally with the zygomatic process of the temporal bone to make the zygomatic arch. The broad articulation inferiorly and medially with the maxilla forms the infraorbital rim and lateral part of the orbital floor. Superiorly and inferiorly, such articulation forms the zygomaticomaxillary buttress, the major buttressing structure between the midface and the cranium.

66. What is the anulus of Zinn?

The anulus of Zinn, or common tendinous ring in the orbit, is the fibrous thickening of the periosteum from which the recti muscles originate.

67. What are the functions of the extraocular muscles?
- **Lateral rectus muscle:** abduction
- **Medial rectus muscle:** adduction
- **Inferior rectus muscle:** depression, adduction, and extorsion (extorsion—the superior pole of the globe moves laterally)
- **Superior rectus muscle:** elevation, adduction, and intorsion (intorsion—the superior pole of the globe moves medially)

- **Superior oblique muscle:** depression, abduction, and intorsion
- **Inferior oblique muscle:** elevation, abduction, and extorsion

68. Which bony structures surround the orbit and protect its contents?
- **Superiorly:** The supraorbital rim is formed by the supraorbital arch of the frontal bone.
- **Inferiorly:** The thick infraorbital rim is formed by the zygoma laterally and the maxilla medially.
- **Medially:** The nasal spine of the frontal bone and the frontal process of the maxilla constitute the anteromedial orbital wall.
- **Laterally:** The frontal process of the zygoma and the zygomatic process of the frontal bone constitute the lateral orbital rim.

69. How many bones form the orbit? Which bones?
Seven bones form the orbit.
The **roof** is composed mainly of the orbital plate of the frontal bone. Posteriorly it receives a minor contribution from the lesser wing of the sphenoid.
The **orbital floor** is composed of the orbital plate of the maxilla, the zygomatic bone anterolaterally, and the orbital process of the palatine bone posteriorly. The orbital floor is equivalent to the roof of the maxillary sinus.
The **lateral wall** is formed primarily by the orbital surface of the zygomatic bone and the greater wing of the sphenoid bone. The sphenoid portion of the lateral wall is separated from the roof by the superior orbital fissure and from the floor by the inferior orbital fissure.
The **medial wall** is quadrangular in shape and composed of four bones: (1) the ethmoid bone centrally; (2) the frontal bone superoanteriorly; (3) the lacrimal bone inferoanteriorly; and (4) the sphenoid bone posteriorly. The medial wall is made of a very thin plate, with the largest component being the ethmoidal portion, which is called the lamina papyracea (paperlike).

70. Which is the only bone that exists entirely within the orbital confines?
The lacrimal bone.

71. Which bone is the keystone of the orbit?
The sphenoid bone. All neurovascular structures to the orbit pass through this bone.

72. Where is the superior orbital fissure located? Which structures pass through it?
The superior orbital fissure is a 22-mm cleft that runs outward, forward, and upward from the apex of the orbit. This fissure, which separates the greater and lesser wings of the sphenoid and lies between the optic foramen and the foramen rotundum, provides passage to the three motor nerves to the extraocular muscles of the orbit—the oculomotor nerve (CN III), trochlear nerve (CN IV), and abducens nerve (CN VI). The ophthalmic division of the trigeminal nerve (CN V1) also enters the orbit through this fissure.

73. What structures pass through the inferior orbital fissure?
The inferior orbital fissure, which separates the greater sphenoid wing portion of the lateral wall from the floor, permits passage of (1) the maxillary division of the trigeminal nerve (CN V2) and its branches (including the infraorbital nerve); (2) the infraorbital artery; (3) branches of the sphenopalatine ganglion; and (4) branches of the inferior ophthalmic vein to the pterygoid plexus.

74. What is Tenon's capsule?
Tenon's capsule is a fascial structure that subdivides the orbital cavity into two halves: an anterior (or precapsular) segment and a posterior (or retrocapsular) segment. The ocular globe occupies only the anterior half of the orbital cavity. The posterior half of the orbital cavity is

filled with fat, muscles, vessels, and nerves that supply the ocular globe and extraocular muscles and provide sensation to the soft tissue surrounding the orbit.

75. Distinguish between intraconal and extraconal fat. Which is important for globe support?

The orbital fat can be divided into anterior and posterior portions. The anterior, extraocular fat is largely **extraconal,** which means that it exists outside the muscle cone. Posteriorly, only fine fascial communications separate the extraconal from the intraconal fat compartments. **Intraconal** fat constitutes three fourths of the fat in the posterior orbit and may be displaced outside the muscle cone, contributing to a loss of globe support from loss of soft tissue volume. The fat on the anterior portion of the orbital floor is extraconal and does not contribute to globe support.

76. Which five bones make up the nose?
1. Maxilla: frontal process of maxilla
2. Frontal bone: nasal process of frontal bone
3. Nasal bones
4. Vomer: contributes to the septum
5. Ethmoid: perpendicular plate of the ethmoid also contributes to the septum

77. With which bones does the zygoma articulate?

Greater wing of the sphenoid and frontal, temporal, and maxillary bones.

78. What are the muscles of mastication?

Muscles of mastication can be divided into two groups of the muscles: primary muscles of mastication and accessory muscles of mastication. Primary muscles of mastication include the temporalis, masseter, the pterygoideus (medial and lateral). Accessory muscles of mastication include the suprahyoid group, infrahyoid group, and platysma. The suprahyoid group includes the digastric, mylohyoid, geniohyoid, and stylohyoid muscles. The infrahyoid group includes the sternohyoid, thyrohyoid, and omohyoid.

79. How do these muscle act to perform the function of mastication?

The muscles of mastication act most of the time as group during functional movement of the jaw. For example, jaw closing is a coordinated function of the elevator muscles, which are the masseter, medial pterygoid, and the temporalis muscles. The jaw closing is a function of the lateral pterygoid, and the suprahyoid muscles. The protrusion is a function of the masseter, medial pterygoid, and lateral pterygoid muscles, whereas retrusion is a function of the digastric and temporalis muscle. The infrahyoid muscles help in the opening of the mouth by fixing the hyoid bone as a stable structure so when the suprahyoid muscles contract, they are able to participate in depressing the anterior portion of the mandible, thus opening the mouth.

80. What is the origin and insertion of each of the muscles of mastication?

With few exceptions, for a skeletal muscle to perform its function, it must originate from a fixed structure in the skeleton and insert into another, mobile part. This rule applies to all muscles of mastication, except for the suprahyoid muscle group (as described previously).

Masseter

Origin: superficial belly from the lower border of the zygomatic arch and the zygomatic process of the maxilla. The deep belly from the posterior third and medial surface of the inferior border of the zygomatic arch.

Insertion: the angle and inferior half of the lateral surface of the ramus of the mandible. The deep portion (belly) of the muscle inserts onto the lateral surface of coronoid process and superior half of the ramus.

Medial Pterygoid

Origin: medial surface of the lateral pterygoid plate and pyramidal process of the palatine bone. A small belly of the muscle arises from the lateral surface of the pyramidal process and tuberosity of the maxilla.

Insertion: inferior and posterior part of the medial surface of the ramus and angle of the mandible

Temporalis

Origin: the temporal fossa of the temporal bone
Insertion: medial surface, apex, and anterior border of the coronoid process of the mandible

Lateral Pterygoid

Origin: the superior belly arises from the inferior part of the lateral surface of the greater wing of the sphenoid and from the infratemporal fossa. The inferior belly arises from the lateral surface of the lateral pterygoid plate.

Insertion: the superior belly inserts into the anterior margin of the articular disc. The inferior belly inserts into a depression on the anterior portion of the neck of the condyle.

Digastric

Origin: digastric fossa of medial side of the lower border of the mandible close to the symphysis. The posterior belly of the muscle arises from the mastoid notch of the temporal bone. Both bellies are united by an intermediate tendon that is connected to the hyoid bone by a loop of fibrous tissue.

The other suprahyoid muscle group originates from different parts of the medial surface of the mandible and inserts into the hyoid bone. The exception is the stylohyoid muscle, which arises from the temporal bone and inserts on the body of the hyoid bone.

Of note is that the origin and insertion of the suprahyoid group (except stylohyoid muscle) are from a mobile origin and insertion. However, because the infrahyoid muscle group functions to stabilize the hyoid bone during mastication, this bone becomes static, allowing the mandible to move when the suprahyoid muscles contract. Inversely, during swallowing, the suprahyoid muscles stabilize the hyoid bone, allowing for swallowing action to be completed with the contraction of the infrahyoid muscles.

81. What are the muscles of the soft palate?

The soft palate is formed by three pair of muscles, all of which fuse at the midline: the uvulus muscle, which runs along the uvula on each side of the midline forming almost one muscle; the levator palatine muscle extending across the midline and forming an arch-shape configuration within the soft palate; and the tensor veli palatine, which loops around the hamulus fusing with the tensor muscle of the opposite side and forming an aponeurosis at the midline.

BIBLIOGRAPHY

1. Abbey SH: Facial nerve disorders. In Jafek BW, Stark AK (eds): ENT Secrets. Philadelphia, 1996, Hanley & Belfus.
2. Abubaker AO, Sotereanos GC, Patterson GT: Use of bicoronal approach to treatment of craniofacial fractures. J Oral Maxillofacial Surg 48:579-586, 1990.
3. Anderson JE (ed): Grant's Atlas of Anatomy. Baltimore, 1983, Williams & Wilkins.
4. Coker NJ: Acute paralysis of the facial nerve. In Bailey BJ (ed): Head and Neck Surgery—Otolaryngology. Philadelphia, 1993, J.B. Lippincott.
5. Cummings CW, Haughey B, Thomas R et al (eds): Otolaryngology: Head and Neck Surgery, 4th ed. St Louis, 2005, Mosby.
6. Demas PN, Sotereanos GC: Incidence of nasolacrimal injury and turbinectomy-associated atrophic rhinitis with Le Fort I osteotomies. J Craniomaxillofac Surg 17:116-118, 1989.

7. Dingman RO, Grabb WC: Surgical anatomy of the mandibular ramus of the facial nerve, based on the dissection of 100 facial halves. Plast Reconstr Surg 29:266-272, 1962.
8. Ellis E, Zide M: Surgical Approaches to the Facial Skeleton. Baltimore, 1984, Williams & Wilkins.
9. Ermshar CB Jr: Anatomy and neuroanatomy. In Morgan DH, Hall WP, Vamvas SJ (eds): Diseases of the Temporomandibular Joint: A Multidisciplinary Approach. St Louis, 1977, Mosby.
10. Frick H, Leanhardt H, Starck D: The Eye and the Orbit. In Human Anatomy 2, 4th ed. Stuttgart, Germany, 1991, Thieme.
11. Haller J: Trauma to the salivary glands. Otolaryngol Clin North Am 32:907-917, 1999.
12. Hollinstead H: Anatomy for Surgeons: The Head and Neck, 3rd ed. Philadelphia, 1982, Harper & Row.
13. Last J: Head and neck. In Last J: Anatomy: Regional and Applied, 6th ed. New York, 1978, Churchill Livingstone.
14. Long CD, Granick MS: Head and neck embryology and anatomy. In Weinzweig J (ed): Plastic Surgery Secrets. Philadelphia, 1996, Hanley & Belfus.
15. Moore KL: Clinically Oriented Anatomy, 2nd ed. Baltimore, 1984, Williams & Wilkins.
16. Ochs M, Buckley M: Anatomy of the orbit. Oral Maxillofac Surg Clin 5:419-430, 1993.
17. Pansky B: The facial (VII) nerve. In Pansky B (ed): Review of Gross Anatomy. New York, 1984, Macmillan.
18. Patrick GH, Bevivino JR: Fractures of the zygoma. In Weinzweig J (ed): Plastic Surgery Secrets. Philadelphia, 1999, Hanley & Belfus.
19. Pitanguy I, Ramus A: The frontal branch of the facial nerve: the importance of its variation in face lifting. Plast Reconstr Surg 38:352-356, 1966.
20. Rees TD, Aston SJ, Thorne CHM: Blepharoplasty and facioplasty. In McCarthy JG (ed): Plastic Surgery. Philadelphia, 1990, Saunders.
21. Schow RS, Miloro M: Diagnosis and management of salivary gland disorders. In Peterson LJ, Ellis E 3rd, Hupp JR et al (eds): Contemporary Oral and Maxillofacial Surgery, 3rd ed. St Louis, 1998, Mosby.
22. Schwember G, Rodriguez A: Anatomic dissection of the extraparotid portion of the facial nerve. Plast Reconstruct Surg 81:183-188, 1988.
23. Sinha U, Ng M: Surgery of the salivary glands. Otolaryngol Clin North Am 32:888-905, 1999.
24. Snell RS: Head and neck anatomy. In Snell RS (ed): Clinical Anatomy for Medical Students, 5th ed. Boston, 1995, Little, Brown.
25. Stuzin JM, Wagstrom L, Kawamoto HK et al: Anatomy of the frontal branch of the facial nerve: the significance of temporal fat pad. Plast Reconstr Surg 83:265-271, 1989.
26. Weinzweig J, Bartlett SP: Fractures of the orbit. In Weinzweig J (ed): Plastic Surgery Secrets. Philadelphia, 1999, Hanley & Belfus.
27. You-ZH, Bell WH, Finn RA: Location of the nasolacrimal canal in relation to the high Le Fort osteotomy. J Oral Maxillofac Surg 50:1075-1080, 1992.
28. Ziarah HA, Atkinson ME: The surgical anatomy of the mandibular distribution of the facial nerve. Br J Oral Surg 19:159-170, 1981.

28. DENTOALVEOLAR SURGERY

James A. Giglio, DDS, MEd

1. Why is it necessary to use a bite block when removing mandibular teeth?

To diminish pressure on the contralateral temporomandibular joint (TMJ).

2. Why is distilled water not used for irrigation?

Distilled water is a hypotonic solution and will enter cells down the osmotic gradient, causing cell lysis and rapid death of bone cells.

3. Why is buccal to lingual movement not efficient when removing mandibular posterior teeth?

Mandibular bone is too dense and does not expand in a fashion similar to that of the maxillary bone.

4. **What anatomic structure can interfere with efficient removal of a maxillary first molar?**
    Root of the zygoma.

5. **Which muscle is pierced by the needle when performing inferior alveolar nerve block anesthesia?**
    Buccinator muscle.

6. **What muscles insert on the pterygomandibular raphe?**
    The buccinator muscle and the superior pharyngeal constrictor muscle.

7. **What two structures form a V-shaped landmark for an inferior alveolar nerve block?**
    Deep tendon of the temporalis muscle and the superior pharyngeal constrictor.

8. **What is the orthodontic indication for removal of an impacted third molar?**
    To facilitate distal movement of the second molar.

9. **What is the "shift rule" as applied to impacted maxillary cuspids?**
    This radiographic technique determines the position of the impacted cuspid. A series of periapical radiographs are made. The film position is kept constant, but the head of the x-ray unit is moved either anteriorly or posteriorly after each exposure. If the impacted tooth seems to move with the x-ray head, it is located on the palate. If it moves opposite to the unit head, it will be found on the buccal. This is also referred to as the SLOB rule: *s*ame *l*ingual (palate), *o*pposite *b*uccal.

10. **What is the advantage of an apically positioned mucoperiosteal flap for exposure of a buccally positioned impacted cuspid?**
    This flap design allows for the impacted tooth to erupt into attached mucosa and minimizes the possible development of periodontal defects and pocket formation.

11. **Where is the inferior alveolar nerve most often located in relation to the roots of a mandibular third molar?**
    Buccal to the roots, and slightly apical.

12. **The root of which tooth is most often dislodged into the maxillary sinus during an extraction procedure?**
    Palatal root of the maxillary first molar.

13. **While trying to remove a root tip of a mandibular third molar, it disappears from view. Where might it be dislodged?**
    - Inferior alveolar canal
    - Cancellous bone space
    - Submandibular space

14. **What is the usually recommended sequence for extractions?**
    Maxillary teeth before mandibular teeth, and posterior teeth before anterior teeth.

15. **What complications are associated with the removal of a freestanding, isolated maxillary molar?**
    Alveolar process fracture and fracture of the maxillary tuberosity.

16. **How do you minimize the chance of dislodging an impacted maxillary third molar into the infratemporal fossa during its surgical removal?**
    Develop a full-thickness mucoperiosteal flap, bringing the incision anterior to the second

molar (add a releasing incision if necessary), to improve visualization of the impacted tooth and place a broad retractor distal to the molar while elevating it.

17. When performing a surgical removal, should you completely section through a mandibular molar?

No. The lingual plate is often thin, and complete sectioning may perforate the plate and injure the lingual nerve.

18. How is bleeding from pulsating nutrient blood vessels controlled following surgery on alveolar bone?

- Burnish bone.
- Crush with rongeurs.
- Apply bone wax.

19. What are some common causes of postoperative bleeding following dental extractions?

- Failure to suture
- Failure to remove all granulation tissue
- Rebound blood vessel dilation following use of local anesthetic with a vasoconstrictor
- Torn tissue
- Torn surgical flaps

20. Why shouldn't a local anesthetic be used with a vasoconstrictor when treating post-operative hemorrhage?

The vasoconstrictor will mask the source of bleeding.

21. Why are mucoperiosteal flaps designed with a broad base?

To ensure an adequate blood supply to the flap margin.

22. What are the two basic flaps used in dentoalveolar surgery?

1. Full-thickness mucoperiosteal flap
2. Split-thickness mucoperiosteal flap

23. What are the two basic types of full-thickness mucoperiosteal flaps?

1. Envelope flap
2. Envelope flap with a releasing component

24. Where are releasing incisions contraindicated?

- Palate
- Lingual surface mandible
- Canine eminence
- Through muscle attachments
- In the region of the mental foramen

25. How do absorbable gelatin sponge (Gelfoam) and oxidized regenerated cellulose (Surgicel) assist with homeostasis?

They form a matrix or scaffold upon which a clot can form. Gelatin sponge does not become as readily incorporated into the clot as does the oxidized regenerated cellulose. Healing is delayed more often with cellulose than with the gelatin sponge, but oxidized regenerated cellulose is the more efficient homeostatic agent.

26. Why is a conventional dental handpiece that expels forced air contraindicated when performing dentoalveolar surgery?

Such an instrument can cause tissue emphysema or an air embolism. An air embolism can be fatal.

27. What are the cardinal signs of a localized osteitis (dry socket)?

- Throbbing pain (often radiating)
- Fetid odor
- Bad taste
- Poorly healed extraction site

28. Why is it contraindicated to curette a dry socket to stimulate bleeding?

Curetting a dry socket can cause the condition to worsen because healing will be further delayed, any natural healing already taking place will be destroyed, and there is a risk of causing the localized inflammatory process to be spread to the adjacent sound bone.

29. What is the treatment for a localized osteitis?

Conservative management is indicated. The wound should be irrigated gently with slightly warmed saline, and a sedative dressing should be placed. The dressing should be removed within 48 hr and replaced until the patient becomes asymptomatic. Systemic antibiotics are generally not indicated. Nonsteroidal antiinflammatory analgesics should be prescribed if necessary.

30. What causes a dry socket?

The etiology of a dry socket is not absolutely clear but is thought to develop because of increased fibrinolytic activity causing accelerated lysis of the blood clot. Smoking, premature mouth rinsing, hot liquids, surgical trauma, and oral contraceptives have all been implicated in the development of a dry socket.

31. Why should flaps be repositioned and sutured over sound bone?

Unsupported flaps can collapse into bony defects, causing tension on the sutures. The sutures subsequently will pull through the tissue, allowing the suture line to open and the wound to dehisce.

32. What percentage of dentoalveolar injuries include the primary maxillary central incisor?

70%.

33. How are avulsed primary teeth treated?

No treatment is necessary; reimplantation is not indicated for primary teeth.

34. How is an extruded primary tooth treated?

If there is a gross interference with the opposing teeth, the tooth should be extracted. Otherwise, the teeth can be pressured and splinted in place.

35. What is the incidence of pulp necrosis after intrusion injuries of teeth?

With intrusion injuries, the risk of pulp necrosis for a tooth with a closed apex is 95% and with an immature apex is 65%. Accordingly, any form of luxation should be followed with routine clinical and radiographic exams.

36. How long should dentoalveolar fractures be splinted?

4-6 weeks.

37. What media can be used to transport avulsed teeth?

Saliva, fresh milk, balanced salt, or Hank balanced salt solution (HBSS). Water is harmful because, as a hypotonic fluid, it may cause periodontal ligament cell death when it enters cells down the osmotic gradient, causing cell lysis and death.

If the tooth is placed in an appropriate medium within 15-20 min, periodontal ligament cells can remain vital for 2 hr in saliva and 6 hr in fresh milk. Balanced salt solution can be used up to 24 hr if the initial dry storage was < 30 min.

38. How long should extruded or avulsed teeth be splinted?
7-10 days.

39. What are the significant radiologic predictions of a close relationship between the inferior alveolar canal and the impacted mandibular third molar?
Signs of close proximity of the mandibular third molar to the inferior alveolar canal are mostly radiographic in nature and include:
- Darkening and notching of the root
- Deflected roots at the region of the canal
- Narrowing of the root
- Interruption of canal outlines
- Diversion of canal from its normal course
- Narrowing of canal outlines on the radiograph

40. What are the most important signs that may increase potential nerve injury with extraction of impacted mandibular third molars?
Of the previously listed signs of close proximity of the canal to impacted third molar, diversion of canal, interruption of canal borders, and darkening of roots are the most reliable signs.

41. What are the possible complications of dentoalveolar surgery?
- Swallowing or aspiration of foreign objects
- Tissue emphysema
- TMJ pain
- Trismus
- Mandibular fracture
- Tuberosity fracture
- Root fracture
- Injuries to adjacent teeth
- Displacement of root and root fragments into the submandibular space, mandibular canal, or maxillary sinus
- Oral-antral communication, bleeding, infection, ecchymosis, and hematoma
- Localized osteitis (dry socket)
- Wound dehiscence
- Inferior alveolar and lingual injuries
  Depending on the location and the nature of the surgery, these complications vary in severity and need for treatment.

42. How are roots or root tips displaced into the submandibular space managed?
Once displacement of a mandibular molar root into the submandibular space is suspected, manual lateral and upward pressure should be applied immediately on the lingual aspect of the floor of the mouth in an attempt to force the root back into the socket. If the root is visualized again in the socket, it may be retrieved from the socket with a root tip pick. If not, a mucoperiosteal soft tissue flap should be reflected on the lingual aspect of the mandible until the root tip is found; ensure that the mylohyoid muscle is sharply detached from its insertion in the mandible. Antibiotic coverage is indicated postoperatively. If the root is not visualized because of its location or uncontrollable bleeding, recovery is best performed as a secondary procedure when fibrosis occurs and stabilizes the tooth in a firm position, usually 4-6 weeks later. The patient should be placed on a short course of antibiotics.

43. How are roots or root tips that are displaced into the inferior alveolar canal managed?
When displacement of a root into the mandibular canal is suspected, periapical and occlusal radiographs should be taken for verification, because the root may be in a large marrow space or

beneath the buccal mucosa. If the root is visualized, careful removal is indicated with a small hemostat after adequate alveolar bone removal. If the root is not visualized, delayed removal is recommended. Delayed removal is also indicated during persistent infection and nerve paresthesia. If the root fragment is small and does not become infected preoperatively, leaving the root in place is a viable and less invasive option.

44. How is a root or root fragment that is displaced into the maxillary sinus managed?

Once the root is suspected to be in the sinus, place the patient in an upright position to prevent posterior displacement and obtain a radiograph of the fractured tooth to determine its location and size. If the fragment is found to be in the sinus, local measures of retrieval should be attempted first, such as:

- Having the patient blow through the nose with the nostrils closed, and observing the perforation for the root to appear in the socket
- Using a fine suction tip to bring the root back into the defect
- Performing antral lavage with sterile isotonic saline in an effort to flush the root out through the defect
- Packing iodoform gauze into the antrum and removing it in one stroke; the root fragment often adheres to the gauze

If local measures are unsuccessful, direct entry into the maxillary sinus via the Caldwell-Luc approach in the area of the canine fossa should be performed. Postoperative management includes a figure-of-eight suture over the socket, sinus precautions, antibiotics, and a nasal spray to keep the sinus ostium open and infection free.

45. How are oral-antral communications managed?

Probing, irrigation, and having the patient blow forcefully with the nostrils occluded are contraindicated because these maneuvers may enlarge an existing opening or create one that did not previously exist. Some will allow patients to blow gently while compressing the nostrils to observe for air bubble formations that will confirm an antral opening. For openings <2 mm, no surgical treatment is necessary, providing adequate hemostasis is achieved. For openings of 2-6 mm, conservative treatment is indicated, including placement of a figure-of-eight suture over the tooth socket and sinus precautions (avoid blowing the nose, violent sneezing, sucking on straws, and smoking). For openings >6 mm, primary closure should be obtained with a buccal flap or a palatal flap procedure. Approximation of the gingiva can be facilitated by removal of a small amount of the buccal alveolar plate and scoring or incising the periosteum on the underside of the flap. Placement of a small piece of absorbable gelatin sponge into the occlusal third of the socket when the gingival margins cannot be coapted is not advisable because it introduces a foreign substance and could lead to subsequent breakdown of the clot. Antibiotics and nasal or oral decongestants are prescribed if there is evidence of acute or chronic sinusitis.

46. What steps should be taken for a tooth (maxillary third molar) that is displaced into the infratemporal fossa?

When a maxillary third molar is displaced into the infratemporal fossa, it is usually displaced through the periosteum and located lateral to the lateral pterygoid plate and inferior to the lateral pterygoid muscle with displacement. If there is good access and adequate light, a single cautious effort to retrieve the tooth with a hemostat can be made. If the effort is unsuccessful, or if the tooth is not visualized, the incision should be closed, the patient should be informed, and prophylactic antibiotics should be prescribed. A secondary surgical procedure is performed 4-6 weeks later after lateral and posteroanterior radiographs are taken to locate the tooth in all three planes. After adequate anesthesia, a long needle—usually a spinal needle—is used to locate the tooth. Careful dissection is performed along the needle until the tooth is visualized and subsequently removed. If no functional problems exist after displacement, the patient may elect not to have the tooth removed. Proper documentation of this is critical.

47. How do you manage postoperative or secondary bleeding from extraction sites?

The first step in managing postoperative bleeding is to carefully examine and visualize the bleeding site to determine the precise source of bleeding. In the case of simple generalized oozing, a damp gauze is held over the site with firm manual pressure for 5 min. If unsuccessful, the area should be anesthetized and examined more closely. If sutures were placed, they should be removed and the existing clot should be curetted from the socket. Hemostatic agents, such as an absorbable gelatin sponge, oxidized cellulose, and oxidized regenerated cellulose, can be placed in the socket and sutured. If hemostasis is not achieved by local measures, lab screening tests should be performed to assist in diagnosis and treatment of the cause.

48. Why is it contraindicated to curette residual pathologic tissue after removing maxillary anterior teeth?

The bony crypt should never be scraped after removal of any tooth. This, however, is especially important in the anterior maxilla, because the veins in this region do not have valves. Consequently, manipulation of infected material and thrombi in the extraction site can force it into the cranial vault to the cavernous sinus, resulting in a cavernous sinus thrombosis.

49. After teeth are removed, when does radiographic evidence of bone formation in the extraction site first become evident?

Because early bone formation in the extraction sites is poorly calcified, radiographs of these regions are generally radiolucent. Evidence of bone formation does not become prominent until the sixth to eighth week. Moreover, there are radiographic differences between the newly formed bone and adjacent alveolar bone for about 4-6 months.

50. Why is it not indicated to scrape the walls of extraction sites after teeth are removed?

Often, after using local anesthesia with a vasoconstrictor, the extraction site appears "dry" and the void does not readily fill with blood. It is unnecessary and not a good practice to scrape the walls of the extraction site to stimulate bleeding or for any other reasons. This practice will delay healing. The remnants of the periodontal ligament (PDL) that are attached to the alveolar crypt are the source of fibroblasts that form fibrin for the rudimentary clot (scaffold) upon which cells necessary for the healing process can migrate. Moreover, the remnants of the PDL provide small capillaries and pluripotential cells that will form osteoblasts necessary for bone formation.

51. Where is the location of the lingual nerve in relation to the mandibular third molar?

The spatial relationship between the lingual nerve and the mandibular third molar region is highly variable. The nerve has been found to be at the level of the lingual plate or higher, in contact with the lingual plate, or intimately attached to the periosteum and the follicular sac of the impacted mandibular third molar.

52. What is the difference between an incisional and excisional biopsy?

An excisional biopsy entails removal of the entire lesion along with at least 2 mm of normal marginal tissue from the sides of the lesion. This technique is usually used for biopsy of a lesion 1 cm or less. An incisional biopsy removes only a representative portion or portions of a lesion along with a representation of adjacent normal tissue.

53. When a biopsy is being performed, why is it necessary to incise parallel to the long axis of any muscle fibers beneath the lesion?

Whenever possible, the incisions should be oriented parallel to lines of muscle tension in order to minimize scarring and wound dehiscence. Biopsy incisions on the face should be oriented to follow Langer's lines.

54. What are the indications for performing a partial odontectomy (coronectomy) of an impacted mandibular molar?

An intentional partial odontectomy is usually performed on an impacted mandibular third molar. This technique is chosen when there is a significant risk of injury to the inferior alveolar nerve, jaw fracture, or in cases where the benefits of root retention outweigh the risks of conventional third molar removal. The roots must be asymptomatic, not associated with pathologic lesions, and must not interfere with future restorative procedures or orthodontic treatment. The technique involves careful sectioning of the crown from the roots at or below the cementoenamel junction. The roots should not be elevated or disturbed as they must remain attached to their apical blood vessels to ensure vitality. The patient must always be informed when this technique is used.

55. On what relationships are the Pell and Gregory impacted mandibular third molar classifications based?

The Pell and Gregory impacted third molar classifications are based on the third molar's relationship to the anterior border of the ascending ramus and to the occlusal plane. A Pell and Gregory Class 1 impaction implies sufficient space between the ramus and the second molar into which the third molar can erupt. A Class 2 impacted third molar is found to be at least half covered by ramus bone. The Class 3 impacted third molar is entirely within the ramus. With regard to the occlusal plane, a Pell and Gregory Class A impaction implies that the occlusal surfaces of the second and third molars are at or about the same level. The occlusal surface of a Class B third molar impaction is between the occlusal surface and cementoenamel junction of the second molar. The Class C impaction is the deepest impaction where the occlusal surface of the third molar is completely below the neck of the second molar.

56. What is low-molecular-weight heparin (LMWH), and how is it used in oral and maxillofacial surgery?

Standard unfractionated heparin (UFH) is formed from a heterogenous combination of sulfated mucopolysaccharides. Its anticoagulant activity is unpredictable, so it must be carefully monitored with the partial thromboplastin time (PTT) test. LMWH (fractionated heparin) is formed from depolymerization of heparin into lower-molecular-weight particles. Because LMWH has increased bioavailability compared with UFH, it can be given as a fixed dose and without the need for monitoring with the PTT.

It is useful in oral and maxillofacial surgery for patients who cannot discontinue oral anticoagulation therapy. Patients stop warfarin therapy and the international normalized ratio (INR) is allowed to normalize while the LMWH is administered to maintain anticoagulation therapy. When the INR returns to an acceptable level, the surgery can be performed and scheduled for early in the day. The LMWH is withheld the day of surgery and resumed in the evening. Warfarin can be resumed the following day and the LMWH continued until the INR returns to the desired therapeutic range.

BIBLIOGRAPHY

1. Alling CC 3rd (ed): Dentoalveolar Surgery. Oral and Maxillofacial Surgery Clinics of North America, 5th vol. Philadelphia, 1993, Saunders.
2. Freedman GL: Intentional partial odontectomy: report of a case. J Oral Maxillofac Surg 50:419-421, 1992.
3. Kiesselbach JE, Chamberlain JG: Clinical and anatomic observations on the relationship of the lingual nerve to the mandibular third molar region. J Oral Maxillofac Surg 42:565, 1984.
4. Lew D: Blood and blood products. In Kwon PH, Laskin DM (eds): Clinician's Manual of Oral and Maxillofacial Surgery, 2nd ed. Carol Stream, Ill, 1997, Quintessence.
5. Peterson L, Ellis E, Hupp J et al: Contemporary Oral and Maxillofacial Surgery, 4th ed. St Louis, 2003, Mosby.

6. Pogrel MA, Renaut A, Schmidt B et al: The relationship of the lingual nerve to the mandibular third molar region: an anatomic study. J Oral Maxillofac Surg 53:1178, 1995.
7. Todd DW, Roman A: Outpatient use of low-molecular weight heparin in an anticoagulated patient requiring oral surgery: case report. J Oral Maxillofac Surg 59:1090-1092, 2001.
8. Whitacre R: Removal of Teeth, 3rd ed. Seattle, 1983, Stoma Press.

29. TRIGEMINAL NERVE INJURY

Kenneth J. Benson, DDS, and A. Omar Abubaker, DMD, PhD

1. What are the two major classifications of nerve injury?
1. Seddon classification
2. Sunderland classification

2. What is the pathophysiology of nerve injury?
Nerve injury is generally described as neurapraxia, axonotmesis, or neurotmesis.

Neurapraxia is Seddon type I nerve injury resulting in conduction deficits without axonal or sheath degeneration. This type of injury is associated primarily with spontaneously reversing paresthesias.

Axonotmesis is a traumatic nerve injury in which there is wallerian degeneration distal to the point of injury, but the endoneural and perineural sheaths are intact. It is Seddon type 2 injury, expanded by Sunderland into second-, third-, and fourth-degree injuries. There is potential for full recovery.

Neurotmesis is a nerve injury with disruption of all axonal and sheath elements producing wallerian degeneration and likely neuroma. This often requires microsurgical repair.

3. What is dysesthesia?
An unpleasant abnormal sensation produced by normal stimuli.

4. What is the difference between analgesia and anesthesia?
Analgesia is an absence of pain in response to stimulation that would normally be painful. Anesthesia is the absence of perception of stimulation by any noxious or nonnoxious stimulation of skin or mucosa. It is divided into general (central), regional, and local types.

5. What is allodynia?
Allodynia is pain due to a stimulus that does not normally provoke pain. Unlike hyperalgesia, hyperpathia, and hyperesthesia, allodynia may include emotionally induced sensations in the nerve-injured patient.

6. What is anesthesia dolorosa?
Anesthesia dolorosa is pain in an area or region that is anesthetic.

7. What is hyperalgesia?
Hyperalgesia is an increased response to a stimulus that is normally painful.

8. What is hyperesthesia?
Hyperesthesia is a increased sensitivity to any noxious or nonnoxious stimulation of skin or mucosa, excluding the special senses; it includes allodynia and hyperalgesia.

9. What are the symptoms of hyperesthesia?
Patients describe a shooting, flashing, burning pain produced by normally nonpainful stimuli.

10. What is hyperpathia?
Hyperpathia is a painful syndrome characterized by increased reaction to a stimulus and increased threshold for response. It commonly is induced by repetitive mechanical pressures and characterized by faulty identification and localization of stimuli.

11. What is hypoalgesia?
Hypoalgesia is diminished pain response to normally painful stimulus.

12. What is paresthesia?
Paresthesia is an abnormal sensation, either evoked or spontaneous, that is not necessarily unpleasant or painful, as in dysesthesia.

13. What is sympathetically mediated pain (SMP)?
SMP is throbbing, diffuse, and hyperalgesic pain perpetuated by abnormal reflex activity in sympathetic pathways following peripheral nerve injury. The classic syndromes of causalgia and reflex sympathetic dystrophy are theorized to involve both peripheral and central mechanisms.

14. What are the symptoms of SMP?
The symptoms are often described as burning, hot, lancinating pain. Patients also complain of increased pain intensity during stressful periods.

15. What is Tinel's sign?
Tinel's sign is a provocative test of regenerating nerve sprouts in which light percussion over the nerve elicits a distal tingling sensation. It is used as a sign of small fiber recovery but is poorly correlated with functional recovery and easily confused with neuroma formation.

16. What is deafferentation pain?
Deafferentation pain is pain in a body region of partial or complete traumatic peripheral nerve deficit in which retrograde central neuropathy has occurred. Deafferentation mechanisms have been implicated in phantom pain, hyperpathia, and allodynia.

17. How many axons and fascicles are in the inferior alveolar nerve?
Approximately 7000-12,000 axons and 10-24 fascicles.

18. What is the incidence of inferior alveolar and lingual nerve injury during removal of third molars?
The incidence of inferior alveolar, lingual, and, less frequently, long buccal nerve injury during mandibular third molar removal ranges between 0.6% and 5.0%. In general, the incidence of inferior alveolar nerve (IAN) injuries is higher than that of the lingual nerve; in one study, incidence was 1.2% for the IAN and 0.9% for the lingual nerve. Factors such as age, surgical technique, and proximity of the nerve to the tooth influence the incidence of these injuries. More than 96% of patients with lingual nerve injuries recover spontaneously.

19. What factors are associated with a higher incidence of lingual nerve injury during the course of third molar removal?
Lingually angled impactions are especially vulnerable to nerve injury during their removal because of the erosion or absence of the lingual cortical plate by infection or cyst exposing the nerve directly to damage during instrumentation to remove the tooth.

20. **What is the average rate of an injured axon's forward growth?**
    Approximately 1-2 mm/day.

21. **What are the potential clinical manifestations of a trigeminal nerve injury?**
    - Nonpainful anesthesia and hypoesthesia
    - Painful anesthesia and hypoesthesia
    - Nonpainful hyperesthesia
    - Painful hyperesthesia

22. **What is the recommended protocol for testing patients with decreased sensation without dysesthesia (Fig. 29-1)?**

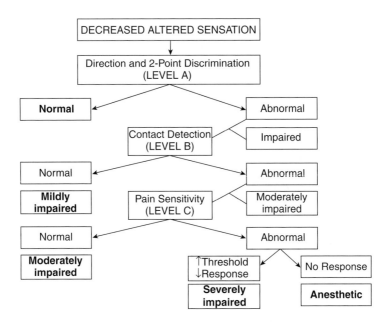

Fig. 29-1 Testing protocol for patients with decreased sensation without dysesthesia. (Modified from Zuniga JR, Essick GK: A contemporary approach to the clinical evaluation of trigeminal nerve injuries. Oral Maxillofac Surg Clin North Am 4:358-367, 1992.)

23. **What is the recommended nonsurgical treatment of chronic trigeminal dysfunction and dysesthesia?**
    See Fig. 29-2.

24. **How should open nerve injuries be managed?**
    If an open injury is observed, it is best managed with immediate primary repair. Delayed primary repair is performed within the first few postoperative days. A delayed secondary repair is performed more than 3 weeks after injury.

25. **When should closed (unobserved) nerve injuries be addressed surgically?**
    Unobserved nerve injuries should be repaired if the patient has:
    - Intolerable anesthesia of more than 3 months
    - Painful symptoms that persist more than 4 months that may be relieved with proximal anesthetic block

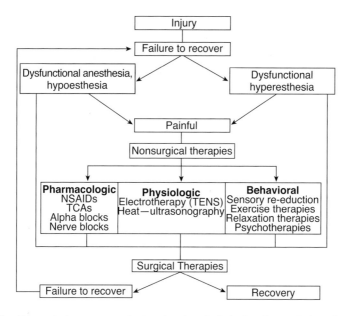

Fig. 29-2 Nonsurgical treatment of chronic trigeminal dysfunction and dysesthesia. *NSAIDs,* Nonsteroidal antiinflammatory drugs; *TCAs,* tricyclic antidepressants; *TENS,* transcutaneous electrical neural stimulation. (Modified from Allig CC, Schwartz E, Campbell RL et al: Algorithm for diagnostic assessment and surgical treatment of traumatic trigeminal neuropathies and neuralgias. Oral Maxillofac Surg Clin North Am 4:555, 1992.)

- Intolerable deterioration of sensation beyond 4 months and no improvement of sensation beyond 4 months

26. What other method of nerve repair can be done if primary repair is not possible?
An interpositional free nerve graft and allogenic nerve guidance.

27. What are the general principles of delayed nerve repair?
Repair must be completed without tension. First, extraneural decompression is performed to remove all irritative, foreign, or compressive forces from nerve contact. Next, the nerve must be inspected for continuity. If nerve continuity is seen, the nerve may be inspected with an epineural incision at the site of injury. Internal decompression (neurolysis) is performed and completed by closing the epineurium. If neuroma-in-continuity is too extensive, excision of neuroma along with part of the nerve is performed. A direct neurorrhaphy is performed in a tension-free manner.

28. What are the types of nerve repair?
- Epineural
- Perineural
- Group fasicular

29. Which type of nerve repair is appropriate for the IAN?
Mixed motor and sensory nerves are best treated with perineural and group fascicular suturing. The sensory IAN can be treated with the epineural suture technique.

30. What does coaptation refer to in nerve repair?

Bringing individual nerve fascicles into the best possible alignment. Direct neurorrhaphy can only be performed when the nerve is tension free.

31. If a defect is too large for a direct neurorrhaphy of the inferior alveolar nerve, which nerves may be considered as donors for free nerve graft?

The sural nerve, greater auricular, and median antebrachial nerves are considered.

32. What factors govern the choice of donor site for free nerve repair?

- Accessibility
- Diameter of donor nerve compared with the host nerve
- Fascicular number and pattern
- Length required
- Patient preference

33. Which nerve is the best donor site for an interpositional graft for an inferior alveolar nerve defect of approximately 25 mm?

The sural nerve graft. The sural nerve can provide up to 30 mm of graft harvest. It provides sensation to the posterior and lateral aspects of the leg and foot. It also has up to 50% fewer axons and smaller axonal size than the inferior alveolar nerve.

34. Which free nerve may be used as a donor site for smaller defects (up to 15 mm long) of the IAN?

The greater auricular nerve can be used for short gaps (up to 15 mm). This nerve graft is a good match with the IAN in terms of axonal size and axonal numbers. However, compared with the host nerve, the greater auricular nerve is half the diameter and has half the fascicles. A cable graft (two parallel strands) may be used to provide a better size match.

35. How much nerve should be harvested for a nerve graft?

Because of primary contracture, the length of the harvested nerve should be at least 25% longer than the defect.

36. When is delayed nerve repair in the maxillofacial region indicated?

If a wound is grossly contaminated or if the mechanism of injury may cause scarring of the proximal and distal ends. Examples of such injuries are blunt, avulsive injuries such as gunshot wounds and injuries sustained in motor vehicle accidents.

37. How is the term *anastomose* applied to nerve injuries?

Trick question. Anastomose is not appropriate nomenclature when discussing nerve repair. Vessels are anastomosed, and nerves are repaired or reconstructed.

38. What type of sutures are most compatible for nerve repair?

Size 8.0 or 10.0 suture on a noncutting needle. Use the least tissue-reactive sutures (polyglycolic provokes less inflammation than nylon).

39. What potential alloplastic nerve conduits may be used in nerve reconstruction?

For guided nerve growth up to 3 mm, the following nerve guides may be used for repair:

- Collagen tubes
- Polytetrafluoroethylene
- Polyglycolic acid tubes

40. What method is used for locating the great auricular nerve?

A line is drawn connecting the mastoid process and angle of mandible. A perpendicular line is then drawn to bisect the mastoid-mandible line. The great auricular nerve approximates this second line.

41. What is the success rate of microsurgical repairs of inferior alveolar and lingual nerve injuries (Table 29-1)?

Table 29-1 *Success Rate of Microsurgical Repairs of Inferior Alveolar and Lingual Nerve Injuries*

	PATIENTS	SUCCESS* (%)	RANGE (%)	SEM
Hypoesthetic				
• IAN	$N = 192$	85.4	66-94	3.68
• Lingual nerve	$N = 131$	87.0	50-91	5.66
Hyperesthetic				
• IAN	$N = 124$	55.6	25-80	7.01
• Lingual nerve	$N = 74$	67.5	50-100	6.82

Adapted from LaBanc JP, Gregg JM: Trigeminal nerve injuries: basic problems, historical perspectives, early success, and remaining challenges. Oral Maxillofac Clin North Am 4:227-283, 1992.
SEM, Standard error of the mean; *IAN,* inferior alveolar nerve.
*Success is defined as (1) minimum recovery of gross touch perception and (2) global pain reduction of > 30%. Overall success rate ($N = 521$) is 76.2%.

BIBLIOGRAPHY

1. Allig CC, Schwartz E, Campbell RL et al: Algorithm for diagnostic assessment and surgical treatment of traumatic trigeminal neuropathies and neuralgias. Oral Maxillofac Surg Clin North Am 4:555, 1992.
2. Donoff R: Surgical management of interior alveolar nerve injuries (part 1): case for early repair. J Oral Maxillofac Surg 53:1327-1329, 1995.
3. Elusten K, Stevens M: Diagnosis and management of interior alveolar nerve injury. Compendium 16:1028-1038, 1995.
4. Greg J: Neurological complications of surgery for impacted teeth. In Alling CC, Helfric JF, Alling RD (eds): Impacted Teeth. Philadelphia, 1993, Saunders.
5. Gregg J: Surgical management of inferior alveolar nerve injuries (part 2): case for delayed management. J Oral Maxillofac Surg 53:1330-1335, 1995.
6. Gregg JM: Nonsurgical management of traumatic trigeminal neuralgia and sensory neuropathies. Oral Maxillofac Surg Clin North Am 4:375-392, 1992.
7. LaBanc J: Reconstructive microneurosurgery of the trigeminal nerve. In Peterson LJ et al (eds): Principles of Oral and Maxillofacial Surgery. Philadelphia, 1992, Lippincott.
8. LaBanc JP, Gregg JM: Glossary. Oral Maxillofac Surg Clin North Am 4:563, 1992.
9. LaBanc JP, Van Bovan RW: Surgical management of inferior alveolar nerve injuries. Oral Maxillofac Surg Clin North Am 4:425-438, 1992.
10. Zuniga JR, Essick GK: A contemporary approach to the clinical evaluation of trigeminal nerve injuries. Oral Maxillofac Surg Clin North Am 4:353-367, 1992.

30. MANDIBULAR TRAUMA

A. Omar Abubaker, DMD, PhD, Kenneth J. Benson, DDS, Ian McDonald, MD, DMD, and Vincent B. Ziccardi, DDS, MD

1. **What are the signs and symptoms that may be associated with mandibular fractures?**

These include pain and tenderness at the fracture site; changes in occlusion; ecchymosis of the floor of the mouth or skin; crepitation on manual palpation; changes in mandibular range of motion; soft tissue bleeding; sensory disturbances (numbness of the lower lip); deviation of the mandible on opening; soft tissue swelling; trismus; step-in occlusion; and palpable fracture line intraorally or at the inferior border of the mandible.

2. **What radiographs are included in a mandible series?**

The mandible film series includes the right and left lateral oblique views, posteroanterior (PA) cephalogram, and reverse Towne's view. The lateral oblique views are useful to evaluate the body or ramus regions of the mandible. The PA view can assess the symphyseal region and evaluate the buccal-lingual displacement of body or angle fractures. The reverse Towne's view is helpful in assessing the mandibular condyles. Panoramic radiographs remain the gold standard for mandible fracture screening. Because these are seldom available in hospital radiology departments, an additional view that is oriented perpendicular to the lateral cortex can be substituted to accurately assess and diagnosis a fracture. A panoramic radiograph combined with a PA or reverse Towne's view is generally adequate for diagnosis.

3. **What is the incidence of fractures in different areas of the adult mandible (Table 30-1)?**

Table 30-1 Fracture Incidences in Different Areas of the Adult Mandible	
AREA OF MANDIBLE	% OF FRACTURE INCIDENTS
Angle	31%
Condyle	18%
Angle (molar) region	15%
Parasymphysis	14%
Symphysis	8%
Cuspid	7%
Ramus	6%
Coronoid process	1%

4. **What is a favorable fracture?**

Favorability is determined by the forces exerted by the masticatory muscles on the fracture segments. A favorable fracture is one that is not displaced by masticatory muscle pull, and an unfavorable fracture occurs when the line of fracture permits the fragments to separate. The four muscles of mastication are the temporalis, masseter, medial pterygoid, and lateral pterygoid. After discontinuity of the mandible due to fracture, these muscles exert their actions on the fragments, leading to malocclusion. Both horizontal and vertical components can be identified. The terms *horizontal* and *vertical* refer to the plane in which the fracture displacement is best visualized. Horizontal favorability is determined by cephalad-caudad stability, whereas vertical favorability is evaluated in the buccal-lingual plane. An example of a horizontally favorable fracture is a body fracture where the inferior border is displaced above the superior border. In this instance, the pull of the pterygomasseteric sling would aid in stabilizing the reduction because of the fracture orientation. At the mandibular angle, unfavorable fracture is caused when the line of fracture runs from anterior-superior to posterior-inferior. However, if the inferior border fracture occurs further anteriorly and the line of fracture extends in a distal direction toward the ridge, a favorable fracture is observed. It should be noted that most angle fractures are horizontally unfavorable fractures. Medial displacement may be considered in a similar fashion. A vertically favorable fracture of the angle occurs when oblique fracture lines form a large buccal cortical fragment that prevents medial displacement. Unfavorable vertical mandibular angle fracture as seen on axial computed tomography [CT] reveals that a vertically unfavorable fractures line extends from a posterolateral point to an anteromedial point. No obstruction counters the action of the lateral pterygoid and mylohyoid muscles, and the posterior fragment is shifted medially.

5. How does muscle pull affect displacement of mandibular fractures?

Muscles involved in displacing mandibular fractures include the medial and lateral pterygoid, temporalis, masseter, digastric, geniohyoid, genioglossus, and mylohyoid. The lateral pterygoid displaces the condyle anteriorly and medially because of its insertion on the pterygoid fovea. Muscles attached to the ramus (i.e., temporalis, masseter, and medial pterygoid) result in superior and medial displacement of the proximal segment. As fractures progress anteriorly toward the cuspid region, the digastric, geniohyoid, genioglossus, and mylohyoid exert a posterior-inferior force on the distal segment.

6. How do pediatric mandibular fractures differ from adult mandibular fractures?

In general, mandibular fractures are less common in children than in adults. When mandibular fractures occur in children, greenstick fractures of the mandible, particularly in the condylar region, are relatively common. Also, the ossification capability of children allows faster healing and distinguishes it from the adult mandible. As a result, many mandibular fractures in children can be treated with immobilization for a shorter period or observation and soft diet only than in an adult. Open reduction and internal fixation in children is reserved for severely displaced fractures. Resorbable plates and screws are often used instead of metallic ones when open reduction and internal fixation is indicated. Problems with osteosynthesis in children include the need to avoid damage to developing tooth buds and the need to remove the plates at a later time if resorbable plates are not used. Another common feature of mandibular fracture in children is the occurrence of high and intracapsular condylar fractures.

7. What factors influence the location of mandibular fractures?

Several factors influence the location of mandible fractures, including site, force, direction of impact, and presence of impacted teeth. The body of the mandible is involved more frequently in mandible fractures (36%) because of the lines of trajectory that pass along the longitudinal axis of the teeth. When a force is distributed to the mandible, the mandible fractures at its weakest point. The weakest points are at the angle of the mandible because of the presence of third molars and at the parasymphyseal region (canine region) because of the length of the root of the canine (26 mm). In some instances, the presence of third molars weaken the mandibular angle via decreased area of bone, and patients with third molars are 3.8 times more likely to develop angle fractures. Accordingly, some suggest that individuals at risk (e.g., contact sport athletes) may benefit from preventive removal of these teeth. Another area of susceptibility of fracture is the mandibular condyle because of the small surface area of bone in this region, especially when force is applied in a trajectory from the opposite side of the mandible or from the midsymphyseal region.

8. **What are some of the common complications associated with mandibular fracture management?**
- Infection
- Delayed union or nonunion, usually resulting from infection or inadequate fixation
- Malocclusion
- Facial or trigeminal nerve injury
- Damage to tooth roots
- Hematoma
- Wound dehiscence
- Tooth injury
- Osteomyelitis

    Of these, infection is one of the most problematic; it is the most frequent complication and is an important cause of nonunion.

9. **What are the risk factors that predispose mandibular fractures to infection?**

    Fractures that occur through the tooth-bearing area should be regarded as contaminated. Infected mandibular fractures are often seen in patients who sustain facial trauma and fail to seek immediate treatment. Mucosal tears and fractures extending through the periodontal ligament produce contamination of the fracture by oral flora. Bony sequestra, devitalized teeth, hematoma, and poor oral hygiene also contribute to infection.

    The most common cause of postoperative infection, however, is movement at the fracture site due to loose, mobile hardware, such as a loose screw in an otherwise stable plate. This may cause infection and drainage intraorally or extraorally or both until the source of infection is removed.

10. **What percentage of mandibular fractures are multiple?**

    More than 50% of mandibular fractures are multiple. Accordingly, detection of one fracture in the mandible should alert the examiner to the possible presence of additional fractures. Radiographic examination should then be directed toward identification of additional fractures.

11. **What percentage of patients with mandibular fractures is associated with concomitant cervical spine injury?**

    Approximately 43% of all patients with mandibular fracture have associated other systemic injuries. Cervical spine fractures were found in 11% of this group of patients. It is imperative to rule out cervical neck fractures, especially in patients who are intoxicated or unconscious and in patients who are involved in vehicular accidents. Posteroanterior, lateral films, and CT of the neck should be reviewed with the radiologist before treatment is initiated in these patients.

12. **What potential fatal outcome can result from bilateral mandibular parasymphyseal fractures?**

    Bilateral parasymphyseal fractures may result in a free-floating anterior mandibular segment. The genial tubercles to which the genioglossus muscle is attached are located on the lingual surface of the mandible. Lack of stability in this area in the presence of a displaced unstable bilateral symphyseal fracture allows for posterior displacement of the tongue with are resultant airway embarrassment and inferior displacement by the suprahyoid musculature. This is known clinically as "gag bite" and can lead to death. In these types of fractures, serious consideration should be given to securing the patient airway in the early phase of management of these patients.

13. **What factors contribute to condylar displacement in patients with a condylar fracture?**

    The lateral pterygoid is the only muscle that inserts directly on the neck of the mandibular condyle. In subcondylar fractures, the forces of this muscle frequently result in anterior and medial displacement of the condyle in the presence of a subcondylar fracture. In higher condylar fractures and in intracapsular fractures above the insertion of the lateral pterygoid fractures, the small fragment can occasionally be seen displaced in a pure horizontal or vertical direction.

14. What is the most likely position of a displaced condylar fracture and why?
Displacement of the proximal segment of the condyle usually occurs in an anteromedial direction because of the pull of the lateral pterygoid muscle. The patient will deviate to the side of the fracture upon opening because of the unopposed action of the contralateral lateralpterygoid muscle.

15. What surgical techniques are available to treat mandible fractures?
The most frequently used treatment modalities available for the management of mandible fractures are:
- Closed reduction and maxillomandibular fixation (MMF) with Ivy loops, arch bars, or transalveolar screw
- Closed reduction and fixation with gunning splints secured to stable osseous structures (circummandibular or perialveolar wires)
- External pin fixation, used principally with comminuted and grossly contaminated fracture
- Open reduction with internal fixation using intraoral or extraoral incisions. With this technique, the segments may be secured across the fracture site with wires, plates, or lag screws with or without concomitant MMF.

16. What is MMF, and how does it differ from intermaxillary fixation (IMF)?
Maxillomandibular fixation (MMF) was previously referred to as **intermaxillary fixation** (IMF) in an era when the mandible was known as the inferior maxilla. Current terminology is MMF and interdental fixation (which is used in the Current Procedural Terminology coding system). MMF is obtained by applying wires or elastic bands between the upper and lower jaws, to which suitable anchoring devices can be attached, such as arch bars or skeletal screws. Alternative to arch bars, Ivy loop wiring embracing only two adjacent teeth to which elastics are secured is another method to achieve MMF. Generally, only one or two Ivy loops are placed in each quadrant, with traction then placed between the jaws in each quadrant.

17. What are the advantages of rigid internal fixation (RIF) in treatment of mandible fractures over other techniques? What are the disadvantages of RIF?
RIF of mandibular fractures allows early mobilization of the jaws, reducing or eliminating the period of MMF. This is a significant benefit to patients, avoiding the potential sequelae of prolonged immobilization, including temporomandibular joint (TMJ) stiffness after removal of IMF, social inconvenience, phonetic disturbance, loss of effective work time, discomfort, and weight loss. In contrast, open reduction of mandibular fractures with wire osteosynthesis requires 4-8 weeks of MMF for satisfactory healing. Closed reduction with MMF requires the patient to be in MMF for 6 weeks or more, with limitation of diet and function, and difficulty in maintaining good oral hygiene. Disadvantages of RIF include surgery incision with possible scars and nerve injury, anesthesia complications, and higher cost of procedure.

18. What are the different options for treatment of mandibular angle fractures?
The treatment of these fractures depends on many factors, including but not limited to the age and medical condition of the patient, severity of the fracture, and displacement. In general, for most angle fractures, superior border plate fixation with a minimum of four screws placed across the fracture line provides adequate stability of the fracture. The patient can be placed in MMF for 1-3 weeks, although that is not always necessary. Plates used range from 1.7-2.0 mm with monocortical screws that range in length (depending on the thickness of the cortical plate

and the positioning of the plate) from 5-7 mm. Other treatment options include inferior border plate and lag screw across the fracture line. If the fracture is nondisplaced, MMF for 3-6 weeks, or even observation and a nonchew diet, represent viable options for treatment. With comminuted fractures of the angle, treatment options include external pin fixation, reconstruction plate and/or MMF.

19. What are the indications for removing a tooth in the line of fracture?

Because mandibular fractures commonly occur through the dental periodontal ligament space, much debate has been focused on whether to extract teeth in the line of fracture. By definition, a fracture that communicates with the oral cavity through the periodontal ligament space is considered a compound fracture. The literature to date does not provide convincing evidence that infection is more likely to occur if a tooth is retained. Nonetheless, current recommendations for removal of teeth in the line of fracture include:

- Presence of obvious pathology, such as caries or periodontal disease
- Gross mobility of involved teeth
- Teeth that prevent adequate reduction of fractures
- Teeth with fractured roots
- Teeth whose root surfaces or apices are exposed in the fracture site

20. What are the indications for open reduction and internal fixation of condylar fractures in adults?

Most fractures of the mandibular condyle are amenable to closed reduction with fixation and immobilization ranging from 7-21 days based on age of the patient, displacement of fracture, and number of other concomitant injuries. Intracapsular condylar fractures are generally treated with a short period of MMF (10-14 days), followed by postfixation physiotherapy to prevent ankylosis of the joint. The mandible will deviate clinically to the side of injury on opening because of unopposed pull of the contralateral lateral pterygoid.

The indications for open reduction of condylar fractures in adults were well described by Zide and Kent and divided into absolute and relative indications.

Absolute Indications

- Inability to obtain adequate occlusion using closed reduction techniques
- Displacement of the condyle into the middle cranial fossa
- Severe angulations of the condyle, lateral extracapsular displacement of the condyle or the condyle outside the glenoid fossa
- Removal of foreign body in the joint capsule (e.g., gunshot pellets)

Relative Indications

- Bilateral condylar fractures with concomitant comminuted midfacial fractures
- Bilateral fractures in an edentulous patient when splints are unavailable or impossible because of severe ridge atrophy
- Displaced condyle fracture in a medically compromised patient (e.g., scizure disorder, psychiatric problems, or alcoholism) with evidence of open bite or retrusion

21. How are dentoalveolar fractures treated?

Alveolar fractures are typically treated with reduction and verification of this reduction by assuring proper occlusion with the opposing arch and proper alignment within the arch. This is often followed by fixation with arch bars or composite or orthodontic splints for 4-6 weeks. MMF is not required and is better avoided unless the fracture is associated with mandibular or maxillary fractures. The patient should be instructed to eat a soft, nonchew diet throughout the period of fixation. Antibiotics and strict instruction of good oral hygiene are recommended.

Endodontic evaluation of the involved teeth is recommended, with possible future need for endodontic treatment because of their possible devitalization after trauma.

22. What is the appropriate management of avulsed primary and permanent teeth?

Avulsed primary teeth usually require no treatment, and no attempt should be made to reimplant them. Radiographs of the injured area are recommended to rule out retained root fragments and assess damage to the developing permanent dentition. Avulsed permanent teeth should be replanted as soon as possible because reimplantation success declines exponentially after 2 hr. If immediate reimplantation is not possible, the tooth should be stored in an appropriate storage media until reimplantation is possible. Ideal media to store such teeth is Hank's balanced salt solution. Cool milk is an acceptable substitute, followed by saline, saliva, and water in decreasing order of utility. The teeth should be inspected for any gross pathology or fractures prior to reimplantation, and the root surfaces and alveolar socket should be irrigated gently with no mechanical manipulation prior to reimplantation. After reimplantation and verification of occlusion, teeth should be splinted with a light passive wire and composite splint for 7-10 days. Antibiotic coverage for 5-10 days is generally recommended, because these are open injuries. Initiation of endodontic therapy should begin 7-14 days after injury to minimize root resorption.

23. When treating mandible fractures, what is a tension band?

During mandibular functioning, stress forces are exerted on the bone in different vectors depending on the location. The superior border is under tension, whereas the inferior border is compressed. A rotational force is found in the parasymphyseal region. A tension band in mandibular fracture management refers to a mechanical means of resisting fracture displacement in the tension zone. This may be accomplished by a superior border plate if teeth are not in the way (i.e., a plate over the external oblique ridge in an angle fracture), an arch bar if stable teeth are present on both sides of the fracture, a superior border wire, or an eccentric dynamic compression plate at the inferior border.

24. What are dynamic compression, eccentric dynamic compression, and passive plating in rigid fixation?

The concept of rigid internal fixation was designed to allow primary bone healing even under functional loading. In an effort to enhance stability, plates were developed that provide compressive forces across fracture lines. Passive plating provides rigid fixation without compression. Dynamic compression plates compress the fracture site by providing axial guiding inclines for the screw heads to slide down as the screw is tightened. The screws first engage the bone, and as they are tightened, they are moved 0.8 mm toward the fracture site by the guiding incline. This produces a compressive force of approximately 300 kPa. Eccentric dynamic compression plates provide compressive forces in more than one direction by changing the direction of the guiding incline in the outer holes of the plate. This concept is useful when plating mandibular body fractures. A compression plate at both the superior and inferior borders would ideally provide compression throughout the fracture, but is usually not possible because of the presence of teeth superiorly, as well as other vital structures. A single eccentric dynamic compression plate placed at the inferior border serves the same purpose by angling the guiding inclines of the outer holes toward the superior border of the mandible and eliminating the need for a superior border tension plate.

25. Which mandibular fractures are likely to be missed on panoramic examination?

Because panoramic radiograph is a flat view taken by a movable x-ray beam that displays the entire mandible as a flat structure, some overlap and blurring is usually seen in the symphysis-parasymphysis region; therefore, fractures of the mandible in this area are frequently missed.

Similarly, and due to the overlap from other cranial and facial structures, fractures of the mandibular condyles can be difficult to detect and, when detected, difficult to ascertain the degree of displacement of the fracture. The combination of panoramic examination, Towne's views and CT scan helps detect almost all mandibular fractures.

26. What is the best treatment for symphyseal and parasymphyseal fractures?

Because the bilateral posterior and lateral pull exerted by the mylohyoid and digastric muscles contributes to displacement of the fragments, symphyseal and parasymphyseal fractures are better treated with open reduction and rigid fixation. Once MMF is obtained, the fracture is exposed through an intraoral or trancutanous incision with care not to injure the mental nerves. The incision into the mucosa is made deep into the labial-alveolar sulcus. The bone fragments are then reduced with bone forceps and secured, if necessary. The plate is then adapted and is slightly overcontoured and secured to the bone with mono- or bi-cortical screws. Two screws are needed on each side of the bony plate to ensure stability.

27. What are the different methods used for management of fractures of the condyles?

Most isolated fractures of the condyles can be treated by MMF alone, usually for 2-4 weeks. Duration of MMF depends on type of dentition, level of the condylar fracture, degree of dislocation of the condylar head, and age of the patient. When unilateral condylar fractures are associated with a fracture in the mandibular body on the contralateral side, longer duration of MMF may be necessary. Condylar fractures differ from mandibular body fractures in that they require shorter duration of MMF to prevent complications related to the TMJ. MMF may not be needed for unilateral condylar fractures in edentulous patients because occlusal discrepancies can be corrected on renewal of the dentures.

The main basis for open reduction is the inability to obtain adequate dental occlusion by closed reduction. This occurs when the condyle is subluxated almost completely in a medial direction, when it is displaced in the opposite direction and projects laterally from the zygoma, and occasionally when the condyle is pushed through the external auditory canal or into the middle cranial fossa.

28. How are edentulous mandible fractures treated?

A distinction should be made when discussing these fractures from fractures of the atrophic mandible. Edentulous but nonatrophic mandible fractures in which there is adequate bone height (15 mm or more in height) are easier to treat than fractures of the atrophic mandible. Treatment of these fractures depends on the location of the fracture, degree of displacement, and whether the patient wears a denture. Nondisplaced fractures can be treated by observation and nonchewing diet with higher degree of success than dentate mandibles. When that is not possible or when there is displacement of the fractures, superior or inferior border plates are needed to adequately stabilize the fracture segments. Compared with using MMF, gunning splints, or the patient dentures, RIF provides the advantage of direct visualization and anatomic reduction, excellent stabilization of the fixed segments, and early return of masticatory function. If a superior border plate is used, monocortical screws should be used in a fashion similar to that of mandibular angle fixation. These plates can be removed later to allow the patient to wear a denture once the fracture has healed. This technique provides the advantage of early and easier dissection and intraoral approach without risk to the facial nerve or scarring of the incision site. Open procedure with inferior border placement allows for lower incidence of injury to the inferior alveolar nerve, which can be located at the superior border if significant resorption of the ridge occurred.

29. How are atrophic mandibular fractures treated?

There is considerable controversy over the choice of treatment methods of these fractures. However, many authors agree that the most important element to the success of the treatment of these fractures is adequate and complete stabilization of the fractured segments. Lack of complete immobilization of the fractured segments is likely to account for most of the commonly reported nonunion of these fractures, especially when nonrigid or semirigid fixation is used (such as wires, miniplates, and denture splints). Nonrigid or semirigid plates will not provide adequate and effective stabilization, and will likely fail with function. There is always the concern for devascularization of the bone from open reduction and reflection of the periosteum of the mandible; open reduction and rigid fixation using a reconstruction plate or a titanium mesh with immediate bone graft provide much more predictable results of healing of these types of fractures. Because atrophic mandible fractures are usually observed in the elderly and unhealthy population (often with respiratory and nutritional problems), early and adequate stabilization and resumption of oral intake provide a better chance of primary bony healing of fractures in these patients.

BIBLIOGRAPHY

1. Aminoff MJ, Greenberg DA, Simon RP: Clinical Neurology, 3rd ed. Stamford, Conn, 1995, Appleton & Lange.
2. Aargon SB, Gardner KE: The mandibular fractures. In Jafeck BW, Murrow BW (eds): ENT Secrets, 2nd ed. Philadelphia, 2001, Hanley & Belfus.
3. Assael LA: Maxillofacial Trauma. Part 1: Applying Science to Practice. Oral and Maxillofacial Surgery Clinics of North America, 10th vol, no. 4. Philadelphia, 1998, Saunders.
4. Deangelis AJ, Backland LK: Traumatic dental injuries: current treatment concepts. J Am Dental Assoc 129:1401-1414, 1998.
5. Ellis E 3rd: Treatment methods for fractures of the mandibular angle. J Craniomaxillofac Trauma 2:28-36, 1996.
6. Fonseca RJ, Walker RV, Betts NJ: Oral and Maxillofacial Trauma, 3rd ed. St Louis, 2005, Saunders.
7. Kaban LB (ed): Oral and Maxillofacial Surgery in Children and Adolescents. Oral and Maxillofacial Surgery Clinics of North America, vol. 6, no. 1. Philadelphia, 1994, Saunders.
8. Polley JW, Flagg JF, Cohen M: Fractures of the mandible. In Weinzweig J (ed): Plastic Surgery Secrets, 2nd ed. Philadelphia, 1999, Hanley & Belfus.
9. Posnick JC (ed): Craniomaxillofacial Fractures in Children. Oral and Maxillofacial Clinics of North America, 6th vol, no. 1. Philadelphia, 1994, Saunders.
10. Smith BR, Ghali GE: Atrophic edentulous mandibular fractures. Oral and Maxillofacial Surgery Knowledge Update, 2nd vol, page Tra/29, 1998.

31. MIDFACIAL FRACTURES: FRACTURES OF THE NOSE, ZYGOMA, ORBIT, AND MAXILLA

A. Omar Abubaker, DMD, PhD, Vincent B. Ziccardi, DDS, MD, and Ian McDonald, MD, DMD

NASAL FRACTURES

1. Where are the most common sites for nasal bones to fracture?

Fractures of the nasal bones occur more commonly in the distal nasal bones, which are broader and thinner. Direct frontal blows to the nasal dorsum usually result in fracture of the thin lower half of the nasal bones. The proximal nasal bones are stronger and thicker and relatively resistant to fracture. However, when the force of the blow is more severe, the fracture may involve the more proximal nasal bones, the frontal process of the maxilla, and frontal bone.

2.   What is the role of radiographs in the diagnosis and treatment of nasal fractures?
Standard facial radiographs are of limited diagnostic and therapeutic value in the treatment of nasal fractures. However, radiographs can serve as a physical record of a nasal fracture, and computed tomography (CT) scans can accurately determine the degree of displacement of nasal fractures and fractures of the orbitoethmoidal region. Therefore although radiographic documentation is recommended for medical-legal reasons, physical exam of the nose should provide the basis for whether surgical intervention is indicated.

3.   When is nasal packing indicated after treatment of nasal fractures?
After successful reduction of a nasal fracture, intranasal packing is often used to serve the following purposes:
- To control bleeding and prevent postoperative septal hematoma
- To splint the nasal septum into position and keep the septal mucosa adapted to the septal cartilage and to provide internal support for reduced bone fragments
- To prevent synechiae if large areas of mucosa are abraded

4.   What are the indications for posterior nasal packing?
A posterior pack is indicated for posterior nasal bleeds. This type of bleeding is often diagnosed when the patient's chief complaint is bleeding into the throat or if a posterior nosebleed is visualized and the bleeding cannot be controlled with a well-placed anterior pack.

5.   How long should a posterior pack be left in place?
For 3-5 days.

6.   What is the treatment of a severely comminuted nasal fracture?
Severely comminuted nasal fractures usually can be reduced primarily and supported with intranasal packing and externally applied splints. Packing is placed underneath the nasal bones so that formation of the bone fragments is sandwiched between and supported by internal and external support mechanisms. The combination of internal and external splinting helps prevent hematoma, compress and narrow the splayed nasal dorsum, and conserve nasal height. Open reduction of a comminuted nasal fracture early after injury risks loss of bone fragments with little soft tissue attachment and should be used with caution or avoided completely.

7.   What are the indications for secondary treatment of nasal fractures?
Even with adequate reduction, postoperative nasal deformity may still occur, and patients should be informed of such a possibility. Late deformities may include a nasal hump or deviation, loss of dorsal height, septal deviation, and nasal obstruction. Secondary treatment of nasal fractures is indicated when any of these deformities is present, especially in the presence of either functional or cosmetic problems.

8.   How are acute septal hematomas treated?
Septal hematomas are treated with an incision along the base or most inferior portion of the hematoma to allow dependent drainage and prevent refilling of the cavity with blood or serum. Bilateral hematomas can be treated with bilateral incisions, maintaining an intact septal cartilage, or with a unilateral incision and resection of a window of cartilage to allow a bilateral communication with the incision. A light nasal packing and prophylactic antibiotics are recommended.

9.   How soon after injury should a nasal fracture be reduced?
Nasal fractures should be reduced within the first few hours after injury. If this is not done within this period, edema makes accurate judgment of the degree of deformity and the decision to operate difficult. The next window of opportunity occurs 3 to 14 days after injury, after the edema has resolved but before bony union of the fractured fragments occurs.

10. What are the late complications of nasal fractures?

The following complications may be seen following nasal fractures with and without treatment:

- Airway obstruction
- Nasal deformity secondary to saddle deformity or dorsal hump
- Nasal deviation and septal perforation
- The formation of synechiae between the septum and turbinates
- Recurrent epistaxis and recurrent sinusitis and headaches

11. What is a nasal septal hematoma, and how is it treated?

A nasal septal hematoma usually presents as a boggy, blue elevation of the septal mucosa. This finding is significant because it requires drainage to prevent secondary infection and necrosis of the septal cartilage leading to perforation and possible saddle nose deformity. Drainage can be accomplished by either needle aspiration or small mucosal incision. Transseptal resorbable sutures and nasal packing can be placed to prevent reaccumulation of blood.

Septal hematomas are treated with an incision along the base or its most inferior point to allow dependent drainage and prevent its refilling with blood or serum. Bilateral hematomas can be treated with bilateral incisions, maintaining an intact septal cartilage, or with a unilateral incision and resection of a window of cartilage. Nasal packing and prophylactic antibiotics are recommended.

12. What is a saddle nose deformity?

Saddle nose deformity is the concave appearance of the nasal dorsum that sometimes follows significant nasal trauma. It results from fracture and inferior displacement of the nasal bones, resulting in buckling of the cartilaginous septum and disruption of the upper lateral cartilage position. Late effects of the injury that amplify the deformity include septal collapse, which may result from septal hematoma formation, asymmetric septal growth, and scar contractures.

13. How is epistaxis managed in the emergency department?

Anterior nasal epistaxis usually involves Kiesselbach's plexus, which is the confluence of the terminal ends of the superior labial, anterior ethmoid, and sphenopalatine arteries. Packing of this area with phenylephrine-soaked cotton pledgets is frequently successful. Direct visualization with a nasal speculum may allow direct cauterization with either electrocautery or silver nitrate sticks to be performed. Excessive cauterization should be avoided, however, to prevent subsequent septal perforation. Most commonly, sterile petrolatum-impregnated gauze is carefully packed in a layered manner and left in place for 2-5 days. Broad-spectrum antibiotic coverage should be initiated to prevent maxillary sinus infections caused by blockage of the middle meatus.

Posterior nose bleeds are more difficult to manage because the lack of posterior stops prevents creating pressure with packing. This frequently is managed by placing a Foley urinary catheter into the affected nares, inflating the balloon with saline, and pulling the balloon back to seal the nasopharynx and to allow packing to be placed around the Foley. Tension is maintained on the catheter by placing an umbilical clip on it at the entrance of the nose. Commercially available posterior nasal balloons are also available.

14. What are the classic clinical findings in a patient with a nasoorbital-ethmoidal (NOE) fracture?

The NOE fracture usually results from a direct blow to the bridge of the nose by a blunt object, such as a steering wheel or dashboard during a motor vehicle accident. Patients classically present with a widened nasal bridge, periorbital edema and ecchymosis, epistaxis, cerebrospinal fluid (CSF) rhinorrhea (42%), and traumatic telecanthus (12%-20%). Epiphora as an early or late finding indicates injury or outflow obstruction to the nasolacrimal apparatus. Treatment goals include restoration of normal intercanthal distance, fixation of the nasal bones, and careful evaluation and possible repair of the bony orbit and nasolacrimal apparatus.

15. What is the difference between telecanthus and hypertelorism?

Telecanthus refers to a widening of the distance between the medial canthi, usually as a result of trauma, such as NOE fractures. The normal Caucasian adult intercanthal distance is approximately 33 mm. **Hypertelorism** is a widening of the orbits themselves and is measured as the interpupillary distance, normally 60 mm. Hypertelorism resulting from trauma is rare because tremendous force is required to fracture and displace the bony orbits. It is more commonly seen in congenital craniofacial deformities, such as craniosynostosis.

16. Why is the placement of a nasogastric tube sometimes contraindicated in a midface fracture patient?

Midface fractures commonly extend through the nasal cavity and may result in soft tissue disruption in the nasopharynx with concomitant cranial injuries. Inadvertent placement of a nasogastric tube in these patients may result in the intracranial placement of the tube or soft tissue dissection in a previously traumatized region.

ORBITAL FRACTURES

17. What are the signs and symptoms of orbital fractures?

The signs and symptoms of orbital fracture depend on the location of the fracture and degree of displacement of the fracture. Orbital fractures generally present with numbness of the infraorbital and lateral nasal area, diplopia, periorbital and subconjunctival hematoma and ecchymosis, and perhaps a visual acuity deficit. The visual acuity deficit is nonspecific to the orbital fracture, but can imply damage to the globe or the optic nerve. Generally, orbital fractures have an early presentation of exophthalmos due to swelling. Enophthalmos is present within 1-3 weeks if the orbital cavity is significantly enlarged and appears as the swelling resolves. An orbital volume enlargement of more than 5%-10% justifies open reduction.

Diplopia with orbital fractures can also be present, especially in downward gaze or upward gaze. Diplopia is due most commonly to muscular contusion, interference with the excursion of the extraocular muscle system, entrapment of fat that is tethered to the muscles by fine ligaments or, less commonly, entrapment of the muscle itself. Only fractures associated with diplopia due to entrapment of muscle or fat should be treated with operative intervention. Diplopia due to muscle contusion usually improves significantly without operative intervention.

18. What is a Marcus Gunn pupil?

It is an afferent pupillary defect resulting from lesions involving the retina or optic nerve back to the chiasm. With this defect a light shone in the unaffected eye produces normal constriction of the pupils of both eyes (consensual response), but a light shone in the affected eye produces a paradoxical dilation rather than constriction of the affected pupil.

19. What is the best radiographic study for diagnosis of orbital fracture?

Axial and coronal CT scans at 2- to 3-mm intervals are ideal to demonstrate abnormalities of the medial and lateral walls and identify fractures of the nasoethmoidal region. Direct or reformatted images demonstrate fractures of the orbital floor, roof, and interorbital space. Less optimally, a Waters view is often sufficient to show an orbital floor fracture, blood in the maxillary sinus as well as orbital floor depression, and herniation of orbital contents.

20. What is the most common site of an isolated intraorbital fracture?

The most frequent intraorbital fracture involves the orbital floor just medial to the infraorbital canal and is usually confined to the medial portion of the floor and the lower portion of the medial orbital wall. Depressed fractures of these regions may cause the orbital soft tissue to be displaced into the maxillary and ethmoid sinuses, leading to an increase in orbital volume.

21. What is the incidence of hypoesthesia or anesthesia in the distribution of infraorbital floor associated with orbital floor fractures?
The incidence is 90%-95%.

22. What causes traumatic enophthalmos, exophthalmos, and ocular dystopia?
Fractures of the lower two thirds of the orbit commonly produce changes in eye position by expansion of the orbit. Fractures of the superior portion of the orbit generally are displaced inward and downward and cause the globe to be driven forward and downward by orbital volume constriction. Fractures of the inferior portion of the orbit may either constrict or expand the orbital cavity. Constriction is most commonly produced by a medially displaced zygoma fracture, which may cause exophthalmos of the globe. In fractures of the zygoma, orbital floor, or medial orbit that expand the volume of the orbit, the globe is displaced posteriorly and medially. The posterior displacement of the globe is termed enophthalmos. Generally, an increase of 1 cc in orbital volume is required for each millimeter displacement of the globe. Inferior globe displacement is called ocular dystopia. Displacement is permitted by expansion of the floor, medial orbital wall, and, in cases of the zygoma, the inferior orbital rim.

23. How can entrapment of orbital contents be diagnosed in an unconscious patient?
Diagnosis of orbital contents entrapment is made by performing a forced duction test. The test involves grasping the insertion of a rectus muscle onto the ocular globe with a forceps approximately 7 mm from the limbus. The globe is then gently rotated in all four directions, and any restriction is noted. The inferior rectus muscle is the most commonly tested muscle, although the superior, medial, or lateral recti muscles may be used as well.

24. What materials are used to reconstruct the orbital floor?
- Autogenous bone grafts (split calvarial, iliac, or split rib)
- Allogenic bone grafts (cranium, rib, iliac crest, anterior wall of the maxillary sinus or the coronoid process)
- Inorganic alloplastic materials (e.g., Medpor, Silastic, Vitallium, stainless steel, Teflon, Supramid, or titanium implants)

25. What are the most frequent complications of inadequately treated or untreated fractures of the orbital floor?
Diplopia and enophthalmos.

26. What complications are associated with fractures of the orbital roof?
Fractures of the orbital roof usually involve the supraorbital ridge, frontal bone, and frontal sinus. The trochlea of the superior oblique muscle is often damaged because of its proximity to the surface of the roof, resulting in transitory diplopia. Another sign is globe displacement and occurs in an inferolateral direction and may result in proptosis. Cranial nerve (CN) VI may be traumatized with orbital roof fractures, resulting in paralysis of the lateral rectus muscle and limitation of ocular abduction. Additional complications include dural tears, anterior cranial base injuries, CSF leaks, cerebral herniation, and pulsatile exophthalmos.

27. What are the different surgical approaches to treatment of orbital fractures?
There are multiple approaches to the orbit. Each has an advantage and disadvantage and the choice often is made based on the amount of surgical exposure needed, the location of the fracture, and operator preference.

The **subciliary lower eyelid incision** begins approximately 2-3 mm below the lash line and extends from the punctum to 8-10 mm lateral to the lateral canthus. This incision is made through the skin, and the dissection is continued to the inferior edge of the tarsus. A skin-muscle flap is then raised from the tarsus; the septum orbitale is followed below the tarsus until the rim of the orbit is reached. An incision is made through the periosteum on the anterior aspect of the orbital rim to avoid damaging the septum. The periosteum is then elevated from the rim and orbital floor. This approach allows easy access to the lateral and medial walls and floor of the orbit.

The **mid-lid incision** is performed within the lower lid crease, approximately 4-5 mm below the ciliary margin. This incision avoids many of the problems associated with the subciliary incision.

The **transconjunctival incision** is made through the conjunctiva, capsulopalpebral fascia, and periosteum to the orbital rim. This incision directly exposes the orbital fat without incising the septum orbitale and avoids an external scar. When combined with a lateral canthotomy incision, this approach provides exposure of all four walls of the orbit.

The **lateral brow incision** or upper blepharoplasty incision provides exposure of the frontozygomatic suture and part of the lateral wall and roof of the orbit.

Medial canthal incisions are usually made in a curvilinear direction. They provide excellent exposure of the medial canthus, medial wall of the orbit, and nasal bones.

The **intraoral approach** provides excellent exposure of the inferior orbital rim, maxilla, and zygoma. It does not allow for adequate exposure of the orbital floor or other orbital walls.

The **bicoronal incision** provides wide access to the orbits, upper portion of the nose, and zygomas as well as the cranium. It is the preferred incision when the exposure of all these areas is necessary, as in treatment of nasoethmoidal fractures, Le Fort III fractures, and frontal sinus fractures, because exposure of the orbital roof must be visualized and the orbital contents must be mobilized 360 degrees.

28. Which incision has the greatest propensity for ectropion?

Scleral show and ectropion are frequent sequelae of the subciliary incision after lower lid surgery and are often due to lid retraction. These conditions improve with time in many patients but may be a permanent deformity that results from permanent scarring within the lower eyelid.

29. What is an NOE fracture?

A severe medial orbital wall fracture usually involving the nasoethmoidal structures. It is sometimes referred to as a nasoethmoidal-orbital fracture or nasoorbital-ethmoidal fracture, or simply an NOE fracture.

30. What is the surgical approach to the treatment of an NOE fracture?

Based on the pattern and comminution of the fracture, one combination of these incisions—coronal, subciliary or mid-lid, and maxillary gingivobuccal sulcus—is usually necessary to expose adequately the nasoethmoidal-orbital region.

31. What is the mechanism of posttraumatic enophthalmos?

Enophthalmos results mostly from displacement of a relatively constant volume of orbital soft tissue contents into an enlarged bony orbital volume caused by disruption and displacement of one or more of the orbital walls. Enophthalmos in excess of 5 mm results in a noticeable deformity.

Diplopia is double vision, often transient, and, if present, only at the extremes of gaze rather than within a functional field of vision. It is commonly attributed to hematoma or edema that causes muscular imbalance by elevating the ocular globe or to injury of the extraocular musculature and temporary effects on the oculorotary mechanism. Diplopia in itself is *rarely* an indication for surgery.

32. What are the etiologies of monocular and binocular diplopia?

Causes of monocular diplopia (double vision) include retinal detachment, dislocated lens, foreign body, uncorrected refractive error, cataract, and corneal opacity. This physical finding warrants immediate ophthalmologic consultation. Binocular diplopia is more common in the traumatic setting and may result from an alteration in globe position, such as proptosis or enophthalmos, or from limitation of globe movement through entrapment of orbital soft tissues. Alternatively, nerve injury may occur intracranially or within the orbit as a result of compression from hematoma or bone fragments. Surgical repair of the bony orbit and decompression of affected nerves result in correction of diplopia.

33. What is a blowout fracture of the orbit?

A blowout fracture of the orbit results from direct trauma to the globe resulting in distortion of the globe and increased intraorbital pressure. The orbital rim generally stays intact, and the force is transmitted to the interior area of the orbital cavity. The force is dissipated by outward fracture of the weaker bones of the orbital floor and medial wall. As force increases, the fractures may extend both posteriorly and circumferentially. A thorough physical exam and diagnostic imaging, specifically CT scanning, are required to evaluate the size of the defect and possible entrapment of orbital structures. Significant defects require operative repair to prevent posttraumatic enophthalmos.

34. What are the differences between superior orbital fissure syndrome and orbital apex syndrome?

Superior orbital fissure syndrome results from compression of the contents found in the superior orbital fissure by hematoma or bony fragment. Clinical findings include:

- Pupillary dilation through dysfunction of CN III innervation of pupillary constrictor muscles
- Ophthalmoplegia secondary to palsy of CNs III, IV, and VI
- Upper eyelid ptosis from levator palpebrae paresis
- Anesthesia of the forehead and loss of corneal reflex from ophthalmic division of the trigeminal nerve compression
- Proptosis secondary to edema from obstruction of the ophthalmic vein and lymphatic system

Orbital apex syndrome usually results from retrobulbar hematoma with compression of the optic canal and superior orbital fissure. Clinical findings include tense proptosis and periorbital swelling, retroorbital pain, pupillary dilation, ophthalmoplegia, and, most importantly, a change in vision. Funduscopy reveals a pale disc with cherry red maculae. Prompt surgical decompression via lateral canthotomy is required to prevent permanent vision loss.

35. What is the bowstring test, and for what type of fracture assessment is it useful?

The bowstring test is a means of assessing the status of the medial canthal ligament in NOE fractures. Commonly, the ligament remains intact and attached to the lacrimal bone, which may be fractured and displaced. The bowstring test is performed by placing gentle lateral traction over the lateral canthus while palpating the medial canthal region to assess mobility. A positive test confirms bony fracture with displacement of the medial canthal ligament or traumatic telecanthus.

36. What is the relationship between orbital volume changes as they relate to orbital trauma?

The normal volume of the bony orbit is approximately 30 cc. Fractures of orbital bones may increase or decrease this volume, with resultant changes in the position of the orbital contents. Fractures that decrease orbital volume compress the orbital contents and may create exophthalmos. Increases in orbital volume provide more room for the globe and may result in dystopia or a change in the vertical position of the globe. Enophthalmos is a change in anterior-posterior position of the globe. Alterations in globe position as a function of orbital volume change are dependent on two factors: disruption of Lockwood's suspensory ligament and the relationship of the change in volume relative to the axis of the globe. The axis is defined as a line connecting the lateral orbital rim to an area just in front of the lacrimal bone. Volume changes behind this line can produce significant alterations in globe position. It is estimated that 1 mL of volume loss behind the axis produces 1.5 mm of enophthalmos. Anterior orbital floor and medial wall fractures are usually in front of the axis and produce minimal changes in globe position.

37. What is a hyphema, and how is it managed?
Hyphema is the layering of blood in the anterior chamber of the globe, usually from the tearing of blood vessels at the root of the iris. It may present with pain, blurred vision, and photophobia. Retinal hemorrhage is also found in more than 50% of hyphemas. Management of hyphema is directed toward prevention of rebleeding, which occurs in 3%-30% of cases. Rebleeds generally occur 3-5 days after injury, are usually more severe than the original injury, and may result in impaired vision, corneal staining, and glaucoma formation. Patients are usually admitted for bed rest and daily ophthalmologic evaluation. An eye patch is applied, and increased intraocular pressure is treated with topical beta blockers and carbonic anhydrase inhibitors or mannitol if necessary. Aspirin is absolutely contraindicated in these patients.

38. What are the possible etiologies of extraocular movement disorders following trauma?
Extraocular movements are controlled by the six extraocular muscles. The inferior, superior, medial rectus, and inferior oblique muscles are all innervated by CN III (oculomotor). The superior oblique muscle is innervated by the trochlear nerve (CN IV), and the lateral rectus muscle is supplied by the abducens nerve (CN VI). Traumatic disruption of either muscle or nerve continuity would likely result in a movement disorder manifested by limited gaze in the direction of affected muscle pull and binocular diplopia. Entrapment of muscle in traumatic bony defects (e.g., orbital floor blowout fracture) also may lead to restricted gaze.

39. What are the causes of traumatic ptosis?
Ptosis refers to the drooping of the upper eyelid. Normal resting eyelid position is mediated by the sympathetic nervous system by the superior cervical ganglion. The muscle end point of these nerves is Mueller's muscle, a smooth muscle that inserts on the upper tarsal plate. Disruption of the sympathetic fibers (e.g., in Horner's syndrome) leads to ptosis. The levator palpebrae superioris is responsible for voluntary eye opening and is innervated by CN III. Injury to this nerve or muscle also results in ptosis. Alteration in globe position may result in the appearance of ptosis despite full function of related nerves and muscles.

ZYGOMATIC FRACTURES

40. What is the pattern of the typical zygomatic or malar complex fracture?
The pattern of zygomatic fracture depends on factors such as the direction and magnitude of the force, the density of the adjacent bones, and the amount of soft tissue covering the zygoma. The natural points of structural weakness in the area of the zygoma also contribute to the pattern of zygomatic complex fractures. Typically, the fracture line travels through the zygomaticofrontal (ZF) suture, into the orbit at the zygomaticosphenoidal suture to the inferior orbital fissure. Anterior to the fissure, the fracture travels through the orbital floor and infraorbital rim, goes through the infraorbital foramen, and continues inferiorly through the zygomaticomaxillary (ZM) buttress. Poteriorly, the fracture extends from the buttress and through the lateral wall of the maxillary sinus. Finally, one of the most frequent pattern of fractures of the zygoma is isolated arch fracture, which occurs at its weakest point, about 1.5 cm posterior to the zygomaticotemporal suture.

41. What is "tripod fracture"?
Tripod fracture has been used more so in the past to consolidate the typical fracture pattern of the zygomatic complex into a concise descriptive term that reflects the configuration of the

complex as it relates to adjacent bone. However, such a term is a misnomer because it wrongly implies that three processes of the zygoma are involved. In reality, the usual zygomatic complex fracture (more accurately now referred to as zygomaticomaxillary complex [ZMC]) involves four major processes: the zygomaticofrontal region, infraorbital rim, ZM buttress, and zygomatic arch.

42. What physical and radiologic findings are associated with orbital ZMC fractures?

Zygomatic fractures are commonly encountered in facial trauma because of their prominent position on the facial skeleton. They are second only to nasal fractures in frequency of involvement. Physical signs and symptoms associated with orbital ZMC fractures include:

- Periorbital ecchymosis and edema
- Subconjunctival hemorrhage that remains bright red for a prolonged period due to continued oxygen saturation of the blood through the oxygen-permeable conjunctiva
- Flattening of the malar prominence or zygomatic arch
- Step deformity and tenderness at the inferior orbital rim, zygomatic arch, frontozygomatic suture, or zygomatic buttress regions
- Pain, especially in mobile fractures
- Epistaxis on the side of fracture due to blood draining from the involved maxillary sinus. Direct nasal injury also must be ruled out.
- Diplopia (double vision), which results from displacement of the globe secondary to entrapment of extraocular muscles, edema, hematoma, neurologic injury, or increased orbital volume due to orbital floor defect or displacement of the lateral orbital wall
- Infraorbital nerve paresthesia due to either direct trauma or impingement from the fractured segments of bone
- Ecchymosis in the maxillary buccal vestibule (Guérin's sign)
- Trismus due to muscle spasm or the physical impingement of the coronoid process by the collapsed zygomatic arch
  Radiologic findings of orbital ZMC fractures include:
- Waters' view or PA oblique demonstrates separation of the frontozygomatic suture, possible distortion of orbital shape, steps in the orbital rim, or opacification of the ipsilateral maxillary sinus.
- Submental vertex view shows fractures of the zygomatic arch, which frequently presents with an "M" configuration. Rotation of the body of the zygoma around a vertical axis can also be assessed with this view.
- CT is the gold standard for assessing fracture location and displacement. Orbital defects, as well as soft tissue injury, can be evaluated accurately using both axial and coronal views.

43. What is the mechanism of limited range of motion of the mandible caused by fracture of the zygoma?

Because of the close proximity of the coronoid process of the mandible to the zygoma and zygomatic process, displaced fractures of the body or arch of the zygoma may impinge on the coronoid process, causing interference with the movement of the mandibile. It should be noted, however, that in the early stages after injury, trismus also may be secondary to edema or spasm of the temporalis or masseter muscles.

44. Which diagnostic images are the most helpful in evaluation and treatment planning for zygomatic complex fractures?

For a long time in the past, posteroanterior oblique (Waters) and submental vertex ("jughandle") roentgenograms were used for evaluating these fractures. However, CT scan (axial and coronal) is currently the diagnostic imaging of choice for evaluating these fractures. This imaging modality shows the location of the fractures, degree of displacement of the bones, and status of the surrounding soft tissues. Axial views are best to evaluate the lateral orbital wall and zygomatic arch, whereas coronal views are necessary to determine the presence and extent of orbital floor fractures.

45. What are the indications for surgical treatment of zygomatic fractures?
Surgical treatment of zygoma fractures should be based on both clinical and radiographic findings. Presence of immediate functional or cosmetic problems should be addressed to prevent long-term sequelae, such as facial dysmorphism, enophthalmos, or orbital dystopia. Other indications for operative treatment include significant displacement or instability of the fracture segments.

46. When is the optimal time to operate on zygomatic fractures?
Ideally, open reduction should be performed before the onset of edema. However, you should always remember that zygomatic fractures are not emergencies, and any associated life-threatening injuries must be addressed first. Even in the absence of such emergencies the patient can be dischanged from the emergency department and readmitted at a later time electively for treatment of these fractures, waiting several days for edema to resolve. Such delay is unlikely to compromise the surgical outcome and often results in better surgical results as long as the delay does not extend beyond 3-4 weeks, at which time reduction of the fracture becomes relatively difficult.

47. What are the different surgical approaches to treat zygoma fractures?
Gingival buccal sulcus incision provides access to the infratemporal surface of the zygoma, allowing for reduction of the zygoma and zygomatic arch fractures with no external surgical scar. Other approaches to reduction of the zygomatic arch fracture include the Gillies approaches. Incisions to treatment of ZMC fracture include infraorbital, a lateral brow, upper blepharoplasty incision, lower eyelid incision, and superior gingivobuccal sulcus incision. Comminuted fractures of the zygoma with the need to reduce and stabilize the fragments are best approached through a coronal incision.

48. What is the most serious complication of surgical treatment of zygomatic fractures?
Although it is a rare complication, blindness is the most feared complication of surgical treatment of zygomatic and orbital fractures. This complication can result from direct damage to the optic nerve due to displacement of a bony fragment or fracture of the optic canal; edema that causes compression of the nerve; or retrobulbar hematoma. Therefore a preoperative ophthalmologic assessment of both eyes is imperative in all patients before treatment of zygomatic and orbital fractures.

49. What is the treatment for ankylosis between the zygomatic arch and coronoid process?
Coronoidectomy.

50. What is the incidence of permanent diplopia after zygomatic fracture?
Initial transient diplopia is present in up to 10% of patients and is commonly evident on upward, downward, and lateral gaze. Permanent diplopia, evident on upward gaze, remains in 5% of patients.

MAXILLARY FRACTURES

51. Who was Le Fort? What are Le Fort fractures?
René Le Fort (ca. 1901) was a French surgeon who at the end of the last century was interested in great lines of weakness in the face and the patterns of midfacial fracture. He performed a number of experiments on cadaver heads using low-velocity impact forces directed against fresh cadavers by dropping them from the top floor of buildings onto a paved courtyard. He determined three basic fault lines along which the face fractured. He observed that fractures of the midface occurred in three typical patterns, were often bilateral, and could be "mixed" (the right or left side of the face). All three types, however, involve a fracture of the pterygoid

plates. In his initial description, the highest facial fracture was referred to as No.1 (separation of the face from the cranium) and the lowest as No. 3 (maxillary fracture) that runs across the maxilla through the piriform rim.

52. What are the types of Le Fort's fractures?

Le Fort I fracture. The fracture line in these types of fractures traverses the maxilla through the piriform aperture above the alveolar ridge, above the floor of the maxillary sinus, and extends posteriorly to involve the pterygoid plates. This fracture allows the maxillae and hard palate to move separately from the upper face as a single detached block. Le Fort I fracture is often referred to as transmaxillary fracture.

Le Fort II fracture: pyramidal disjunction. Superiorly, this fracture traverses the nasal bones at the nasofrontal sutures. It extends laterally through the lacrimal bones, crossing the floor of the orbit, fracturing the medial and inferior orbital rims, and fracturing the pterygoid plates posteriorly. In this fracture, the attachment of the zygomatic bones to the skull at the lateral orbital rims and at the zygomatic arches is preserved. As a result of this fracture, the maxillary and nasal regions are movable relative to the rest of the midface and skull. Because of its triangular pattern, this fracture is often referred to as a pyramidal fracture.

Le Fort III fracture: craniofacial disjunction. This fracture line involves fracture of all the buttress bones linking the maxilla to the skull. In this type, the fractures run at the midline either across the nasal bones or across the nasofrontal suture, across the frontoethmoidal suture. Laterally the fractures run though the medial orbital wall and superior orbit, involving the frontozygomatic suture, extending through the root of the zygomatic bone, and crossing the temporal fossa to involve the pterygomaxillary space. The pterygoid plates are usually fractured free from the base of the skull. This fracture allows the entire upper face (nasal, maxillary, and zygomatic regions) to move relative to the skull. In this fracture, there is a craniofacial disjunction with a separation at the frontozygomatic suture, nasofrontal junction, orbital floor, and zygomatic arch laterally.

53. What are the clinical manifestations of midface fractures?

- Clinical diagnosis of midface fractures is reasonably easy to make when there is a displacement of the fracture, which is often manifested by presence of malocclusion, mainly an anterior open bite.
- Pain and swelling are other signs of midface fracture.
- Mobility of the midface, which can be detected by movement elicited while holding the patient's head stable with the one hand while palpating the nasofrontal junction, lateral orbital rim, and infraorbital rims with the other hand
- Nasal bleeding, subconjunctival ecchymosis, maxillary hypoesthesia, and tenderness of the bony buttresses of the midface are other signs and symptoms of midfacial and maxillary fractures.

54. What diagnostic imaging studies should be used for evaluation of maxillary fractures?

A maxillofacial CT scan, including direct or formatted coronal cuts, is the most commonly used radiographic exam for assessment of maxillary fractures in particular and midfacial fractures in general. Such studies give significantly more information than any type of conventional radiographic exam. When a fracture of the orbit is suspected, CT with coronal views is added to obtain the most accurate means to determine the degree of displacement.

55. Why is the placement of a nasogastric tube sometimes contraindicated in a midface fracture patient?

Midface fractures commonly extend through the nasal cavity and may result in soft tissue disruption in the nasopharynx with concomitant cranial injuries. Inadvertent placement of a nasogastric tube in these patients may result in the intracranial placement of the tube or soft tissue dissection in a previously traumatized region.

56. What is Battle's sign, and what is its clinical significance?

Battle's sign is ecchymosis posterior to the ear. It is generally indicative of a basilar skull fracture involving the middle cranial fossa. It is a relatively late sign presenting approximately 24 hr after injury. "Raccoon eyes" (bilateral periorbital ecchymosis) are commonly seen after fracture of the base of the anterior cranial fossa or maxillary fractures.

BIBLIOGRAPHY

1. Colton JJ, Beekhuis GJ: Management of nasal fractures. Otolaryngol Clin North Am 19:73-85, 1986.
2. Dodson BT: Zygomatic, maxillary, and orbital fractures. In Jafek BW, Murrow BW (eds): ENT Secrets, 3rd ed. Philadelphia, 2005, Hanley & Belfus.
3. Dufresne CR, Manson PN: Pediatric facial trauma. In McCarthy JG (ed): Plastic Surgery. Philadelphia, 1990, Saunders.
4. Ellis E 3rd: Fractures of the zygomatic complex and arch. In Fonseca RJ, Walker RV (eds): Oral and Maxillofacial Trauma. Philadelphia, 1991, Saunders.
5. Evans G, Manson PN, Clark N: Identification and management of minimally displaced nasoethmoidal orbital fractures. Ann Plastic Surg 35:469-471, 1995.
6. Fenner GC, Wolfe SA: Maxillary fractures. In Weinzweig J (ed): Plastic Surgery Secrets. Philadelphia, 1999, Hanley & Belfus.
7. Graper C, Milne M, Stevens MR: The traumatic saddle nose deformity: etiology and treatment. J Craniomaxillofac Trauma 2:37-49, 1996.
8. Harken AH, Moore EE (eds): Abernathy's Surgical Secrets, 5th ed. Philadelphia, 2005, Mosby.
9. Illum P: Long-term results after treatment of nasal fractures. J Laryngol Otol 100:273-277, 1986.
10. Jafek BW: Nasal trauma. In Jafek BW, Murrow BW (eds): ENT Secrets, 3rd ed. Philadelphia, 2005, Hanley & Belfus.
11. Kawamoto HK: Late posttraumatic enophthalmos: a correctable deformity? Plast Reconstr Surg 69:423-432, 1992.
12. Knight JS, North JF: The classification of malar fractures: an analysis of displacement as a guide to treatment. Br J Plast Surg 13:325-339, 1961.
13. Lenhart DE, Dolezal RF: Fractures of the nose. In Weinzweig J (ed): Plastic Surgery Secrets. Philadelphia, 1999, Hanley & Belfus.
14. Manson PN: Facial fractures. In Aston SJ, Beasley RW, Thorne CHM (eds): Grabb and Smith's Plastic Surgery, 5th ed. Philadelphia, 1997, Lippincott-Raven.
15. Manson PN: Facial fractures. In Grotting J (ed): Reoperative Aesthetic and Reconstructive Surgery. St Louis, 1994, Quality Medical.
16. Manson PN: Facial injuries. In McCarthy JG (ed): Plastic Surgery. Philadelphia, 1990, Saunders.
17. Manson PN: Midface fractures. In Georgiade N, Riefhohl R, Barwick W (eds): Plastic, Maxillofacial and Reconstructive Surgery, 2nd ed. Baltimore, 1992, Williams & Wilkins.
18. Manson PN, Clark N, Robertson B et al: Comprehensive management of panfacial fractures. J Craniomaxillofac Trauma 11:43-56, 1995.
19. Manson PN, Iliff N: Management of blow-out fractures of the orbital floor. II. Early repair for selected injuries. Surv Ophthalmol 35:280-292, 1991.
20. Markowitz B, Manson P, Sargent L et al: Management of the medial canthal ligament in nasoethmoidal orbital fractures. Plast Reconstr Surg 87:843-853, 1991.
21. Nguyen PN, Sullivan P: Advances in the management of orbital fractures. Clin Plast Surg 19:87-98, 1992.
22. Pastrick H, Bevivino BR: Zygomatic fractures. In Weinzweig J (ed): Plastic Surgery Secrets. Philadelphia, 1999, Hanley & Belfus.
23. Pollock RA: Nasal trauma: pathomechanics and surgical management of acute injuries. Clin Plast Surg 19:133-147, 1992.
24. Romano JJ, Manson PN, Mirvis WE et al: Le Fort fractures without mobility. Plast Reconstr Surg 85:355-362, 1990.
25. Schendel SA (ed): Orbital Trauma. Oral and Maxillofacial Surgery Clinics of North America, 5th vol, No. 3. Philadelphia, 1993, Saunders.
26. Weinzweig J, Bartlett SP: Fractures of the orbit. In Weinzweig J (ed): Plastic Surgery Secrets. Philadelphia, 1999, Hanley & Belfus.
27. Whitaker L, Yaremchuk M: Secondary reconstruction of posttraumatic orbital deformities. Ann Plast Surg 25:440-449, 1990.
28. Wolfe SA, Baker S: Facial Fractures. New York, 1993, Thieme.
29. Wolfe SA, Berkowitz S: Maxilla. In: Plastic Surgery of the Facial Skeleton. Boston, 1989, Little, Brown.

32. FRONTAL SINUS FRACTURES

A. Omar Abubaker, DMD, PhD

1. What are the signs of frontal sinus fracture?
History of a blow to the forehead resulting in lacerations, contusions, or hematoma should be suspected to be associated with a possible injury of the frontal sinus. Palpable or visible depression of the brow or the forehead should raise suspicion of frontal sinus involvement, although a visible or palpable depression is not always appreciated initially after injury because of swelling, edema, or hematoma. Supraorbital numbness, subconjunctival hematoma, eyelid ecchymosis, and subcutaneous air crepitus and cerebrospinal rhinorrhea are other signs of possible frontal sinus fracture.

2. What is the best radiographic modality used for diagnosis of frontal sinus fractures?
Although plain radiographs and Waters' view of the skull may show displaced frontal sinus fractures by depicting cortical malalignment or air fluid levels, they frequently miss smaller fractures and involvement of the nasofrontal duct. Conventional radiographs can also fail to show the severity of the fracture or the degree of displacement. The computed tomography (CT) scan has become the standard for evaluation of frontal sinus fractures because it allows for visualization of even small and minimally displaced fractures of the floor, septum, and anterior or posterior tables of the frontal sinus (Fig. 32-1). Direct visualization of the ducts and possible injury to the ducts also can be determined by visualizing fractures of the floor that run near the midline, cross the midline, or involve the nasoethmoidal complex. Coronal CT and three-dimensional reconstruction images may allow direct visualizing of the duct involvement in the fractures.

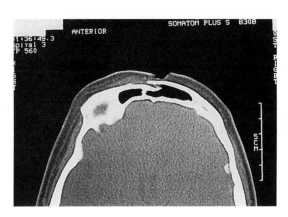

Fig. 32-1 Computed tomography scan showing an isolated outer table fracture. (From Gonty AA: Management of frontal sinus fractures and associated injuries. In Fonseca RJ [ed]: Oral and Maxillofacial Surgery, 3rd vol. Philadelphia, 2000, Saunders.)

3. What are the possible complications associated with frontal sinus fractures?
Most of the complications associated with frontal sinus injury are secondary to interference with drainage of the sinus due to obstruction of the nasofrontal duct, entrapment of mucosa in the fracture lines, or dural tears. Most complications of frontal sinus fractures occur in patients in

whom such fractures go undetected or untreated. These complications can be divided into early and late complications. Early complications include epistaxis, cerebrospinal fluid (CSF) leakage, sinusitis, mucoceles, meningitis, and intracranial hematomas. Early complications occurr within weeks after the injury. Late complications, which may appear many years later, include osteomyelitis, mucopyoceles, intracranial abscesses, and orbital abscesses.

4. What are the indications for surgical intervention in treatment of frontal sinus fractures?

The decision to operate to treat frontal sinus fractures, or merely observe these fractures, is mostly based on degree of displacement of the anterior and posterior tables and the status of the nasofrontal ducts. Nondisplaced or minimally displaced anterior table fractures can be safely observed. However, displaced anterior table fractures may require surgery if the displacement is determined to cause a cosmetic deformity at the time of presentation or later, after the swelling resolves. Similarly, minimally or nondisplaced posterior table fractures can be observed if there is no CSF leak or if the displaced posterior table fracture is less than the thickness of the cortical plate of the sinus wall. Fractures of the posterior wall that are greater than the thickness of the cortical bone, those associated with CSF leak, or those with suspicion of nasofrontal duct injury may merit surgical exploration and reduction.

5. What are the surgical approaches to exploration and repair of frontal sinus fractures?

Coronal incision provides the best access to the whole frontal sinus and frontal bone, as well as the ethmoidal, orbital, and intracranial regions, and provides the most cosmetic results. Exploration and reduction of anterior table fractures alone usually can be performed through this approach, allowing unroofing of the remaining anterior table for complete access to the sinus and reduction and fixation of the fractured segments. Posterior table fractures may require a frontal craniotomy in conjunction with a neurosurgical team to assess and repair dural or parenchymal injuries if necessary.

If the frontonasal duct is involved, and the sinus needs to be obliterated with material such as fat, muscle, or bone, cornoal approach also provides access to harvest cranial bone, temporalis muscle, fat, or fascia to be used for such purpose. Other approaches to the treatment of frontal sinus fractures include presence of a forehead laceration overlying the fractures and open sky approach. These approaches, however, are mostly useful when only the anterior table is involved.

6. What are the different management considerations for treatment of frontal sinus fractures?

Management considerations following frontal sinus fractures include assessment of the following: degree of fracture displacement; injury to the nasofrontal duct; and presence of CSF leak.

- Fractures of the anterior table alone without involvement of the nasofrontal duct can be simply reduced and stabilized with microplates to prevent cosmetic deformities.
- Fractures involving the nasofrontal duct have historically been treated with obliteration of the sinus. This procedure consists of removing all sinus mucosa from the sinus and upper duct with a high-speed burr, then packing the duct and the entire sinus with material that encourages scarring and ossification of the sinus and the duct. Many materials have been used, including autologous tissue such as bone, muscle (temporalis), fat (temporal or abdominal), fascia, and periosteal flaps; alloplastic materials such as Gelfoam and synthetic bone have also been used. All methods have been shown to have comparable success, but cancellous iliac bone and abdominal fat remain the two most popular tissues used.
- Fractures that involve a displaced or comminuted posterior table can be associated with dural tear or parenchymal brain injury and may require a craniotomy. Fractures involving only the inner table with no CSF leak are seldom treated. If a CSF leak is present, cranialization and repair of the dura are recommended. In this procedure, after any neurosurgical repair of the

dura is completed, the posterior table is removed, the floor is reduced and stabilized, the remaining mucosa and inner cortices of the sinus and duct are burred, the duct is packed with an appropriate material, as mentioned. The brain is then allowed to resume its proper location in a newly enlarged anterior cranial fossa. Finally, the anterior table is then reduced and stabilized with microplates and screws.

7. How is the risk for fracture of the frontal sinuses in children compared with adults?
The frontal sinus starts at birth and begins to appear as a pneumatic expansion at age 7 from the nasal cavity, with complete development by ages 18-20. The remnants of this embryonic connection between sinuses are the nasofrontal ducts. These bilateral structures (foramina ducts) drain the frontal sinus from its posteromedial aspect, through the ethmoidal air cells and out to the nasal cavity, usually at the middle meatus ducts. The small or nonexistent frontal sinuses in children and young adolescents make it less likely to be involved in a fracture in this age group.

BIBLIOGRAPHY

1. Disa JD, Robertson BC, Metzinger SE et al: Transverse glabellar flap for obliteration/isolation of the nasofrontal duct from the anterior cranial base. Ann Plast Surg 36:453-457, 1996.
2. Ioannides C, Freihofer HP, Friens J: Fractures of the frontal sinus: a rationale of treatment. Br J Plast Surg 46:208-214, 1993.
3. Minniti JG, Harshbarger M: Fractures of the frontal sinus. In Weinzweig J (ed): Plastic Surgery Secrets. Philadelphia, 1999, Hanley & Belfus.
4. Rohrich RJ, Hollier LH: Management of frontal sinus fractures: changing concepts. Clin Plast Surg 19:219-232, 1992.
5. Rohrich RJ, Mickel TJ: Frontal sinus obliteration: in search of the ideal autogenous material. Plast Reconstr Surg 95:580-585, 1995.
6. Wolfe SA, Johnson P: Frontal sinus injuries: primary care and management of late complications. Plast Reconstr Surg 82:781-789, 1988.

33. SOFT TISSUE INJURIES

Bashar M. Rajab, DDS, and A. Omar Abubaker, DMD, PhD

1. What are the two important mechanisms involved in protecting the human body against microbiologic invasion?
Mechanical barrier: includes the epithelium of the skin and mucous membrane. The skin provides a chemical protection in the form of surface lipids, and the mucous membranes provide protection by surface immunoglobulin (IgA) and acidic pH. The skin and oral mucosa surfaces are also inhabited by normal flora that can compete with potential microbial pathogens.
Biological barrier: provided by the activation of the kallikrein-kinin system, the release of amines, and an increase in the vascular permeability that allows for influx of humoral and cellular immunologic elements. These elements are ultimately responsible for the recognition of the organisms involved and their subsequent phagocytosis.

2. What are the classifications of soft tissue injuries?
- Contusions
- Abrasions
- Lacerations
- Flaplike lacerations
- Avulsion injuries

3.   What are the different types of soft tissue repair?
- Primary closure
- Healing with secondary intention
- Local flap
- Distance flap
- Free flap
- Specialized flap

4.   What are the types of wound closures?
- Primary closure and healing by primary intention
- Leaving the wound open, treating it with frequent dressing changes, and allowing it to heal by secondary intention and wound contracture
- Delayed primary closure, in which the wound is splinted in a position of rest with an occlusive dressing and is closed in 3-5 days when it is free of infection and necrotic tissue

The timing of wound closure has a direct correlation to the risk of infection. In general, wounds with a high risk of infection should be closed as soon as possible (within the first 6-8 hr), whereas wounds with low risk of infection, such as those in the head and neck area, can be closed primarily within the first 18-24 hr after injury. After 24 hr, for most wounds, consideration should be given to packing them open and performing a secondary repair 4-8 days later.

5.   What are the risk factors for posttraumatic soft tissue wound infections?
Factors related to the wound and patient: (1) size, configuration, and depth of the wound; (2) location of the injury; (3) mechanism of injury; (4) type and amount of contamination, including presence of foreign body; (5) time between injury and wound closure; (6) care of the wound between injury and definitive care; and (7) age and systemic condition of the patient.

Technical risk factors: (1) inadequate debridement of foreign bodies, bacterial contamination, and presence of devitalized tissues; (2) inadvertent introduction of foreign material into the wound during cleansing; (3) inadequate hemostasis and failure to eliminate dead space, which provides an environment for bacterial colonization; (4) using an excessive number of sutures to close the wound; and (5) placing excessive tension on the sutures used to approximate the tissue edges and compromising local tissue perfusion.

6.   In which area of soft tissue injury should we avoid local anesthesia with vasoconstrictor?
In areas of skin or tissue flaps of doubtful viability, where the use of vasoconstrictors might cause further impairing circulation.

7.   What is the role of irrigation with wound preparation?
Irrigation is essential in preventing infection because it removes debris, dirt, micro-organisms, and devitalized tissue from the wound, which results in a reduction in infection rate. High-pressure irrigation with normal saline has been shown to decrease the bacterial count of wounded tissues and decrease the rate of infection. The use of concentrated povidone-iodine, hydrogen peroxide, and detergents may cause significant tissue damage and should be avoided.

8.   What are the five phases to treat a posttraumatic soft tissue wound infection in head and neck?
1. Early recognition of infection
2. Rapid resuscitation and initiation of empiric antibiotics
3. Immediate surgical debridement
4. Hemodynamic and nutritional support
5. Early wound closure

9.   What are the different types of organisms isolated from a bite wound, and what is the optimal therapeutic agent for these injuries?
Dog bites: *Pasteurella canis*
Cat bites: *Pasteurella multocida* and *Pasteurella septica*

Human bites: *S. aureus, Eikenella corrodens, Haemophilus influenzae*, and beta-lactamase–producing oral anaerobic bacteria

The optimal therapeutic agents include a combination of beta-lactam antibiotic and beta-lactamase inhibitor. Oral amoxicillin-clavulanic acid will provide excellent coverage of the suspected pathogens. Ertapenem also has an excellent potency against the full range of animal and human bite pathogens.

10. **In order, what are the layers of the skin? What is the relation of the muscles of facial expression to the layers of the skin?**
1. The epidermis (stratified squamous epithelium)
   - Stratum corneum
   - Stratum lucidum
   - Stratum granulosum
   - Stratum spinosum
   - Stratum germinativum
2. The dermis
   - Papillary layer
   - Reticular layer

A thin subcutaneous layer supports the facial dermis. The muscles of facial expression are within the subcutaneous layer and insert into the reticular layer of the dermis.

11. **What is the interaction of the suture material and tissue healing process?**
Wound healing is a process that can be divided into three phases:
1. Initial lag phase (0-5 days): There is no gain in wound strength, and the wound is primarily dependent on sutures and epidermal cellular adhesion.
2. Fibroblastic phase (5-15 days): This phase has a rapid increase in wound strength.
3. Maturation phase (14 days and onward): This phase is characterized by further connective tissue remodeling.

As the tissue reduces the suture strength with time, the relative rates at which the suture material loses strength and the wound gains strength are important. Because wounds do not gain strength until 4-6 days, the entire burden of tissue approximation depends on the suture.

12. **What are the indications of a skin graft for traumatic wounds? Which areas can accept a skin graft?**
   Indications:
- To limit the amount of contractions and tissue deformity following a large skin loss
- Temporary coverage before definitive treatment

Tissues that support a skin graft are muscle, fat, fascia, dura, and periosteum. Tissues that cannot support a skin graft are cortical bone denuded of its periosteum, tendons, nerves, or cartilage.

13. **What are the classification types of free skin grafts?**
Free skin grafts are classified according to the thickness of the graft.
Split-thickness graft, which consists of the epidermis and portion of the dermis:
   - Thin (0.008-0.012 inch)
   - Medium (0.012-0.018 inch)
   - Thick (0.018-.030 inch)
Full-thickness skin graft, which includes both the epidermis and the dermis.

14. **What are the properties of both a split-thickness and full-thickness skin graft?**
   Split-thickness skin graft:
- Thin graft, which rapidly vascularizes and survives under less optimal conditions
- Can be expanded
- Multiple donor sites that heal with minimal scarring
- Thicker split-thickness skin graft closely resembles the qualities of color, texture, and limited contractions of a full-thickness skin graft.

- Usually harvested with a dermatome
    Full-thickness skin graft:
- Provides a good color, and texture match
- Optimal wound condition required
- Limited tissue contraction
- The donor site must be closed primarily.
- Usually harvested by dissection

15. What are the most common causes of graft failure?

Hematoma formation and failure of immobilization are the most common causes of graft failure.

16. What is the treatment process of a through-and-through lip laceration?

- Reapproximation of the muscular layer
- Closure of the dermis and subcutaneous layer
- Skin closure with careful alignment of the vermillion border
- Closure of the mucosal layer

17. What are the treatment options for an avulsive lip injury?

With avulsive lip injuries, one fourth of the upper lip and up to one third of the lower lip can be lost without a functional or a cosmetic defect. In these situations, tissue margins should be straightened, with the removal of a tissue wedge for primary closure.

In an extensive avulsive injury, the Abbe-Estlander flap or the Karapandzic flap can be used for lip closure.

18. What are the types of eyelid injury, and how are they managed?

Simple lacerations: should be closed in layers, restoring the orientation of the skin, muscle, tarsal, and conjunctival layers. Careful attention in approximating the lid margins should be done to avoid functional or cosmetic defects.

Upper lid lacerations: may involve detachment of the levator muscle and Muller's muscle from the tarsal plate. The muscles should be identified and reattached to the tarsal plate to prevent ptosis and restore levator function.

Laceration of the medial third of the lid: may involve the lacrimal canaliculus.

Avulsive injuries: Full-thickness avulsion of < 25% of the lid length can be repaired primarily as a simple laceration. Otherwise, avulsive injures are treated with a full-thickness skin graft from the postauricular region or the other upper eyelid.

19. What is the treatment of an eyelid injury that involves the lacrimal drainage system?

The lower canaliculus is more commonly injured than the upper canaliculus. The treatment begins with identifying the two segments of the canaliculus. A silicon tube is passed through the punctum and lateral portion of the canaliculus through the remaining medial canaliculus into the lacrimal sac, nasolacrimal duct, and the nose beneath the inferior turbinate. The other end of the tube is passed into the uninvolved punctum, traveling through the nasolacrimal duct to exit beneath the inferior turbinate. The free ends are then tied and secured in the nose. The tube is left in place for 2-3 months if epiphora persists.

20. What is the course of the parotid duct?

The duct exits from the anterior portion of the gland and passes interiorly superficial to the masseter muscle parallel with a plane drawn from the tragus of the ear to the midpoint of the upper lip. One cm anterior to the anterior border of the masseter muscle, the duct turns medially and penetrates the buccinator muscle, opening into the mouth at the level of the second maxillary molar.

21. What are the ways to diagnose a parotid duct injury?
- Attempt to identify the location of the clear fluid in the wound after pressing the gland to express saliva.
- Direct inspection ductal with a lacrimal probe cannulation of the distal aspect of the duct
- Injection of methylene blue or milk into the duct in a retrograde fashion
- Radiographic exam (sialogram or computed tomography [CT] imaging)

22. How is a parotid ductal injury managed?
- Place an Intracath stent through the distal portion of the duct from the oral orifice.
- Identify the proximal portion of the duct, which can be facilitated by massaging the gland to express saliva. The proximal end is then cannulated.
- Close the ends of the duct over the Intracath with small nylon or Prolene sutures.
- Secure the Intracath to the buccal mucosa.
- Layer the closure of the wound and place an external pressure dressing for 24-48 hr.
- Leave the catheter left in place for 10-14 days.

If the repair of the ductal injury is determined to be impossible, the proximal portion of the duct should be ligated. This will result in physiologic death of the gland.

23. What is the treatment process of parotid duct injury in relation to the location of the injury?
- Within the parotid gland: closure of the parotid capsule and application of pressure dressing
- Over the masseter muscle: primary anastomosis
- Anterior to the masseter muscle: If primary anastomosis is impossible, the proximal portion of the duct can be drained directly into the mouth by creating a new opening.

24. What is the etiology and treatment of ear hematomas?
The etiology of auricular hematoma is most commonly a blunt trauma. The extravasated blood is replaced by fibrous tissue or new cartilage, if not evacuated, resulting in the "cauliflower ear." The hematoma also caries the risk of secondary infection.

Treatment: evacuation of the hematoma by needle aspiration if done soon after the injury, or incision and drainage may be required in late treatment of the hematoma. Application of an external pressure dressing (bolster dressing) after hematoma evacuation will prevent reformation of the hematoma.

25. What are the ear injury classifications? What are their most common treatments?
Lacerations: The wound should be closed primarily, preserving and maintaining all attached tissue due to the rich blood supply to the auricle.

Avulsive injuries: Avulsion of the skin can be addressed by a pedicle posterior auricular flap. Exposed cartilage will not accept a skin graft. Full-thickness tissue and loose or severely damaged tissue may require full-thickness excision with primary closure and reducing the auricle size.

Total avulsion:
- Simple reattachment as a composite graft. The ear is cleansed and sutured directly into the vascular bed. Small incisions are made in the skin to decrease venous congestion. Administration of dextran or heparin to decrease blood viscosity might be helpful. Most clinicians believe that the greatest success is seen with reattachment within 4 hr.
- The pocket principle. The ear is thoroughly dermabraded, a posterior auricular incision is made, and a pocket is created into which the auricle is tucked. After 10-14 days, the auricle is retrieved and allowed to reepithelialize.

26. What craniofacial injuries are accompanied by facial nerve palsy?

Fractures of the temporal bone as a part of skull-base fractures may cause facial nerve palsy. In absence of facial laceration, a CT scan of the temporal bone may show such injury. High-dose steroids and decompression are considered for certain injuries. The prognosis varies with the site of the fracture.

27. What are the causes of traumatic transection of the lacrimal system? How is it diagnosed, and how is it treated?

It is usually caused by a laceration in the vicinity of the medial canthus or accompanies Le Fort or nasoethmoidal fractures. The lacrimal punctum may be dilated and saline squirted through the punctum into the system. Appearance of saline in the wound is diagnostic of a canalicular laceration.

Treatment of these transections can be accomplished by placement of tubes into the nose, through the lacerated canaliculus to splint the repair. Both upper and lower canalicular lacerations should be explored and repaired if needed. Repair and repositioning of the fracture fragments often permit adequate function of the system. Repair of a chronically obstructed nasal lacrimal duct is accomplished with a dacryocystorhinostomy.

28. Do facial lacerations require debridement before their repair?

The facial blood supply is excellent, and often areas of contused tissue will heal but with increased scarring. Therefore the zone of contusion should be excised, if permitted by flexibility and availability of soft tissue. However, excision should not be performed in the upper and lower eyelid areas because the eyelids may not be able to close completely over the globe. In general, excision also should not be performed in eyelid or eyelid margin lacerations, nostril rim lacerations, or lacerations of the lip margins or ear because distortion may be noticeable even with minimal tissue deficiency at the suture line. In other areas, resection of the contused skin allows conversion to a primary surgically created wound with more predictable healing and generally improved appearance. A layered repair of the facial soft tissue should be performed.

29. What is the appropriate management of tongue lacerations?

The tongue has a very rich blood supply that can lead to significant bleeding. At the same time, the tongue has a remarkable ability to heal in a very short period. Therefore small tongue lacerations, especially in children, often do not warrant primary repair. However, large lacerations, especially in the presence of bleeding and possible dislodgement of foreign bodies, are worthy of exploration and repair. After local anesthesia administration, the wound is closed in layers with resorbable sutures. Large lacerations merit a thorough evaluation of the airway because of the possibility of significant swelling and posterior displacement of the tongue. Wounds should be explored and radiographs taken to rule out the presence of foreign bodies, such as dental fragments.

30. What management considerations are required in repairing an ear laceration?

A complete physical exam evaluating the pinna, external auditory canal, tympanic membrane, and hearing is essential before treatment of external ear injuries. The pinna is the most frequently lacerated component of the ear, consisting of a relatively avascular cartilage layer covered by a thin, but richly vascular, skin layer. Management includes local anesthesia without vasoconstrictor, conservative debridement, and placement of 6.0 nylon skin sutures aligning known landmarks and reapproximating the soft tissue envelope. Suturing the cartilaginous framework is seldom required; however, fine, permanent tacking sutures may be used. Hematoma formation requires drainage, either through fine-needle aspiration or a small incision. Some type of pressure dressing is required to prevent reaccumulation of blood; this can be most easily accomplished using a transcartilaginous horizontal mattress suture and bolster dressing.

31. What anatomic structures need to be evaluated in a patient with a large through-and-through laceration of the cheek?

Cheek lacerations may involve several underlying vital structures, including the parotid gland and duct, facial nerve branches, facial artery and its branches, and the buccal fat pad. Careful exam of the wound to identify these structures is warranted. Laceration of the parotid duct requires the placement of a stent and careful suturing of the cut ends with 6.0 nylon suture under magnification. Overlying tissues are then closed in layers. Gland injuries without duct involvement should be closed routinely and followed for sialocele or parotid fistula formation, which may be treated using pressure dressings or antisialagogues. Facial nerve lacerations proximal to a vertical perpendicular line through the lateral canthus are amenable to surgical repair. The buccal fat should be preserved and replaced, if possible, to prevent cosmetic deformity or cheek hollowing.

32. What percentage of tissue can be lost without a significant cosmetic defect after primary closure in an avulsive injury of the upper and lower lips?

Avulsive injuries to the upper lip can involve 20%-25% of lip structure and still be closed primarily without significant functional or cosmetic deformity. The lower lip is even more forgiving, allowing primary closure of defects involving 30%-35% of lip structure. In all lip repairs, attention must be given to proper alignment of the vermilion border and orbicularis oris muscles. Significant avulsive injuries may be amenable to repair via Abbe or local rotational flaps.

33. How do animal and human bites differ from other traumatic injuries?

Animal and human bites differ from other traumatic injuries because they are contaminated by the oral flora. Thorough cleansing and debridement of the wound with the use of copious normal saline irrigation is essential before closure. Facial wounds can then be closed in routine layered fashion. Wound infections from human bites are frequently caused by *Streptococcus* and *Staphylococcus* organisms. Serious infections may also be associated with *Eikenella*. Prophylactic antibiotic coverage with penicillin or amoxicillin-clavulanic acid is recommended. Unlike human bites, 50%-75% of infections in animal bites are caused by *P. multocida*. Amoxicillin-clavulanic acid is recommended for prophylaxis in animal bites. Tetanus immunization is required for all bites, and rabies prophylaxis may be required when animals exhibit suspicious behavior.

34. What are the zones of the neck, and how are they assessed in penetrating neck injuries?

Penetrating trauma to the neck carries significant risk of vascular injury. In an attempt to standardize management, three zones of the neck have been defined. Zone 1 extends from the clavicle to cricoid cartilage, zone 2 extends from the cricoid cartilage to the mandibular angle, and zone 3 extends from the mandibular angle to the base of the skull. Diagnosis of vascular injury by physical exam or exploratory surgery is most easily accomplished in zone 2, whereas zone 1 and 3 injuries often remain obscure. Similarly, surgical repair of zone 2 injuries is frequently successful, whereas repair of zones 1 and 3 is often fraught with danger. Consequently, arteriography and possible embolization are the recommended treatment modalities for wounds in zones 1 and 3.

35. What distinguishes facial from other lacerations?[*]

Appearance is clearly of primary importance. Quality of the final result depends on strict adherence to basic principles of wound management and painstaking technique. Copious irrigation,

---

*Reprinted from Ketch LL: Facial lacerations. In Harken AH, Moore EE (eds): Abernathy's Surgical Secrets, 5th ed. Philadelphia, 2005, Mosby.

judicious debridement, gentle tissue handling, meticulous hemostasis, and minimization of sutures combined with early stitch removal are critical to an optimal result. Fine suture and sharp instruments should be used; eversion of the wound margin with layered closure, obliteration of dead space, and lack of tension are mandatory.

36. How are clean lacerations repaired?*

They should be irrigated with normal saline or Ringer's lactate. Only the surrounding skin should be prepared, and no antiseptic should be introduced into the wound. Regional anesthesia is preferred because of the potential for spread of contamination with direct injection of the wound margin. Epinephrine should be avoided because it devitalizes tissue and potentiates infection. Wounds should be repaired in layers with absorbable suture in deep tissue. The smallest number of sutures necessary to overcome the natural resting wound tension should be used. Sutures should be removed within 3-5 days, and the wound margin should be subsequently supported with Steri-Strips.

37. How are dirty lacerations repaired?*

Heavily contaminated wounds should remain open after irrigation and debridement to undergo delayed closure. Because of cosmetic considerations, however, this approach is unacceptable in the face. For this reason, meticulous debridement of devitalized tissue and removal of all foreign material is essential. The wound should be cultured before copious irrigation, and a broad-spectrum antibiotic should be instituted prophylactically. The patient must be informed of the potential of a postrepair infection.

38. What factors influence suture selection?*

Any method of suturing provokes tissue damage, impairs host defense, increases scar proliferation, and invites infection. Presence of a single silk suture in a wound lowers the infective threshold by a factor of 10,000. Therefore fine monofilament suture, just strong enough to overcome the resting wound tension, should be used. Use as few sutures as possible. Wounds with little or no retraction may be closed with tape alone.

39. Which wounds are suitable for closure with tissue adhesives?*

N-butyl-2-cyanoacrylate may suffice for cutaneous closure of low-tension lacerations in children (preferred method) and adults. This adhesive effectively closes low-tension lacerations. This method is fast and relatively painless. It has a low complication rate and produces excellent cosmetic outcomes. In many instances, if initial wound orientation is against Langer's lines, it may, in fact, offer an advantage over conventional manual suturing.

40. Should eyebrows be shaved when facial lacerations are repaired?*

No. They provide a landmark for realignment of disrupted tissue edges and do not always grow back.

41. Should skin grafts or flaps be used for primary closure of a wound?*

Complicated tissue transfer techniques have no place in the acute treatment of facial wounds. Closure should be achieved in the simplest way possible and complex reconstructive efforts should be deferred until the scar has matured (months). When tissue loss prevents closure, it may be necessary to use a thin split-thickness skin graft for coverage.

42. When are antibiotics indicated in the treatment of facial lacerations?*

Copious irrigation, debridement, and gentle tissue handling are more pertinent to the prevention of infection than the use of antibiotics in clean and clean-contaminated wounds. Antibiotic coverage is indicated, however, in crush avulsion injuries, bites, and heavily contaminated injuries.

43. When should scars be revised?[*]

A scar usually has its worst appearance at 2 weeks to 2 months after suturing. Scar revision should await complete maturation, which may take 4-24 months. A good rule of thumb is to undertake no revisions for at least 6-12 months after initial repair. The maturation of the wound may be assessed by its degree of discomfort, erythema, and induration.

BIBLIOGRAPHY

1. Amiel GE, Sukhotnik I, Kawar B et al: Use of *N*-butyl-2-cyanoacrylate in elective surgical incisions: long-term outcomes. J Am Coll Surg 189:21-25, 1999.
2. Farion KJ, Osmond MH, Hartling L et al: Tissue adhesives for traumatic lacerations: a systematic review of randomized controlled trials. Acad Emerg Med 10:110-118, 2003.
3. Hollander JE, Richman PB, WerBlud M et al: Irrigation in facial and scalp lacerations: does it alter outcome? Ann Emerg Med 31:73-77, 1998.
4. Ketch LL: Facial lacerations. In Harken AH, Moore EE (eds): Abernathy's Surgical Secrets, 5th ed. Philadelphia, 2005, Mosby.
5. Mitchell RB, Nanez G, Wagner JD et al: Dog bites of the scalp, face, and neck in children. Laryngoscope 113:492-495, 2003.
6. Quinn J, Wells G, Sutcliffe T et al: A randomized trial comparing octylcyanoacrylate tissue adhesive and sutures in the management of lacerations. JAMA 277:1527-1530, 1997.
7. Simon HK, Zempsky WT, Burns TB et al: Lacerations against Langer's lines: to glue or suture? J Emerg Med 16:185-189, 1998.

34. OROFACIAL INFECTIONS AND ANTIBIOTIC USE

A. Omar Abubaker, DMD, PhD

1. What is the source of the bacteria that cause most odontogenic infections?

Odontogenic infections are caused mostly by indigenous bacteria that normally live on or in the host. When such bacteria gain access to deeper tissues, they cause odontogenic infection.

2. What are the predominant bacteria found in the oral cavity?

See Box 34-1.

3. Which species of bacteria cause odontogenic infection?

Most of the microorganisms associated with odontogenic infections are gram-negative rods (fusobacteria, bacteroides). Some are gram-positive cocci (streptococci and peptostreptococci), and 25% are aerobic, mostly gram-positive streptococci. About 60% are anaerobic bacteria. Almost all odontogenic infections are caused by multiple bacteria (an average of five species). *Fusobacterium* sp. is associated with severe infections (Fig. 34-1 and Table 34-1).

4. Which staphylococci are clinically important to orofacial infections?

Of the 23 species of staphylococci, only three are clinically important to orofacial infections: *Staphylococcus aureus*, *Staphylococcus epidermidis*, and *Staphylococcus saprophyticus*.

5. What is coagulase? Which *Staphylococcus* species produces coagulase?

Coagulase is an enzyme that coats the bacteria with fibrin and reduces the ability of the host cell to phagocytize it. *S. aureus* is the only coagulase-positive staphylococcus.

Box 34-1	*Predominant Bacteria Found in the Oral Cavity*
AEROBES	ANAEROBES
Gram-positive rods	Gram-positive rods
Corynebacterium	*Actinomyces*
Rothia	*Lactobacillus*
Diphtheroids	*Propionibacterium acnes*
Gram-negative rods	*Bifidobacterium*
Eikenella corrodens	*Eubacterium*
Haemophilus	*Clostridia*
Enterobacteriaceae	Gram-negative rods
Klebsiella	*Bacteroides*
Pseudomonas	*B. gingivalis*
Escherichia	*B. intermedius*
Gram-positive cocci	*B. endontalis*
Streptococcus	*B. oralis*
Alpha-hemolytic	*B. melaninogenicus*
Strep. salivarius	*Fusobacterium*
Strep. mitior	*F. nucleatum*
Strep. sanguis	*Wolinella*
Strep. mutans	*Capnocytophaga*
Strep. milleri	Gram-positive cocci
Beta-hemolytic	*Peptostreptococcus*
Strep. pyogenes	*Streptococcus*
Enterococci	Gram-negative cocci
Staphylococcus	*Veillonella*
Staph. aureus	
Staph. epidermidis	
Gram-negative cocci	
Neisseria	
Branhamella	
Spirochetes	
Treponema	
Fungi	
Candida	

Adapted from Peterson LJ: Microbiology of head and neck infections. Oral Maxillofacial Surg Clin 3:247-258, 1991.

6.   What is the basis for microbiologic diagnosis of odontogenic infection?
Initially, an empirical diagnosis of the causative organism of odontogenic infection is made, based on the presumption of involvement of bacteria typical for the site (oral flora). The microbiologic diagnosis stems from this presumption and can be confirmed via Gram stain and culture.

7.   What is Gram staining? What is its clinical significance?
Each specimen obtained from a patient with an infectious process initially should be stained according to the protocol developed by Hans Christian Joachim Gram. The process involves staining, decolorizing, and restaining the specimen with a different stain. The organisms are

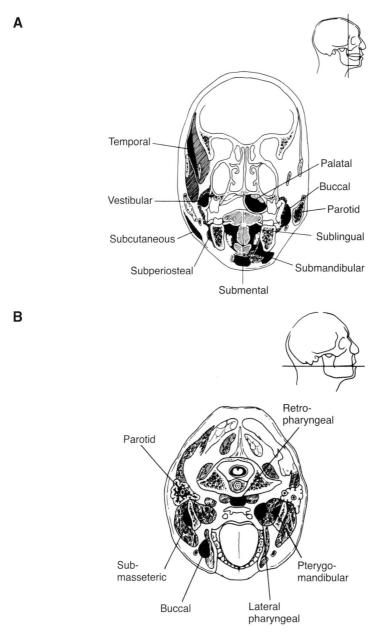

Fig. 34-1 Anatomy of the deep space infections. **A**, Coronal, and **B**, Axial sections of the head showing most of the deep fascial spaces of the head and neck. (From Eycleshymer AC, Schoemaker DM: Cross-Section Anatomy. New York, 1911, D. Appleton & Company.)

Table 34-1 *Species of Bacteria Responsible for Odontogenic Infections*

ORGANISM	PERCENTAGE
Aerobic[*]	25
Gram-positive cocci	85
Streptococcus spp.	90
Streptococcus (group D) spp.	2
Staphylococcus spp.	6
Eikenella spp.	2
Gram-negative cocci (*Neisseria* spp.)	2
Gram-positive rods (*Corynebacterium* spp.)	3
Gram-negative rods (*Haemophilus* spp.)	6
Miscellaneous and undifferentiated	4
Anaerobic[†]	75
Gram-positive cocci	30
Streptococcus spp.	33
Peptococcus spp.	33
Peptostreptococcus spp.	33
Gram-negative cocci (*Veillonella* spp.)	4
Gram-positive rods	14
Eubacterium spp.	
Lactobacillus spp.	
Actinomyces spp.	
Clostridia spp.	
Gram-negative-rods	50
Bacteroides spp.	75
Fusobacterium spp.	25
Miscellaneous	6

Adapted from Peterson LJ: Principles of management and prevention of odontogenic infection. In Peterson LJ, Ellis E, Hupp J et al (eds): Contemporary Oral and Maxillofacial Surgery, 2nd ed. St Louis, 1998, Mosby.
[*]49 different species.
[†]119 different species.

categorized into one of four groups based on their stain retention and morphology: gram-positive cocci, gram-negative cocci, gram-negative rods, or gram-positive rods. Because Gram staining can be completed within a few minutes, it usually narrows the list of likely causative organisms immediately, whereas culture and sensitivity testing and biochemical identification may take 1-5 days to complete.

8. What is the Gram stain process?
- The smear of specimen is heat-fixed to the slide and stained with crystal violet. The cells will appear dark blue or purple.
- The slide is placed in a dilute solution of iodine, which further fixes the violet stain to the cell by forming a crystal-violet-iodine complex.
- The slide is rinsed in a 95% solution of alcohol, or alcohol and acetone. The cell walls of microorganisms with high lipid contents develop porosities, allowing for loss of the violet stain. In organisms with more carbohydrates in their cell walls, the violet stain-iodine complex is further fixed by the alcohol.
- The specimen is counterstained with a red dye, safranin. Organisms that retained their initial

stain will remain violet (gram-positive), whereas those that lost the initial stain will be restained red (gram-negative).

9. **How do morphologic findings relate to bacterial categories (Table 34-2)?**

Table 34-2   *The Relation of Morphologic Findings to Bacterial Categories*

MORPHOLOGIC FINDINGS	BACTERIAL SPECIES
Gram-positive cocci, single or clumps	*Micrococcus, Peptococcus, Staphylococcus*
Gram-positive cocci, pairs and chains	*Enterococcus, Peptostreptococcus, Streptococcus*
Gram-positive rods, large	*Bacillus, Clostridium*
Gram-positive rods, small	*Arachnia, Bacterionema, Bifidobacterium, Corynebacterium, Erysipelothrix, Eubacterium, Lactobacillus, Listeria, Propionibacterium*
Gram-positive rods, branching	*Actinomyces, Nocardia*
Gram-negative rods, large	Enterobacteriaceae
Gram-negative rods, thin, uniform	*Pseudomonas*
Gram-negative rods, small, coccobacillary	*Bacteroides, Bordetella, Brucella, Capnocytophaga, Cardiobacterium, Eikenella, Fusobacterium, Haemophilus, Pasteurella*
Gram-negative rods, nonspecific morphology	*Alcaligenes, Campylobacter, Cardiobacterium, Flavobacterium, Pectobacterium, Chromobacterium, Helicobacter, Vibrio, Yersinia*
Gram-negative cocci, pairs	*Acinetobacter, Moraxella, Neisseria*
Gram-negative cocci	*Veillonella*

Adapted from Bartlett RC: Laboratory diagnostic techniques. In Tobazian RG, Goldberg MH (eds): Oral and Maxillofacial Infections, 3rd ed. Philadelphia, 1994, Saunders.

10. **What is the progression of odontogenic infections?**
    Early infection is often initiated by high-virulence aerobic organisms (commonly streptococci), which cause cellulitis, followed by mixed aerobic and anaerobic infections. As the infections become more chronic (abscess stage), the anaerobic bacteria predominate, and eventually the infection becomes exclusively anaerobic.

11. **What is cellulitis?**
    Cellulitis is a warm, diffuse, erythematous, indurated, and painful swelling of the tissue in an infected area. Cellulitis can be easy to treat but can also be severe and life threatening. Antibiotics and removal of the cause are usually sufficient. Surgical incision and drainage are indicated if no improvement is seen in 2-3 days, or if evidence of purulent collection is identified.

12. **What is an abscess?**
    An abscess is a pocket of tissue containing necrotic tissue, bacterial colonies, and dead white cells. The area of infection may or may not be fluctuant. The patient is often febrile at this stage. Cellulitis, which may be associated with abscess formation, is often caused by anaerobic bacteria.

13. What is the difference between an abscess and cellulitis (Table 34-3)?

Table 34-3   *A Comparison of Cellulites and Abscess*

	CELLULITIS	ABSCESS
Duration	Acute	Chronic
Pain	Severe and generalized	Localized
Size	Large	Small
Localization	Diffuse borders	Well circumscribed
Palpation	Doughy to indurated	Fluctuant
Presence of pus	No	Yes
Degree of seriousness	Greater	Less
Bacteria	Aerobic	Anaerobic

Adapted from Peterson LJ: Principles of management and prevention of odontogenic infection. In Peterson LJ, Ellis E, Hupp J et al (eds): Contemporary Oral and Maxillofacial Surgery, 2nd ed. St Louis, 1998, Mosby.

14. What are the signs and symptoms of a serious orofacial infection?
Serious infection occurs when the infection extends beyond the local area of infection and presents life-threatening systemic manifestations, including airway compromise, bacteremia, septicemia, fever, lethargy, fatigue, malaise, and dehydration. Swelling, induration, fluctuation, trismus, rapidly progressing infection, involvement of secondary spaces, dysphagia, odynophagia, and drooling are also signs and symptoms of serious orofacial infection.

15. What factors influence the spread of odontogenic infection?
- Thickness of bone adjacent to the offending tooth
- Position of muscle attachment in relation to root tip
- Virulence of the organism
- Status of patient's immune system

16. What are the *primary* fascial spaces?
The spaces directly adjacent to the origin of the odontogenic infections. Infections spread from the origin into these spaces, which are:
- Buccal
- Canine
- Sublingual
- Submandibular
- Submental
- Vestibular

17. What are the *secondary* fascial spaces?
Fascial spaces that become involved following spread of infection to the primary spaces (Fig. 34-2). The secondary spaces are:
- Pterygomandibular
- Infratemporal
- Masseteric
- Lateral pharyngeal
- Superficial and deep temporal
- Retropharyngeal
- Masticator
- Prevertebral

18. What is the danger space?
Also called space 4 of Grodinsky and Holyoke, it is the potential space between alar and prevertebral fascia. Its superior limit is the skull base, and it extends inferiorly into the posterior mediastinum.

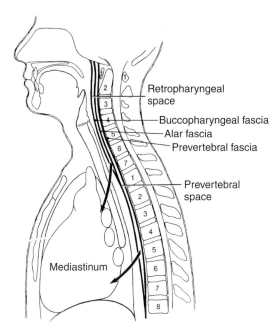

Fig. 34-2 Retropharyngeal and prevertebral spaces, with the potential for spread of infection to the mediastinum from these spaces. (From Peterson LJ: Odontogenic infections. In Cummings CW, Fredrickson JM, Harker LA et al [eds]: Otolaryngology: Head and Neck Surgery, 3rd ed. St Louis, 1998, Mosby.)

Retropharyngeal space

Buccopharyngeal fascia
Alar fascia
Prevertebral fascia

Prevertebral space

Mediastinum

19. What are the seven spaces of Grodinsky and Holyoke in the head and neck?
1. Space 1: between platysma and investing fascia
2. Space 2: between investing and infrahyoid fascias
3. Space 2a: space among infrahyoid muscles
4. Space 3: the pretracheal and retrovisceral spaces
5. Space 4: danger space and between prevertebral and alar fascia
6. Space 4a: between prevertebral and investing fascia above clavicle
7. Space 5: space within prevertebral fascia

20. Which teeth are likely to be the cause of space infections? What are the surgical approaches for incision and drainage of these spaces?
See Table 34-4 and Fig. 34-3.

21. What imaging and lab studies are used for diagnosis of odontogenic infections?
- Radiographs to identify the cause of infection: periapical, occlusal, and panoramic views
- Imaging studies to identify the extent of infection and presence of purulent collection: computed tomography (CT), magnetic resonance imaging (MRI), soft tissue films, and ultrasound
- Lab studies to evaluate the immune system: white cell and differential counts

22. What are the principles of therapy for odontogenic infection?
The important components in treatment of odontogenic infection are:
- Determining the severity of infection
- Determining whether the infection is at the cellulitis or abscess stage
- Evaluating the state of the patient's host defense mechanisms

Text continued on p. 306

Table 34-4 *Teeth Likely to Cause Fascial Space Infections, with Surgical Approaches*

FASCIAL SPACE	ANATOMIC BOUNDARIES OF SPACE	LIKELY SOURCE OF INFECTION	SWELLING SITE	SITE OF I&D
Canine	Between canine fossa, zygomaticus, orbicularis oris, levator labii superioris and levator anguli oris	Maxillary canines, especially with very long roots and apex situated above attachment of muscles. May also be caused by central, lateral or premolar teeth.	Extraoral swelling just lateral to nose, obliterating nasolabial fold and may extend upward, causing periorbital cellulites. May be in labial sulcus.	Intraoral incision in horizontal direction in mucobuccal fold. Rarely, space is drained extraorally.
Buccal	Check area between buccinator and buccopharyngeal fascia medially, overlying skin laterally, zygomatic muscle and depressor muscles anteriorly, zygomatic arch superiorly, lower border of mandible inferiorly, and pterygomandibular raphe posteriorly	Upper premolars Upper molars and lower premolars	Extraoral swelling over cheek area between inferior border of mandible and zygomatic arch. Typically, if inferior border of mandible palpable, it is buccal space; if inferior border is not palpable, then involved space is submandibular.	Intraoral by a transverse incision to depth of buccinator muscle passing through mucosa, submucosa, and buccinator muscle, avoiding injury to important anatomic structures, such as parotid duct. Drainage also accomplished by extraoral incision near point of fluctuance below Stensen's duct.
Sublingual	Above mylohyoid muscle. Roof of space is mucosa of floor of mouth; floor is made by mylohyoid, genioglossus, geniohyoid, and styloglossus muscles, tongue, and lingual	From teeth of root apices above mylohyoid muscle attachment, namely lower premolars and sometimes first molars	Infection spread lingual in floor of mouth causing sublingual swelling involving contralateral side (because barrier between two sides is	Intraoral incision parallel to Worton's duct and lingual cortex in anteroposterior direction, as close as possible (within 1 cm) to lingual

I&D, Incision and drainage.

Table 34-4 Teeth Likely to Cause Fascial Space Infections, with Surgical Approaches—cont'd

FASCIAL SPACE	ANATOMIC BOUNDARIES OF SPACE	LIKELY SOURCE OF INFECTION	SWELLING SITE	SITE OF I&D
	frenum (medial raphe).		very weak)	cortical bone because sublingual fold contains sublingual gland and ducts of submandibular gland. Intraoral-extraoral approach may be used.
Submandibular	Below mylohyoid muscle. Lies inferior to mylohyoid muscle; inferior boundary is anterior and posterior bellies of digastric muscles. Medially, mylohyoid hyoglossus, and styloglossus muscles bound space. Lateral boundary is skin, superficial fascia, platysma muscle, superficial layer of deep cervical fascia, and lateral border of mandible.	Lower molars, especially lower second and third molars	Swelling mostly extraoral due to pus accumulation between skin and mylohyoid muscle. Swelling begins by obliterating inferior border of mandible, then extends medially to anterior belly of digastric and posterior to hyoid bone.	Through extraoral incision parallel to inferior border of mandible, kept at least 1 cm from border to avoid injury to mandibular branch of facial nerve, submandibular gland, facial artery, and lingual nerve
Submental	Between hyoid bone and symphysis, at site of attachment of anterior belly of digastric muscle. Roof of space is mylohyoid muscle, floor is skin, laterally is anterior belly of digastric muscle.	Lower incisors and canines, or from trauma such as symphyseal fracture	Mostly extraoral. Chin and submental areas swollen. Pus situated between digastric muscle, mylohyoid muscle, and skin. Rarely, there is submental swelling only. Usually submental and submandibular swelling because boundaries between	Extraoral transverse incision midway between symphysis and hyoid bone

Continued

Table 34-4 Teeth Likely to Cause Fascial Space Infections, with Surgical Approaches—cont'd

FASCIAL SPACE	ANATOMIC BOUNDARIES OF SPACE	LIKELY SOURCE OF INFECTION	SWELLING SITE	SITE OF I&D
			two spaces are not definitive (only digastric muscle), so pus travels posteriorly to submandibular region.	
Masseteric	Between outer surface of ascending ramus medially and masseter muscle laterally	Can spread from a buccal space infection site of attachment of buccinator muscle. Also from pericoronitis of lower third molars, or from fracture of angle of mandible.	Extraoral swelling over area occupied by masseter muscles, which is over ascending ramus and angle of mandible. Infection of this space characterized by trismus due to involvement of muscles of mastication.	Approximately 4-cm-long incision made below and behind angle of ascending ramus. Dissection carried through skin, superficial fascia, and platysma muscles. When inserting, artery forceps should remain in contact with outer aspect of ascending ramus. Incision can be used to approach two spaces (masseteric and pterygoid mandibular). Masseteric space can also be drained through an intraoral incision or a combined intraoral extraoral approach.
Pterygo-mandibular	Between ascending ramus and medial pterygoid muscle medially; laterally	Can result from infection of molar teeth, especially third molar; spread from	Intraoral swelling of mucosa over medial aspect of the ascending	Can be drained extraorally at angle of mandible. When inserting, artery

Table 34-4   Teeth Likely to Cause Fascial Space Infections, with Surgical Approaches—cont'd

FASCIAL SPACE	ANATOMIC BOUNDARIES OF SPACE	LIKELY SOURCE OF INFECTION	SWELLING SITE	SITE OF I&D
	is inner surface of ascending ramus. Superiorly, space bound by lateral pterygoid muscle, posteriorly by parotid gland, and anteriorly by pterygomandibular raphe and superior constrictor of pharynx.	infratemporal space, which communicates freely with pterygomandibular space; septic inferior dental nerve block with contaminated needle or solution; pericoronitis; spread from submandibular space infection; spread from sublingual space	ramus. Extraorally, swelling is extremely rare, but if seen is found near mandibular angle area. Sometimes no extraoral swelling at all, only trismus due to involvement of medial pterygoid muscle, especially when infection is caused by inferior dental nerve block.	forceps should remain in contact with inner surface of ascending ramus. This space can also be drained through intraoral incision placed just medial to pterygomandibular raphe and by dissecting posteriorly along medial surface of ramus of mandible. Incision can also be used to drain lateral pharyngeal space and inferior portion of infratemporal space.
Temporal	Muscle divides into two spaces: superficial temporal between temporalis muscle and temporal fascia, and deep temporal space (infratemporal space) between temporalis muscle and bony wall of skull medially. Temporal space is contiguous pterygomandibular and masseteric spaces.	Infection usually originates from upper and lower molars, or from extension of infection from masseteric or pterygomandibular spaces through infratemporal space, or from spread of infection from posterior superior alveolar nerve block	Extraoral swelling just behind lateral orbital rim and above zygomatic arch	Infection of this space is almost always associated with trismus; thus is difficult to approach intraorally. Extraoral approach more practical, but intraoral is preferred. Intraoral site for I&D is placed at anterior border of ascending ramus, with forceps inserted on outer aspect of ascending ramus

Continued

Table 34-4   *Teeth Likely to Cause Fascial Space Infections, with Surgical Approaches—cont'd*

FASCIAL SPACE	ANATOMIC BOUNDARIES OF SPACE	LIKELY SOURCE OF INFECTION	SWELLING SITE	SITE OF I&D
				and directed up. Extraoral incision is through transverse incision starting slightly superior to zygomatic arch and extending posteriorly between lateral orbital rim and hairline. Incision is made parallel to it to avoid zygomatic branch of facial nerve.
Lateral pharyngeal	Inverted cone shape extending from base of skull to hyoid bone. Situated just medial to pterygomandibular space. Lateral wall made up of medial pterygoid muscle and superior constrictor muscle. Posteriorly, boundary is parotid gland, and anteriorly is pterygomandibular raphe. Medial wall is continuous with carotid sheath. Styloid process divides this space into two compartments:	Infection can result from infection of lower and upper molars by way of neighboring spaces, such as submandibular or pterygomandibular spaces. Can also result from nonodontogenic sources, such as palatine tonsils, infected parotid gland, and infected lymph nodes. If infection of this space is not treated at early stage, it can readily spread to retropharyngeal and	Most common site is an intraoral swelling of lateral pharyngeal wall (very characteristic). Medial displacement of uvula and palatal draping may also be present. Extraoral lateral swelling of neck immediately below angle of mandible and anterior to anterior border of sternocleidomastoid muscle also possible.	Intraoral drainage of anterior compartment via a similar incision to that of intraoral incision for drainage of pterygomandibular space. Incision made through mucosa, and dissection directed medially and posteriorly along medial side of medial pterygoid muscle. Extraoral approach through horizontal incision made at level of hyoid bone just anterior to sterno-

Table 34-4   Teeth Likely to Cause Fascial Space Infections, with Surgical Approaches—cont'd

FASCIAL SPACE	ANATOMIC BOUNDARIES OF SPACE	LIKELY SOURCE OF INFECTION	SWELLING SITE	SITE OF I&D
	anterior compartment, which contains mainly muscles, and posterior compartment, which contains several important structures, namely carotid sheaths inside which are external carotid artery, internal jugular vein, and CN X. Outside sheaths are CN IX, XI, and XII.	prevertebral spaces.		cleidomastoid. Dissection made superiorly and medially between submandibular gland and posterior belly of digastric muscle until medial surface of medial pterygoid muscle reached. Dissection carried along surface of muscle into space. Space can also be drained using through-and through drainage.
Retropha-ryngeal	Extending from base of skull superiorly to upper mediastinum inferiorly (level of C6 or T1 behind posterior pharyngeal wall). Anteriorly, space is bounded by posterior wall of pharynx and posterior to it lies "danger space," which communicates with posterior mediastinum.	Spreads from upper and lower molars by extension from lateral pharyngeal space by way of pterygomandibular, submandibular, or sublingual spaces. Retropharyngeal and lateral pharyngeal spaces separated by thin layer of fascia, which can easily rupture and cause spread of infection.	If able to visualize pharynx, bulge of posterior pharyngeal wall will be noticed—usually unilateral. Lateral soft tissue radiographs or CT will better delineate extent of swelling.	Extraoral approach by incision parallel to and along anterior border of sternocleidomastoid muscle below hyoid bone. Muscle and carotid sheath are retracted laterally, and a finger is inserted posterior to inferior constrictor. A soft noncollapsible rubber drain is preferred because of deep location of this space.

Continued

CN, Cranial nerve; *CT,* computed tomography.

Table 34-4 *Teeth Likely to Cause Fascial Space Infections, with Surgical Approaches—cont'd*

FASCIAL SPACE	ANATOMIC BOUNDARIES OF SPACE	LIKELY SOURCE OF INFECTION	SWELLING SITE	SITE OF I&D
		Infection of retropharyngeal space may also result from nasal and pharyngeal infection in children, esophageal trauma, foreign bodies, and tuberculosis.		

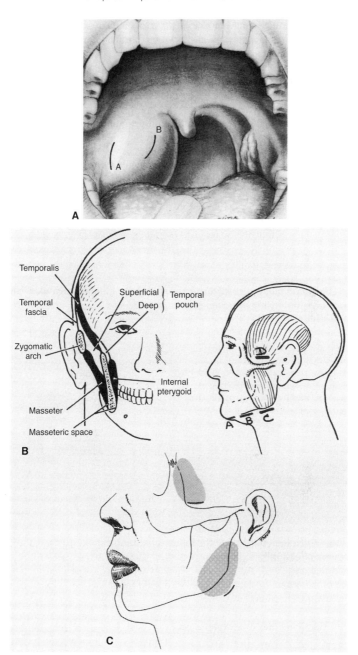

Fig. 34-3 Typical sites of incision and drainage for various fascial space infections. **A**, Intraoral drainage of pterygoid compartment of masticator space *(A)* and lateral pharyngeal space *(B)*. **B**, Masseteric, pterygoid, and temporal compartments of the masticator space. Incisions at *B* and *C* can be used to drain the submandibular space. **C**, Suggested locations for incision for extraoral drainage of temporal and lateral pharyngeal space infections. (From Goldberg MH, Topazian RG: Odontogenic infections and deep fascial space infections of dental origin. In Topazian RG, Goldberg MH [eds]: Oral and Maxillofacial Infections, 3rd ed. Philadelphia, 1994, Saunders.)

Odontogenic infection is treated surgically, pharmacologically, or by medical support of the patient, including removing the source of infection; incision and drainage; and use of antibiotics, fluids, analgesics, and nutritional support.

23. How is the severity of odontogenic infection determined?
By analyzing the history, physical findings, and results of lab and imaging studies.

24. What are the different methods of drainage of odontogenic infections?
- Endodontic treatment
- Extraction of the offending tooth
- Incision and drainage of soft tissue collection

25. What are the surgical principles of incision and drainage?
- Before incision, obtain fluid for culture through aspiration of pus using a syringe and needle.
- Incise the abscess in healthy skin or mucosa and in a cosmetically or functionally acceptable place, using blunt dissection and thorough exploration of the involved space.
- Use one-way drains in intraoral abscesses; use through-and-through drainage in extraoral cases.
- Remove the drain gradually from deep sites.

26. What is the percentage of oral bacteria resistant to commonly used antibiotics for treatment of odontogenic infection (Table 34-5)?

Table 34-5   *Percentage of Oral Bacteria Resistant to Commonly Used Antibiotics*

	ORAL BACTEROIDES	FUSOBACTERIA	ANAEROBIC COCCI	ALPHA-STREPTOCOCCI
Penicillin	15-30	6	4	0
Erythromycin	0	85	18	0
Clindamycin	4	0	2	0
Metronidazole	0	0	24	100
Cephalexin	10	0	6	18

Adapted from Peterson LJ: Microbiology of head and neck infections. Oral Maxillofacial Surg Clin 3:255, 1991.

27. What should you look for during the follow-up appointment after treating a patient for odontogenic infection?
- Response to treatment
- Recurrence of infection
- Presence of allergic reactions
- Toxicity reactions to antibiotics
- Secondary infection (e.g., *Candida*)

28. What are the principles of antibiotic use?
When choosing a specific antibiotic as part of treatment of odontogenic infection, adhere to the following principles:
- Use the correct and narrow-spectrum antibiotic.
- Use the least toxic drug with the fewest side effects.
- Use bactericidal drugs whenever possible.
- Be aware of drug cost.
- Ensure effective oral administration through the use of proper dose and proper dosage interval.
- Continue the antibiotic for an adequate length of time.
- Administer the antibiotics through the proper route.

29. What are the most commonly used antibiotic formulations for oral and maxillofacial infections (Table 34-6)?

	Table 34-6	*Formulations for Antibiotics Commonly Used in Oral and Maxillofacial Infections*	
DRUG	TYPES	FORMULATIONS	UNIT DOSE
Penicillin G			
• Potassium	Generic, Pfizerpen	Vial for IM, IV	1-, 5-, and 20-million U
• Sodium	Generic	Vial for IM, IV	5-million U
• Repository	Bicillin CR	Vial for IM	300-600,000 U/mL
Penicillin V	Generic, Betapen VK, Pen Vee K, Veetids	Tablets Oral solution	250, 500 mg 125, 250 mg/5 mL
Ampicillin	Generic, Omnipen, Polycillin, Principen	Capsules Oral suspension Pediatric drops Vial	250, 500 mg 250 mg/5 mL 100 mg/mL 125, 250, 500, 1000, 2000 mg
Amoxicillin	Generic, Amoxil, Polymox, Trimox, Wymox	Capsule Oral suspension Pediatric drops	250, 500 mg 125, 250 mg/5 mL 50 mg/mL
Amoxicillin-clavulanate	Augmentin	Tablets Tablets (chewable) Oral suspension	250, 500 mg 125, 250 mg 125, 250 mg/5 mL
Oxacillin	Generic, Prostaphlin	Capsules Oral solution Vials for IM, IV	250, 500 mg 250 mg/5 mL 250, 500, 1000 mg
Dicloxacillin	Generic, Dynapen, Pathocil	Capsules Oral suspension	250, 500 mg 62.5 mg/5 mL
Cephalexin	Generic, Keflex	Capsules/Pulvules Tablets Oral suspension Pediatric drops	250, 500 mg 250, 500, 1000 mg 125, 250 mg/5 mL 100 mg/mL
Cephradine	Generic, Anspor, Velosef	Capsules Oral suspension Vial for IM, IV	250, 500 mg 125, 250 mg/5 mL 250, 500, 1000 mg
Cefazolin	Generic, Ancef, Kefzol	Vial for IM, IV	250, 500, 1000 mg
Cefaclor	Ceclor	Pulvules Oral suspension	250, 500 mg 125, 250 mg/5 mL
Cefoxitin	Mefoxin	Vial for IM, IV	1000 mg
Erythromycin			
• Base	Generic, ERYC, Ilotycin, E-mycin, Ery-Tab	Tablets	250, 500 mg

Adapted from Hupp JR: Antibacterial, antiviral, and antifungal agents. Oral Maxillofacial Surg Clin 3:273-286, 1991.
IM, Intramuscular; *IV,* intravenous.

Continued

Table 34-6 *Formulations for Antibiotics Commonly Used in Oral and Maxillofacial Infections—cont'd*

DRUG	TYPES	FORMULATIONS	UNIT DOSE
• Estolate	Generic, Ilosone	Tablets	250, 500 mg
		Tablets (chewable)	125 mg
		Oral suspension	125, 250 mg/5 mL
		Pediatric drops	100 mg/mL
• Ethylsuccinate	Generic, EES, Ery	Tablets	400 mg
	Ped, Eryzole,	Tablets (chewable)	200 mg
	Pediamycin	Oral suspension	200, 400 mg/5 mL
		Pediatric drops	100 mg/2.5 mL
Clindamycin	Generic, Cleocin	Capsules	75, 150, 300 mg
		Oral solution	75 mg/5 mL
		Vial for IM, IV	250, 500, 750 mg
Chloramphenicol	Chloromycetin	Capsule	250 mg
		Oral suspension	150 mg/5 mL
		Vial for IV	1000 mg
Vancomycin	Generic, Vancocin	Capsules	125, 250 mg
		Oral solution	250 mg/5 mL
		Vial for IV	500, 1000 mg
Metronidazole	Generic, Flagyl,	Tablets	250 mg
	Protostat	Vial for IV	500 mg
Nystatin	Generic, Mycostatin,	Tablets	500,000 U
	Nilstat	Oral suspension	100,000 U/mL
		Pastilles	200,000 U
Clotrimazole	Mycelex	Troche	10 mg
Ketoconazole	Nizoral	Tablets	200 mg
Acyclovir	Zovirax	Capsules	200 mg
		Ointment	5% concentration
		Vial for IV	500 mg

30. What is the minimal inhibitory concentration (MIC) of antibiotics?

MIC is a measure of sensitivity of bacteria. For an antibiotic to have maximum antibiotic efficacy in treatment of specific infections, the concentration of the antibiotic at the site of infection should be 3-4 times the MIC. Concentrations >4 times the MIC are not more effective.

31. What is the beta-lactam group of antibiotics?

These antibiotics, which have in common a beta-lactam ring in their structures, comprise three classes: penicillins, cephalosporins, and carbapenems. Penicillins and cephalosporins encompass many different antibiotics that are commonly used for odontogenic infection. Imipenem is an example of the carbapenems.

32. What was the first carbapenem to be used clinically?

Imipenem was the first clinically available carbapenem. It has the broadest antibacterial activity of any currently used systemic antibiotic and therefore is reserved for use in treatment of severe head and neck infections.

33. What is the mode of action of penicillin?
Penicillin affects bacteria by two mechanisms:
1. It inhibits bacterial cell wall synthesis.
2. It activates endogenous bacterial autolytic processes that cause cell lysis. The bacteria must be actively dividing, and the cell wall must contain peptidoglycans for this action. Penicillin inhibits enzymes necessary for cell wall synthesis.

34. How do bacteria build up resistance to antibiotics?
An antibiotic's ability to penetrate cell walls and bind to enzymes plays an essential role in resistance of antibiotics. Specifically, bacteria build resistance by two mechanisms:
1. Alteration in cell wall permeability to prevent antibiotics from inhibiting peptidoglycan synthesis
2. Bacterial production of beta-lactamase that causes beta-lactams to become ineffective

35. What are the pediatric and adult dosages for the most commonly used antibiotics (Table 34-7)?

Table 34-7 *Pediatric and Adult Antibiotic Dosages*

ANTIBIOTIC	ROUTE(S) OF ADMINISTRATION	ADULT DOSE	PEDIATRIC DOSE/DAY
Penicillin G	IM, IV	6-12 × 10 U/4 hr	100,000 U/kg ÷ 3
Penicillin V	PO	500 mg qid	50 mg/kg ÷ 3 or 4
Ampicillin	PO, IM, IV	500 mg qid PO	25 mg/kg ÷ 4
Amoxicillin	PO	250 mg qid PO	25 mg/kg ÷ 3
Amoxicillin-clavulanate	PO	250-500 mg tid	20 mg/kg 3
Oxacillin	IM, IV	500-1000 mg q6h	50-200 mg/kg ÷ 4
Dicloxacillin	PO	250-500 mg q6h	12.5-50 mg/kg ÷ 4 or 5
Cephalexin	PO	500 mg qid	25-50 mg/kg ÷ 4
Cephradine	PO, IV	500 mg qid	25-50 mg/kg ÷ 3
Cefazolin	IM, IV	1 g q8h	25-50 mg/kg ÷ 3 or 4
Cefaclor	PO	500 mg q6h	20 mg/kg ÷ 3
Cefoxitin	IM, IV	500 mg q6h	80-160 mg/kg ÷ 4 or 5
Erythromycin	PO, IV	500 mg qid	40 mg/kg ÷ 4
Clindamycin	PO, IM, IV	300-450 mg q6h	10-20 mg/kg ÷ 4
Chloramphenicol	PO, IV	500-750 mg q6h PO	75-100 mg/kg ÷ 4
Vancomycin	IV	500 mg q6h	50 mg/kg ÷ 4
Metronidazole	PO	500 mg tid	30-40 mg/kg
Nystatin	Topical, PO	0.5-2 million U/ day ÷ 2-4	Infants: 800,000 U ÷ 4 Older children: 1.6 million U ÷ 4

Adapted from Hupp JR: Antibacterial, antiviral, and antifungal agents. Oral Maxillofacial Surg Clin 3:273-286, 1991.
IM, Intramuscular; *IV,* intravenous; *PO,* orally; *qid,* four times a day; *tid,* three times a day; *q6h,* every 6 hours; *q8h,* every 8 hours

Continued

Table 34-7   *Pediatric and Adult Antibiotic Dosages—cont'd*

ANTIBIOTIC	ROUTE(S) OF ADMINISTRATION	ADULT DOSE	PEDIATRIC DOSE/DAY
Clotrimazole	Topical	10 mg 5 times/day	<3 yr: safety not established ≥3 yr: 10 mg 5 times/day
Ketoconazole	PO	200-400 mg qd	3.3-6.6 mg/kg
Acyclovir	Topical, PO, IV	600 mg ÷ 3 PO 15 mg/kg ÷ 3 IV	Safety in children not established

qd, Daily.

36. What is the antimicrobial spectrum of the most common antibiotics used in treatments for oral and maxillofacial infections (Table 34-8)?

Table 34-8   *Antimicrobial Spectrum of Common Antibiotics Used in the Treatment of Oral and Maxillofacial Infections*

ANTIBIOTIC	SPECTRUM	ANTIBIOTIC	SPECTRUM
Penicillin	*Streptococcus* (except group D) *Staphylococcus* (non–beta-lactamase producing) *Treponema* *Actinomyces* Oral anaerobes	Erythromycin	*Streptococcus* *Staphylococcus* *Mycoplasma* *Haemophilus influenzae* *Legionella*
Ampicillin and amoxicillin	Same as penicillin plus: *Escherichia coli* *H. influenzae* *Proteus mirabilis*	Clindamycin	Oral anaerobes *Streptococcus* *Staphylococcus* *Actinomyces* *Bacteroides fragilis*
Amoxicillin plus clavulanate	Same as ampicillin plus: *Klebsiella* *Staphylococcus aureus* *Staphylococcus epidermidis* *Enterococci* *Gonococci*	Chloramphenicol	Oral anaerobes *Streptococcus* *Staphylococcus* *H. influenzae* *E. coli* *Salmonella* *Shigella* *Rickettsia*

Adapted from Peterson LJ: Principles of antibiotic therapy. In Tobazian RG, Goldberg MH (eds): Oral and Maxillofacial Infections, 3rd ed. Philadelphia, 1994, Saunders.

Table 34-8 *Antimicrobial Spectrum of Common Antibiotics Used in the Treatment of Oral and Maxillofacial Infections—cont'd*

ANTIBIOTIC	SPECTRUM	ANTIBIOTIC	SPECTRUM
Oxacillin and dicloxacillin	Beta-lactamase–producing staphylococci		*Bacteroides fragilis* Oral anaerobes
Cephalexin, cephradine, and cefazolin	*Streptococcus* (except group D) *Staphylococcus* *E. coli* *Proteus mirabilis* *Klebsiella*	Vancomycin Metronidazole	*Streptococcus* *Staphylococcus* Oral anaerobes
Cefaclor	Same as cephalexin plus: *H. influenzae*		
Cefoxitin	Same as cephalexin plus: *Enterobacter* *Bacteroides fragilis* Oral anaerobes		

37. When should antibiotics be used?
- Acute-onset infection
- Diagnosed osteomyelitis of the jaw
- Infection with diffuse swelling
- Involvement of fascial spaces
- Patients with compromised host defenses
- Severe pericoronitis

38. When are prophylactic antibiotics for prevention of odontogenic infections not necessary?
Antibiotics have minimal or no benefits in the treatment of chronic well-localized abscess, minor vestibular abscess, dry socket, and root canal sterilization.

39. What are the indications for prophylactic antibiotics?
- To prevent local wound infection
- To prevent infection at the surgical site causing local wound infection
- To prevent metastatic infection at a distant susceptible site due to hematogenous bacterial seeding from the oral flora (e.g., subacute bacterial endocarditis, prosthetic joint replacement) following oral surgical procedures

40. When are prophylactic antibiotics indicated for prevention of local wound infection?
- When the procedure to be performed has a high incidence of infection
- When infections may have grave consequences
- When the patient's immune system is compromised
- When the surgical procedure lasts longer than 3 hr
- When the surgical procedure has a high degree of contamination

41. What is the antibiotic of choice for treatment of odontogenic infection?
The empiric therapy is **penicillin** or penicillin plus metronidazole, if the patient is not allergic to antibiotics and is not immunocompromised. In patients who are allergic to penicillin, **clindamycin** is an excellent alternative. Definitive antibiotic therapy should be based on culture and sensitivity.

42. What is the mechanism of action, route of excretion, and spectrum of the most commonly used antibiotics for oral and maxillofacial infection (Table 34-9)?

Table 34-9 Profiles of the Most Commonly Used Antibiotics for Oral and Maxillofacial Infection

	PENICILLIN V	ERYTHROMYCIN	CLINDAMYCIN	CEPHALEXIN	CEFADROXIL	METRONIDAZOLE	DOXYCYCLINE	AMOXICILLIN	NYSTATIN
Bactericidal or bacteriostatic	Bactericidal	Bacteriostatic	Both	Bactericidal	Bactericidal	Bactericidal	Bacteriostatic	Bactericidal	Bactericidal
Spectrum	Streptococci, oral anaerobes	Gram-positive cocci, oral anaerobes	Gram-positive cocci, anaerobes	Gram-positive cocci, some gram-negative rods, oral anaerobes	Gram-positive cocci, some gram-negative rods, oral anaerobes	Anaerobes	Gram-positive cocci, some gram-negative rods, oral anaerobes	Gram-positive cocci, *E. coli, H. influenzae,* oral anaerobes	Candida organisms
Dose-interval	250-500 mg qid	250-500 mg qid	150-300 mg q6h	500 mg qid	500 mg bid	250 mg qid	100 mg bid	250 mg tid	200,000 U lozenge qid
Metabolized	Kidney	Liver	Liver	Kidney	Kidney	Liver	Liver	Kidney	
Toxicity and side effects	Allergy	Nausea, vomiting, cramping, diarrhea	Nausea, vomiting, cramping, diarrhea, antibiotic-associated colitis	Allergy, antibiotic-associated colitis	Allergy, antibiotic-associated colitis	Nausea, vomiting, cramping, diarrhea, disulfiram-like effect	Teeth coloration, photo-sensitivity, nausea, vomiting, diarrhea	Allergy, antibiotic-associated colitis	
Primary indication	Drug of choice	Useful alternative for mild infection	Useful alternative, especially for resistant anaerobes	Bactericidal drug required	Bactericidal drug required	Only anaerobic bacteria involved	Broad-spectrum in mild infections	Broader spectrum needed	Candidosis

Adapted from Peterson LJ: Principles of management and prevention of odontogenic infection. In Peterson LJ, Ellis E, Hupp J et al (eds): Contemporary Oral and Maxillofacial Surgery, 2nd ed. St Louis, 1993, Mosby.

qid, Four times a day; *bid,* twice a day; *q6h,* every 6 hours; *tid,* three times a day.

43. What are the possible causes of failure of antibiotic therapy?
- Inadequate surgical treatment
- Depressed host defenses
- Presence of foreign body
- Problems associated with use of antibiotics (e.g., patient compliance, inadequate dose, antibiotic-related infection, use of wrong antibiotic)

44. What is antibiotic-associated colitis (AAC)?
AAC is a toxic reaction associated with the use of an antibiotic that causes alteration of colonic flora leading to the overgrowth of *Clostridium difficile*. The toxins from *C. difficile* cause pseudomembranous colitis or AAC, which is manifested clinically as profuse, watery diarrhea that may be bloody; cramping; abdominal pain; fever; and leukocytosis.

45. What are the risk factors for AAC?
Risk factors associated with AAC are related to the type of antibiotic and patient-related factors. Clindamycin, which originally was thought to be the main antibiotic associated with AAC, has now been recognized to be associated with only one third of cases. Ampicillin is associated with one third, and the cephalosporins are associated with the last third. Patient-related factors for AAC include previous gastrointestinal procedures, medically compromised patients, advanced age, female gender, inflammatory bowel disease, cancer chemotherapy, and renal disease.

46. What is the diagnosis of and treatment for AAC?
In addition to the clinical signs and symptoms, the diagnosis of AAC is usually made based on positive *C. difficile* culture and *C. difficile* toxin in the patient's stool. Sigmoidoscopy is occasionally used to confirm the diagnosis. Treatment includes discontinuation of the causative antibiotics, use of alternate antibiotics if necessary, restoration of fluid and electrolyte balance, and administration of anticlostridial antibiotics. The usual choice is oral vancomycin or oral metronidazole.

47. What is Ludwig's angina?
Ludwig's angina is bilateral, brawny, boardlike induration of the submandibular, sublingual, and submental spaces due to infection of these spaces. The term *angina* is used because of the respiratory distress caused by the airway obstruction. This obstruction can occur suddenly owing to the possible extension of the infection from the sublingual space posteriorly to the epiglottis, causing epiglottis edema.

48. How is Ludwig's angina treated?
The principles of treatment of Ludwig's angina are early diagnosis, prompt surgical intervention, and definitive airway management. After securing an airway, surgical drainage of each individual space should begin even before fluctuance becomes palpable externally. Appropriate antibiotics and management of the host defense mechanism are also important.

49. What is erysipelas?
Erysipelas is a superficial cellulitis of the skin that is caused by beta-hemolytic streptococci and by group B streptococci. It usually presents with warm, erythematous skin and spreads rapidly from release of hyaluronidase by the bacteria. It is associated with lymphadenopathy and fever and has an abrupt onset with acute swelling. It may affect the skin of the face. Treatment consists of parenteral penicillin.

50. What is cervicofacial necrotizing fasciitis?
Cervicofacial necrotizing fasciitis is a very aggressive infection of the skin and superficial

fascia of the head and neck and is commonly seen in diabetic and immunocompromised patients. It carries a mortality rate of 30%-50% from sepsis of the dead tissue in the affected area. The etiologic factors of cervicofacial necrotizing fasciitis include odontogenic infections; burns; cuts; abrasions; contusions; peritonsillar abscess and boils of the head and neck region; surgery; and trauma.

51. Which organisms are involved in necrotizing fasciitis of the head and neck?

The causative organisms of necrotizing fasciitis include aerobes and obligate anaerobes in synergistic combinations. In a study of 16 patients with necrotizing fasciitis, two distinctive types of bacterial findings were found. Both types had identical clinical presentations. **Type I** patients had anaerobic and facultative anaerobic bacteria, such as Enterobacteriaceae and streptococci other than group A. **Type II** patients had group A streptococci (pyogenous) alone or in combination with anaerobic bacteria. Group A streptococci and staphylococci were not isolated from type I patients.

52. What are the clinical features of necrotizing fasciitis of the head and neck?

The initial presentation of necrotizing fasciitis is usually deceivingly benign, although the extent of tissue and fascial destruction far exceeds the external evidence of infection. The rate of infection is usually rapid, and the patient often has a concomitant systemic disease, such as diabetes mellitus, arteriosclerosis, obesity, malnutrition, or alcoholism.

The clinical features of this condition are usually manifested as smooth, tense, and shiny skin, with no sharp demarcation in the area involved. As the disease progresses, the pathognomonic signs of the condition include dusky purplish discoloration of the skin, small purplish patches with ill-defined borders, formation of blisters or bullae, subcutaneous fat, necrosis of the fascia, and gangrene of the overlying skin. Typically, the drainage in these patients yields "dishwater"—a purplish, foul-smelling discharge. Systemic features of necrotizing fasciitis include sepsis, hypotension, hypertension, hyperpyrexia, jaundice, and hemoglobinuria.

53. What is the treatment for necrotizing fasciitis?

Treatment for necrotizing fasciitis includes antibiotics, fluid replacement, nutrition, and daily debridement to remove devitalized tissues. However, the cornerstone of treatment is debridement of the necrotic tissue and daily monitoring to assure adequate removal. Appropriate antibiotics and medical support are also important. Medical support includes fluid and electrolyte replacement, monitoring of the intravascular volume, and management of the underlying medical condition. Hyperbaric oxygen treatment has also been suggested for promotion of vascularization of infected tissue.

After resolution of infection, the resulting soft tissue defect is reconstructed with a skin graft and/or regional or local tissue flaps. Penicillin, clindamycin, and aminoglycosides are effective antimicrobial agents for this condition.

54. What are the common granulomatous infections with recognized head and neck manifestations?

See Table 34-10.

55. What are the classifications of salivary gland infections?

Salivary gland infection can be classified based on clinical, microbiologic, or mechanical causes. Accordingly, they are classified as **acute or chronic,** bacterial or viral, obstructive or nonobstructive (involvement by systemic granulomatous diseases). The **bacterial and viral** infections include mumps and acute, chronic, and recurrent sialadenitis. The **obstructive** infections include sialolithiasis, mucous plugs, stricture/stenosis, and foreign bodies. Systemic granulomatous infections **(nonobstructive)** include tuberculosis, actinomycosis, fungal infections, and sarcoid.

Table 34-10   *Common Granulomatous Infections with Head and Neck Manifestations*

DISEASE	CAUSATIVE ORGANISM	TYPICAL CLINICAL APPEARANCE
Actinomycosis	*Actinomyces israelii* (anaerobic gram-positive bacillus)	Painless, slowly enlarging soft tissue cervicofacial infection with fistulae
Cat scratch disease	Unnamed gram-negative bacillus	Indolent regional lymphadenitis
Glanders	*Pseudomonas mallei* (gram-negative bacillus)	Farcy: draining facial abscesses, lymphadenopathy
Leishmaniasis	Leishmania (protozoal parasite)	Mucocutaneous ulcerations
Leprosy	*Mycobacterium leprae* (acid-alcohol-fast bacillus)	Facial leproma, nasomaxillary destruction, paresthesia of V2 and VII
Scleroma	*Klebsiella rhinoscleromatis* (gram-negative bacillus)	Chronic destructive lesion of nasomaxillary complex
Syphilis (tertiary)	*Treponema pallidum* (spirochete)	Gumma of soft tissue or bone
Tuberculosis	*Mycobacterium tuberculosis* (acid-fast aerobic bacillus)	Scrofula: indolent cervical lymphadenitis, ulcerations of palate or tongue
Tularemia	*Francisella tularensis* (gram-negative coccobacillus)	Oropharyngeal ulcerations

Adapted from Wood RS: Chronic granulomatous infections. Oral Maxillofacial Surg Clin 3:405-422, 1991.

56. Which studies should be included in evaluation of chronic salivary gland infection?

Complete blood count with differential, Gram stain, and culture and acid-fast staining of the salivary secretions are all useful in evaluating patients with salivary gland infection. Plain films (occlusal and panoramic view), sialography, CT, MRI, ultrasonography, and scintigraphy of the gland are useful in showing tissue changes of the salivary gland tissue. Chest x-ray, tuberculin test, and salivary gland biopsy may be necessary when involvement of the gland by systemic disease is suspected.

57. What is the treatment of sialadenitis?

If stones are present in the submandibular gland duct, a ductoplasty is indicated. If the stones are large, beyond the mylohyoid flexure of the duct, or intraglandular, the gland must be removed. Parotid gland infection is more serious and must be drained or treated by superficial parotidectomy. Antibiotics should be administered to cover *Streptococcus* and *Staphylococcus* spp. *Escherichia coli* and *Haemophilus influenzae* are also occasionally implicated. Hydration with intravenous (IV) fluid, especially in the elderly and children, is often a necessary part of the treatment of acute sialadenitis.

58. What are the most commonly used antibiotics for treatment of salivary gland infection?

Empirically, or if Gram stain shows gram-positive cocci, administration of penicillinase-resistant antistaphylococcal antibiotics, such as methicillin, is advisable. In patients who have a history of allergy to penicillin, cephalosporins can be used. Aminoglycosides (gentamicin) could also be used. Antibiotics should be administered in high doses and intravenously in patients who are hospitalized or seriously ill.

59. Which cranial nerves pass through the cavernous sinus?

Cranial nerves III, IV, V (ophthalmic division of V), and VI pass through the cavernous sinus.

60. What is the cavernous sinus thrombosis?

It is an uncommon but potentially lethal extension of odontogenic infection. Valveless veins in the head and neck allow retrograde flow of the infection from the face to the sinus. The pterygoid plexus of veins and angular and ophthalmic veins may contribute to retrograde flow. The first clinical signs of cavernous sinus thrombosis include vascular congestion in periorbital, scleral, and retinal veins. Other clinical signs include periorbital edema, proptosis, thrombosis of the retinal vein, ptosis, dilated pupils, absent corneal reflex, and supraorbital sensory deficits.

61. What are the pathways of odontogenic infection to the cavernous sinus?

An orofacial infection can reach the cavernous sinus through two routes: an **anterior route** via the angular and inferior ophthalmic veins, and a **posterior route** via the transverse facial vein and the pterygoid plexus of veins.

62. What is the flora of acute and chronic sinusitis?

Acute sinus infections are caused by *Streptococcus pneumoniae* (30%-50%) and *H. influenzae* (20%-40%). Other organisms associated with acute sinusitis include *Moraxella catarrhalis, S. aureus, Streptococcus pyogenes,* and beta- and alpha-hemolytic streptococci.

Chronic sinusitis is due to *S. aureus,* alpha hemolytic streptococci, *Peptostreptococcus, Pseudomonas, Proteus,* and *Bacteroides.* The flora of chronic sinusitis is usually a mixture of aerobic and anaerobic organisms.

63. What is the treatment for maxillary sinus infections?

Treatment for maxillary sinus is based on a combined approach of medical treatment and, if necessary, surgical treatment. The medical treatment includes use of antibiotics, topical or oral decongestants, antihistamines, and topical or oral steroids. Commonly prescribed antibiotics for the treatment of maxillary sinusitis include ampicillin, amoxicillin, amoxicillin plus clavulanic acid, cefaclor, cefuroxime axetil, and trimethoprim-sulfamethoxazole.

Surgical treatment is indicated when the underlying cause of the infection cannot be corrected with medical therapy. The goal is to reestablish drainage and remove the underlying cause (if identified) using minimally invasive techniques, such as functional endoscopic surgery.

64. What are the most common bacterial and fungal infections affecting patients with diabetes mellitus?

Mucormycosis (phycomycosis) is the most common infection in patients with diabetes mellitus, especially those with diabetic ketoacidosis. Of patients with rhinocerebral mucormycosis, 75% have ketoacidosis. Mucormycosis is a fungal disease, possibly caused by phycomycetes organisms of the Zygomycetes class.

65. Which organisms are associated with infections from a human and animal bite?

Approximately 25% of animal bite infections are caused by *Pasteurella multocida.* Approximately 10% are caused by *S. aureus,* 40% are caused by alpha-hemolytic streptococci, and 20% are caused by bacteroides and fusobacteria. About 25% of human bite infections are caused by *S. aureus* from the skin of the victim; 10% are caused by alpha-hemolytic streptococci; 50% are caused by anaerobic bacteria including gram-positive cocci, fusobacteria, and *Bacteroides* species; and 15% are caused by *Eikenella corrodens.* The latter organisms are mostly associated with severe infections.

66. What is the treatment for animal and human bites?

Treatment includes antibiotic therapy and surgical intervention. Good surgical technique involves debridement of the devitalized tissue and thorough irrigation with copious quantities of saline. Oral ampicillin and amoxicillin are the antibiotics of choice for both types of bites. Also provide prophylaxis against rabies virus, if deemed necessary.

67. What is actinomycosis?

Actinomycosis is a bacterial infection caused by a gram-positive, facultative, anaerobic rod bacteria called *Actinomyces israeli*. The organism is part of the normal oral flora. The infection presents as a hard swelling of the jaw and drainage characterized by sulfur granules. The treatment of actinomycosis includes 10-20 million U of penicillin daily for 2-4 weeks, followed by 5-10 million U for 3-4 months. Surgical debridement of the area may accelerate resolution of the infection.

68. Which diseases are associated with Epstein-Barr virus?

Mononucleosis, Burkitt's lymphoma, nasopharyngeal carcinoma, and hairy leukoplakia are associated with the Epstein-Barr virus.

69. What is a Jarisch-Herxheimer reaction?

It is a transient, increased discomfort in an erythematous skin lesion plus temperature elevation occurring within 2 hr after starting antibiotic therapy in treatment of secondary syphilis and Lyme disease (penicillin or tetracycline).

70. What are the various fungal infections that may affect the head and neck?

The various fungal infections of the head and neck include candidiasis, zygomycosis, histoplasmosis, blastomycosis, aspergillosis, and coccidiomycosis.

71. What are the common *antifungal* agents?

The most common antifungal agents are nystatin, clotrimazole, ketoconazole, and amphotericin B.

72. What are the common *antiviral* agents?

The common antiviral agents are acyclovir, zidovudine, vidarabine (ara-A), and idoxuridine.

73. What are the most common agents used in HIV-positive patients?

See Table 34-11.

74. Is the following statement true or false? Osteomyelitis can be classified into three major groups.

False. Osteomyelitis is generally classified as two major groups: suppurative and nonsuppurative.

75. What is the most common classification of osteomyelitis of the jaws?

Suppurative osteomyelitis is classified as acute, chronic, or infantile osteomyelitis. Non-suppurative osteomyelitis is classified as chronic sclerosing (focal and diffuse), Garré's sclerosing osteomyelitis, and actinomycotic osteomyelitis.

76. What is Garré's osteomyelitis?

Garré's osteomyelitis is characterized by localized, hard, nontender, bony swelling of the lateral and inferior aspects of the mandible. It is primarily present in children and young adults and is usually associated with carious molar and low-grade infection. The radiographic features of Garré's osteomyelitis include a focal area with proliferative periosteal formation, most often seen as a carious mandibular molar opposite the hard bony mass, and periosteal bony outgrowth

Table 34-11	*Common Drugs Used to Treat HIV-Positive Patients*	
DRUG	MAIN ACTION	COMPLICATIONS
Immunosuppressive		
Glucocorticoids	Decrease circulating lymphocytes Impair delayed hypersensitivity Alter lymphocyte-macrophage interaction Cause monocytopenia Impair neutrophil chemotaxis	Infection Diabetes mellitus Adrenal suppression Peptic ulcer disease Impaired wound healing
Azathioprine	Interferes with DNA/RNA synthesis, leading to lymphocytopenia	Hepatitis Agranulocytosis Infection
Antithymocyte globulin	Lymphocyte-selective immunosuppression	Infection Predisposition to tumor development Thrombocytopenia Hemolysis Leukopenia
Cyclosporine	Inhibits T-cell proliferation and activation	Nephrotoxicity Hepatotoxicity Lymphoma Gingival hyperplasia
Cyclophosphamide	Depletes circulating T-lymphocyte pools Inhibits T-cell function and proliferation	Leukopenia

Adapted from Miyasaki SH, Perrott D, Kaban LB: Infections in immunocompromised patients. Oral Maxillofacial Surg Clin 3:393-402, 1991.

seen on occlusal films. Treatment of this condition includes extraction of the tooth and removal of potential sources, which leads to gradual remodeling of the area involved. Long-term postoperative antibiotics generally are not necessary.

77. Which conditions are associated with periosteal thickening?
In addition to Garré's osteomyelitis, infantile osteomyelitis, cortical hyperostoses (Caffey's disease), syphilis, leukemia, Ewing's sarcoma, metabolic neuroblastoma, and fracture callus are all associated with periosteal thickening.

78. What are the general treatment principles of osteomyelitis of the jaws?
Treatment of osteomyelitis of the jaws usually includes both surgical intervention and medical management of the patient, as well as sensitivity testing. Medical management involves administration of empirical antibiotics, performing Gram stain, administration of culture-guided antibiotics, use of appropriate imaging to rule out other causes such as tumors, and evaluation and correction of the patient's immune defenses. Surgical treatment includes removal of loose teeth and foreign bodies; sequestrectomy; debridement; decortication; resection; and reconstruction, if necessary.

79. What is meant by generations of antibiotics, as in third-generation cephalosporins?[*]

The earliest antibiotics were bacteriostatic, largely through interference in protein synthesis, so that they might keep a microorganism from reproducing even if they did not kill it. The difference between **infestation** (presence of living microbes in the host) and **infection** (replication and spread of microorganisms in the host) may be useful in understanding how earlier drugs possibly controlled infection but were less capable of eliminating organisms in any brief period of therapy.

Penicillin changed all that. It may be the first antibiotic with a legitimate claim to the title "wonder drug," because it has the microbicidal capability of eradicating sensitive organisms. Penicillin was the first generation of the beta-lactam antibiotics, joined by the congener first-generation cephalosporins (e.g., cefazolin). They shared beta-lactam structure and had good gram-positive coverage with less range in any effect over gram-negative microbes.

The second-generation beta-lactam antibiotics (e.g., cefoxitin) covered new classes of microbes beyond gram-positive aerobes, such as many of the *Bacteroides* species, but had little effect on gram-negative aerobic microbes. Because the third-generation cephalosporins covered some of the latter microbes, they were touted as single-agent therapy for all principal-risk flora.

As with penicillin, the original wonder drug, the wonderment waned with failures of the new agents because of rapidly induced antimicrobial resistance. The most easily measured and calculated difference in the generations is cost: wholesale values are about $2.00/g for the first generation, $5.00/g for the second, and $30.00/g for the third. Despite this bracket creep in cost, the higher generations lose some of their potency against the original gram-positive organisms for which the first-generation agents were truly wonderful. Therefore it takes 2 g of moxalactam to be half as good as 1 g of cefazolin for gram-positive coverage. It does not take a pharmacoeconomist to ask, "What have I got in return for this sixtyfold surcharge?"

80. Are two prophylactic doses better than one in preventing infection? Are three doses better still?[*]

Only one dose of prophylactic antibiotic can be proved, beyond statistical or clinical doubt, to be efficacious—the dose in systemic circulation at the time of the inoculum. Whether the dose needs to be repeated one or more times during the 24 hr after the inoculum depends on the blood levels of the drug, which are largely a function of protein binding and clearance rate. We also know for sure that 10 days of the same prophylactic drug that is efficacious if given immediately before the inoculum results in a higher risk of infection than no antibiotic at all.

81. What factors determine the timing of antibiotic administration under the criteria of prophylaxis?[*]

The one immutable principle has been set out above—the most important element in timing of prophylaxis is that the drug be **circulating** before the inoculum. When should it stop? When the reduction in infection risk is no longer provable and before continued use will defeat the prophylactic purpose (as explained above). To summarize with an arbitrary rule of thumb: *There is no justification for prophylactic antibiotic 24 hr after the inoculum of an invasive procedure.*

What does this rule imply? Should we not continue prophylaxis for weeks to cover the presence of a prosthetic hip joint? Presumably, the prosthetic hip will be in the patient for many years, but surely you do not argue that the antibiotic should continue on a daily basis as long as the hip is in place. What is "prophylaxed" is not the prosthetic hip but the procedure of implantation. And it is not only implantation that poses a risk to the patient with a prosthesis— so does hemorrhoidectomy done years later, for which prophylaxis is made mandatory by the presence of the hip prosthesis.

The prosthetic or rheumatic heart valve is a risk, but the indication for the use of

[*]Reprinted from Geelhoed GW: Surgical infectious disease. In Harken AH, Moore EE (eds): Abernathy's Surgical Secrets, 5th ed. Philadelphia, 2005, Mosby.

prophylactic antibiotics is an invasive procedure; a root canal is an example in which an inoculum is unavoidable. *Operations are covered by prophylactic antibiotics; the conditions that are risk factors during the operation are not.*

82. To be safe, why not administer prophylactic antibiotics to all patients undergoing any kind of operation?*

Can you give me the indication for a prophylactic antibiotic in a patient undergoing a clean elective surgical procedure that implants no prosthesis, such as hernia repair?

"Sure," one of my brighter students once responded, "the patient who has a serious impairment in host response, such as acute granulocytic leukemia in blast crisis."

I responded, "Why on earth are you fixing his hernia? That is a clean error (hopefully not a clean kill) in surgical judgment that has nothing to do with antibiotics at all. A patient with that degree of host impairment does not undergo an elective surgical procedure."

Rule of thumb: If you can provide the indication for a prophylactic antibiotic to cover a clean elective nonprosthetic operation for a patient, you have provided the contraindication for the operation.

83. What is the drug of choice for the treatment of an abscess?*

A knife. Surgically drain the abscess. Abscesses have no circulation of blood within them to deliver an antibiotic. The antibiotic, even if injected directly into the abscess, would be worthless because the abscess contains a soup of dead microorganisms and white blood cells (WBCs). Even if the organisms were barely alive, they would not be reproducing and incorporating the antibiotic. The drug most likely would not work at all at the pH and pKa conditions of the abscess environment.

If there is an indication for an antibiotic, it would be in the circulation around the compressed inflammatory edge of the abscess and the cellulitis (at the vascularized "peel of the orange") and uncontaminated tissue planes through which the necessary drainage must be carried out. A *focal* infection is managed by a *local* treatment, which is both *necessary* in all abscesses and *sufficient* treatment in many. Adjunctive systemic antibiotics are occasionally indicated for protection of the tissues through which drainage is carried out. If it helps to make this fundamental surgical principle clear, here is the rule of thumb for management of abscesses: *Where there is pus, let there be steel.* Perhaps one of the most gratifying procedures in all of medicine is the drainage of pus with immediate relief of local and systemic symptoms (e.g., a perirectal abscess).

84. Are antibiotic drug combinations always superior to a single antibiotic agent?*

Monotherapy is superior to combination antibiotic treatment regimens, but this is provable probably only in the highest-risk patients. With the carbapenem-class antibiotic agents, a large multicenter clinical trial proved imipenem therapy superior to aminoglycoside and a macrolide antibiotic, with survival demonstrably superior only in the patients with the highest APACHE scores. Ertapenem monotherapy was the equivalent of ceftriaxone and metronidazole in a smaller, more recent trial.

More is not always better, and the R and S on culture reports does not translate directly to the M and M (morbidity and mortality) at the Death and Complications Conference reports. It is not just important that the effective antibiotic regimen kills the bacteria; also important are *how* this microbicidal effect is carried out and what effect it may have on the patient in quenching or prolonging the systemic inflammatory response.

85. What are triple antibiotics? What are the doses?†

†Reprinted from Harken AH: What does postoperative fever mean? In Harken AH, Moore EE (eds): Abernathy's Surgical Secrets, 5th ed. Philadelphia, 2005, Mosby.

A shotgun approach to potentially life-threatening infections when the patient is seriously ill and the surgeon is seriously concerned:

1. Gram-positive coverage (e.g., ampicillin): 1 g every 6 hr IV in adults; 40 mg/kg every 6 hr IV in children
2. Gram-negative coverage (e.g., gentamicin): 7 mg/kg IV every 24 hr (this single daily dose is less nephrotoxic than 2 mg/kg IV every 8 hr)
3. Anaerobic coverage (e.g., metronidazole [Flagyl]): 500 mg IV every 6 hr in adults; 7.5 mg/kg IV every 6 hr in children

To avoid overgrowth of yeast and resistant bacteria, focus on the culprit bacteria as soon as the cultures define it.

86. How do I use antibiotics correctly to prevent surgical wound infection?[‡]

First by knowing what organism you are targeting, then choosing an appropriate antibiotic and delivering it at the appropriate time via the appropriate route. Because you usually will not have a preoperative culture to guide therapy, you need to base your choice of antibiotic on predicted organisms. Staphylococci are the most common skin organism and the most common etiologic agent in surgical site infections (SSIs). Cefazolin, a first-generation cephalosporin, is usually the recommended antibiotic for prophylaxis in clean surgical procedures. In circumstances in which known contamination has occurred, initial antibiotics should be tailored based on the violated organ's common flora. If the gut was entered, Enterobacteriaceae and anaerobes are common; biliary tract and esophageal incisions yield these organisms plus enterococci. The urinary tract or vagina may contain group D streptococci, *Pseudomonas,* and *Proteus.*

87. If prophylactic antibiotics are used, how and when should they be administered?[‡]

Maximal benefit is obtained when tissue concentrations are therapeutic at the time of contamination. Efficacy is enhanced when prophylactic antibiotics are administered IV 20-30 min before surgical incision; late administration is similar to no administration. Multiple-dose regimens have no proven benefit over single-dose regimens. Indiscriminate antibiotic selection outside recommended hospital protocols may increase the incidence of SSIs. In special circumstances, administration routes other than IV may be indicated.

88. What can the patient do to help decrease surgical wound infection?[‡]

Stop smoking. Although obesity, poor nutritional status, advanced age, and diabetes are risk factors for SSIs, cigarette smoking is probably the leading preventable patient factor for SSIs, just like it is the leading preventable cause of death and disability in the United States. Half of all people who smoke eventually die from a smoking-related illness. Smoking not only kills, but also more than triples the risk of incisional wound breakdown; in one study, smoking increased the incidence of SSIs in clean operative procedures sixfold, from 0.6%-3.6%. Tobacco use results in decreased blood flow and decreased oxygen delivery to the wound. Toxic tobacco by-products also directly impede all stages of wound healing. Despite this knowledge, surgeons continue to operate electively on smokers, and most smokers continue to smoke up until the day of surgery.

BIBLIOGRAPHY

1. Barie PS: Modern surgical antibiotic prophylaxis and therapy: less is more. Surg Infect 1:23-29, 2000.
2. Bartlett RC: Laboratory diagnostic techniques. In Tobazian RG, Goldberg MH (eds): Oral and Maxillofacial Infections, 3rd ed. Philadelphia, 1991, Saunders.

‡Reprinted from Peterson SL: Surgical wound infection. In Harken AH, Moore EE (eds): Abernathy's Surgical Secrets, 5th ed. Philadelphia, 2005, Mosby.

3. Ciftci AO, Tanyei FC, Buyukpamukcu N et al: Comparative trial of four antibiotic combinations for perforated appendicitis in children. Eur J Surg 163:591-596, 1997.
4. Falagas ME, Barefoot L, Griffith J et al: Risk factors leading to clinical failure in the treatment of intraabdominal or skin/soft tissue infections. Eur J Clin Microbiol Infect Dis 15:913-921, 1996.
5. Flynn TR: Anatomy and surgery of deep fascial space infections of the head and neck. Oral Maxillofac Surg Knowl Update 1:79-105, 1994.
6. Geelhoed GW: Surgical infectious disease. In Harken AH, Moore EE (eds): Surgical Secrets, 5th ed. Philadelphia, 2005, Mosby.
7. Geelhoed GW: Preoperative skin preparation: evaluation of efficacy, timing, convenience, and cost. Infect Surg 85:648-669, 1985.
8. Hupp JR: Antibacterial, antiviral and antifungal agents. Oral Maxillofac Surg Clin 3:273-286, 1991.
9. Kluytmans J, Voss A: Prevention of postsurgical infections: some like it hot. Curr Opin Infect Dis 15:427-432, 2002.
10. Krueger JK, Rohrich RJ: Clearing the smoke: the scientific rationale for tobacco abstention with plastic surgery. Plast Reconstr Surg 108:1063-1073, 2001.
11. Lieblich SE: Clinical microbiology and taxonomy. Oral Maxillofac Surg Knowl Update 1:11-21, 1994.
12. Miyasaki SH, Perrott DH, Kaban LB: Infections in immunocompromised patients. Oral Maxillofac Surg Clin 3:393-402, 1991.
13. Peterson LJ: Microbiology of head and neck infections. Oral Maxillofac Surg Clin 3:247-258, 1991.
14. Peterson LJ: Principles of management and prevention of odontogenic infection. In Peterson LJ, Ellis E, Hupp J et al (eds): Contemporary Oral and Maxillofacial Surgery, 2nd ed. St Louis, 1998, Mosby.
15. Peterson SL: Surgical wound infection. In Harken AH, Moore EE (eds): Surgical Secrets, 5th ed. Philadelphia, 2005, Mosby.
16. Rogerson KC: Microbiology of the maxillary sinus antrum: treatment of infections. Oral Maxillofac Surg Knowl Update 1:49-60, 1994.
17. Topazian RG: Osteomyelitis of the jaws. In Topazian R, Goldberg M (eds): Oral and Maxillofacial Infections, 3rd ed. Philadelphia, 1994, Saunders.
18. Wood RS: Chronic granulomatous infections. Oral Maxillofac Surg Clin 3:405-422, 1991.

35. TEMPOROMANDIBULAR JOINT ANATOMY, PATHOPHYSIOLOGY, AND SURGICAL TREATMENT

Renato Mazzonetto, DDS, PhD, Steven G. Gollehon, DDS, MD, FACS, Daniel B. Spagnoli, DDS, PhD, and Gregory M. Ness, DDS

1.   What is the main function of cartilage?
Cartilage is aneural, avascular, and alymphatic. Its main function is to withstand compressional forces during frictional joint loading. The articular cartilage functions to resist forces of compression and joint friction between the condyle and fossa. Chondrocytes within the cartilage also secrete important biochemicals for joint function, such as lubricin, which acts to maintain joint integrity and reduce functional wear.

2.   What is the difference between temporomandibular joint (TMJ) articular cartilage and cartilage of other synovial joints?
Most synovial joints have hyaline cartilage on their articular surface; however, a number of joints, such as the sternoclavicular, acromioclavicular, and TMJs, are associated with bones that develop from intramembranous ossification. These have fibrocartilage articular surfaces.

3.   What are the unique properties of the TMJ and its articular disc?
The articular disc is tightly attached to the lateral and medial poles of the condyle. Therefore

during mouth opening, the condyle-articular disc complex moves in a sliding movement relative to the temporal bone to or beyond the apex of the articular eminence, whereas the condyle rotates underneath the disc. Because the TMJ has characteristics of both a hinge joint (ginglymus) and a gliding joint (articulatio plana), it is classified as a ginglymoarthrodial joint. A unique feature of the TMJ is that it is rigidly connected to both the dentition and the contralateral TMJ.

4. What are the main protective and functional responsibilities of the articular disc of the TMJ?

The main functions of the disc are to absorb shock and to resist stretching and compressional forces by transforming them into tension stresses in the collagen fibers. These stresses are dispersed throughout the collagen network and consequently reduced. Another function of the articular disc is to establish joint stability while translatory movements of the condyle occur.

5. What is synovium?

Synovium is the thin epithelioid tissue lining nonarticular surfaces of diarthrodial joints. In the healthy TMJ, the anterior and posterior recesses of both the superior and inferior joint spaces are lined with synovium. The synovium contains specialized cell types A and B. Type A cells are derived from the monocyte/macrophage lineage and are phagocytic, filling an important role in the catabolic metabolism of articular cartilage. Type B cells are more fibroblastic in nature and secrete hyaluronic acid and proteoglycans, components of synovial fluid. Synovial fluid is a dialysate of blood plasma containing hyaluronate and proteoglycans, and it is important for joint surface nutrition, oxygenation, and lubrication.

6. What are the external causes of internal derangements of the TMJ?

External causes of internal derangements are classified as macrotrauma or microtrauma. External factors such as clenching, grinding, bruxing, nail biting, and other parafunctional habits can cause excessive joint loading and lack of motion. These actions lead to inflammatory biochemical alterations in the joint that promote degradation, synovial inflammation, and formation of adhesions.

7. What is the relationship between osteoarthritis and TMJ disc displacement?

The relationship between osteoarthritis and disc displacement is a subject of debate. Disc displacement may be a sign, as well as a cause, of TMJ osteoarthritis. However, it often is a concomitant phenomenon with an initial disturbance of molecular and cellular processes leading to osteoarthritis in cartilaginous tissues. The concomitant manifestation of both osteoarthritis and disc displacement comprises a substantial portion of all TMJ disorders, although both conditions may manifest separately and may be mutually independent. Currently, osteoarthritis, alone or in combination with disc displacement, is one of the most prevalent TMJ disorders.

8. How do external factors lead to anatomic alterations in the TMJ?

Acute **macrotrauma** to the joint, such as direct or coup-contrecoup injuries, may result in displacement, contusion, hemorrhage, and irreversible deformation of the joint tissues with the potential for intracapsular interferences, restrictive fibrosis, and inflammation.

Functional overload, or **microtrauma,** is another frequent cause of internal derangements. Chronic microtrauma is associated with parafunctional activities such as chronic clenching habits, grinding, nail biting, and gum chewing that alter the lubricating properties of the joint; introduce friction between the disc and the condyle, causing degenerative changes; and result in gradual anterior displacement and eventual perforation of the disc.

9. What is the sensitive balance between anabolism and catabolism that exists in the TMJ synovium and articular disc?

Because the articular cartilage is avascular and alymphatic, nutrition and elimination of waste products are dependent on diffusion through the cartilage matrix from and to the synovial fluid. Joint loading significantly stimulates disc diffusion and is essential to chondrocyte nutrition. Because cartilage is avascular, chondrocytes have to function under almost anaerobic conditions. Consequently, they have relatively low metabolic activity, which renders them vulnerable to toxic influences. Chondrocytes are unable to regenerate after major trauma, but they have considerable recuperative abilities. Although once thought of as an inert tissue, articular cartilage is now recognized as a dynamic system that is capable of remodeling under functional demands and turnover of extracellular matrix components. As long as the environment of the TMJ synovium and articular cartilage exists in a balance between net breakdown and net buildup, most destructive processes in the TMJ remain subclinical. It is when the net catabolism (breakdown) exceeds the anabolic buildup (reparative processes) that most chronic inflammatory conditions begin to become symptomatic.

10. What is synovitis, and how does it occur?

Synovitis is an inflammatory disorder of the synovial membrane that is characterized by hyperemia, edema, and capillary proliferation in the synovial membrane. Synovitis occurs when the level of cellular debris and the concentration of biochemical mediators of inflammation and pain produce levels that the synovial membrane is unable to ingest, absorb, or process.

11. Biochemically, what compounds have been linked to the pathogenic pathway in TMJ osteoarthritis?

In osteoarthritic cartilage, which is characterized by tissue degradation, an imbalance between protease and protease inhibitor levels or activities has been postulated as a possible pathogenic pathway in osteoarthritis. In support of this, high levels of active metalloproteases, in particular MMP-2, MMP-9, and MMP-3, were found in lavage fluids of affected TMJs.

12. What is "weeping lubrication"? What is its origin and function in maintaining TMJ homeostasis?

Loading of cartilage during joint movement results in an increase of the internal hydrostatic pressure. If the hydrostatic pressure exceeds the osmotic pressure exerted by the proteoglycans, water is squeezed out of the extracellular matrix, contributing to the lubrication of the joint surfaces during joint movement. This so-called weeping lubrication occurs particularly under high loads. Under low loads, the so-called boundary lubrication functions through a lubricating glycoprotein, lubricin. The proteoglycans, in collaboration with the collagen network, determine the viscoelastic properties of the cartilage and provide it with its resilience, elasticity, shear strength, and self-lubrication. In addition, proteoglycans can function as internal membrane receptors.

13. What are the goals of nonsurgical management of TMJ disorders?

Some patients with TMJ disorders can be managed successfully without surgery. Between 2% and 5% of all patients treated for TMJ disorders undergo surgery. Physical therapy, occlusal splint therapy, pharmacologic therapy, occlusal adjustments, and patient counseling can treat joint pain and limitation in mouth opening. The goals are:
- To eliminate pain or at least decrease it to a level that the patient can manage
- To decrease or eliminate jaw dysfunction and to increase masticatory ability
- To restore jaw movement to a normal range of motion
- To counsel the patient about habits that tend to decrease TMJ function

14. What are the indications to proceed with TMJ surgery?

Patients with pain and dysfunction whose signs and symptoms do not respond satisfactorily to nonsurgical therapy within a period of 3 months may be candidates for surgery, particularly if they are diagnosed with advanced internal derangement caused by ankylosis, rheumatoid arthritis, or severe degenerative osteoarthritis. Patients with no improvement in range of motion and mouth opening despite conservative treatment are also candidates for surgical therapy. Some clinicians recommend earlier (within days or weeks) invasive management by arthrocentesis of conditions such as acute closed lock.

15. When is TMJ arthrocentesis indicated?

Arthrocentesis is used to manage TMJ problems in patients who do not respond well to nonsurgical therapy. The major indications for its use are (1) acute or chronic limitation of motion owing to an anterior displaced disc without reduction and (2) hypomobility resulting from restriction of condylar translation in the upper joint space. Patients with normal range of motion despite an anterior disc displacement with reduction who nonetheless have chronic pain also respond favorably to arthrocentesis. Arthrocentesis also may be used to manage pain and dysfunction in patients who have undergone previous invasive procedures that have failed to relieve pain with limitation of function. The alteration of the biochemical environment within the intracapsular space by arthrocentesis to relieve various vasoactive pain mediators is also another strong indication for treatment. Arthrocentesis may bridge the gap between nonsurgical therapy or nonsurgical and pharmacologic therapy and invasive TMJ surgery.

16. What are the major advantages of TMJ arthroscopic surgery over open joint surgery?

A minimally invasive surgical procedure, arthroscopy allows direct visualization of the anatomic structures of the TMJ, biopsy of pathologic tissue, and removal of osteoarthritic fibrillation tissue, as well as direct injection of steroid into inflamed synovial tissues and correlation of clinical findings with the actual joint pathology or previous imaging studies. Patients experience decreased morbidity, faster recovery time, and less intraarticular inflammation and destruction than with open joint procedures.

17. When is arthroscopic surgery contraindicated?

Contraindications to arthroscopy are similar to those for other elective procedures, such as any medical condition that places the patient at an increased risk from general anesthesia or the surgical procedure itself. Local contraindications include skin or ear infections, and severe or advanced fibrous ankylosis resulting in severe limitations and movement of the condyle. Emotional instability, obesity that prevents the joints from being palpated adequately, and other circumstances unique to the patient are also considerations.

18. Why is preservation of the synovial membrane, articular cartilage, and disc important during TMJ surgery?

The synovial membrane must be maintained to provide joint lubrication. Excessive removal of synovial tissue with shavers, cautery, or laser should be avoided to prevent scar formation and the subsequent formation of dense connective tissue. Articular cartilage should be preserved when possible to maintain resiliency and compressibility of the joint; moreover, only the fibrillated osteoarthritic tissue should be removed conservatively during arthroscopy. Disc preservation is important because it gives the joint a biochemical advantage by facilitating intracapsular boundaries and hydrostatic weeping lubrication. Many surgeons achieve favorable results using arthroscopic lysis and lavage alone, removing no tissues at all.

19. What role does disc repositioning play in achieving successful TMJ surgery outcomes?

There is debate over this question among surgeons. Most would advocate preservation of as much normal joint structure and architecture as possible for the reasons listed previously. Patients who undergo disc removal develop radiographic changes, such as condylar flattening and osteophyte formation, similar to those seen in advanced osteoarthritis, although these postsurgical changes are often asymptomatic. On the other hand, procedures such as meniscectomy have high clinical success rates, and disc repositioning has been found to be temporary in many cases following arthroscopy or meniscoplasty procedures, suggesting that the clinical benefit is not dependent on restoring a reduced disc position.

20. Do lasers have advantages over conventional rotary instruments in arthroscopic procedures?

Yes. The effectiveness of joint surgery has improved greatly with the application of laser technology. Diseased tissues can be removed without mechanical contact, thus minimizing trauma to the articular cartilage and surrounding synovial surfaces. Coagulation of bleeding occurs instantly without thermal damage. Bone spurs are easily removed, minimizing the use of larger mechanical instruments in narrow places, which further reduces local tissue insult.

21. What are the indications for total joint reconstruction?

- Fibrous or bony ankylosis with severe anatomic abnormalities
- Failed autogenous grafts in multiply operated patients
- Destruction of autogenously grafted tissues by pathology
- Failed Proplast-Teflon implants that result in severe anatomic joint mutilation
- Failed Vitek-Kent total or partial joints
- Severe inflammatory disease, such as rheumatoid arthritis, that results in anatomic mutilation of the joint components and functional destabilization

22. In the total joint reconstruction surgery, what is the best way to reproduce the patient's anatomy and create an accurate and long-lasting custom joint prosthesis?

Currently, conventional computed tomography (CT) is used to create a three-dimensional stereolithographic model from epoxy resin material that reproduces a functional model of the patient's cranium, temporal bones, and mandible. Recontouring "model surgery" can be done to simulate the surgical changes needed to provide a stable, accurate replica of the patient's anatomy and increase the chances for successful fit and placement of prosthetic components. Accurate reproduction of the patient's occlusion and centric relation positions of the mandible can be obtained, and prosthetic joint components can then be fabricated using diagnostic wax-ups. Once accuracy is maintained and diagnostic wax-ups are verified, customized TMJ prostheses using chrome, cobalt, and molybdenum can be fabricated with or without high-molecular-weight polyethylene fossa components. In total TMJ reconstruction, these techniques have become the standard of care for providing a long-lasting, stable prosthesis in patients who require total joint rehabilitation.

23. What are the stages of osteoarthritis?

1. Initial stage
2. Repair stage
3. Degradation stage
   - Early
   - Progressive
4. Late stage

24. What occurs during the initial and repair stages of osteoarthritis?

If a primary insult, whether biochemical, biomechanical, inflammatory, or immunologic, disturbs the chondrocyte control balance between synthesis and degradation of extracellular matrix components in normal tissue turnover, cartilage degradation ensues. Initially, cartilage degradation caused by increased proteolytic activity will be counteracted by attempts at repair. In the repair stage, an increased degradation of extracellular matrix components by protease is counteracted by an increased anabolic cytokine-mediated synthesis of these components by chondrocytes. This results in a new balance between increased degradation and increased synthesis of extracellular matrix components. Histologically, the repair stage is characterized by the proliferation of chondrocytes. Clinically, the cartilage changes in the repair stage of osteoarthritis may remain asymptomatic for many years. In general, osteoarthritis is progressive and ultimately manifests clinically. However, what causes the established balance to tip, resulting initially in a focal net degradation of extracellular matrix components, still is not known.

25. **How does the early degradation stage of osteoarthritis differ from the initial and repair stages?**

In early stages of osteoarthritis, the degradation caused by the increased synthesis and activity of protease exceeds the increases of extracellular matrix components by the chondrocytes. This results in an initial focal degradation and loss of articular cartilage. The key feature of disease progression is the enzymatic breakdown of the cartilage. Consequently, the content of several extracellular matrix components is reduced focally, whereas the composition and distribution of the other extracellular matrix components are altered. The collagen network shows signs of electron-microscopic disorganization. The fibrils, of the articular surface in particular, appear disoriented and separated more widely than normal. In addition, the histochemical stains for proteoglycans show uneven staining with focally increased affinity, especially in areas of swelling and focal loss of metachromasia. Also, the chondrocytes may produce free radicals that will cause cleavage of extracellular matrix molecules. The content of proteolytic enzymes, including acid phosphatase, serine protease, and metalloprotease such as collagenase and stromelysin-1, is increased in early osteoarthritic cartilage proportional to the severity of the disease process.

26. **What role does synovial clearance play in the initial clinical manifestations of osteoarthritis?**

The degradation products of the extracellular matrix components are further degraded by the chondrocytes or diffused into synovial fluid, where they are removed by the circulation or are phagocytosed by synovial A lining cells. This latter phenomenon is called synovial clearance and frequently induces a secondary synovitis. Often, the osteoarthritic process becomes manifest only when a secondary synovitis develops, causing joint pain and, frequently, a limitation of joint movement. Moreover, the involvement of the synovial tissues in the osteoarthritic process initiates a cascade of secondary events, creating a vicious circle that leads to further cartilage damage by the synthesis of inflammatory and pain mediators.

27. **What is the clinical importance of interleukin-1 and prostaglandins in the early breakdown stages of osteoarthritis?**

Interleukin-1 induces increased synthesis of prostaglandins, prostaglandin E_2 (PGE_2) in particular, by synoviocytes. This increase in prostaglandins may be responsible for several of the symptoms observed in this stage of osteoarthritis. Prostaglandins and leukotrienes are mediators of inflammation. In response to inflammatory changes, nonmyelinated sensory neurons in the synovial tissues may release substance P and other pain mediators. Among other effects, substance P may enhance the synthesis of collagenase and PGE_2 by the synovial lining cells, thereby perpetuating the catabolic process.

28. **What occurs during the progressive degradation stage of osteoarthritis?**

In this stage, the anabolic process has become increasingly defective relative to catabolic effects. The synthesis of extracellular matrix components fails or, as the synthesis and activity of protease remains increased, results in a progressive degradation, erosion, and loss of articular cartilage. Histologically, the progressive degradation stage of osteoarthritis is characterized by fibrillation, detachments, and thinning of the cartilage from mechanical wear. Irregularities and reduplication of the tide mark have been observed, although less often in the TMJ than in other osteoarthritic synovial joints.

29. **What are the hallmark arthroscopic features of the progressive degradation stages of osteoarthritis?**

Arthroscopically, the articular cartilage of the TMJ may appear fibrillated or eroded. Fibrillation of the cartilage of the articular eminence may be focal or extensive. Articular disc displacement, either reducing or nonreducing, is frequently seen. Angiogenesis in the cartilage of the articular eminence may be observed, whereas creeping synovitis may be seen on the posterior wall of the glenoid fossa and the articular disc. The synovial tissues may appear hypervascularized and redundant or may show fibrotic changes in local areas. In addition, adhesion formation may result in a reduction of the anterior and posterior joint recesses.

30. What occurs during the late stages of osteoarthritis?

The content of several extracellular matrix components, including water, proteoglycans and collagen is further reduced. The synthesis and activity of protease may remain increased or may be finally reduced when the articular cartilage is nearly destroyed, resulting in so-called residual osteoarthritis. Histologically, the late stage of osteoarthritis is characterized by an extensive fibrillation of the cartilage, eventually resulting in severe thinning of the articular cartilage layer or even denudation of the subchondral bone. Chondrocyte necrosis often occurs. The collagen network is severely disorganized and disintegrated, whereas histochemical stains for proteoglycans show severe depletion of proteoglycans. Biochemically, the late stage of osteoarthritis is characterized by continuous increased syntheses of protease or by decreased synthesis of protease in the case of residual osteoarthritis. The content of several extracellular matrix components is further reduced to levels in residual osteoarthritis.

31. What arthroscopic findings are seen in the late stage of osteoarthritis?

Cartilage may appear severely fibrillated and eroded. Denudation of subcondylar bone is seen, and angiogenesis of the cartilage of the articular eminence may be present. Disc displacement or disc perforation may have developed. The synovial tissues may appear hypervascularized and redundant or may have become fibrotic. In the latter stages of this disease, adhesion formation with opposing surfaces frequently results in limited joint recesses.

32. What are the clinical manifestations of the late stages of osteoarthritis?

- Clinically, the late stages of osteoarthritis may be manifest by joint pain and limitation of joint movement.
- Joint noises may be present if the disc displacement or proliferation has developed, or may be caused by articular cartilage surface irregularities.
- In the case of residual osteoarthritis of the TMJ, clinical signs and symptoms may have ceased.

33. What serious complications may arise from arthroplasty for TMJ bony ankylosis?

Injury to the middle ear with loss of hearing, damage to the facial nerve (specifically the temporal or zygomatic branches), and severe intraoperative bleeding, usually from the internal maxillary artery are significant risks of this operation.

BIBLIOGRAPHY

1. Dijkgraaf LC, Milam SB: Osteoarthritis: histopathology and biochemistry of the TMJ. Oral Maxillofac Surg Knowledge Update 3:1-20, 2000.
2. Dijkgraaf CL, Spijkervet FK, de Bont LG: Arthroscopic findings in osteoarthritic temporomandibular joints. J Oral Maxillofac Surg 57:255-268, 1999.
3. Frost DE, Kendell BD: The use of arthrocentesis for treatment of temporomandibular joint disorders. J Oral Maxillofac Surg 57:583-587, 1999.
4. Hall DH: The role of discectomy for treating internal derangements of the temporomandibular joint. Oral Maxillofac Surg Clin North Am 6:287-296, 1994.
5. Hoffmann KD: Differential diagnosis and characteristics of TMJ disease and disorders. Oral Maxillofac Surg Knowledge Update 1:43-66, 1994.
6. Israel HA: The use of arthroscopic surgery for treatment of temporomandibular joint disorders. J Oral Maxillofac Surg 57:579-582, 1999.
7. Laskin DM: Etiology and pathogenesis of internal derangements of the temporomandibular joint. Oral Maxillofac Surg Clin North Am 6:217-229, 1994.
8. Quinn JH: Arthroscopic histopathology. Oral Maxillofac Surg Knowledge Update 1:115-132, 1994.
9. Sanders B: Arthroscopic management of internal derangements of the temporomandibular joint. Oral Maxillofac Surg Clin North Am 6:259-269, 1994.

10. Spagnoli DB: Anatomy of the TMJ. Oral Maxillofac Surg Knowledge Update 1:1-41, 1994.
11. Wilkes CH: Internal derangements of the temporomandibular joint. Pathological variations. Arch Otolaryngol Head Neck Surg 115:469-477, 1989.

36. TEMPOROMANDIBULAR DISORDERS AND FACIAL PAIN: BIOCHEMICAL AND BIOMECHANICAL BASIS

Steven G. Gollehon, DDS, MD, FACS, Daniel B. Spagnoli, DDS, PhD, and Gregory M. Ness, DDS

1. How are the treatment modalities to manage temporomandibular joint (TMJ) pain and dysfunction classified?

The treatment of TMJ pain and dysfunction is divided into irreversible and reversible modalities. Reversible therapy consists of patient education, medication, physical therapy, and splint therapy. Occlusal adjustments, prosthetic restoration, orthodontic treatment, orthognathic surgery, and TMJ surgery are irreversible therapies that involve permanent changes in the function or morphology of the masticatory system.

2. What is the most common form of pain and discomfort associated with TMJ disorders?

Masticatory myalgia or myofascial pain.

3. How is the etiology of muscle pain categorized?

- Muscle hyperactivity (functional and dysfunctional)
- Muscle inflammation (myositis) secondary to injury or infection
- Myalgia associated with muscle hyperactivity

In contrast to episodic myofascial pain, myofascial pain dysfunction (MPD) syndrome is chronic and self-perpetuating. Sustained muscular hyperactivity results in increased loading of the articular surfaces, and microtrauma leads to inflammation, arthralgia, reflex muscle splinting, and continued myospasm.

4. What clinical sign is pathognomonic for the first stage of internal derangement of the articular disc?

Reciprocal clicking is considered pathognomonic for the first stage of disc displacement. In the first stage of internal derangement, clicking begins suddenly and spontaneously or after an injury. The noise is often loud and may be audible to others, but it is rarely associated with severe pain. The patient may be aware of a feeling of obstruction within the joint during movement until the click occurs. The mandible frequently deviates toward the affected side until the click occurs and then returns to the midline after the click.

5. What are the hallmarks of the second stage of internal derangement?

The second stage of disc derangement is reciprocal clicking with intermittent locking. The typical patient complains that the jaw becomes locked and there is usually, but not always, severe pain over the affected joint. Patients may describe a feeling of obstruction to opening within the joint. Patients may be able to manipulate the joint to restore function. In some cases, the jaw may unlock spontaneously. In nearly all cases, there is a prior history of clicking of the affected joint.

6. How does stage 3 of internal derangements of the articular disc differ?

The third stage of disc derangement is associated with limited opening and has been termed closed lock. A limited opening of <27 mm and severe pain over the affected joint are characteristic findings. A deviation of the mandible on opening is also seen. Again, the patient often describes a feeling of fullness or obstruction. In contrast to stage 2, few patients are able to unlock or relocate their closed lock and restore normal function.

7. Why is the fourth stage of internal derangement less painful when compared with earlier stages of disc derangement?

The fourth and final stage in the classification of internal derangement involving the articular disc is characterized by an increase in opening and crepitus occurring within the joint during movement due to degenerative changes in the disc and articular surfaces. This stage appears to be less painful than previous stages because the neurovascular tissue is no longer impinged between the condyle and the glenoid fossa.

8. What is the relationship between disc displacement and clinical symptoms of pain and discomfort?

Despite the clinical evidence supporting the existence of TMJ disc derangement, many questions remain unanswered, raising doubts about its clinical significance. Because pain is usually aggravated by functional and parafunctional movements, it would appear that pain originates from pressure and traction on the disc attachments. However, many, and perhaps the majority of, patients with displaced discs have no pain, whereas some have severe pain. Studies by Kircos et al. (1987) and Westesson et al. (1989) show a 30% incidence of disc displacement in asymptomatic patients with normal TMJ exams and an 88% incidence of disc displacement in the contralateral asymptomatic joint in patients with unilateral pain and discomfort, respectively. These findings make it clear that disc displacement is not necessarily related to pain.

9. Does "preemptive" analgesia reduce postsurgical pain and chronic pain following surgery in patients with TMJ disorders?

Recent studies have demonstrated that dynamic processing by neurons in the affected pathway may facilitate nociception. The old view that nociceptive pathways are merely static conductors of signals generated by noxious stimuli appears to be invalid. As a result, preemptive analgesic techniques may reduce postsurgical pain and, perhaps, reduce the possibility of chronic pain in the operated patient.

10. What is the main goal in the postoperative management of patients with TMJ dysfunction?

Chronic pain and restricted jaw movement are the most common complaints of multiply operated TMJ dysfunction patients. Typically, pain restricts the patient's ability to comply with postsurgical physical therapy, contributing to a gradual decline in jaw mobility. Therefore the major management objective should be adequate pain control coupled with effective physical therapy to maintain jaw function.

11. What are the management strategies used to treat pain and discomfort in the multiply operated patient with TMJ dysfunction?

Strategies include pharmacologic approaches, behavioral modification techniques, psychiatric counseling, and physical therapy. Obviously, the success of any approach will depend on an accurate assessment of the patient's physical and emotional status. Furthermore, combination therapies (provided by a coordinated, multidisciplinary team of qualified health care providers) are often required to optimize the patient's condition. Further surgery is ineffective at reducing pain in the multiply operated patient and is not indicated unless a specific mechanical obstruction to function is identifiable and amenable to surgical correction (e.g., ankylosis). In such cases, the patient must understand that improvements in range of motion and function are not likely to be accompanied by pain reduction.

12. What is peripheral sensitization? What is its role in hyperalgesia in facial pain?

According to Hargreaves and Wardle, small-diameter group III and IV afferent nerve fibers innervate joints and muscles and respond to stimuli that can be perceived as noxious, such as pressure, algesic chemicals, and inflammatory agents. Ischemia also is an effective stimulus if present for significant amounts of time and is associated with muscle contractions. These nociceptors may be excited by a variety of stimuli, and their sensitivity may be increased following mild, persistent injury. As a result, this "peripheral sensitization" is thought to be a major factor in the production of hyperalgesia. In conjunction with central sensitization, peripheral sensitization explains the persistent, chronic nature of myofascial pain and the pain of TMJ disorders.

13. What subnucleus of the trigeminal tract seems to be related to reception and processing as a second-order sensory neuron in the modulation of facial and TMJ-derived pain?

Electrophysiologic data acquired in the last two decades generally support the view that subnucleus caudalis of the V spinal tract nucleus is an essential V brainstem relay for orofacial pain. Neurons responsive to noxious mechanical stimuli or to algesic chemicals applied to articular and muscular tissues predominate in the superficial and deep laminae of the subnucleus caudalis, where anatomic studies indicate projections of deep afferent inputs terminate. Evidence is emerging that the role of the subnucleus caudalis in pain is related primarily to processing of nociceptive information from facial skin and deep tissues, whereas the more rostral components, such as the subnucleus oralis, may be more involved in intraoral and perioral pain mechanisms.

14. What are the main types of neurons that perceive and transmit nociceptive stimuli from the orofacial region?

Second-order nociceptive-specific and wide dynamic range neurons in the nucleus caudalis of V receive nociceptive input from peripheral nociceptors in skin and deep muscle tissues. The transmission, interaction, and feedback mechanisms at the level of higher order sensory neurons in the thalamus and somatosensory cortex remain unknown and are an intense area of research.

15. What molecular events may contribute to degenerative disease in the TMJ?

The inflammatory, catabolic changes that lead to osteoarthritis of the TMJ may be provoked by oxidative stress triggered by several possible mechanisms. A variety of potentially injurious cytokines, neuropeptides, cartilage matrix degrading enzymes, and arachidonic acid metabolites have been identified in the synovial fluid of diseased TMJs. Oxidative stress is the accumulation of reactive free radical molecules that may then injure tissues both directly and indirectly by stimulating production of these molecules. The free radical formation may be initiated (1) by direct mechanical stress to cartilage, erythrocytes, or other tissues, (2) by cyclic hypoxia-reperfusion injury to tissues within the joint, or (3) as a direct result of neurogenic inflammation, in which free radicals may modulate cytokine production.

16. What role does estrogen play in the female predilection for TMJ dysfunction?

In general, women tend to report more pain and exhibit a higher incidence of joint noise and mandibular deflection with movement than do men. Functional estrogen receptors have been identified in the female TMJ but not in the male TMJ. Estrogen may also promote degenerative changes in the TMJ by increasing the synthesis of specific cytokines, whereas testosterone may inhibit these cytokines. It is likely that sex hormones profoundly influence several cell activities that may be associated with remodeling or degenerative processes in the human TMJ.

17. What is the incidence of TMJ dysfunction and pain in patients with rheumatoid arthritis?

The occurrence of TMJ pain caused by rheumatoid arthritis depends on the severity of the systemic disease. According to several clinical investigations, about one third to one half of patients with rheumatoid arthritis will experience pain in this joint at some time, with nearly 60% of patients suffering from bilateral joint dysfunction. For more than one third of patients, temporomandibular dysfunction symptoms begin within 1 year after the onset of general disease. Fifteen percent to 16% of these patients will develop great functional disability.

18. What occurs during progression of rheumatoid arthritis in the TMJ?
The target tissue of rheumatoid arthritis is the synovial membrane. Progression in the TMJ follows a general scheme with exudation, cellular infiltration, and pannus formation. The articular surfaces of the temporal and condylar components are destroyed, the disc becomes grossly perforated, and the subchondral bone is resorbed. Complete ankylosis of the joint seldom occurs, although most persons have reduced mandibular mobility and loss of posterior height, resulting in apertognathia. The progression of rheumatoid arthritis is slow in most people, although a few experience severe joint destruction within a few months. The presence of a high erythrocyte sedimentation rate is a negative prognostic factor.

19. How is chondromalacia defined as it applies to the TMJ?
Chondromalacia is a term used rather loosely by the medical profession to describe a clinically distinctive posttraumatic softening of the articular cartilage of the patella in young people. The term is now also applied to the TMJ and mimics lesions of early osteoarthritis. Osteoarthritis starts focally in a joint; clinical symptoms occur when it is present to a certain degree or when a certain area is affected.

20. How do primary and secondary osteoarthritis differ as they apply to the TMJ?
Primary osteoarthritis will result in degenerative changes, disc displacement, and finally changes in joint morphology. All signs and symptoms seem to be the result of this primary, idiopathic process. Secondary osteoarthritis shows degenerative changes due to joint afflictions, such as rheumatoid arthritis, but also may be due to disc displacement. Osteoarthritis of the TMJ deals with synovial joint pathology, primarily with a connective tissue disease.

BIBLIOGRAPHY

1. Dolwick MF: Temporomandibular joint disk displacement: clinical perspectives. In Sessle BJ, Bryant PS, Dionne RA (eds): Temporomandibular Disorders and Related Pain Conditions: Progress in Pain Research and Management, 4th ed. Seattle, 1995, IASP Press.
2. Hargreaves AS, Wardle JJ: The use of physiotherapy in the treatment of temporomandibular disorders. Br Dent J 155:121-124, 1983.
3. Hoffmann KD: Differential diagnosis and characteristics of TMJ disease and disorders. Oral Maxillofac Surg Knowl Update 1:43, 1994.
4. Kircos LT, Ortendahl DA, Mark AS et al: Magnetic resonance imaging of the TMJ disc in asymptomatic volunteers. J Oral Maxillofac Surg 45:852-854, 1987.
5. Kopp S: Degenerative and inflammatory temporomandibular joint disorders: clinical perspectives. In Sessle BJ, Bryant PS, Dionne RA (eds): Temporomandibular Disorders and Related Pain Conditions: Progress in Pain Research and Management, 4th ed. Seattle, 1995, IASP Press.
6. Lambert GM: Degenerative and inflammatory temporomandibular joint disorders: basic science perspectives. In Sessle BJ, Bryant PS, Dionne RA (eds): Temporomandibular Disorders and Related Pain Conditions: Progress in Pain Research and Management, 4th ed. Seattle, 1995, IASP Press.
7. Milam SB: Nonsurgical management of the multiply operated TMD patient. Selected Readings Oral Maxillofac Surg 6:4, 1999.
8. Milam SB: Articular disk displacements and degenerative temporomandibular joint disease. In Sessle BJ, Bryant PS, Dionne RA (eds): Temporomandibular Disorders and Related Pain Conditions: Progress in Pain Research and Management, 4th ed. Seattle, 1995, IASP Press.
9. Milam, SB, Zardeneta G: Oxidative stress and degenerative temporomandibular joint disease: a proposed hypothesis. J Oral Maxillofac Surg 56:214-223, 1998.
10. National Institutes of Health: Management of Temporomandibular Disorders: National Institutes of Health Technology Assessment Conference Statement. Bethesda, Md, 1996, NIH.

11. Sessle BJ: Masticatory muscle disorders: basic science perspectives. In Sessle BJ, Bryant PS, Dionne RA (eds): Temporomandibular Disorders and Related Pain Conditions: Progress in Pain Research and Management, 4th ed. Seattle, 1995, IASP Press.
12. Stohler CS: Clinical perspectives on masticatory and related muscle disorders. In Sessle BJ, Bryant PS, Dionne RA (eds): Temporomandibular Disorders and Related Pain Conditions: Progress in Pain Research and Management, 4th ed. Seattle, 1995, IASP Press.
13. Westesson PL, Eriksson L, Kurita K: Reliability of a negative clinical temporomandibular joint examination: prevalence of disk displacement in asymptomatic temporomandibular joints. Oral Surg Oral Med Oral Pathol 68:551-554, 1989.

37. DENTOFACIAL ABNORMALITIES

A. Omar Abubaker, DMD, PhD, and Bashar M. Rajab, DDS

1. What are the two types of anteroposterior (AP) mandibular deficiencies?
1. Low mandibular plane angle type
2. High mandibular plane angle type
    Each has distinct morphologic and occlusal presentations, but in both types the mandible is small.

2. What are the features of AP mandibular deficiencies?
The features of the **low mandibular plane angle** type include small mandible, short facial height, curled-over lower lip, and deep labiomental crease. The angles of the mandible and the masseters are usually well developed and well defined, and the maxilla may be vertically deficient. The occlusion shows a curve of Spee, which is generally excessive in both arches. The mandibular anterior teeth may occlude with the palate, along with an excessively deep bite. Radiographically, the ramus height is usually normal, and the angular and linear cephalometric measurements are usually smaller than normal.

The **high mandibular plane angle** variety is characterized by normal or excessive face height, a small and retropositioned chin, flattened labiomental fold, and excessive activity of the mentalis muscles. The mandibular ramus is short, the condyles are usually small, and the angles of the mandible are obtuse and hypoplastic. The occlusion is characterized by protrusive maxillary teeth, narrow arch form, constricted mandibular arch, and Class II canine and molar relationships. There may be an open bite, which is indicative of conditions such as rheumatoid arthritis, temporomandibular joint (TMJ) ankylosis, and condylar resorption. If AP mandibular deficiency of the high mandibular plane angle type exists along with vertical maxillary excess, all the features of vertical maxillary excess are present, and the features of mandibular deficiency are exaggerated.

3. How is mandibular deficiency treated?
Treatment of isolated mandibular deficiency usually involves mandibular advancement. Bilateral sagittal split osteotomy (BSSO) with rigid fixation is the most frequently performed procedure to accomplish this advancement, whereas inverted L osteotomy with rigid fixation and bone grafting is recommended for advancement >1 cm. In general, stability of mandibular advancement is better with smaller amounts of advancements than with large ones. Augmentation genioplasty procedures using an alloplastic or osteoplastic technique with and without BSSO technique occasionally is used to disguise significant mandibular deficiency. Also, mandibular subapical osteotomy may help in leveling the mandibular arch.

4.   What are the features of mandibular prognathism?

Although isolated mandibular prognathism is a rare condition, mandibular prognathism often is associated with maxillary deficiency. When the two conditions are present together, the appearance of mandibular prognathism is exaggerated. Overclosure of the vertical dimension and centric relation-centric occlusion slides also may coexist and exaggerate such appearance. The chin and lower lip in patients with these conditions are forward relative to the upper lip, often making them the dominant facial feature. The mandibular body and mandibular angle are well defined, often with an obtuse angle. The occlusion is Class III, and often the skeletal discrepancy is greater than the occlusal discrepancy because of the dental compensations. Such compensation is manifested as flared maxillary anterior teeth and upright mandibular anterior teeth.

5.   How is mandibular prognathism treated?

Sagittal split osteotomy with rigid fixation is the procedure of choice for correction of mandibular prognathism. Transoral vertical ramus osteotomy is advocated by some, especially for large posterior movement and when there is a need for an asymmetric setback. However, problems with control of the proximal segment and adverse postsurgical occlusal changes have been reported with this procedure. Surgery should be undertaken only after dental compensations are eliminated with presurgical orthodontics and, preferably, after mandibular growth is completed.

6.   What are the clinical and radiographic features of condylar hyperplasia?

Condylar hyperplasia (hemimandibular elongation) is typically a postpubertal-onset, gradually developing asymmetry. The clinical features of this condition include asymmetry affecting the lower facial third, deviation of the mandible away from the affected side, and a secondary compensatory vertical growth of the maxilla on the affected side. There is also a shift of the mandibular dental midline away from the affected side, with asymmetric canine and molar relationships and lateral crossbite. The canine and molars are always in Class III occlusion on the affected side. Associated mandibular prognathism or maxillary deficiency also may be present.

The radiographic features include a longer condylar neck on the affected side with a condylar head that may or may not be normal in morphology, depending on the rate of growth when the condition begins. The cephalometric radiograph always demonstrates asymmetry of the mandibular ramus and angle with varying degrees of dental compensation. Similarly, the AP cephalogram often shows mandibular asymmetry, with varying degrees of dental compensation and enlargement of the affected ramus and condyle.

7.   How is mandibular condylar hyperplasia treated?

An important component of planning the treatment of condylar hyperplasia is determining the status of growth of the mandibular condyle before intervention. This can be done by eliciting a careful history of asymmetric growth. A history of recent change suggests active growth, whereas a history of lengthy presence without change indicates inactivity. Scintigraphic studies also are helpful in confirming active growth, although false-positive interpretations of this study are possible.

Once growth status of the mandibular condyle is determined, a decision on the treatment and its timing should be made. If active growth is present, the condylectomy may be either performed or delayed until growth has ceased. When condylectomy is performed, reconstruction of the ramus may be necessary. Maxillary and mandibular osteotomies, with and without condylectomy, to correct the facial asymmetry and malocclusion often are also part of the treatment of this condition.

8.   What is hemimandibular hypertrophy?

Hemimandibular hypertrophy, like condylar hyperplasia, causes facial asymmetry. Unlike condylar hyperplasia, however, development of hemimandibular hypertrophy usually occurs earlier, sometimes even during childhood. With this condition the maxilla can be affected secondarily, with a downward cant of the occlusion on the affected side. Depending on the degree of compensation, there may or may not be a malocclusion or shifting of the mandibular dental midline. The nonaffected side of the face is commonly small, and, therefore, the exact pathology is difficult to identify. The major distinguishing feature of this condition is an overall elongation of the side of the face, affecting both the osseous and soft tissue components.

The radiographic features of hemimandibular hypertrophy always show an enlargement of all parts of the mandible on the affected side, including the condyle, ramus, body of the mandible, and sometimes even the teeth. The enlargement may terminate short of the facial midline or may cross the midline and gradually taper with an abrupt stop in the inferior mandibular border. The inferior alveolar neurovascular bundle is often displaced inferiorly toward the inferior border of the mandible.

9. What is the treatment of hemimandibular hypertrophy?

As with condylar hyperplasia, a careful history of the growth pattern is necessary. Scintigraphic studies may be helpful in identifying growth activity and are critical for planning treatment. Surgical treatment generally consists of combined maxillary and mandibular osteotomies, to elongate the short side and shorten the long side of the face, and inferior border osteotomy and bone grafting. Condylectomy with reconstruction of the ramus also may be indicated if the condyle is actively growing.

10. What are the clinical features of vertical maxillary excess (VME)?

VME is characterized by excessive tooth display at lip repose, excessive gingival exposure on smiling, and lip incompetency. An open bite is almost always present, especially when there are steps in the maxillary occlusal plane. The face height is always long, and the chin is rotated downward and posteriorly. This condition is exaggerated by the presence of a short upper lip or maxillary protrusion. VME can be seen with Class I, II, or III occlusions.

11. How is VME treated?

VME can be treated with orthodontic intervention early in life (ages 8-12) with high-pull head gear or open bite Bionater to control vertical growth of the maxilla. If successful, such treatment may resolve the skeletal abnormalities, and ultimately the soft tissues and other facial structures grow accordingly. However, when an adult presents with this condition, it usually is treated with Le Fort I osteotomy and superior repositioning of the maxilla.

12. Are there any special factors that should be considered when treating VME?

Yes. Because the vertical growth of the maxilla is the last vector to cease, the excessive vertical development may continue growing later than expected. If significant vertical growth occurs, postsurgical relapse can result. Accordingly, as with most deformities characterized by excessive growth, delaying surgery until growth has slowed or completed is recommended. However, if VME is severe, early surgery may be justified on the basis of psychosocial benefits.

13. What are the causes of posterior VME?

• When opposing posterior mandibular teeth have been extracted, passive eruption of the maxillary teeth results.
• Posterior VME also may be caused by excessive maxillary vertical growth, which is usually associated with anterior open bite.

14. What are the clinical and radiographic features of posterior VME?

A distinct step in the maxillary occlusal plane is usually present. When posterior maxillary vertical excess occurs due to passive eruption of teeth, the condition is usually associated with inadequate interarch space, which poses a serious prosthetic challenge. Facial change is not apparent because the passive eruption ceases when the teeth contact the mandibular ridge. When posterior VME occurs in the dentate state, there is an increased facial height with lip incompetency secondary to downward and backward rotation of the mandible. The maxillary incisor-to-lip relationship may be normal, but during animation excessive gingiva shows in the posterior region.

Radiographic features of both conditions include excessive distance from the palatal plane to the first molar cusp. In the partially edentulous patient, excessive pneumatization of the maxillary sinus may be seen.

15. How is posterior VME treated?

Treatment of posterior VME involves an interdental osteotomy and superior positioning of the posterior segment. If inadequate space exists between the teeth, orthodontic movement or extraction of a tooth is necessary to avoid damage to adjacent teeth.

In the partially edentulous patient, the anterior occlusion should not change if isolated posterior maxillary osteotomy is performed. In the dentate state, superior repositioning of the posterior maxilla results in closure of the open bite, shortening of the face height, improved lip competency, improved mandibular rotation, and forward projection of the chin.

16. What are the clinical and cephalometric features of maxillary vertical deficiency?

- Maxillary vertical deficiency is often present with other skeletal abnormalities, such as AP or transverse maxillary deficiency or mandibular prognathism.
- The lower face height is always reduced, and the freeway space is excessive.
- Often, the maxillary incisors are completely covered by the upper lip at rest, with only a portion of the crowns exposed when smiling, and a proper-sized mandible will appear prognathic because of the overclosed position.
- The occlusion is typically Class III with differences between centric relation-centric occlusion.
- Cephalometrically, the palatal plane to first molar distance is always reduced.

17. How is vertical maxillary deficiency treated?

Treatment of vertical maxillary deficiency usually involves Le Fort I osteotomy with down-grafting, often in combination with mandibular osteotomy.

18. What are the features of maxillary AP deficiency? How is it treated?

AP deficiency of the maxilla is typically characterized by paranasal deficiencies, deficiency of the infraorbital region, and lack of zygomatic prominence. The upper lip behind the lower lip is the soft tissue characteristic. The occlusion is Class III with compensatory flaring of the maxillary anterior incisors in the true condition and is overly retracted if premolars have been removed previously to compensate orthodontically for mandibular deficiency.

Cephalometrically, the maxillary unit length measurements may confirm the diagnosis.

Treatment of maxillary AP deficiency usually consists of Le Fort I advancement with or without bone grafts, depending on the extent of advancement.

19. What are the possible complications of a Le Fort I osteotomy?

Intraoperative Complications

- Unfavorable osteotomy
- Improper maxillary repositioning
- Inability to stabilize the maxilla
- Bleeding
- Other minor technical difficulties

Postoperative Complications

- Relapse
- Bleeding
- Ophthalmic injury (rare)
- Condylar malpositioning (rare)

- Neurologic dysfunction
- Unfavorable facial aesthetics

- Avascular necrosis of segment (rare)

20. What are the possible complications of a BSSO?

As with maxillary procedures, complications of BSSO are classified as either intraoperative or postoperative. The most common complications of mandibular procedures in general—and BSSO in particular—include unfavorable osteotomy splits, nerve injury, bleeding, proximal segment malpositions, mandibular dysfunction (including TMJ dysfunction symptoms), and relapse. Wound infection, wound dehiscence, and vascular injury are some other possible complications.

21. What is the incidence of neurosensory dysfunction after Le Fort I osteotomy?

Injury to cranial nerve V2 is the most common injury, with 25% of patients experiencing reduced nociceptive response to pinpricks. Injury also has been reported to cranial nerve IV and the parasympathetic fibers of the lacrimal gland.

22. What is the incidence of unfavorable split osteotomy during BSSO? How is this complication treated?

An unfavorable split between the proximal and distal segments occurs in 3.1%-20% of cases. The use of heavy osteotome and twisting technique is believed to be the main cause. An unfavorable split should be treated by completing the osteotomy and using plates and screws to fix the fractured segments.

23. What is the incidence of neurosensory deficits following BSSO?

Neurosensory deficits of the inferior alveolar nerve following BSSO is one of the most significant concerns with this procedure. Complications occur in 20%-85% of surgeries. However, the incidence is only 9% at 1 year after surgery. This complication is more common in patients older than age 40 and in patients who undergo simultaneous genioplasty.

24. What are the different mandibular procedures for correction of mandibular deficiency and prognathism?

For treatment of mandibular deficiency, BSSO and inverted L osteotomy with bone grafting are the preferred procedures. For treatment of mandibular prognathism, BSSO and vertical subcondylar osteotomy are the most widely used procedures. Other procedures for treatment of mandibular deficiency and prognathism include C-ramus, subapical, and segmental osteotomies. More recently, distraction osteogenesis has become a popular procedure for treatment of mandibular deficiency and hypoplasia.

25. Which orthognathic procedure has the highest degree of relapse?

According to Proffit et al., transverse expansion of the maxilla is the most unstable orthognathic procedure. The greatest relapse is seen in the second molar region with an average of 50% loss of surgical expansion. After 1 year, inferior maxillary positioning and mandibular setbacks were also found to be less predictable than in other surgical techniques.

26. What is idiopathic condylar resorption?

Idiopathic condylar resorption of the mandibular condyle is a progressive dissolution of the condylar head without a history of apparent direct cause. The condition is seen mostly after orthognathic surgery, although it has been reported in patients who are undergoing or who have finished orthodontic treatment.

27. What are the causes of idiopathic condylar resorption?

Several clinical and radiographic risk factors have been reported in the literature, but the exact causes and pathogenesis of the condition remain unclear.

Patient-Related Risk Factors

- Age (young)
- Gender (female)
- Preoperative TMJ dysfunction symptoms
- Mandibular hypoplasia

- High mandibular plane angle
- Short posterior height
- Small posterior-to-anterior facial height ratio

Surgery-Related Risk Factors

- Counterclockwise rotation of the proximal and distal segments
- Surgically induced posterior condylar displacement in patients with extremely high mandibular plane angle
- Type of fixation (wire osteosynthesis and intermaxillary fixation; controversial)
- Direction and degree of mandibular movement (severe magnitude mandibular advancement; controversial)
- Condylar displacement after orthognathic surgery (controversial)

28. What are the clinical manifestations of condylar resorption?

The clinical signs of occlusal relapse after orthognathic surgery or orthodontic treatment develop before the radiographic sign of condylar resorption. The resorptive process can occur unilaterally or bilaterally and usually starts within the first year after treatment. Clinically, idiopathic condylar resorption is manifested by progressive development of anterior open bite and posterior rotation of the mandible with Class II canine and molar relation. The patient often begins to appear retrognathic and occludes mostly on the posterior teeth. The patient may have pain or changes in range of motion. In some patients, the clinical presentation of condylar resorption is similar to that of rheumatoid arthritis. If pain is present, it usually is mild in proportion to the degree of radiographic changes in the joint.

The radiographic features of condylar resorption include generalized resorption of the condylar head, often bilaterally, with anterior rotation of the condylar stump in the glenoid fossa. The resorption process often continues regardless of treatment until the entire condylar head resorbs. Bone scintigraphy often shows an increased uptake throughout the resorptive process that may not be interrupted by a period of decrease or cessation of uptake.

29. What are the treatment options of condylar resorptions?

As with other progressive condylar changes, a critical step in treatment planning for condylar resorption is to determine whether the condition is still progressing or has ceased. A history of recent occlusal changes and scintigraphy is important to determine the stage of the condition. Most authors agree on delaying surgical intervention, especially orthognathic surgery, until the resorptive activity has stopped. During such activity, nonsurgical measures, such as nonsteroidal antiinflammatory drugs (NSAIDs) and splint therapy are recommended. Once the resorptive process ceases, orthognathic surgery or condylar replacement with alloplastic or costochondral graft (the two most common surgical modalities) is performed. Recent reports show higher stability after costochondral graft than with orthognathic surgery alone.

30. What are the commonly used systems of cephalometric bony analysis?

- Arnett
- Harvold
- McNamara
- Ricketts

- Sassouni
- Steiner
- Tweed
- Witts

31. What are the most common soft tissue facial measurements?

- Facial contour angle
- Nasolabial angle
- Upper lip length

- Lower lip length
- Ricketts E-line
- Upper face height–to–total face height ratio

32. **What is the most likely source of profuse bleeding during internal vertical ramus osteotomy (IVRO)?**
- Internal maxillary artery, which lies just deep to the ramus at the level of the condylar neck (most likely)
- Masseteric artery
- Inferior alveolar artery
- Retromandibular vein

33. **What is the most likely source of profuse bleeding following Le Fort I incision but before bony osteotomy?**
    The posterior superior alveolar artery, which is located at the posterolateral surface of the maxilla, is often encountered during reflection of the periosteum off the bone before making the bony cut. If these vessels are lacerated, they bleed profusely. This bleeding can easily be controlled with pressure packing.

34. **What muscles are freed with a suprahyoid myotomy and advancement of the mandible?**
- Genioglossal
- Geniohyoid
- Anterior fibers of the mylohyoid
- Anterior bellies of the digastric

35. **What are the different types of genioplasty procedures?**
- Horizontal osteotomy with advancement: for correction of pure horizontal microgenia
- Double-sliding horizontal osteotomy: for the correction of significant microgenia
- Horizontal osteotomy with anterior posterior reduction: for correction of an isolated chin excess
- Vertical reduction genioplasty by a horizontal resection: for correction of an isolated vertical excess
- Oblique osteotomy and advancement caudally, or caudally and inferiorly, with placement of interposition graft: for correction of pure vertical deficiency or a combination of vertical and horizontal deficiency
- Alloplastic augmentation

36. **How would you describe the procedure of the horizontal osteotomy (genioplasty)?**
    The incision should be started at halfway between the depth of the vestibule and the wet-dry line. The mucosa is incised, then undermined, followed by beveled incision of the mentalis muscle inferiorly toward bone. The periosteum should be left intact on the inferior border and the anterior mandible to maintain the soft tissue support and blood supply to the distal segment. Identify the mental nerves bilaterally. Inscribe a midline and paramidline lines to facilitate the repositioning following any symmetric or asymmetric movements. The osteotomy line should be 5 mm below the canine roots, as well as 10-15 mm above the inferior border. The orientation of the osteotomy should extend 4-5 mm below the mental foramina. After complete stabilization of genioplasty, the incision must be closed in 2-3 layers, with special emphasis placed on accurately suturing and reattaching the mentalis muscle into its anatomic position. A pressure dressing should be applied to minimize hematoma formation and help with soft tissue reattachment.

37. **How can the angles of the osteotomy influence the movement of the distal segment?**
    The more parallel the osteotomy line with the occlusal plane and the mandibular plane, the more pure the AP movement. If vertical shortening is desired, the angle of the osteotomy should become more acute compared with the mandibular plane.

38. **What are the possible complications of the alloplastic chin augmentation?**
- Infection
- Extrusion and rejection
- Bone resorption beneath the implant
- Less predictable and stable

- Dehiscence
- Malposition

- Less versatile

39. What are the possible complications of osseous genioplasty?
- Wound dehiscence and infection
- Hematoma
- Tooth devitalization
- Neurosensory loss

- Soft-tissue chin ptosis
- Root exposures
- Asymmetry
- Irregularities and step-type deformities

40. What are the clinical characteristics of transverse maxillary deficiency? What is the best radiographic method of diagnosis of this deficiency?

The clinical indicators of transverse maxillary deficiency include unilateral or bilateral palatal crossbite; crowded, rotated, and palatally or buccally displaced teeth; a narrow tapering maxillary arch form; and a narrow high palatal vault. The soft tissue features are limited to a degree of paranasal hallowing, narrow nasal base, deepened nasolabial folds, and zygomatic hypoplasia. When sagittal and vertical dysplasia exist concomitantly with a maxillary transverse deficiency, they often mask the transverse deficiency. Patients who present with crossbite should be examined closely to determine whether such finding represents a displacement of the teeth relative to the basal bone or a true skeletal bite due to a wide mandible or narrow maxilla. Generally, if a crossbite involves more than one or two teeth, the crossbite is probably skeletal.

For diagnosis and determination of transverse maxillary deficiency, posterior-anterior (PA) cephalogram is the most readily available and reliable radiograph for identification and evaluation of transverse skeletal discrepancy.

41. What are the treatment methods of transverse maxillary deficiency?

The method of correction used depends on several factors, including whether the deficiency is skeletal or dental, or both; the patient's skeletal growth; the magnitude of the transverse discrepancy; and the periodontal status of the dentition. The treatment commonly used is either orthopedic maxillary expansion or surgically assisted maxillary expansion (SME). SME is indicated when the maxillary transverse deficiency is > 5 mm; when there is a significant transverse maxillary deficiency associated with a narrow maxilla and wide mandible; in failed orthodontic/orthopedic expansion; if there is extremely thin, delicate gingival tissue; in the presence of significant buccal gingival recession in the maxillary canine–premolar region; and, finally, when the skeletal age is 15 years or older.

42. What are the components of technique of SME?

Although several techniques have been described to accomplish the expansion of the transversely deficient maxilla, most authors agree on the following steps of the technique:
1. Bilateral osteotomy of the maxilla from the piriform rim to the pterygomaxillary fission
2. Release of the nasal system
3. Midline palatal osteotomy
4. Osteotomy of lateral nasal walls
5. Bilateral osteotomy of pterygoid plates from the maxillary tuberosity
6. Activation of the maxillary appliance to a total widening of 1.0-1.5 mm to assure mobility of both sides of the maxilla
7. Soft tissue closure in a similar fashion to that of Le Fort I osteotomy, preferably using alar cinch and V-Y closure

BIBLIOGRAPHY

1. Abubaker A, Strauss R: Genioplasty: a case for advancement osteotomy. J Oral Maxillofac Surg 58:783-787, 2000.
2. Arnett GW, Tamborello JA: Progressive class II development: female idiopathic condylar resorption. Oral Maxillofac Surg Clin North Am 2:699, 1990.

3. Bell WH, Profitt WR, White RP: Surgical Correction of Dentofacial Deformities, 2nd vol. Philadelphia, 1980, Saunders.
4. Crawford FG, Stoelinga PJ, Blijchop PA et al: Stability after reoperation for condylar resorption after orthognathic surgery: report of 7 cases. J Oral Maxillofac Surg 52:460-466, 1994.
5. Epker BN, Wolford LM: Surgical Correction of Dentofacial Deformities. St Louis, 1980, Mosby.
6. Guyuron B: Genioplasty. Bahman Guyuron, 1993, Library of Congress.
7. Hoppenreijs TJ, Freihfer M, Stoelinga PJ et al: Condylar remodeling and resorption after Le Fort I and bimaxillary osteotomies in patients with anterior open bite. A clinical and radiographic study. Int J Oral Maxillofac Surg 27:81-91, 1998.
8. Huang YL, Pogrel MA, Kaban LB: Diagnosis and management of condylar resorption. J Oral Maxillofac Surg 55:114-119, 1997.
9. Hwang SJ, Haers PE, Zimmermann A et al: Surgical risk factors for condylar resorption after orthognathic surgery. Oral Surg Oral Med Oral Pathol Oral 89:542-552, 2000.
10. O'Ryan F: Complications of orthognathic surgery. Oral Maxillofac Surg Clin North Am 2:593-613, 1990.
11. Proffit W, Turvey TA, Phillips C: Orthognathic surgery: a hierarchy of stability. Int J Adult Orthodont Orthognath Surg 11:191-204, 1996.
12. Turvey TA, Simmons KE: Recognition and management of dentofacial and craniofacial abnormalities. In Kwon PH, Laskin DM (eds): Clinician Manual of Oral and Maxillofacial Surgery, 2nd ed. Chicago, 1996, Quintessence.

38. THE CLEFT LIP AND CLEFT PALATE PATIENT

A. Omar Abubaker, DMD, PhD

1. How many pharyngeal arches are in the human embryo?

There are six pharyngeal arches: arch I, or the maxillomandibular arch; arch II, or the hyoid arch; arches III and IV; and arches V and VI, or the rudimentary arches.

2. What structures (including muscles and nerves) are derived from each arch?

First arch: all muscles of mastication; the mylohyoid, anterior digastric, tensor veli palatini, and tensor tympani muscles; and the fifth cranial nerve. **Second (hyoid) arch:** the muscles of facial expression; posterior digastric, stylohyoid, and stapedius muscles; and the facial nerve, including the chorda tympani to the anterior two thirds of the tongue. **Third arch:** the stylopharyngeus and the glossopharyngeal nerves. **Fourth arch:** the pharyngeal constrictors; levator veli palatini; cricothyroid; larynx; and vagus nerve. **Fifth arch:** laryngeal muscles and recurrent laryngeal branch of the vagus nerve.

3. Which processes merge to form the upper lip and anterior maxillary alveolus, the nose, and the mouth?

The merger of the maxillary and medial nasal processes forms the upper lip and anterior maxillary alveolus. The merger of maxillary and mandibular processes forms the mouth, whereas the merger of the lateral nasal process forms the ala of the nose.

4. What structures are formed by the merger of the medial nasal process and the inter-maxillary segment?

This merger forms the philtrum of the lip, the premaxilla, and the primary palate.

5. What does the merger of the mandibular processes form?
The merger of the mandibular processes forms the mandible, lower lip, and lower part of the face.

6. What are the primary and secondary palates?
The primary palate comprises the lip, alveolar arch, and palate anterior to the incisive foramen (the premaxilla). The secondary palate comprises the soft palate and hard palate posterior to the incisive foramen. The primary and secondary palates are separated by the incisive foramen (Fig. 38-1).

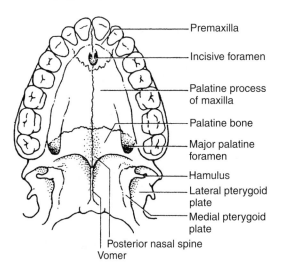

Premaxilla

Incisive foramen

Palatine process of maxilla

Palatine bone

Major palatine foramen

Hamulus

Lateral pterygoid plate

Medial pterygoid plate

Posterior nasal spine

Vomer

Fig. 38-1 Anatomy and divisions of the palate into primary and secondary palates. (From Randall P, LaRosa D: Cleft palate. In McCarthy JG [ed]: Plastic Surgery. Philadelphia, 1990, Saunders.)

7. How is the secondary palate formed?
The secondary palate is formed by fusion of the palatine processes of the maxillary arches, which involves fusion of the palatine processes of the maxilla, fusion of the palatine bones, the soft palate, and uvula.

8. How does cleft lip develop?
Cleft lip develops from failure of fusion of the medial nasal process and the maxillary process.

9. What is the anatomy of cleft lip and palate?
A cleft lip and palate is a disruption of the facial anatomy that may involve the lip and its muscles, nose, alveolar segments, palate (hard and soft), nose septum, and the soft palate palatini muscles.

10. Embryologically, when do cleft lips and/or palates develop?
The upper lip, nose, and palate form in two phases. Anterior to the incisive foramen, the upper lip, nose, and premaxilla develop during the second month of gestation. Posterior to the incisive foramen, the palate develops during the third month. Accordingly, the time when a cleft develops depends on the type of cleft.

11. Which orofacial muscles are anatomically abnormal in cleft lip and palate?
In cleft lip, the main muscle involved is the orbicularis oris muscle. In cleft palate, several muscles are usually involved, depending on the extent of the cleft. In *complete* cleft palate, the

levator veli palatini, tensor veli palatini, uvular, palatopharyngeus, and palatoglossus muscles are involved (Fig. 38-2).

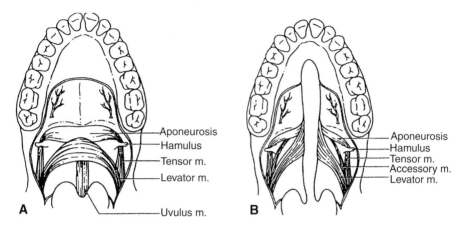

Fig. 38-2 Musculature of the normal (**A**) and cleft (**B**) soft palate. Note that in the normal musculature, the elevator muscles are oriented transversely and insert in the midpalate. In the cleft palate, the musculature is disrupted and the muscles are oriented more longitudinally, inserting on the posterior edge of the palatal bone and along the bony edges of the cleft. (From Randall P, LaRosa D: Cleft palate. In McCarthy JG [ed]: Plastic Surgery. Philadelphia, 1990, Saunders.)

12. What are the most common nasal deformities associated with cleft lip?

Most patients with cleft lip have nasal deformities that become more apparent and severe with age. These deformities include:

- A shortened columella with its base angled to the noncleft side
- Septal deviation and distortion to the noncleft side, with a similar deflection of the caudal septum toward the noncleft side and a compensatory hypertrophy of inferior turbinate on the cleft side
- Collapse of medial crura of lower lateral cartilage inferomedially on the cleft side
- Lateral crura of lower lateral cartilage collapsed and buckled on the cleft side
- Flaring of the alar base

13. What are the most common skeletal jaw deformities in the cleft palate patient?

The skeletal deformities associated with cleft lip and palate vary but generally include one or more of the following: midface deficiency, maxillary transverse deficiency, Class III skeletal and occlusal deformity, and prognathic mandible.

14. What is Passavant's ridge?

Passavant's ridge is a transverse ridge or a bulge produced by the forceful contraction of the superior pharyngeal constrictor on the posterior pharynx opposite the arch of the atlas. This ridge is observed during gagging and pronunciation of vowels. It is an important mechanism in velopharyngeal closure.

15. Why are left-sided secondary or palatal clefts more common than right-sided clefts?

Up to the seventh week of gestation, the two palatal shelves of the human embryo lie almost vertically. As the neck straightens from its flexed position, the tongue drops posteriorly, and the shelves rotate superiorly to the horizontal position; they fuse from anterior to posterior to form the palate by 12 weeks. In rodents, the right palatal shelf reaches the horizontal position before the left one, leaving the left side susceptible to developmental interruption for a longer period than the right. It is believed that this sequence of changes occurs in humans as well and may account for the higher incidence of left-sided clefts.

16. How can clefts be classified?

Clefts can be described as **complete** or **incomplete,** and prepalatal (cleft of the primary palate) or palatal (cleft of the secondary palate). **Prepalatal** can be further divided into unilateral or bilateral; each may be further subdivided into involving one third, two thirds, or all (complete cleft) of the lip. Similarly, **palatal** clefts may be described as involving one third, two thirds, or all of the soft palate and one third, two thirds, or all of the hard palate, extending up to the incisive foramen (Fig. 38-3).

A cleft can also be classified as a submucosal cleft palate or a bifid uvula (see questions 18 and 19).

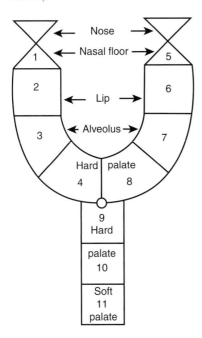

Fig. 38-3 Millard's modified classification of Kernahan's and Elsahy's classification of cleft lip and palate. The small circle indicates the incisive foramen. (Modified from Randall P: Cleft palate. In Smith JW, Aston SJ [eds]: Grabb and Smith's Plastic Surgery, 4th ed. Boston, 1991, Little, Brown.)

17. What are complete and incomplete cleft lips?

A complete cleft lip is a cleft of the entire lip and the underlying premaxilla, or alveolar arch. An incomplete cleft lip involves only the lip.

18. What is a submucous cleft?

A submucous cleft is a deficiency in the musculature of the palate due to failure of the levator muscle fibers to fuse completely in the midline. However, clinically the palate looks intact because the overlying oral and nasal mucous membranes are present. A submucous cleft is characterized by a bifid uvula, loss of the posterior nasal spine, and a bluish midline streak on the soft palate due to muscular diastases. A notch may be present in the posterior hard palate.

This type of cleft usually leads to difficulties with speech and to velopharyngeal incompetence (VPI) because the muscles of the soft palate are unable to function normally. A congenital absence of the muscularis uvulae may also occur—with or without a bifid uvula—and is often associated with palatal incompetence.

19. What is a bifid uvula?

A bifid uvula is a variation of cleft palate seen in 2% of the normal U.S. population. It may be associated with palatal incompetence, and patients should be followed for possible speech problems.

20. What factors are known to cause cleft deformities?

Less than 40% of clefts of lip and palate are of genetic origin, and less than 20% of isolated cleft palates are of genetic origin. Corticosteroids and diazepam taken during the first 8 weeks of pregnancy are also believed to be etiologic factors. Viral infections, lack of certain vitamins, and other factors during the first trimester of pregnancy are suspected as well.

21. What is the incidence of cleft lip with or without cleft palate in the general population? In different ethnic groups?

The incidence of cleft lip worldwide is approximately 1 in every 700-800 live births. Incidence is highest in the Japanese, about 2.1-3.2 in every 1000 births. In Caucasians, incidence is 1.4 in every 1000 births; in Africans, it is 0.3-0.43 in every 1000 births.

The incidence of isolated cleft palate in general is 1:2000.

22. What is the familial risk for developing cleft palate?

Newborns are at greatest risk when both parents are affected. Risk for a newborn developing cleft palate when one parent has cleft vs. neither parent with cleft varies depending on the number of normal siblings. When one parent and one child are affected, the chance of a second child having a cleft palate is 13%. When both parents are normal (without cleft) but two of the children have clefts, the chance of a third child being affected is 19%. When one parent has a cleft palate and two offspring are normal, the chance of the third child being born with a cleft palate is the lowest (3.5%).

23. When is a cleft palate associated with a cleft lip?

The most frequent combination is a unilateral cleft of the lip and palate, which is seen more often in boys than girls, and predominantly on the left side. The hereditary incidence in these patients is fairly high. The next most common cleft is isolated cleft palate, which is seen more frequently in girls; the hereditary incidence in these patients is fairly low. Bifid uvula has an incidence of about 2%, but most cases are asymptomatic. However, as many as 20% of patients with bifid uvula have some degree of VPI.

24. What is the incidence of clefts affecting the left side vs. the right side, and males vs. females?

Cleft palate alone occurs in females 2:1 compared with males. The cleft occurs on the left side 2:1 vs. on the right side. The incidence of cleft lip *and* palate is 2:1 in males vs. females.

25. Which disciplines should be included in a cleft palate team?

The team should include a pediatrician, a surgeon experienced in cleft management, such as a plastic and/or maxillofacial surgeon, a speech pathologist, a pediatric otolaryngologist, an orthodontist, a pediatric dentist, and an audiologist. The team also should have access to a geneticist, a prosthodontist, an ophthalmologist, a clinical psychologist and/or psychiatrist, a social worker, and a nurse experienced in cleft problems.

26. What are the criteria for timing of cleft lip repair?

Surgical repair of cleft lip is generally carried out at 10-14 weeks of age. However, traditionally the time of repair of cleft lip often is based on the **Rule of Tens.** According to this rule, cleft lip can be closed when the infant is ≥ 10 weeks old, the hemoglobin is ≥ 10 g/dL, and the child's weight is ≥ 10 lb.

27. At what age should cleft palate be surgically repaired?
Some authors advocate repair at 6-9 months of age. Others even suggest a slight improvement with closure at 3-6 months of age. However, in most centers, repair of cleft palates is carried out when the child is 10-18 months of age, the age at which articulate speech skills are beginning to develop. In contrast, some centers prefer repair to be delayed until 18-24 months of age, after eruption of the first molars. The differences in timing of cleft palate repair are mostly based on different opinions regarding the balance between needs for normal speech vs. normal palate growth and occlusion.

28. What are the goals of successful cleft palate repairs?
- Separation of the nasal and oral cavities through closure of both mucosal surfaces
- Construction of a water-tight velopharyngeal valve
- Preservation of facial growth
- Good development of aesthetic dentition and functional occlusion

29. What are the basic techniques for repairing cleft lip?
These techniques are lip adhesion procedure, the Millard rotation-advancement flap, and the Tennison-Randall triangular flap.

30. What is the lip adhesion procedure?
This technique is most commonly used for a wide, internal cleft with protrusive premaxilla and when there is inadequate tissue available for primary repair. The primary repair is completed after 6 months. The advantage of this procedure is that it turns a wide, complete cleft into an easier-to-correct incomplete cleft.

31. What is the Millard rotation-advancement flap?
The Millard rotation-advancement flap is a modified Z-plasty technique placed at the top of the cleft so that the point of greatest tension is placed at the base of the nares. It is the most popular method of cleft lip repair. It is used for complete, incomplete, and wide cleft repairs and is ideal for closing incomplete or narrow clefts. The technique involves downward rotation of the philtrum of the lip as a flap into normal symmetric position, while the lateral lip segment is advanced across the cleft and into the space behind the central lip. The final scar from the suture line closely recreates the philtrum of the lip on the cleft side (Fig. 38-4).

32. What is the Tennison-Randall method?
This technique uses a Z-plasty of the cleft lip edges to position the Cupid's bow. It produces an unnatural lip scar across the philtrum column and partial flattening of the philtrum dimple.

33. What are the basic techniques of cleft palate closure?
The V-Y pushback and two-flap palatoplasties are the most commonly used techniques for repairing incomplete and complete clefts of the palate, respectively. Other techniques include the von Langenbeck operation, the vomer flap, four-flap palatoplasty, Furlow palatoplasty, Wardill-Kilner operation, and Schweckendiek's primary veloplasty.

34. What is the V-Y pushback repair?
It is used for repair of complete and incomplete clefts of the palate. The procedure involves elevation of most of the palatal mucosa as posteriorly based flaps over the greater palatine vessels and repositioning of these flaps posteriorly. This technique provides adequate closure of the palate and additional palatal length (Fig. 38-5).

35. What is the von Langenbeck operation?
The von Langenbeck operation involves long, relaxing incisions laterally, with elevation of large mucoperiosteal flaps from the hard palate, which is bipedicled anteriorly and posteriorly.

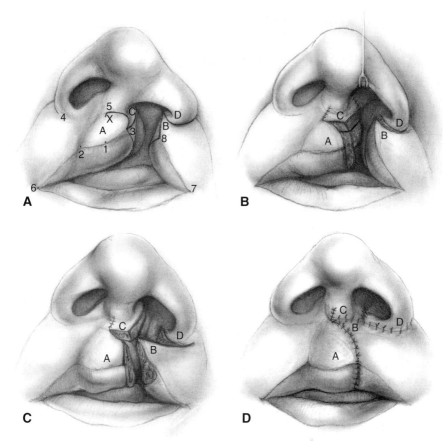

Fig. 38-4   Rotation advancement cleft lip repair (Millard, 1958, 1976). **A,** An incision is made at right angles to the vermilion borders into the medial edge of the cleft lip at a point corresponding to the potential height of Cupid's bow on the cleft side *(3).* From this point superiorly the cleft-edge vermilion is trimmed. The full-thickness incision is then carried upward following the curvature and position of the philtrum on the normal side until it reaches the base of the columella. The incision is cut to preserve as much muscle as possible on the flap. Without crossing into the normal philtrum, the incision curves under the base of the columella and extends toward the normal side as far as is necessary to rotate Cupid's bow *(flap A)* into a normal horizontal plane. A small back-cut *(X)* directed obliquely downward facilitates this rotation. **B,** A hook is used to exert upward traction on the cleft-side alar rim. This results in a defect at the base of the cleft-side columella to be filled with flap C. An incision is made into the membranous septum following the posterior border of flap C. This flap is subsequently undermined and advanced into position to balance the columella. The medial aspect of flap C is tailored and sewn into the superior aspect of the defect created by the downward rotation of flap A. **C,** Flap B is then developed to preserve as much muscle on the flap as possible. The vermilion is trimmed by making an incision at a right angle to the vermilion border at a point *(8)* at which the vermilion becomes attenuated to preserve the length of the lateral element when sutured to the medial element *(flap A).* The distance between this point *(8)* and the ipsilateral oral commissure *(7)* corresponds to the distance between the apex of Cupid's bow *(2)* and the oral commissure on the noncleft side *(6).* The incision is carried up along the vermilion border to include the most superomedial usable lip tissue and then curved laterally around the alar base. Once this is completed, and through an incision in the upper gingivobuccal sulcus, the lateral element is then dissected from the maxilla. At the same time the cleft-side alar base *(flap D)* is released from its pyriform aperture attachment. The orbicularis oris muscle bundles are then carefully dissected, freeing them subcutaneously and submucosally so that when approximated across the cleft, the orientation of their fibers will be changed from a near-vertical direction to the normal horizontal direction. Flap B is then advanced medially and sewn into the defect created by the downward rotation of flap A, and the lip is closed in three layers: muscle, skin, and mucosa. Flap D is then advanced medially to close the nostril floor. A portion of this flap may be deepithelialized and sewn to the base of the nasal septum anteriorly with a permanent suture as a unilateral alar cinch. **D,** The completed repair. (From Perry RJ, Loré JM Jr: Cleft lip and palate. In Loré JM, Medina JE [eds]: An Atlas of Head and Neck Surgery, 4th ed. Philadelphia, 2005, Saunders.)

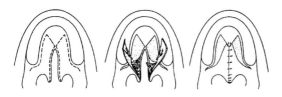

Fig. 38-5   The V-Y pushback palatoplasty. (From Randall P, LaRosa D: Cleft palate. In McCarthy JG [ed]: Plastic Surgery. Philadelphia, 1990, Saunders.)

The cleft margins of both the hard and soft palates are approximated at the midline. The levator muscles are completely detached from their abnormal bony insertion, and the soft palate musculature is repaired in the midline (Fig. 38-6). A palatal lengthening procedure is not included in this operation.

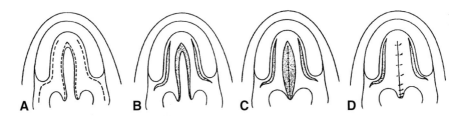

Fig. 38-6   The von Langenbeck operation. **A,** Flap design. **B,** The relaxing incisions. **C,** Elevation of the mucoperiosteal flap. **D,** Closure of the nasal mucosa and closure of the oral mucosa. (From Randall P, LaRosa D: Cleft palate. In McCarthy JG [ed]: Plastic Surgery. Philadelphia, 1990, Saunders.)

36. What is a vomer flap?
This procedure consists of elevation of a wide, superiorly based flap of nasal mucosa from the vomer to close the hard palate. In bilateral clefts, vomer flaps can be obtained from each side of the vomer. This technique avoids the need for elevating large mucoperiosteal flaps from the hard palate and the potential risk of resultant maxillary growth disturbances.

37. What are the most common postoperative complications of cleft palate?
Hypernasal speech is the most common complication following cleft palate repair, occurring in up to 30% of patients. Oral-nasal fistulas are the second most common complication and occur in 10%-21% of cleft repairs. These fistulas typically occur at either end of the hard palate (i.e., at the anterior alveolus or at the junction of the soft and hard palate).

38. What are the major sequelae of an unrepaired cleft palate?
The problems associated with an unrepaired cleft palate are numerous, and they begin at birth and continue for the patient's lifetime:
• An inability to build up suction and nasal regurgitation
• Poor eustachian tube function, which may lead to fluid in the middle ear space and inclination toward recurrent otitis media
• Breathing problems, particularly if the chin is short and the tongue falls backward, causing inspiratory obstruction, as in Pierre Robin sequence
• Speech problems, including hypernasality with vowel sounds and distortion of the pressure consonants
• Adjacent teeth angled into the cleft and possibly malformed or absent, if the alveolar ridge is involved
• Dental caries and severe malocclusion

39. What are the goals of successful alveolar grafting?

The goals of alveolar grafting are providing alveolar continuity for eruption of the maxillary anterior teeth and/or for fabrication of acceptable prosthesis; establishing continuity of the maxillary arch; and providing bony support for the nasal structures. In addition, any residual oronasal fistula, if present, is often successfully closed during the alveolar grafting.

40. What is the ideal age for alveolar cleft repair?

Most studies indicate that the bone graft should be placed before the eruption of the permanent canine and when the canine root is one fourth to one half or one half to two thirds developed. Root resorption and graft failure are common when bone grafts are placed after eruption of the canine. Traditionally, bone grafts are placed at ages 9-11, although early grafting at ages 5-7 is becoming more popular. Orthodontic treatment to stimulate growth and tooth eruption should be instituted within 3 months before bone graft. Orthodontic expansion of the maxillary arch *after* grafting instead of before grafting, at approximately ages 7-12, has also been advocated.

41. Which is the ideal bone for alveolar cleft repair?

Particulate bone with cancellous marrow is the best choice for grafting an alveolar cleft because its osteoinduction and osteoconduction qualities are most predictable.

42. What is velopharyngeal incompetence (VPI)?

VPI is the inability of the soft palate to make contact with the posterior pharyngeal wall to achieve full velopharyngeal closure. Such deficiency leads to speech problems and hypernasality. Evaluation of palatal function should begin as speech development occurs and continue through puberty. Various diagnostic tools are used to evaluate VPI, including speech articulation tests, cinefluoroscopy, lateral neck x-rays, manometry, and nasopharyngoscopy.

43. Which muscles are the most important in achieving VP closure?

The levator palatini muscles contribute the most to VP closure by pulling the middle third of the soft palate superiorly and posteriorly to produce firm contact with the posterior pharyngeal wall at about the level of the adenoidal pad. Other muscles that contribute to VP closure include the paired palatopharyngeus muscles, which pull the soft palate posteriorly; the muscularis uvulae, which cause the uvula to thicken centrally with contraction; and the superior pharyngeal constrictors, which move the lateral pharyngeal walls medially or the posterior pharyngeal wall anteriorly with contraction.

44. How is VPI managed?

Speech therapy usually begins with parental counseling when the child is 6 months old, and individual child therapy should begin when the child is about age 4 or when the definitive diagnosis is made. Dental prosthesis may also be helpful. About 20%-25% of VPI cases require surgery. Surgical methods include secondary palatal lengthening, pharyngeal augmentation using soft tissue or implants, and pharyngeal flaps. Such flaps convert the incompetent nasopharynx into two lateral "ports" and are most successful in patients with good lateral pharyngeal wall motion.

45. What is the traditional sequence of treatment for cleft lip and palate?

- At birth, the cleft lip and palate team evaluates the child.
- At 10 weeks old, the cleft lip is repaired.
- At age 1 year, the child is reevaluated by the cleft lip and palate team.
- At 12-18 months, the soft and hard palates are repaired.
- At 5-8 years, interceptive orthodontics are used.
- At 5-7 years, the pharyngeal flap (if necessary) is done.

- At 7-8 years, maxillary expansion is done, if needed.
- At 9-11 years, alveolar cleft bone grafting is performed.
- At 12-13 years, comprehensive orthodontics are initiated.
- At 14-16 years, orthognathic surgery and nasal surgery are done, if needed.

BIBLIOGRAPHY

1. American Cleft Palate-Craniofacial Association: Parameters for evaluation and treatment of patients with cleft lip or palate and other craniofacial anomalies. In Philips BJ, Warren DW (eds): The Cleft Palate and Craniofacial Team. Chapel Hill, NC, 1993, American Cleft Palate Association.
2. Grabb WC, Rosenstein SW, Bzoch KR (eds): Cleft Lip and Palate: Surgical, Dental, and Speech Aspects. Boston, 1971, Little, Brown.
3. Hendrick DA: Cleft lip and palate. In Jafek BW, Stark AK (eds): ENT Secrets. Philadelphia, 1996, Hanley & Belfus.
4. Johnson MC, Bronsky PT, Millicorsky G: Embryogenesis of cleft lip and palate. In: McCarthy JG (ed): Plastic Surgery. Philadelphia, 1990, Saunders.
5. Kernahan DA: The striped Y—a symbolic classification for cleft lip and palate. Plast Reconstr Surg 47:469-470, 1971.
6. Millard DR Jr: Combining the Von Langenbeck and the Wardill-Kilner operations in certain clefts of the palate. Cleft Palate J 29:85-86, 1992.
7. Millard DR Jr: Cleft lip. In Weinzweig J (ed): Plastic Surgery Secrets. Philadelphia, 1996, Hanley & Belfus.
8. Millard DR Jr, Latham RA: Improved primary surgical and dental treatment of clefts. Plast Reconstr Surg 86:856-871, 1990.
9. Natsume N, Kawai T: Incidence of cleft lip and palate in 39,696 Japanese babies born in 1983. Int J Oral Maxillofac Surg 15:565-568, 1986.
10. Randall P: Cleft palate. In Smith JW, Aston SJ (eds): Grabb and Smith's Plastic Surgery, 4th ed. Boston, 1991, Little, Brown.
11. Randall P, LaRosa D: Cleft palate. In Weinzweig J (ed): Plastic Surgery Secrets. Philadelphia, 1996, Hanley & Belfus.
12. Randall P, LaRosa D: Cleft palate. In McCarthy JG (ed): Plastic Surgery. Philadelphia, 1990, Saunders.

39. CRANIOFACIAL SYNDROMES AND SYNDROMES AFFECTING THE OROMAXILLOFACIAL REGION

A. Omar Abubaker, DMD, PhD, and Kenneth J. Benson, DDS

1. What are the different types of craniomaxillofacial anomalies?

It is important to distinguish craniomaxillofacial anomalies from each other because they differ clinically, prognostically, and in recurrence risk.

Malformation—morphologic defect of an organ, part of an organ, or larger region of the body resulting from an intrinsically abnormal development

Example—cleft lip (palate), craniosynostosis

- Time of occurrence—embryonic
- Frequency—3%

Deformation—abnormal form or position of part of a body caused by nondisruptive mechanical forces. Most common cause is intrauterine molding.

- Time of occurrence—fetal

- Frequency—1%-2%
  Disruption—morphologic defect of an organ, part of an organ, or larger region of the body resulting from breakdown of or an interference with an originally normal developmental process.
- Time of occurrence—embryonic or fetal
- Frequency—1%-2%

2. **What are the general malformations, deformations, and disruptions (Table 39-1)?**

Table 39-1   *General Comparison of Malformations, Deformations, and Disruptions*

FEATURES	MALFORMATIONS	DEFORMATIONS	DISRUPTIONS
Time of occurrence	Embryonic	Fetal	Embryonic/fetal
Level of disturbance	Organ	Region	Area
Perinatal mortality	+	–	+
Clinical variability of any given anomaly	Moderate	Mild	Extreme
Multiple causes for any given anomaly	Very frequent	Less common	Less common
Spontaneous correction	–	+	–
Correction by posture	–	+	–
Correction by surgery	+	–/+	+
Relative recurrence risk	Higher	Lower	Extremely low
Approximate frequency in newborns	2%-3%	1%-2%	1%-2%

Data from Cohen MM Jr: The Child with Multiple Defects, 2nd ed. New York, 1997, Oxford University Press.

3. **What is a syndrome?**
   A syndrome is a set of symptoms that occur together. A particular syndrome may have three, four, or ten manifestations, but a key sequence of symptoms leads to the diagnosis of a particular syndrome.

4. **Are all syndromic children destined to develop a learning deficiency?**
   Although it is clear that not all syndromic patients have a learning deficiency, such issues are not well settled, especially in regard to the role of surgical intervention and its timing on such issues. For example, mental retardation occurs in < 5% of patients with Crouzon's syndrome. Apert's syndrome, which is similar to Crouzon's in its craniofacial abnormalities, has a much higher rate of mental retardation (more than 50% of patients). Timing of surgical intervention to improve the incidence of severity of mental retardation is controversial. To date, no evidence proves or disproves any theory.

5. **What are the features associated with Treacher Collins syndrome?**
   Treacher Collins syndrome is a syndrome with an autosomal dominant transmission and variable expression. The systemic features of the syndrome may include mental deficiency (which may be secondary to deafness) and ventricular septal defect and other cardiac malformations. The craniomaxillofacial features include downward sloping of the palpebral fissures, possible coloboma in the outer third of eyelid, depressed cheekbones, dysplastic ears, receding chin, downturned mouth, symmetric and grossly underdeveloped malar bones with

nonfusion of the zygomatic arches, small or completely absent paranasal sinuses, and ear deformity (crumpled forward, or displaced). Many patients may have absence of the auditory canal or have a defect of the ossicles causing conductive deafness. Nasofrontal angle is usually obliterated, the bridge of the nose is raised, and the nose may appear large secondary to underdevelopment of malar complex. The mandible is often hypoplastic with obtuse gonial angles or deficient ramus or may be concave, producing antegonial notching. The oral features may include cleft palate, crossbite, open bite, and macrostomia. Malocclusion, when present, is usually secondary to maxillary underdevelopment or to cleft palate or high-arched palate. Teeth may be widely spaced, hypoplastic, or displaced.

6.   What is a coloboma, and in what syndromes may it be present?
Coloboma is a notch on the lower eyelid and it occurs in about 75% of Treacher Collins patients.

7.   What are the features of Apert's syndrome?
Apert's syndrome is characterized by craniosynostosis, symmetric syndactyly of hands and feet (which always involves the second, third, and fourth digits of the hands), and, in some patients, mental deficiency, although normal intelligence is often observed. Many patients have congenital heart defects and polycystic kidneys. The familial transmission of Apert's syndrome suggests autosomal dominant transmission.

The craniomaxillofacial features of Apert's syndrome include irregular early obliteration of cranial sutures, especially the coronal suture. Craniofacial appearance and degree of asymmetry are variable depending on the degree of sutural involvement. Commonly observed features include oxycephaly, flattened occiput, steep forehead, "parrot beak" appearance, hypertelorism, proptosis, downslanting of palpebral fissures, strabismus, and variable incidence of hydrocephalus. Most patients also have midface hypoplasia resulting in relative mandibular prognathism. Oral features of Apert's syndrome include highly constricted arched palate, which may also have a median furrow, bifid uvula in > 30% of cases, and Class III malocclusion with anterior open, unilateral, or bilateral posterior crossbite. The maxillary dental arch is frequently V-shaped with crowded occlusion (also called Byzantine arch).

8.   What features distinguish Apert's syndrome from other craniofacial anomalies?
Syndactyly (fusion of digits 2, 3, and 4) is present in Apert's syndrome, but not in other craniofacial anomalies. Differential diagnoses include Crouzon's, Carpenter-Pfeiffer, and Jacobson-Weiss syndromes.

9.   What is Ellis–van Creveld syndrome?
Ellis–van Creveld syndrome is found mostly in the Amish population and includes dwarfism, hidrotic ectodermal dysplasia, and fusion of the mid upper lip. The syndrome is also called chondroectodermal dysplasia. It is the most common cause of dwarfism among the Amish population.

10.   What is Hallermann-Streiff syndrome?
The systemic features of Hallermann-Streiff syndrome include mental deficiency (15%), winglike scapulae, decreased body height, osteoporosis, syndactyly, lordosis, scoliosis, and spina bifida. The craniomaxillofacial features include dyscephaly, beaked nose, mandibular hypoplasia, hypotrichosis, and blue sclera. Brachycephaly is often accompanied by frontal bossing, narrow upper airway passages, and short ascending ramus; the mandibular condyle may be missing, or the glenoid fossa is hypoplastic. There also may be small paranasal sinuses and microphthalmia; bilateral congenital cataracts are nearly always present. Patients may have strabismus and/or nystagmus. The oral features include anodontia, retained primary teeth, or the palate is high and narrow. The syndrome has a sporadic genetic transmission.

11. What are the congenital and acquired causes of macroglossia?

Congenital and hereditary conditions causing macroglossia include vascular lesions, such as lymphangioma and hemangioma, hemihypertrophy, cretinism, Beckwith-Wiedemann syndrome, Down syndrome, neurofibromatosis, and multiple endocrine neoplasia syndrome (MENS) type III. Acquired causes include long-term edentulous state, amyloidosis, myxedema, acromegaly, angioedema, and tumors of the tongue.

12. What is Crouzon's syndrome (craniofacial dysostosis)?

This is a syndrome with premature craniosynostosis that usually occurs by age 2 or 3. Syndactyly is *not* present (Apert's syndrome is a craniofacial dysostosis with syndactyly). The patient may have hypertelorism and divergent strabismus, exophthalmus secondary to shallow orbits, protuberant frontal region (triangular frontal defect), maxillary hypoplasia, mandibular prognathism, high-arched palate, and a parrot beak nose. It is an autosomal dominant syndrome.

13. What are the features of Crouzon's syndrome?

General features of Crouzon's syndrome include increased intracranial pressure and mental deficiency in some cases. The craniomaxillofacial features include craniosynostosis beginning during the first year of life and completed by ages 2-3. Cranial malformation is dependent on rate and progression of craniosynostosis. Ocular features include proptosis secondary to shallow orbits, divergent strabismus, and hypertelorism. Most patients (80%) have optic nerve involvement. Maxillary hypoplasia is usually accompanied by relative mandibular prognathism and parrot beaked nose. Brachycephaly, trigonocephaly, and scaphocephaly also may be seen in this syndrome. Oral features of Crouzon's syndrome include highly arched and constricted palate with a median furrow, Class III malocclusion, anterior open, and unilateral or bilateral posterior crossbite. The syndrome has autosomal dominant transmission and no limb deformities.

14. What are the features of hemifacial microsomia?

The majority of cases of hemifacial microsomia are sporadic in occurrence, with the exact etiology not yet determined. The general features include a malformation complex that may occur as an isolated finding or as part of various malformation syndromes. The systemic features include congenital heart defects (50%) and mitral regurgitation (10%). The patient may have asymmetric facial involvement that is sometimes bilateral (10%). The craniomaxillofacial features include unilateral microtia, failure of formation of mandibular ramus and condyle, and flattened gonial angle. The maxillary, temporal, and malar bones on the involved side may be reduced in size and flattened, and the ipsilateral eye may be at a lower level than the unaffected side. There may be hypoplastic or nondeveloped muscles of facial expression, frontal bossing (right side is affected more frequently than the left), ear tags, conduction deafness, and coloboma. The oral features may include macrostomia, narrowed palate, and, occasionally, cleft lip and palate. Muscles of the tongue and the palate may be hypoplastic or paralyzed on the affected side.

15. What is Goldenhar's syndrome?

Goldenhar's syndrome with microsomia (oculo-auriculo-vertebral syndrome) is a variant of hemifacial microsomia, which includes vertebral anomalies and epibulbar dermoids along with features of hemifacial microsomia.

16. What is Pfeiffer's syndrome?

Pfeiffer's syndrome is an autosomal dominant, complete-penetrance, and variably expressed syndrome. The systemic features of the syndrome may include normal intelligence, but deficiency may be seen. The thumbs and great toes are broad, with variable mild soft tissue syndactyly of the hands. The craniomaxillofacial and oral features are similar to those in Apert's syndrome. Other features may include highly arched and constricted palate with possible median furrow and Class III malocclusion with anterior open and unilateral or bilateral posterior crossbite.

17. **What are the features of Stickler's syndrome?**

Stickler's syndrome is an autosomal dominant, variably expressed syndrome. The general features of the syndrome involve connective tissue dysplasia in the form of generalized skeletal abnormalities, including slender body habitus, hyperextensibility of joints, prominence of large joints, arthropathy, and mild epiphyseal dysplasia. Orofacial features may include midfacial flattening, cleft lip and palate, isolated cleft palate, or submucosal cleft and hearing loss. Ocular features include myopia, retinal detachment, and cataracts. Craniomaxillofacial features in general may resemble Crouzon's syndrome or Pierre Robin sequence.

18. **What is Pierre Robin sequence/syndrome?**

Genetically, the sequence can occur as (1) micrognathia, (2) a component of various syndromes, many of which are genetic, or (3) in association with various anomalies that are not currently recognized as constituting syndromes of known genesis. The majority of cases occur as an isolated complex. Some patients with the sequence may have heart defects or heart murmurs. The oral and craniomaxillofacial features include mandibular hypoplasia, cleft palate, and glossoptosis (often causing airway problems). The pathogenesis of the syndrome include arrested development of mandible preventing the normal descent of the tongue, which in turn prevents fusion of palatal shelves and closure of the palate. Mandibular catch-up growth can be seen by ages 10-11.

19. **Which craniofacial syndromes affect the limbs?**

Several craniofacial syndromes affect the limbs. Among the more common is Apert's syndrome, which involves syndactyly of the feet and hands. Crouzon's syndrome, which has similar facial features to Apert's syndrome, does not involve hand anomalies. Other syndromes in which the limbs are affected include Saethre-Chotzen syndrome (brachydactyly), Pfeiffer's syndrome (large, broad great toes and thumbs), Carpenter's syndrome (short hands and poly-syndactyly of the feet) and Nager's syndrome (missing digits, syndactyly, and either hypoplastic or aplastic thumbs and/or radius).

20. **Are all craniosynostoses associated with a syndrome?**

Syndromes are present only in 10%-20% of patients with primary craniosynostosis. Usually single-suture synostoses are isolated, sporadic anomalies, whereas multiple-suture synostoses are syndromic.

21. **What is Binder's syndrome (nasomaxillary dysplasia)?**

Binder's syndrome includes hypoplasia of nasal bones and maxilla with a convex lip, vertical nose, absent frontal nasal angle, absent anterior nasal spine, atrophied nasal mucosa, and hypoplastic frontal sinus. It is not associated with any brain abnormalities and is not considered a true syndrome.

22. **What are the features of achondroplasia?**

Achondroplasia is a disease with >80% sporadic genetic incidence representing point mutations. Risk factors for the disease include advanced paternal age at time of conception, and > 20% are familial, showing autosomal dominant mode of transmission. Systemic features of this syndrome include short limbs, short stubby hands, lordotic lumbar spine, prominent buttocks, protuberant abdomen, and predilection for obesity. The craniomaxillofacial features include macroencephaly (enlarged head), frontal bossing, depression of nasal bridge, midface hypoplasia with relative mandibular prognathism, and otitis media. Otitis media in these patients is common during the first 6 years of life, which can lead to hearing loss if untreated. Oral features include anterior dental crowding and Class III malocclusion.

23. **What syndromes are associated with mandibular prognathism?**

Mandibular prognathism may be present in the following syndromes: basal cell nevus syndrome

(Gorlin's syndrome), Klinefelter's syndrome, Marfan's syndrome, osteogenesis imperfecta, and Waardenburg's syndrome.

24. What common malformation syndromes are associated with midface deficiency?
The following syndromes may be associated with midface deficiency: achondroplasia, Apert's syndrome, cleidocranial dysplasia, Crouzon's syndrome, Marshall's syndrome, Pfeiffer's syndrome, and Stickler's syndrome.

25. What common malformation syndromes are associated with median cleft?
Any of the following syndromes can be accompanied by a median cleft: frontonasal dysplasia, oral-facial-digital syndrome, oral-facial-digital syndrome II (premaxillary agenesis), Pierre Robin complex, Treacher Collins syndrome, Nager's acrofacial dysostosis, hemifacial microsomia (Goldenhar's syndrome), Möbius' syndrome, and Hallermann-Streiff syndrome.

26. What syndromes in the first column correspond to features in the second column?

Syndromes	Features
A. Treacher Collins	A. Glossoptosis
B. Acrofacial dysostosis	B. Chondroectodermal dysplasia
C. Pierre Robin	C. Mandibulofacial dysostosis
D. Crouzon's	D. Absent thumb
E. Ellis–van Creveld	E. Ocular proptosis
F. Hallermann-Streiff	F. Aplastic clavicles
G. Cleidocranial dysplasia	G. Blue sclera

ANSWERS: A-C; B-D; C-A; D-E; E-B; F-G; G-F

27. What syndromes are often associated with hyperdontia/hypodontia (Box 39-1)?

Box 39-1 *Syndromes Associated with Hyperdontia and Hypodontia*	
SYNDROMES ASSOCIATED WITH HYPERDONTIA	**SYNDROMES ASSOCIATED WITH HYPODONTIA**
Cleidocranial dysplasia	Crouzon's
Gardner's	Down
Hallermann-Streiff	Ectodermal dysplasia
Sturge-Weber	Ehlers-Danlos
Oral-facial-digital, type I	Ellis–van Creveld
Fabry-Anderson	Goldenhar's
	Gorlin's
	Hallermann-Streiff
	Hurler's
	Oral-facial-digital, type I
	Witkop tooth and nail
	Sturge-Weber
	Turner's

28. In what diseases are café au lait spots seen?
Café au lait spots are seen in patients with neurofibromatosis (von Recklinghausen's disease) and in McCune-Albright syndrome.

29. What is von Recklinghausen's disease?

Von Recklinghausen's disease is a neurofibromatosis disease. Eight forms are recognized, but 85%-90% are type I (skin related). The disease is autosomal dominant, and occurrence is 1 in 3000 with no sex predilection. The majority of cases exhibit café au lait spots of the skin (melanin pigmentation). The presence of six or more spots that are > 1.5 cm in diameter is pathognomonic for the disease. Axillary freckling is called Crow's sign and is often present in this disease. Type I of the disease most frequently involves the skin and oral mucosa. Café au lait spots have smooth borders (coastline of California). The disease is thought to arise from Schwann's cells, fibroblasts, and perineural cells. Histologically, proliferation of delicate spindle cells with thin wavy nuclei and myxoid matrix is often seen. There is no curative treatment for the disease. Radiotherapy is ineffective and can be associated with transformation of the lesions into sarcomas.

30. What is neurilemoma (schwannoma)?

Neurilemoma is a slow-growing tumor thought to be derived from Schwann's cells. It is an uncommon disease, and 25%-48% occur in head and neck areas. The tongue is the most common intraoral location. Histologically the lesions usually show characteristic palisaded cell pattern known as Verocay bodies. This is called Antoni type A. Antoni type B shows a disorderly arrangement of cells and fibers. The treatment of neurilemoma is surgical excision with a low rate of recurrence.

31. What is Albright's syndrome?

Albright's syndrome is a severe type of fibrous dysplasia that involves nearly all bones of the skeleton. It is also associated with pigmented lesions of the skin (café au lait spots) and sexual precocity. Café au lait spots here have very irregular (coastline of Maine) borders. Radiographically, the bone usually has ground-glass or orange-peel appearance. Histologically, the lesions show a considerable variation, including loose arrangement of fibrous stroma with irregularly shaped trabeculae of immature (woven) bone.

32. What is the differential diagnosis of a newborn with a crusty lower lip that wipes off easily, leaving areas of indentation?

The differential diagnosis of this condition includes Stevens-Johnson syndrome, herpetic gingivostomatitis, epidermolysis bullosa, dermatitis herpetiforms, herpes zoster, and toxic epidermal necrolysis (Lyell's disease).

33. What are the clinical features of basal cell nevus syndrome?

The syndrome is also known as Gorlin's syndrome. It is an autosomal dominant syndrome with very complex and highly variable abnormalities. It has several orofacial and systemic abnormalities, including:

- Cutaneous anomalies, including basal cell carcinoma, palmar and plantar pitting
- Dental and osseous anomalies, such as multiple odontogenic keratocysts (OKCs) in 75% of patients, mandibular prognathism, rib anomalies (bifid ribs), vertebral anomalies such as kyphoscoliosis in 50%, and brady metacarpalis
- Ophthalmologic and frontal abnormalities, such as ocular hypertelorism (40%), and frontal and temporoparietal bossing
- Neurologic anomalies in the form of mental retardation, and calcification of falx cerebri
- Sexual abnormalities in the form of ovarian fibromas and medulloblastomas
- Oral manifestations, including OKCs, which are indistinguishable from those not associated with the syndrome. The treatment of these cysts is similar to that for other OKCs.

34. What is gustatory sweat (Frey's) auriculotemporal syndrome?

Frey's syndrome is sweating of the temporal cutaneous region upon eating. It usually occurs due to surgical damage to the auriculotemporal nerve during temporomandibular joint (TMJ) or parotid surgery. The damaged nerve regenerates in misdirected fashion and the parasympathetic salivary nerve supply carried along the auricular region and nerve reconnect along sympathetic pathways that innervate the sweat glands. After salivary, gustatory, or psychic stimulation of the parasympathetic fibers, sweating occurs. Confirmation of the diagnosis consists of using Minor's starch iodine test to detect sweating. The treatment for this condition includes topical anticholinergic and local atropine injections, severing of the auriculotemporal nerve, or transplantation/interposition of fascia lata graft under the skin in the involved area. This syndrome should be differentiated from a similar condition called crocodile tears, which is a lacrimation that occurs during eating and generally following Bell's palsy, herpes zoster, or head injury.

35. What is Ramsay Hunt syndrome?

Symptoms of Ramsay Hunt syndrome include facial nerve paralysis, otalgia, and vesicular eruption on the external ear, vertigo, and hearing deficits. It is caused by herpes zoster virus infection of an ipsilateral geniculate ganglion.

36. What is Reiter's syndrome?

Reiter's syndrome is a triad of urethritis, conjunctivitis, and arthritis. The disease is also called keratodermal blennorrhagicum. It usually affects young males (male to female ratio is 9:1). Urethritis usually is the first sign, although rare. The joint pain may affect the TMJ, leading to TMJ dysfunction symptoms. The syndrome is of unknown etiology. Treatment for this condition—indicated only in symptomatic patients—consists of a course of doxycycline and nonsteroidal antiinflammatory drugs for arthritis.

37. What is Heerfordt's syndrome?

Heerfordt's syndrome also is called uveoparotitis or uveoparotid fever. It is associated with acute sarcoidosis. It is characterized by firm painless enlargement of the parotid gland with uveal inflammation of the tracts of the eyes (conjunctivitis, keratitis) and cranial nerve (CN) involvement (usually CN VII nerve paralysis in half the cases).

38. What are the clinical features of Ascher's syndrome?

There are three features associated with Ascher's syndrome:
1. Acquired double lip: seen when lips are tensed, resembling a Cupid's bow
2. Blepharochalasis: drooping of tissue between the eyebrow and edge of upper lid so the tissue hangs loosely over lid margin
3. Thyroid enlargement, which is not a consistent finding and may not appear until many years after eyelid involvement

39. What are the types of polyostotic fibrous dysplasia?

There are the two distinct types of polyostotic fibrous dysplasia. The first is Jaffe's type, in which a variable number of bones is affected, and most of the skeleton is normal. The second type is Albright's syndrome. In this type, there is a severe fibrous dysplasia involving nearly all bones in the skeleton, accompanied by pigmented skin lesions (café au lait), and varying endocrine disturbances are present.

40. What are the clinical features of the benign lymphoepithelial lesion?

This condition is also referred to as Mikulicz's disease. It is typically seen as a unilateral or bilateral parotid or submandibular gland enlargement. Some cases include mild local discomfort and xerostomia. The onset of the disease can be associated with fever, oral infection, upper respiratory tract infection, or other local inflammatory conditions.

41. What is Melkersson-Rosenthal syndrome?

Recurrent attacks of facial paralysis, noninflammatory painless facial edema, cheilitis granulomatosa, and fissured tongue. Facial palsy may begin suddenly in childhood and precede facial edema by many years.

42.   Which muscles are most commonly affected in Möbius' syndrome?

Möbius' syndrome is caused by a defect, with secondary degeneration of sixth and seventh nerve nuclei. The lateral rectus is most commonly affected by paralysis with defects of the abducent nerve.

43.   What is the most common human chromosomal abnormality?

Down syndrome, also called trisomy 21 syndrome. Clinically, the patient has a flat face, large anterior fontanel, open sutures, fissured tongue, frequent prognathism, and hypermobility of the joints.

44.   Which syndrome used to be referred to as "hysterical dysphagia"?

Plummer-Vinson syndrome, which usually occurs in the fourth and fifth decades of life. Most commonly seen in women. This syndrome is a manifestation of iron deficiency anemia. Symptoms include cracks at commissures, lemon-tinted skin color, red and smooth painful tongue, and dysphagia from esophageal stricture.

45.   What is Papillon-LeFèvre syndrome?

It is juvenile periodontitis with associated skin lesions. It is manifested as severe destruction of alveolar bone involving deciduous and permanent teeth, deep periodontal pockets, boggy gingiva, and fetid breath. Skin lesions may be present and include keratotic lesions of palmar and plantar surfaces.

46.   What is Möbius' syndrome (congenital occlusofacial paralysis)?

Möbius' syndrome involves, at a minimum, CN VI and VII palsies but may also include other CNs, especially III, V, IX, and XII. The patients may have limb defects (50%), mild mental retardation (10%-15%), syndactyly, or absence of the pectoralis major. The craniomaxillofacial features may also include masklike facies, unilateral or bilateral paralysis of the lateral rectus muscles, high and broad nasal bridge, and a frequently hypoplastic mandible. The oral features include droop of angles of the mouth, unilateral tongue hypoplasia, poor palatal mobility, inefficient sucking and swallowing, and speech impairment.

47.   Which syndrome is associated with lower lip pits?

Lower lip pits are a common manifestation of van der Woude's syndrome (lip pit–cleft lip syndrome). Lower lip pits are present in 80% of patients with this syndrome. Patients may also be missing the central and lateral incisors, canines, or bicuspids. In addition, these patients often have a cleft lip, but may or may not have a cleft palate or cleft uvula. Van der Woude's syndrome is an autosomal dominant disorder.

48.   What is Parkes Weber syndrome?

Parkes Weber syndrome is a neoplastic syndrome associated with arteriovenous fistulas. The craniofacial manifestations of this syndrome include asymmetric facial hypertrophy, hemangiomata, microcephaly, and intracranial calcifications. Other findings include enlarged abdominal viscera, limb hypertrophy and disturbed major blood vessels. Patients are usually mentally impaired and may be prone to seizures.

49.   What is Horner's syndrome?

Horner's syndrome is a combination of ptosis of the upper eyelid, myosis of the pupil, and anhidrosis of the forehead caused by interruption of the cervical sympathetic trunk to the orbit. The ptosis is a result of interruption of the innervation to the superior tarsal muscle, leading to constant ptosis and interference with maintenance of normal elevation of the upper lid. This should be distinguished from the inability to open the eye voluntarily, which usually results from paralysis of the oculomotor nerve, and from the inability to close the lids tightly, which is a result of facial nerve paralysis. The myosis is a result of the unopposed action of the parasympathetic nerves on the ciliary muscles, whereas the anhidrosis is the result of interruption of sympathetic flow to the sweat glands. Isolated Horner's syndrome may be caused by trauma to the neck and by tumors involving the carotid artery or may even be the first sign of lung cancer.

50. What is superior orbital fissure syndrome?

Superior orbital fissure syndrome is a combination of symptoms that result from direct or indirect pressure on the structures passing through the superior orbital fissure. This mostly occurs as a rare complication of orbital fracture, although it can result from neoplastic or inflammatory conditions affecting the superior orbital fissure. The clinical presentation varies in severity, depending on the number of structures involved. The complete presentation of the syndrome includes subconjunctival ecchymosis; proptosis; ptosis; persistent periorbital edema; ophthalmoplegia; loss of corneal, direct, consensual, and accommodation reflexes; and loss of sensation over the forehead extending to the vertex.

BIBLIOGRAPHY

1. Bell W, Proffit W, White R: Surgical Correction of Dentofacial Deformities. Philadelphia, 1980, Saunders.
2. Cohen M: Anomalies, syndromes and medical genetics. In: Oral and Maxillofacial Surgery Update, 2nd vol. Rosemont, Ill, 1998, AAOMS.
3. Cohen MM Jr (ed): Craniosynostosis: Diagnosis, Evaluation, and Management. New York, 1986, Raven Press.
4. Goodrich JJ, Hall CD: Craniofacial Anomalies: Growth and Development from a Surgical Perspective. New York, 1995, Thieme Medical.
5. Gorlin R, Cohen M, Levin L: Syndromes of the head and neck, 3rd ed. New York, 1990, Oxford Press.
6. Lettieri S, Vander Kolk CA: Craniofacial syndromes. In Weinzweig J (ed): Plastic Surgery Secrets. Philadelphia, 1996, Hanley & Belfus.
7. Neville B, Damm D, Allen C et al: Anomalies of the teeth. In: Oral and Maxillofacial Pathology, Philadelphia, 1995, Saunders.
8. Salmon AM: Developmental Defects and Syndromes. Aylesbury, England, 1978, HM+M Publications.

40. SALIVARY GLAND DISEASES

Chris A. Skouteris, DMD, PhD

1. What are the signs and symptoms of salivary gland malignancy?

Rapid tumor growth or a sudden growth acceleration in a long-standing salivary mass, pain, and peripheral facial nerve paralysis.

2. Can peripheral facial nerve paralysis be a sign of nonmalignant conditions affecting the parotid gland?

Yes. It has been reported that peripheral facial nerve paralysis can be associated with acute suppurative parotitis, nonspecific parotitis with inflammatory pseudotumor, amyloidosis, and sarcoidosis of the parotid.

3. What are the appropriate diagnostic methods in evaluating salivary obstruction?

Clinical exam
- Palpation of the gland
- Bimanual palpation along the course of the duct
- Visual confirmation of diminished or absent salivary flow
- Assessment of the type of any ductal discharge

Sialoendoscopy (used for diagnosis and treatment of sialolithiasis)

Imaging techniques
- Plain films: occlusal, frontal, lateral, lateral oblique, and panoramic views
- Sialography: contraindicated in the presence of acute sialadenitis and when sialoliths have been positively identified on clinical exam and plain films
- Ultrasonography
- Computed tomography (CT): useful in identifying parenchymal or extraparenchymal masses that can cause obstruction by pressure or ductal invasion
- Radionuclide scanning: evaluates the effect of the obstruction on glandular dynamics and function

4. Are sialoliths always visible on radiographs?

No. Sialoliths in the early stage of development are quite small and not adequately mineralized to be visible radiographically. It has also been reported in the literature that 30%-50% of parotid and 10%-20% of submandibular sialoliths are radiolucent. These radiolucent sialoliths can be visualized indirectly by the imaging defect that they produce on sialography, or directly through sialoendoscopy.

5. What methods are used for the treatment of sialolithiasis?

Transoral removal of palpable sialoliths should be considered as the treatment of choice in patients suffering from submandibular stones located within either the floor of the mouth or the perihilar region of the gland. Methods include:
- Stone removal through sialoendoscopy
- Extracorporeal shock-wave lithotripsy
- Intracorporeal shockwave lithotripsy (endoscopically controlled, stone fragmentation via laser or pneumoballistic energy)
- Fluoroscopically guided basket retrieval
- Laser surgery for sialolithiasis (sialolithectomy with CO_2 laser)

There is increasing evidence to show that the submandibular gland regains function after stone removal, and sialoadenectomy may not be the treatment of choice for proximal calculi. In cases of severely impacted hilar calculi or intraparenchymal calculi that are associated with frequent recurrent episodes of sialadenitis, excision of the submandibular gland or superficial parotidectomy is warranted. Submandibular sialoadenectomy can be accomplished through the conventional cervical approach or, more recently, by intraoral or extraoral endoscopic excision.

6. Is fine-needle aspiration (FNA) biopsy efficacious in the diagnosis of salivary gland pathology?

Refinements in sampling techniques and specimen preparation, as well as improvements in cytologic interpretation, have considerably increased the diagnostic value of FNA biopsy in the evaluation of salivary pathology. The specificity of the procedure ranges from 88%-99%, and the sensitivity is 71%-93%.

7. What are the contemporary imaging modalities for visualizing tumors of the major salivary glands?
- CT
- CT sialography
- Magnetic resonance imaging (MRI)
- MR sialography
- Positron emission tomography (PET)
- Ultrasound

8.   Is there an association between salivary disease and AIDS?

Yes. Conditions affecting the salivary glands in AIDS patients include parotid lympho-epithelial lesions, cysts, lymphadenopathy, Kaposi's sarcoma, AIDS-related intraglandular lymphoma, salmonella and cytomegalovirus parotitis, and a Sjögren's syndrome–like condition with xerostomia.

9.   What is the incidence of tumors affecting the sublingual salivary glands?

Sublingual salivary gland tumors comprise < 1% of all salivary gland neoplasms. These tumors are predominantly malignant (>80%) and are usually adenoid cystic or mucoepidermoid carcinomas.

10.   Are there any imaging techniques for visualization of the facial nerve?

High-resolution MRI using a three-dimensional Fourier transform gradient-echo sequence is able to visualize the facial nerve in its course from the stylomastoid foramen to the level of the retromandibular vein. However, this technique, as well as others, has not been successful in visualizing the intraparotid divisions and course of the nerve, which are of great clinical importance.

11.   Can ultrasonography, CT, MRI, and PET scanning distinguish between benign and malignant salivary gland tumors?

Ultrasonography can be useful in differentiating between benign and malignant tumors. Recent evidence suggests that malignant tumors (with the exception of lymphomas) are charac-terized sonographically by attenuation of posterior echoes, whereas benign tumors exhibit distal echo enhancement. CT can effectively differentiate among benign, malignant, and inflammatory lesions in approximately 75% of cases. MRI appears to be the most suitable for evaluation of salivary gland tumors, especially malignant tumors. However, PET scanning is not able to distinguish between benign and malignant tumors.

12.   What is the role of radionuclide imaging in the diagnosis of salivary gland pathology?

In addition to assessing salivary function, salivary scintigraphy can be useful in the diagnosis of acute and chronic sialadenitis of specific or nonspecific etiology, abscesses, lymphomas, and tumors. In salivary neoplasia, radionuclide imaging can identify glandular masses > 1 cm in diameter, distinguish between certain tumor types based on their specific uptake characteristics, and, in some instances, differentiate benign from malignant disease.

13.   What are the most common nonneoplastic salivary gland pathoses in children?

- Acute viral sialadenitis
- Acute bacterial sialadenitis
- Sialolithiasis
- Mucoceles

14.   How can you differentiate between viral and bacterial parotitis?

Viral parotitis infection is bilateral and is preceded by prodromal signs and symptoms of 1-2 days' duration, including fever, malaise, loss of appetite, chills, headache, sore throat, and preauricular tenderness. Purulent discharge from Stensen's duct is rare but, if present, might be the result of the development of secondary bacterial sialadenitis. Lab investigations reveal elevated serum titers for mumps or influenza virus, leukopenia, relative lymphocytosis, and high levels of serum amylase.

15.   What syndromes can affect the salivary glands?

Primary Sjögren's syndrome is usually characterized by parotid and lacrimal gland enlarge-ment, xerostomia, and xerophthalmia. Secondary Sjögren's syndrome involves autoimmune parotitis that occurs with rheumatoid arthritis, lupus, systemic sclerosis, thyroiditis, primary biliary cirrhosis, and mixed collagen disease. Sarcoidosis may involve the parotid gland. Sarcoidosis of the parotid gland, along with fever, lacrimal adenitis, uveitis, and facial nerve paralysis is called

Heerfordt's syndrome. Recently, a sicca syndrome–like condition has been recognized in HIV-positive children. This condition presents with parotid gland enlargement, xerostomia, and lymphadenopathy.

16. What is the incidence of metastatic neck disease in patients with malignant salivary tumors?

In a large series of patients with malignant tumors of the parotid, submandibular, sublingual, and minor salivary glands, the reported overall incidence of metastatic cervical lymphadenopathy was 15.3%. Parotid cancer is associated with metastatic lymph node involvement in 18%-25% of cases.

17. How is acute bacterial parotitis diagnosed?
- History, with emphasis on diabetes, dehydration, malnutrition, immunosuppressive therapy, antisialic drugs, debilitating systemic disease, and recent surgery
- Physical exam, including palpation and observation for purulent ductal discharge
- Imaging, including ultrasound and CT
- Culture of purulent discharge and antibiotic sensitivity testing

18. What types of lesions can result from mucus escape?

Mucoceles and ranulae.

19. What are the different types of clinical presentation of a ranula?

A ranula can present as a floor-of-the-mouth swelling, as a plunging ranula with an intraoral and a cervical component, and as a purely cervical ranula without an intraoral component. An extreme case of ranula is the thoracic ranula, which can originate in the submandibular area and extend into the subcutaneous tissue planes of the anterior chest wall.

20. What are the treatment modalities for the different types of ranulae?
Intraoral ranula:
- Excision (for small lesions) ± excision of sublingual salivary gland
- Marsupialization (for larger lesions) ± excision of the sublingual salivary gland
- Cryotherapy
- Laser ablation (CO_2) or laser excision (diode)
- Hydrodissection
- Intracystic injection of the streptococcal preparation OK-432

Excision, wherever feasible, or marsupialization with excision of the sublingual salivary gland is the most preferred method for the treatment of floor of the mouth ranulae, especially in recurrent cases.
Plunging ranula:
- Intraoral marsupialization with excision of the sublingual gland (preferred method)
- Extraoral removal of lesion with excision of the sublingual gland
- Intraoral fenestration and continuous pressure
- Intralesional injection of OK-432

Cervical ranula: excision of lesion and sublingual salivary gland through a cervical approach

21. What are the most common causes of xerostomia?

Xerostomia can be idiopathic, drug-induced, radiation-induced, or the principal manifestation of primary and secondary Sjögren's syndrome.

22. Is incisional biopsy indicated for the diagnosis of pathologic conditions of the parotid gland?

Yes, it is indicated for the diagnosis of suspected systemic disease with parotid involvement particularly when FNA biopsy findings are inconclusive. Systemic conditions in which incisional parotid biopsy can be of great diagnostic value include sarcoidosis, Sjögren's syndrome, lymphoma, and sialosis.

23. What are the clinical manifestations of a tumor involving the deep lobe of the parotid?
Tumors of the deep parotid lobe can grow undetected until they are large and clinically evident. In cases in which the tumor has grown into the lateral pharyngeal space, a bulging in the lateral pharyngeal wall can be seen. Extensive tumors in this anatomic location can displace the soft palate and uvula, with resultant difficulties in speech, breathing, and deglutition.

24. What is the most common benign tumor of minor and major salivary glands?
Pleomorphic adenoma.

25. What are the most important histologic features associated with the incidence of recurrence of pleomorphic adenoma?
Hypocellular pleomorphic adenomas often have a thin capsule and constitute the most frequently encountered histologic type in recurrence. Pseudopodia—fingerlike tumor extensions outside the pseudocapsule—are considered to be an additional factor in recurrence.

26. What are the most common malignant tumors of minor and major salivary glands?
- Mucoepidermoid carcinoma in the parotid gland
- Adenoid cystic carcinoma in the submandibular, sublingual, and minor salivary glands

27. Which are the most common salivary neoplasms in children?
Hemangiomas and lymphangiomas of the salivary glands, followed by pleomorphic adenomas, are the most common benign tumors. Malignant neoplasms are very rare, but the rate of malignancy in children is much higher than in adults. The most common malignant salivary tumor is mucoepidermoid carcinoma, followed by acinic cell carcinoma.

28. Is it possible to determine accurately the actual clinical extent of an adenoid cystic carcinoma? Why?
No. Adenoid cystic carcinoma tends to invade nerves and spread perineurally. Therefore it can extend well beyond its primary location.

29. Are there central (intraosseous) salivary tumors?
Yes. Although rare, salivary tumors arising in the maxilla and mandible have been reported. These tumors are thought to derive from heterotopic salivary gland inclusions and are mostly mucoepidermoid carcinomas. However, other salivary malignancies, such as acinic cell carcinoma, clear cell carcinoma, and myoepithelial carcinoma in pleomorphic adenoma, have also been reported to occur centrally within the jaws.

30. Is there a role for intraoperative frozen-section evaluation of tumors of the major salivary glands?
Yes. When FNA biopsy is inconclusive and because open biopsy is not indicated, intraoperative frozen sections might provide information that can modify the treatment plan. Frozen section is more accurate in the evaluation of benign tumors, whereas its sensitivity for malignancy is 61.5% and its specificity is 98%.

31. What types of surgical procedures can be used for the management of benign and malignant tumors of the parotid?
- Extracapsular excision or lumpectomy—tumor removal with a safety margin without facial nerve dissection
- Partial superficial parotidectomy—with no need for dissection of the full facial nerve or excision of the entire superficial lobe

- Superficial parotidectomy—with preservation of the facial nerve
- Deep lobe parotidectomy—with facial nerve preservation

Malignant tumors, based on their tumor, node, metastasis (TNM) stage and histology, can be managed by superficial or total parotidectomy, which can be combined with selective or radical neck dissection. When the facial nerve is involved or is in close proximity to the tumor, its sacrifice is inevitable, and repair may be followed by immediate or late reconstruction.

32. What are the most reliable anatomic landmarks in locating the main trunk of the facial nerve during parotid surgery?

Recent studies have shown that the tympanomastoid fissure is the most reliable landmark in locating the main trunk of the facial nerve. Its average distance to the main trunk of the facial nerve in cadaver dissections was found to be 2.7 mm. An almost equally dependable anatomic landmark is the tragal cartilage pointer. The distance from the tragal pointer to the main trunk of the facial nerve has been recently estimated to be less than the previously accepted standard of 1 cm. In general, the facial nerve will be found running deep to the tissue between the pointer and the mastoid attachment of the posterior belly of the digastric muscle.

33. What is the role of radiation and chemotherapy in the management of malignant salivary gland tumors?

Postoperative radiation therapy should be administered when the tumor is high stage or high grade, the adequacy of resection is in question, or the tumor has ominous pathologic features. Neutron beam therapy shows promise in controlling locoregional disease but requires further study. Currently, chemotherapy is clearly indicated only for palliation in patients with recurrent or unresectable disease.

34. What is considered an effective method for the treatment of salivary duct stenosis?

Strictures of the submandibular or parotid duct can be treated by balloon dilatation of the duct under fluoroscopic guidance (per oral balloon sialoplasty).

35. What methods have been used for the surgical management of drooling?

- Bilateral submandibular duct relocation to the posterior tonsillar pillar (most preferred)
- Bilateral parotid duct relocation to the posterior tonsillar pillar
- Bilateral parotid duct diversion with autogenous venous grafts
- Bilateral submandibular duct relocation plus parotid duct ligation
- Bilateral submandibular and parotid duct ligation
- Bilateral submandibular gland excision with parotid duct ligation, if the problem is very severe
- Chorda tympani neurectomy (only as an adjunct procedure in carefully selected cases)

    Note: The purpose of duct ligation is to ultimately establish gland atrophy.

BIBLIOGRAPHY

1. Arzoz E, Santiago A, Esnal F et al: Endoscopic intracorporeal lithotripsy for sialolithiasis. J Oral Maxillofac Surg 54:847-850, 1996.
2. Baurmash H: Laser surgery for sialolithiasis. J Oral Maxillofac Surg 54:1479, 1996.
3. Braun TW, Sotereanos GC: Cervical ranula due to an ectopic sublingual gland. J Maxillofac Surg 10:56-58, 1982.
4. Cannon CR, Replogle WH, Schenk MP: Facial nerve in parotidectomy: a topographical analysis. Laryngoscope 114:2034-2037, 2004.
5. Carlson ER: The comprehensive management of salivary gland pathology. Oral Maxillofac Clin North Am 1:387-430, 1995.
6. Carvalho MB, Soares JM, Rapoport A et al: Perioperative frozen section examination in parotid gland tumors. Sao Paolo Med J 117:233-237, 1999.
7. Choi TW, Oh CK: Hydrodissection for complete removal of a ranula. Ear Nose Throat J 82:946-951, 2003.

8. de Ru JA, van Benthem PP, Bleys RL et al: Landmarks for parotid gland surgery. J Laryngol Otol 115:122-125, 2001.
9. Drage NA, Brown JE, Escudier MP et al: Balloon dilatation of salivary duct strictures: report on 36 treated glands. Cardiovasc Intervent Radiol 25:356-359, 2002.
10. Fukase S, Ohta N, Inamura K et al: Treatment of ranula with intracystic injection of the streptococcal preparation OK-432. Ann Otol Rhinol Laryngol 112:214-220, 2003.
11. Greensmith AL, Johnstone BR, Reid SM et al: Prospective analysis of the outcome of surgical management of drooling in the pediatric population: a 10-year experience. Plast Reconstr Surg 116:1233-1242, 2005.
12. Guerrissi JO, Taborda G: Endoscopic excision of the submandibular gland by an intraoral approach. J Craniofac Surg 12:299-303, 2001.
13. Iizuka K, Ishikawa K: Surgical techniques for benign parotid tumors: segmental resection vs. extracapsular lumpectomy. Acta Otolaryngol Suppl 537:75-81, 1998.
14. Komatsuzaki Y, Ochi K, Sugiura N et al: Video-assisted submandibular sialadenectomy using an ultrasonic scalpel. Auris Nasus Larynx 30 Suppl:S75-S78, 2003.
15. McGurk M, Escudier MP, Brown JE: Modern management of salivary calculi. Br J Surg 92:107-112, 2005.
16. Nahlieli O, Shacham R, Bar T et al: Endoscopic mechanical retrieval of sialoliths. Oral Surg Oral Med Oral Pathol Oral Radiol Endod 95:396-402, 2003.
17. Niccoli-Filho W, Morosolli AR: Surgical treatment of ranula with carbon dioxide laser radiation. Lasers Med Sci 19:12-14, 2004.
18. Pang CE, Lee TS, Pang KP et al: Thoracic ranula: an extremely rare case. J Laryngol Otol 19:233-234, 2005.
19. Paris J, Facon F, Chrestian MA et al: Recurrences of pleomorphic adenomas of the parotid: development of concepts. Rev Laryngol Otol Rhinol 125: 75-80, 2004.
20. Shintani S, Matsuura H, Hasegawa Y: Fine-needle aspiration of salivary gland tumors. Int J Oral Maxillofac Surg 26:284-286, 1997.
21. Skouteris CA, Sotereanos GC: Plunging ranula: report of a case. J Oral Maxillofac Surg 45:1069-1072, 1987.
22. Spiro RH: Management of malignant tumors of the salivary glands. Oncology 12:671-680, 1998.
23. Spiro RH: Treating tumors of the sublingual glands, including a useful technique for repair of the floor of the mouth after resection. Am J Surg 170:457-460, 1995.
24. Witt RL: Facial nerve function after partial superficial parotidectomy: an 11-year review (1987-1997). Otolaryngol Head Neck Surg 121:210-213, 1999.

41. ORAL AND MAXILLOFACIAL CYSTS AND TUMORS

Chris A. Skouteris, DMD, PhD

1. What is the current treatment of solid mandibular ameloblastoma?

Small lesions can be managed effectively by curettage with peripheral ostectomy or marginal resection. Large tumors require block resection. Supraperiosteal resection should be performed in cases of cortical bone perforation.

2. What methods have been used for the surgical treatment of calcifying epithelial odontogenic tumor (CEOT)?

Tumor behavior and, consequently, type and extent of surgical treatment seem to be associated with certain histologic features of CEOT. Tumors with more amyloid and calcified content tend to behave better than those of the clear cell variant. For small lesions, enucleation followed by vigorous curettage is considered adequate treatment. For larger lesions, resection with 1 cm of disease-free bone margin is recommended.

In general, maxillary lesions should be treated more aggressively than mandibular tumors.

3.   Is there a nonsurgical treatment for aneurysmal bone cysts of the jaw?
Yes. Human calcitonin is administered subcutaneously (100 IU/day) for a period of 6 months. If the cyst shows evidence of osseous regeneration and a decrease in size at the end of this period, treatment is continued for 12-18 months until complete resolution of the lesion is accomplished.

4.   Is there a nonsurgical alternative to the treatment for central giant cell lesions of the jaws?
These lesions have been treated nonsurgically by intralesional injections of a mixture of equal parts of triamcinolone acetonide (10 mg/mL) and a local anesthetic (bupivacaine 0.5% with epinephrine 1:200,000). Antiangiogenic therapy with systemic administration of interferon alpha-2a has been reported to be effective in controlling recurrent lesions. Radiation therapy has been used in rare instances, primarily in elderly patients.

5.   How are odontogenic keratocysts treated?
Evidence suggests that these cysts can be managed effectively by a conservative approach. Good results have been achieved with decompression or marsupialization with or without later cystectomy, enucleation combined with excision of overlying mucosa and Carnoy solution application to the bony defect, and enucleation combined with liquid nitrogen application to the osseous cavity. It appears that although odontogenic keratocysts are notorious for their capricious nature relative to their tendency to recur, block resection of these lesions is hardly justifiable.

6.   Is suction drainage required after removal of jaw cysts?
Although vacuum drainage is not a common practice in the postsurgical management of cysts of the jaws, it does not seem to adversely affect primary wound healing at the surgical site.

7.   What is the incidence of development of cystic lesions around retained, asymptomatic, impacted mandibular third molars?
According to various literature reports, it ranges from 0.3%-37%.

8.   Does ultrasonography have a role in the evaluation of intraosseous lesions of the jaws?
Yes. Ultrasound has been found to be a useful complementary imaging technique, particularly for the diagnosis of bone lesions of the jaws that are not surrounded by dense cortex. Ultrasound can correctly identify solid tumors in radiolucent lesions 92.4% of the time, fluid-filled cystic lesions 73.9% of the time, and lesions with both solid and cystic areas 92.8% of the time.

9.   Is it possible to assess osseous resection margins during removal of aggressive mandibular tumors?
Yes. Frozen section analysis of cancellous bone is possible and has been shown to be a good predictor of osseous surgical margins.

10.   What is the mechanism of "recurrence" in bone grafts following resection of benign, locally aggressive tumors?
Recurrence can result from positive osseous resection margins and from residual tumor attached to periosteum in cases in which, although tumor perforation of cortical bone is present, a subperiosteal resection is performed.

11.   What are the clinical signs that should alert the clinician to the possible presence of a central vascular lesion in the mandible?
"Floating" teeth associated with spontaneous gingival bleeding and audible bruit.

12. **What lab values should be assessed in patients scheduled for resection of a large central arteriovenous malformation that has been pretreated with embolization?**
   Complete coagulation profile with special emphasis on platelet count and bleeding time. The incidence of transient thrombocytopenia and precipitous consumption coagulopathy has been reported following preoperative embolization, particularly in lesions that contain significant shunting or dilated venous channels.

13. **What are the most common soft tissue cysts and benign tumors in children?**
   Thyroglossal duct, dermoid, and epidermoid cysts are the most common soft tissue cysts in children. The most common benign soft tissue tumor is hemangioma.

14. **What are the most common benign intraosseous tumors in children?**
   Odontoma is the odontogenic tumor with the highest incidence; ossifying fibroma is the most common nonodontogenic tumor in children.

15. **Is it necessary to remove teeth that are in close association with a cyst?**
   Appropriate imaging techniques should be obtained to ascertain that teeth are indeed involved by the lesion. Usually teeth with displaced but intact roots can be treated endodontically and preserved. Teeth showing root resorption should be extracted. The removal of teeth associated with odontogenic keratocysts is appropriate to prevent recurrence.

16. **What is the surgical treatment of mandibular giant cell lesions?**
   In most cases, removal of the lesion with marginal removal of bone provides cure for the patient.

17. **What osseous resection margin is considered safe for odontogenic myxoma of the jaws?**
   The lesion should be resected with a 1-cm margin of normal bone.

18. **Is there anything that can be done intraoperatively to prevent a stress fracture from occurring in the remaining mandible at the site of a marginal resection that has been performed for the removal of a benign but locally aggressive tumor?**
   The remaining mandible can be reinforced by plates and screws. In addition, a stress fracture is less likely to occur when resection borders are rounded off instead of being perpendicular to the preserved inferior border of the mandible.

19. **What types of cervical lymphoepithelial (branchial) cysts have been identified based on intraoperative findings?**
   These cysts have been classified into four types. Type I cysts lie superficially beneath the platysma and cervical fascia along the anterior border of the sternocleidomastoid muscle. The type II cyst, which is the most common, lies on the great vessels of the neck. A type III lesion extends through the carotid bifurcation to the lateral wall of the pharynx, occasionally exhibiting a prolongation to the skull base. Type IV is a cyst, usually lined by columnar epithelium, lying against the pharyngeal wall.

20. **What should be suspected when a lesion giving the impression of a branchial cyst is noted in the neck of a patient older than age 50?**
   The possibility of cystic lymph node metastasis should be ruled out. Carcinoma of the tonsil is known to be associated with cystic metastases in cervical lymph nodes. Therefore a thorough clinical exam of the patient that might even require a diagnostic tonsillectomy is of utmost importance.

21. **Is it possible to preserve the inferior alveolar nerve during surgical ablation of benign cysts and tumors of the mandible?**

Yes. Cysts and slowly expanding, well-encapsulated neoplasms usually displace the inferior alveolar nerve without invading it. The relation of the nerve to the lesion can be determined preoperatively by contemporary imaging techniques such as Dentascan. In certain cases in which the nerve is encompassed by the tumor, microdissection and exposure of the neurovascular bundle are completed along its course through the neoplasm. The tumor is then resected after the neurovascular bundle has been isolated and protected. Potential disadvantages of this technique are the presence of tumor remnants on the neurovascular sheath and the dissemination of tumor cells in the surrounding tissues.

22. How should fibrous dysplasia be treated?

Recontouring is usually performed in cases in which aesthetic and functional improvement is required, but it is more effective when the dysplastic site has undergone maturation. Although complete resection of fibrous dysplasia has been decried in the past, current refined instrumentation and craniofacial surgical techniques allow a more aggressive, nondisabling approach, particularly when vital anatomic structures are affected by the lesion.

23. Can maxillary or mandibular osteotomies be performed in patients with fibrous dysplasia?

Yes. Recent evidence suggests that osteotomy sites can heal without complications. Fixation plates and screws seem to be well tolerated by the dysplastic bone.

24. Is fine-needle aspiration (FNA) biopsy efficacious in the diagnosis of benign intraosseous lesions?

FNA biopsy can accurately distinguish between benign and malignant tumors, but it is not as accurate in making a definitive diagnosis of benign lesions.

25. What is the method of choice in the treatment of cervicofacial lymphangiomas?

When technically feasible, total removal is the treatment of choice. Aspiration and decompression should be performed only to secure the airway in emergencies.

26. How should the surgeon approach cyst-associated teeth when marsupialization is contemplated for the treatment of dentigerous cysts in preadolescents?

In this setting, cyst-associated teeth should not be removed and should be allowed to erupt with or without orthodontic traction.

27. What is the appropriate treatment for peripheral ameloblastoma?

Conservative surgical removal by local excision.

28. What diagnostic methods can be used for the evaluation of a cystic jaw lesion?

- Aspiration for cytology and culture
- Auscultation for bruits
- Computed tomography scan
- Dentascan
- Fiberoptic endoscopy
- Open biopsy
- Panorex and plain films
- Ultrasonography

29. Does the treatment of cystic ameloblastomas differ from that of solid lesions?

Yes. Evidence suggests that unilocular or multilocular cystic ameloblastomas can be adequately treated initially by marsupialization that is later followed by enucleation with peripheral ostectomy when the lesion has attained a much smaller size.

30. Is it possible to assess intraoperatively and in follow-up extensive cystic lesions, particularly dentigerous cysts for which marsupialization has been selected as a treatment modality?

Yes. This can be accomplished through fiberoptic endoscopy. The lining epithelium of dentigerous cysts is known to possess neoplastic potential and can give rise to tumors such as ameloblastomas, primary intraosseous epidermoid carcinomas, adenocarcinomas, and primary intraosseous mucoepidermoid carcinomas, among others. Suspicious luminal growths, erosions, and ulcerations can be identified and histologically examined through endoscopic biopsies that can alter the diagnosis and eventually modify the final treatment plan.

31. What is a Sistrunk procedure?

This is a surgical procedure used for the excision of thyroglossal duct cysts. In this operation, the central portion of the hyoid bone is always excised. The retrohyoid cyst tract is dissected and excised at the base of the tongue together with the area of the foramen cecum.

BIBLIOGRAPHY

1. Assael LA: Benign lesions of the jaws. Oral Maxillofac Clin North Am 7:73-126, 1991.
2. Germanier Y, Bornstein MM, Stauffer E et al: Calcifying epithelial odontogenic (Pindborg) tumor of the mandible with clear cell component treated by conservative surgery: report of a case. J Oral Maxillofac Surg 63:1377-1382, 2005.
3. Josephson GD, Spencer WR, Josephson JS: Thyroglossal duct cyst: the New York Eye and Ear Infirmary experience and a literature review. Ear Nose Throat J 77:642-651, 1998.
4. Lauria L, Curi MM, Chammas M et al: Ultrasonography evaluation of bone lesions of the jaw. Oral Surg Oral Med Oral Pathol 82:351-357, 1996.
5. Marker P, Brondum N, Clausen PP et al: Treatment of large odontogenic keratocysts by decompression and later cystectomy: a long-term follow-up and a histologic study of 23 cases. Oral Surg Oral Med Oral Pathol Oral Radiol Endod 82:122-131, 1996.
6. Meara JG, Shah S, Li KK et al: The odontogenic keratocyst: a 20-year clinicopathologic review. Laryngoscope 108:280-283, 1998.
7. Motamedi MHK: Aneurysmal bone cysts of the jaws: clinicopathological features, radiographic evaluation, and treatment analysis of 17 cases. J Craniomaxillofac Surg 26:56-62, 1998.
8. Patino B, Fernandez-Alba J, Garcia-Rozado A et al: Calcifying epithelial odontogenic (Pindborg) tumor: a series of four distinctive cases and a review of the literature. J Oral Maxillofac Surg 63:1361-1368, 2005.
9. Pogrel AM: Treatment of keratocysts: the case for decompression and marsupialization. J Oral Maxillofac Surg 63:1667-1673, 2005.
10. Rapidis AD, Stavrianos SD, Andressakis D et al: Calcifying epithelial odontogenic tumor (CEOT) of the mandible: clinical therapeutic conference. J Oral Maxillofac Surg 63:1337-1347, 2005.
11. Sampson DE, Pogrel MA: Management of mandibular ameloblastoma: the clinical basis for a treatment algorithm. J Oral Maxillofac Surg 57:1074, 1999.
12. Sato M, Tanaka N, Sato T et al: Oral and maxillofacial tumors in children: a review. Br J Oral Maxillofac Surg 35:92-95, 1997.
13. Skouteris CA: Fiberoptic endoscopy of a marsupialized dentigerous cyst. J Oral Maxillofac Surg 46:74-77, 1988.
14. Skouteris CA, Patterson GT, Sotereanos GC: Benign cervical lymphoepithelial cyst: report of cases. J Oral Maxillofac Surg 47:1106-1112, 1989.
15. Stoelinga PJW: The treatment of odontogenic keratocysts by excision of the overlying attached mucosa, enucleation, and treatment of the bony defect with Carnoy solution. J Oral Maxillofac Surg 63:1662-1666, 2005.

42. CANCER OF THE ORAL CAVITY

Chris A. Skouteris, DMD, PhD, and Kiki C. Marti, DMD, MD, PhD

1. What is the usual clinical presentation of squamous cell carcinoma?

Oral squamous cell carcinoma usually presents as an indurated ulcer with poorly defined borders. The lesion is characteristically painless, unless inflammation from superinfection or chronic mechanical irritation is present. An indolent clinical presentation in the form of a small superficial ulceration, leukoplakia, or erythroplakia is also likely, especially in the early stages of development.

2. What is the current staging system for oral cancer?

The TNM (tumor, node, metastasis) staging system (Tables 42-1 to 42-4).

Some inherent inadequacies of this system have prompted the proposal of certain modifications and revisions in an effort to enhance its prognostic significance.

3. Which factors indicate a poor prognosis in oral cancer?

The most important poor prognostic factors include:

- Site
- Tumor diameter
- Tumor thickness and invasion
- Degree of histologic differentiation
- Lymph node metastasis
- Level of lymph node involvement
- Number of affected lymph nodes
- Extranodal spread
- Distant metastasis

Local or locoregional recurrence and nonresponse to radiation and chemotherapy are also factors that adversely influence prognosis of overall patient survival.

4. What is the most common anatomic site for oral cancer?

The tongue and floor of the mouth. Other sites might be more common in different parts of the world through certain predisposing ethnic, cultural, or other factors.

5. What is the most common form of oral cancer?

Squamous cell carcinoma.

6. What is the main difference between carcinoma in situ and invasive carcinoma?

Carcinoma in situ is an epithelial dysplasia that includes all the layers of the epithelium but does not extend beyond the basal layer. Once the malignant cells have penetrated the basal layer

Table 42-1	*Tumor Classification of Cancer of the Oral Cavity*
CLASS	TUMOR SIZE
T_1	≤ 2 cm at greatest dimension
T_2	> 2 cm but ≤ 4 cm at greatest dimension
T_3	> 4 cm at greatest dimension
T_4	Tumor invades adjacent structures

Data from Sobin LH, Wittekind CK: TNM Classification of Malignant Tumors, 6th ed. Hoboken, NJ, 2002, John Wiley & Sons.

Table 42-2 *Node Classification of Cancer of the Oral Cavity*

CLASS	DESCRIPTION
N_X	Regional lymph nodes cannot be assessed
N_0	No regional lymph node metastasis
N_1	Metastasis in a single ipsilateral lymph node, ≤ 3 cm at greatest dimension
N_2	Metastasis in a single ipsilateral lymph node, more than 3 cm but not more than 6 cm at greatest dimension *or* Multiple ipsilateral lymph nodes, none more than 6 cm at greatest dimension *or* Bilateral or contralateral lymph nodes, none more than 6 cm at greatest dimension
N_{2a}	Metastasis in a single ipsilateral lymph node, > 3 cm but ≤ 6 cm at greatest dimension
N_{2b}	Metastasis in multiple ipsilateral lymph nodes, none > 6 cm at greatest dimension
N_{2c}	Metastasis in bilateral or contralateral lymph nodes, none > 6 cm at greatest dimension
N_3	Metastasis > 6 cm at greatest dimension in a lymph node

Data from Sobin LH, Wittekind CK: TNM Classification of Malignant Tumors, 6th ed. Hoboken, NJ, 2002, John Wiley & Sons.

Table 42-3 *Metastasis Classification of Cancer of the Oral Cavity*

CLASS	DESCRIPTION
M_X	Distant metastasis cannot be assessed
M_0	No distant metastasis
M_1	Distant metastasis

Data from Sobin LH, Wittekind CK: TNM Classification of Malignant Tumors, 6th ed. Hoboken, NJ, 2002, John Wiley & Sons.

into the lamina propria, early invasive squamous cell carcinoma has been established. If tumor invasiveness extends deeper into the tissues, involving fat, muscle, or other structures, then true invasive squamous cell carcinoma has evolved.

7. Which is the best imaging modality to diagnose invasive squamous cell carcinoma?

Soft tissue invasion is best assessed by magnetic resonance imaging (MRI). Osseous invasion is best assessed by conventional computed tomography (CT) or Dentascan imaging.

8. What features are characteristic of lip carcinoma?

Squamous cell carcinoma usually affects the lower lip and rarely the upper lip. This occurrence has been attributed to greater exposure of the lower lip to sunlight. Lip carcinoma commonly presents as an ulcer. In many cases, a keratin crust covers the ulcer. The rest of the lip vermilion may show actinic changes.

Table 42-4 *Stage Grouping of Cancer of the Oral Cavity*

STAGE	TUMOR CLASS	NODE CLASS	METASTASIS CLASS
Stage 0	Tis[*]	N_0	M_0
Stage I	T_1	N_0	M_0
Stage II	T_2	N_0	M_0
Stage III	T_3	N_0	M_0
	T_2	N_1	M_0
	T_3	N_1	M_0
Stage IVA	T_4	N_0	M_0
	T_4	N_1	M_0
	Any T	N_2	M_0
Stage IVB	Any T	N_3	M_0
Stage IVC	Any T	Any N	M_1

Data from Sobin LH, Wittekind CK: TNM Classification of Malignant Tumors, 6th ed. Hoboken, NJ, 2002, John Wiley & Sons.
*In situ.

9. **Which feature best describes the degree of malignancy of a tumor?**
The degree of histologic differentiation. Malignant neoplasms are histologically classified as (1) well differentiated, (2) moderately differentiated, or (3) poorly differentiated (anaplastic) tumors. From a histologic point of view, poorly differentiated tumors have the highest degree of malignancy. However, that does not necessarily correlate with the clinical behavior of a neoplasm or its response to treatment.

10. **What are the most common routes of spread of oral carcinoma?**
Local spread is achieved by direct invasion and infiltration of adjacent structures. Perineural invasion and spread is particularly important because it can adversely influence the actual extent of the tumor. Regional spread to the neck lymph nodes occurs by the lymphatic route. Usually, the higher echelon nodes that mainly drain the area of the lesion are affected. Widespread nodal involvement can also occur, as well as direct involvement of a lower level of nodes, by skipping all other intermediate levels through the so-called fast tracks. Midline lesions affect nodes on both sides of the neck. Spread to distal organs follows the hematogenous route.

11. **What is the most appropriate management of a small, painful, ulcerative lesion on the posterolateral aspect of the tongue that has been present for several weeks?**
Remove any suspected source of trauma or irritation. Traumatic ulcers heal within 10-14 days. Ulcers that persist for more than 2 weeks should undergo biopsy, as should deep-seated large ulcers, particularly those with rolled borders.

12. **What are the roles of the three major treatment modalities (surgery, radiation, and chemotherapy) in the management of oral cancer?**
Surgery, with the recent advances in reconstructive techniques, remains the mainstay of treatment for oral carcinoma. The primary site is resected, and the cervical lymph nodes are removed through different types of neck dissections.
Radiation therapy can be the primary treatment modality in certain cases in the form of external beam radiation or brachytherapy. Radiation therapy also can be combined with surgery. In such instances, radiation therapy can be delivered preoperatively (neoadjuvant), intraoperatively, or postoperatively (adjuvant).

Chemotherapy is not suitable as the primary treatment modality for oral carcinoma. However, it can be combined with surgery and radiation in different treatment protocols, particularly for the management of patients with advanced disease. Chemotherapy, in general, may be administered as induction, primary or neoadjuvant, adjuvant, and palliation therapy.

13. **Which are the most advanced stereotactic radiosurgery (SRS) treatment delivery techniques?**
   SRS has been introduced in the treatment of head and neck cancer. These techniques include the Gamma Knife; linear accelerator-based stereotactic techniques using circular collimators or using micro multileaf collimators (mMLCs); the CyberKnife, using an x-band linear accelerator mounted on a robotic arm; and serial and spiral tomotherapy.

14. **What are the most common adverse effects of radiation therapy on the oral and paraoral tissues?**
   - Rampant caries
   - Radiation mucositis
   - Xerostomia
   - Difficulty in swallowing
   - Varying degrees of trismus
   - Radiation dermatitis

   Osteoradionecrosis does not develop unless the patient's oral condition is not optimized before radiation therapy, and postirradiation dental procedures are performed without proper precautions.

15. **What is the proper management of postmaxillectomy defects?**
   Some controversy exists over the best way to manage postmaxillectomy defects. One school of thought holds that immediate reconstruction of such defects is inappropriate because it prevents inspection for possible recurrence. An obturator is used for 1 year, and if recurrence is not detected, a delayed reconstruction is performed.
   Other surgeons prefer immediate defect reconstruction after intraoperative frozen section assessment of resection margins. Defect reconstruction can be performed successfully by nonvascularized grafts, local flaps, regional flaps, and free tissue transfers. The most frequently used methods include the temporalis muscle flap as a simple or composite flap with attached calvarial bone, the buccal fat pad, and free composite flaps that can be combined with osseointegrated implants for oral rehabilitation.

16. **Which tests should be included in the metastatic work-up for oral cancer?**
   Blood and biochemical profiles, chest x-ray, liver ultrasound, and bone scan. In the case of equivocal results, CT scanning or MRI also may be required to clarify the findings.

17. **What is the best way to manage a highly suspicious lesion that is biopsied and determined by the pathologist to be noncancerous?**
   The lesion should be rebiopsied. Tissue sampling should be obtained from multiple sites of the lesion. If this action does not solve the diagnostic problem, a second opinion from another pathologist might be appropriate before any final treatment decision is reached. However, it cannot be overemphasized that all pertinent clinical information and the findings of other diagnostic modalities must be provided to the pathologist at the time of the initial submission of the specimen.

18. **Which is the most appropriate imaging study for evaluation of a maxillary sinus neoplasm?**
   CT.

19. **What conditions should be suspected (a) when a patient who has undergone marginal mandibulectomy and postoperative radiation therapy for squamous cell carcinoma**

presents with a fracture in the area of the marginal mandibulectomy and (b) when a patient who has been treated surgically for carcinoma of the posterior maxilla develops trismus?
a. Osteoradionecrosis and, most importantly, tumor recurrence
b. Tumor recurrence

20. What are radical neck dissection, modified radical neck dissection, and selective neck dissection?

Radical neck dissection (RND) is the en bloc removal of the lymph-node-bearing tissues of one side of the neck, from the inferior border of the mandible to the clavicle and from the lateral border of the strap muscles to the anterior border of the trapezius. Included in the resected specimen are the spinal accessory nerve, the internal jugular vein, and the sternocleidomastoid muscle.

Modified radical neck dissection (MRND) differs from RND in that one, two, or all three of the major anatomic structures that are removed during RND (spinal accessory nerve, internal jugular vein, sternocleidomastoid muscle) are preserved in MRND. Thus three types of MRND have evolved from these modifications: type I (preservation of the spinal accessory nerve); type II (preservation of the spinal accessory nerve and internal jugular vein); and type III (preservation of the spinal accessory nerve, internal jugular vein, and sternocleidomastoid muscle).

Selective neck dissection (SND) entails the removal of only those lymph node groups that are at highest risk of containing metastases according to the location of the primary tumor, preserving the spinal accessory nerve, internal jugular vein, and sternocleidomastoid muscle. Currently, the most frequently used SND is the anterolateral neck dissection (supraomohyoid neck dissection and the expanded supraomohyoid neck dissection). In both operations, nodal regions I (submental, submandibular nodes), II (upper jugular, jugulodigastric, and upper posterior cervical nodes), and III (midjugular nodes) are removed en bloc together with the lymph nodes found within the fibroadipose tissue located medial to the sternocleidomastoid muscle. The expanded supraomohyoid neck dissection also includes the nodes in region IV (lower jugular, scalene, and supraclavicular lymph nodes located deep to the lower one third of the sternocleidomastoid muscle).

21. What is the definition of the sentinel node?

The sentinel node is any lymph node receiving direct lymphatic drainage from a primary tumor site.

22. What is the procedure for sentinel node biopsy (SNB)?

A radiotracer (usually 99mTc-labeled small-particle radiocolloid) is injected in the area of the primary site 24 hr before surgery. The area of radiotracer uptake is identified with a handheld gamma probe. In the immediate preoperative period, blue dye (isosulphan blue) is injected in the area of the primary site. The area of the radiotracer uptake is dissected, and any stained node or nodes are identified. The stained node or nodes are assessed again for radiotracer uptake with the handheld gamma probe. Any node that is "hot" and stained represents the sentinel node or nodes. The sentinel node is removed and is sent for frozen section. Based on the findings of SNB studies in melanoma and breast cancer cases, if the sentinel node is negative for micrometastasis no further lymph node dissection is required. If the sentinel node is positive, the appropriate type of lymph node dissection is then performed.

23. What is the role of SNB in head and neck cancer?

SNB has been introduced in recent years as a very promising procedure aiding in the proper management and staging of the N_0 neck.

24. What is the validity of SNB in head and neck cancer?

The results of a recent multicentric study on 379 patients with N_0 disease showed that the sentinel node was identified in 97% of the patients and most importantly that the negative predictive value of a negative sentinel node for the remaining neck was 96%.

25. What is the incidence of cervical lymph node metastasis from an unknown primary site?

The incidence of cervical lymph node metastasis in patients with squamous cell carcinoma of unknown primary site has been reported to be 5%-10%.

26. What is the appropriate diagnostic work-up in the assessment of a patient with cervical lymph node metastases of squamous cell carcinoma from an unknown primary site?

Clinical

- Thorough intraoral and extraoral exam (include the scalp, facial skin, and external auditory meatus)
- Panendoscopy (rhinoscopy, pharyngoscopy, laryngoscopy, esophagoscopy, bronchoscopy with bronchial washings)

Imaging

- Orthopantomogram
- Ultrasound
- CT scan
- MRI
- Positron emission tomography (PET) scan
- Combined PET-CT
- FDG (2-[fluorine-18]fluoro-2-deoxy-D-glucose) SPECT (single photon emission computed tomography)

Invasive

- Multiple "blind" biopsies
- Diagnostic tonsillectomy

27. What patient characteristics are suggestive of a malignant neoplasm of the oral cavity?

The following characteristics suggest, but are not conclusive of, advanced disease:

- Malnourishment
- Halitosis
- Drooling
- Difficulty in speech and deglutition

BIBLIOGRAPHY

1. Black RJ, Gluckman JL, Shumrick DA: Screening for distant metastases in head and neck cancer patients. Aust N Z J Surg 54:527-530, 1984.
2. Calabrese L, Jereczek-Fossa BA, Jassem J et al: Diagnosis and management of neck metastases from an unknown primary. Acta Otorhinolaryngol Ital 25:2-12, 2005.
3. Davison SP, Sherris DA, Meland NB: An algorithm for maxillectomy defect reconstruction. Laryngoscope 108:215-219, 1998.
4. Eversole LR: Oral Medicine: A Pocket Guide. Philadelphia, 1996, Saunders.
5. Howaldt HP, Kainz M, Euler B: Proposal for modification of the TNM staging classification for cancer of the oral cavity. J Craniomaxillofac Surg 27:275-288, 1999.
6. Jereczek-Fossa BA, Jassem J, Orecchia R: Cervical lymph node metastases of squamous cell carcinoma from an unknown primary. Cancer Treat Rev 30:153-164, 2004.
7. Medina JE, Rigual NR: Neck dissection. In Byron J, Bailey J (eds): Head and Neck Surgery—Otolaryngology. Philadelphia, 1993, J.B. Lippincott.
8. Menda Y, Graham MM: Update on 18F-fluorodeoxyglucose/positron emission tomography and positron emission tomography/computed tomography imaging of squamous head and neck cancers. Semin Nucl Med 35:214-219, 2005.
9. Mendenhall WM, Mancuso AA, Parsons JT et al: Diagnostic evaluation of squamous cell carcinoma metastatic to cervical lymph nodes from an unknown head and neck primary site. Head Neck 20:739-744, 1998.

10. Nakayama B, Matsuura H, Ishihara O et al: Functional reconstruction of a bilateral maxillectomy defect using a fibula osteocutaneous flap with osseointegrated implants. Plast Reconstr Surg 96:1201-1204, 1995.
11. Stoeckli SJ, Pfaltz M, Ross GL et al: The second international conference on sentinel node biopsy in mucosal head and neck cancer. Ann Surg Oncol 12:919-924, 2005.
12. Yu C, Shepard D: Treatment planning for stereotactic radiosurgery with photon beams. Technol Cancer Res Treat 2:93-104, 2003.

43. LASERS IN ORAL AND MAXILLOFACIAL SURGERY

Robert A. Strauss, DDS, MD

1. What does the term *laser* mean?

The word *laser* is derived from the acronym for *l*ight *a*mplification by *s*timulated *e*mission of *r*adiation.

2. What is the most common laser used in oral and maxillofacial surgery (OMS) practice?

Carbon dioxide (CO_2) laser.

3. CO_2 laser wavelength is absorbed principally by what tissue component?

At a wavelength of 10,600 nm, the CO_2 laser is almost completely absorbed by water (98%). Its use in OMS is based on the fact that all soft tissues are composed mainly of water, and therefore they absorb this wavelength exceedingly well.

4. What are the four basic tissue interactions associated with lasers?

1. Reflection (bouncing off the tissue)
2. Transmission (going through the tissue)
3. Scatter (breaking up inside the tissue)
4. Absorption

Of these, only absorption has any significant beneficial effects on tissue. Therefore a laser is usually chosen by its percentage of absorption into the intended target tissue.

5. What are the four main reactions seen in tissue after laser energy absorption?

1. Photothermal
2. Photochemical
3. Photoablative
4. Photoacoustic

6. What is a photothermal reaction?

When laser energy is absorbed into a target tissue, one possible result is the generation of heat. This change in energy from light to heat is termed a photothermal reaction and results in tissue vaporization. This reaction is used to perform most soft tissue surgeries in OMS.

7. What is a photoablative reaction?

When laser energy is absorbed into a target, another possible result is fragmentation of the chemical bonds of the target, resulting in vaporizing of the tissue. Unique to this reaction is that little or no heat is generated within the target, allowing surgery without lateral thermal damage. For example, this reaction is used in ophthalmology to ablate the cornea for vision correction without damaging the eye.

8.   Which basic tissue interaction is used by the CO_2 and Er:YAG lasers?

Both of these lasers are primarily absorbed by tissue water, with a resultant generation of heat. This *photothermal* reaction then causes the intracellular water to vaporize, generating steam that expands and eventually disrupts the cell membrane.

9.   What are the two most common lasers used for cosmetic skin resurfacing?

Because of their high affinity for tissue water found in the epidermis and dermis, the CO_2 and Er:YAG lasers are the most common lasers used for skin resurfacing techniques.

10.   What is power density (irradiation)?

Power density is a measure of the amount of laser power applied to a given area. Measured in watts per square centimeters (W/cm^2), it determines how deep the laser's effect will go into the tissue in any given time unit (e.g., 1 sec). Therefore greater power or a smaller spot size causes a deeper laser effect in tissue for each sec of use. As the power is diminished or the spot size is increased, the laser's effect becomes more superficial for each sec of use.

11.   What is energy density (fluence)?

Energy density is a measure of the total amount of laser energy applied to a given unit of tissue during a complete laser pulse. Essentially, this represents the power density over the course of time of the entire laser pulse and is measured as $W/cm^2 \times$ time (in sec). In other words, the total depth of effect will be greater for a given power density (power and spot size) the longer the laser is applied. As an example, a 2-sec pulse will create twice the total effect depth in tissue as a 1-sec pulse.

12.   What is thermal relaxation time?

Thermal relaxation is the process by which heat diffuses through tissue by thermal conduction. Thermal relaxation time is the time required for a given tissue to dissipate 50% of the heat absorbed from the laser pulse. Any pulse that is longer than the thermal relaxation time for the target tissue would therefore lead to some amount of lateral thermal damage.

13.   What is coagulation necrosis?

Coagulation necrosis refers to the area surrounding the intended surgical site that is both reversibly and irreversibly damaged by lateral thermal conduction. The longer the laser energy is applied, the greater the zone of lateral thermal damage that occurs through conduction. Conversely, this principle does have the positive effect of contracting blood vessel wall collagen, thereby sealing any blood vessel that is within this zone (300-500 μm diameter for a continuous-wave CO_2 laser). This leads to bloodless surgery in many cases.

14.   What is the significance of the thermal relaxation time of approximately 700-1000 μsec for skin?

If a laser can provide a pulse of energy that is shorter in duration than the thermal relaxation time for the target tissue, there will be little or no thermal damage to adjacent and underlying tissue. It is this effect that makes skin resurfacing possible. The time on tissue is maintained below the thermal relaxation time for skin, ensuring that there will be little or no damage to the underlying dermal tissues and allowing rapid reepithelialization from intact dermal adnexal structures.

15.   What three delivery systems for lasers are used currently?

The ideal delivery system is a fiberoptic guide. Unfortunately, many laser wavelengths useful in OMS cannot be transmitted through fiberoptics. Articulated arm lasers use a series of connecting hollow metal tubes with prism articulations to transmit the beam, but this is sometimes cumbersome in intraoral use. More recently, hollow wave guide technology using internal mirrored and bendable hollow metal fibers has facilitated the use of lasers in the oral cavity.

16. What is the difference between a focused and a defocused laser beam?

A laser beam can be focused down to a very small spot size or backed away from the target, allowing the spot size to increase. Because spot size is a determinant of power density, the smaller the spot size the greater the power density and the deeper the laser affects tissue during each pulse. A larger spot size will cause a larger but more superficial effect as the power density diminishes. A high-power density and a small spot size are used to make incisions, whereas a large spot size with lower power density is generally used for tissue ablation.

17. What is tissue ablation?

Tissue ablation, or tissue vaporization, is the removal of the surface layers of tissue over a wide area, such as would be used to remove a superficial leukoplakia. This is accomplished by applying the laser at a large spot size, thereby lowering the power density and creating a large but superficial effect in tissue. This technique allows for removal of large surface lesions with little damage to underlying structures but does preclude obtaining an excisional specimen for histologic exam.

18. How is a particular laser chosen?

In general, laser choice is determined by matching the wavelength of the laser with the absorption of that wavelength by the intended target tissue. The greater the absorption, the greater the effect in that tissue.

19. What is the effect of a laser beam on supplemental oxygen being delivered to the patient?

Although oxygen is not flammable, it does support combustion. Hence in higher concentrations (approximately over 30%), the oxygen would support rapid combustion with disastrous consequences if anything in the surgical field caught fire (e.g., endotracheal tube, hair, gauze). Keeping everything but the target wet, protecting endotracheal tubes, and minimizing exposed oxygen supplementation can help diminish the risk.

20. What is an aiming beam?

Lasers that are not within the visible spectrum of light, such as the CO_2 laser, cannot be seen. Therefore to aim and focus the beam, a secondary laser that is within the visible spectrum (e.g., helium neon [HeNe] or diode) is sent coaxially along with the CO_2 to act as a visible aiming beam.

21. What are YAG lasers?

The crystal of these lasers is made of *yttrium, aluminum,* and *garnet* and is doped with a rare earth element (e.g., neodymium [Nd], holmium [Ho], or erbium [Er]) as the active lasing medium.

22. What is the typical zone of coagulation necrosis surrounding the CO_2 laser wound?

Using a continuous-wave CO_2 laser, the zone of coagulation necrosis is generally around 500 microns or less. Manipulating the speed of the pulse (e.g., Superpulse or Ultrapulse) can decrease this to less than 100 microns.

23. What is coherent light?

Coherent light is a state in which all light waves are temporally and spatially in phase. In other words, the light is monochromatic (one wavelength), collimated (all the waves are parallel), and uniform of phase (all the peaks and troughs line up on top of one another).

24. What is IPL, and what are its main uses?

IPL, the acronym for *intense pulsed light,* duplicates or improves on some effects of the laser using monochromatic, but not coherent, light. Some generalized and deep vascular and pigmented lesions, for example, can be treated effectively using noncoherent light, which has a greater degree of scatter than most laser light sources.

25. What is a chromophore?

A chromophore is a target tissue for a specific laser wavelength. The primary chromophore for the CO_2 and Er:YAG lasers is water, whereas the argon laser is absorbed well by hemoglobin and tissue pigments (which are its chromophores), but not by water. It is important to match the intended target with the chromophore for the particular laser being used.

26. What are "Superpulsing" and "Ultrapulsing"?

Because the amount of time a laser is applied to tissue is directly related to the amount of lateral thermal damage, when it is important to limit this effect (as in skin resurfacing procedures), it is critical to have very short, but very high energy, laser exposures. This is most easily accomplished using flashlamp pulsed lasers. Some lasers, although desirable for their absorption properties, cannot be optically pulsed (such as the continuous-wave CO_2). In this situation, continuous-wave lasers can be "overpumped" with excess power (e.g., 90-250 watts using a 30-60–watt laser tube) and computer controlled to limit their time to below the thermal relaxation time of the target. This leads to very limited lateral thermal damage in tissue.

27. What is Q-switching?

Even true pulsed lasers can be manipulated to have exceptionally short pulse times, thereby limiting lateral damage in tissues with short thermal relaxation times. Q-switching is a mechanism to do this with some lasers, such as the ruby laser, used for tattoo removal.

28. What is the chromophore for the Nd:YAG laser?

The Nd:YAG wavelength is not well absorbed by any particular chromophore but has some absorption for multiple chromophores. This leads to deep penetration in most tissues unless the beam is attenuated in some manner (e.g., using a contact tip). The most common chromophore that is targeted by this wavelength is tissue pigment, making it useful for hair removal as one example.

29. How can a laser produce dual or multiple wavelengths?

It is a basic principle of lasers that only a single wavelength can be produced by any laser tube *at any moment in time*. However, some lasers can produce multiple different wavelengths, which then allows the user to choose the particular wavelength desired. For example, the argon laser can produce wavelengths at either 488 or 514 nm (but not both at one time). Before use, the surgeon selects the desired wavelength. The pulsed dye uses a series of colored flowing dyes as the lasing medium. By choosing the particular dye that flows into the tube, one can choose the wavelength produced. Some lasers can produce multiple wavelengths by incorporating more than one laser tube in the same physical box.

BIBLIOGRAPHY

1. Atkinson T: Fundamentals of the carbon dioxide laser. In Catone G, Alling C (eds): Laser Applications in Oral and Maxillofacial Surgery. Philadelphia, 1997, Saunders.
2. Holmes JD, Diers EJ: Oral cancer. In Miloro M (ed): Peterson's Principles of Oral and Maxillofacial Surgery. Hamilton, London, 2004, B.C. Decker.
3. Monheit GD: Skin rejuvenation procedures. In Miloro M (ed): Peterson's Principles of Oral and Maxillofacial Surgery. Hamilton, London, 2004, B.C. Decker.
4. Strauss RA: Laser management of discrete lesions. In Catone G, Alling C (eds): Laser Applications in Oral and Maxillofacial Surgery. Philadelphia, 1997, Saunders.

44. PATIENTS IRRADIATED FOR HEAD AND NECK CANCER

A. Omar Abubaker, DMD, PhD

1. What are the principles of management of irradiated patients?

The overall goals of the treatment of patients who have undergone or who are about to receive radiation therapy are:
- Better understanding of radiation effects and the pathogenesis of osteoradionecrosis (ORN)
- Better prevention and management of the radiation effects
- Minimizing postradiation complications by use of hyperbaric oxygen (HBO) therapy
- Functional bony reconstruction and total oral rehabilitation of radiation patients using dental implants

2. What is the incidence of oral cancer?

According to 1996 statistics, the estimated annual number of new cases of head and neck cancer in the United States is 29,490. This accounts for 3% of all new cancer cases in men and 2% in women. The most common head and neck cancer is squamous cell carcinoma. The most common sites for oral carcinoma are the floor of the mouth, retromolar trigone, pharynx, tongue, and lips.

3. What are the methods of treating head and neck cancer?

In the early stages of the disease, surgery or radiotherapy is often used as the sole therapy. In more advanced stages of the disease, therapies combining surgery, radiotherapy, and chemotherapy are usually used to minimize recurrence of the disease and to improve the survival rate.

4. What are the types of radiotherapy?
- External radiation sources, which include supervoltage and megavoltage (cobalt 60 and linear accelerator)
- Low-dose brachytherapy, which includes radium needles and cesium and iridium wires

5. What is the mechanism of action of radiotherapy?

The radiation interacts with the atoms and molecules of the cells and produces free radicals, which diffuse a short distance into the cell to damage critical targets such as DNA. It affects all phases of the cell cycle.

6. How is radiation measured?

The measurement of dose of radiation has changed from rads (100 ergs/g) to grays (Gy; 1 joule/kg): 1 Gy = 100 rads = 100 cGy.

7. What cell types are most affected by radiation therapy?

Radiation affects all rapidly dividing cells, including neoplastic cells, epithelial cells, endothelial cells, and reticuloendothelial cells.

8. Which orofacial tissues are affected by radiation therapy?
- Bone
- Cartilage
- Peripheral and cranial nerves
- Pituitary gland

- Lymphatics
- Muscles of mastication
- Nasolacrimal drainage system
- Oral flora
- Oral mucosa
- Paranasal sinuses
- Salivary glands
- Skin
- Subcutaneous tissue
- Teeth
- Temporomandibular joint (TMJ)
- Thyroid and parathyroid glands

9. What are the effects of radiation on teeth and periodontium?

The most common manifestations of radiation therapy on oral tissues are erythema of the oral mucosa and friable and easily injured gingival tissue. The gingival tissue also becomes less cellular and fibrotic. The effects on teeth are mostly in the form of radiation caries.

10. What is radiation caries?

Radiation caries is characterized by circumferential decay of the cervical portion of numerous teeth. It is believed that radiation caries is related, at least in part, to xerostomia. Another possible contributing factor is change in the oral flora. Radiation caries also may be related to pulpal death, dentine dehydration, and enamel loss (similar to dentigerous imperfecta). Radiation caries is most severe within the radiation field.

11. How does radiation affect the oral mucosa?

Long-term changes include decreased keratinization, decreased vascularity, easy ulceration, and delayed healing. Short-term effects include taste changes and mucositis.

12. What is irradiation mucositis?

Painful erythema of the oral mucosa, pharynx, and larynx. It usually develops after 1 week of radiation therapy, may become severe after 3 weeks of beginning treatment, and subsides 2-3 weeks after completion of treatment. Its duration and severity are greatly influenced by daily dose. The most common sites affected are the soft palate, tonsillar pillars, buccal mucosa, lateral border of the tongue, and the larynx and pharyngeal walls. Mucositis usually does not develop at the hard palate, alveolar ridges, dorsum of the tongue, or true vocal cords.

13. What are the effects of radiation on oral flora?

Radiation causes long-term changes in the microbiologic population of oral flora, including increased fungal and anaerobic organisms, and a high incidence of candidiasis.

14. Does radiation affect the TMJ and muscles of mastication?

Changes in these areas are uncommon with irradiation for oral cancer because the TMJ is often outside the field of radiation. When the TMJ and muscles of mastication are within the field of radiation, trismus and fibrosis of the muscles of mastication are seen, along with fibrous ankylosis of the TMJ and myofascial pain.

15. What are the effects of radiation on bone?

The decreased vascularity of the bone causes delayed healing after any trauma to the bone. These effects, which are the most serious, are significant after 4 months and progress with time. They are chronic, can occur as late as 30 years after radiation, and occasionally result in ORN.

16. What is the dental management of patients before radiation treatment?
- Complete oral/dental exam and treatment plan
- Any necessary extraction and surgery
- Maintenance of teeth and caries control
- Restoration of restorable teeth
- Prosthetic exam to prevent postradiation trauma from ill-fitting dentures

17. What factors should be considered in evaluation of patients before radiation of the head and neck?

- Age of the patient
- Condition of the dentition
- Level of oral hygiene and patient attitude
- Radiation field and dose
- Urgency of radiation treatment

18. What are the methods of caries control and prevention in the preradiation patient?

The goal of preradiation management is prevention of dental and oral diseases, which consists of:

- Prophylactic care before and at the end of therapy
- Oral hygiene instructions
- Daily administration of fluoride
- Weekly follow-up during therapy and every 3-4 weeks afterward

19. What are some guidelines for extraction before radiation therapy?

- All carious mandibular teeth in the field of radiation (more than 6000 cGy) should be extracted, except in patients with particularly good oral hygiene and excellent dental condition.
- All questionable teeth should be extracted.
- Full bony impacted teeth can be left in place.
- Optimal time for extraction is 21 days before beginning of radiotherapy (no less than 2 weeks).
- Less optimally, extraction can be done within 4 months after completion of therapy.
- Perform radical alveolectomy with primary soft tissue closure following extraction.

20. How should a patient be managed during radiation therapy?

Management of the radiation patient at this phase should be mainly palliative, including only pulpectomy, pulpotomy, incision and drainage, analgesics, and antibiotics. Extractions should not be performed during radiation therapy, and definitive treatment should be delayed until after completion of radiation therapy.

21. What is the management of a patient who has undergone head and neck radiation?

Patients who have a history of radiation therapy should be managed carefully to prevent ORN, which may result from any dental or surgical trauma. Obtaining records of radiation fields and dose is essential to determine the best approach to these patients. Once such records are available, the following guidelines should be followed:

- Recall for prophylaxis and home care evaluation every 3 months.
- The patient should continue daily fluoride application for the rest of his or her life.
- Restorative dental procedures may be performed as needed.
- Prosthetic appliances may be constructed as early as 3 months, if mucositis has cleared.
- Prosthetic appliances must be adjusted carefully to prevent irritation and trauma to the underlying mucosa.
- Invasive procedures involving the irradiated bone should be avoided, if at all possible.
- Within 4 months of completion of radiation therapy and after resolution of the mucositis, minor surgical procedures, such as extraction and minor preprosthetic surgery and vestibuloplasty, can be performed.
- If an invasive procedure is necessary within the field of radiation (receiving more than 6000 cGy) 4 months after radiation or thereafter, the procedure should be performed after HBO therapy.

22. What is the management of a postradiation patient who needs oral and maxillofacial surgery (OMFS)?

Four months after completion of therapy (more than 6000 cGy), all surgical procedures in the field of radiation should be done after prophylactic HBO treatment.

23. How are irradiation mucositis and xerostomia managed?

Treatment of mucositis and xerostomia in patients who received radiation therapy is mostly symptomatic:

- Keep mouth and teeth moist and plaque-free.
- Avoid using petrolatum-based lip balms, commercial mouthwashes, peroxide rinses for longer than 3 days, denture adhesives, and citrus and spicy foods.
- Sugarless candy and gum chewing are encouraged.
- Do not drink alcohol excessively or use tobacco.
- Use a saliva substitute (e.g., Xero-lube, Saliva-lube, Saliva-aide, Moi-stir, Salivart).
- Thin foods with liquid to aid in swallowing.
- Keep dentures out if mucositis is present.
- Filter smoke from room with filtering appliances.
- Use water, beeswax, or vegetable oil–based lubricant or hydrous lanolin to moisten the mouth.
- If toothpaste is irritating, use baking soda.

24. How should pain caused by irradiation mucositis and xerostomia be managed?

- Viscous lidocaine 2%, half an hour before meals
- Benadryl syrup and Kaopectate mixed in equal parts
- Ulcers may be coated with sucralfate suspension.
- Analgesics, starting with ibuprofen and progressing to narcotics, as needed

OSTEORADIONECROSIS

25. What is ORN?

After completion of radiation treatment, an area of exposed, nonviable bone at the field of radiation that fails to show any evidence of spontaneous healing is diagnosed as ORN. The bone, which is exposed because of mucosal or cutaneous ulceration, must be at least 3-5 mm in size and must be present in the field of irradiation for at least 6 months (although some authors require only 3 months for diagnosis).

26. What are the risk factors for ORN (Box 44-1)?

Box 44-1 *Risk Factors for Osteoradionecrosis*		
PATIENT-RELATED FACTORS	TUMOR-RELATED FACTORS	TREATMENT-RELATED FACTORS
Presence of teeth	Anatomic location of the tumor	Field of radiation
Presence of active dental disease	Clinical stage of the tumor	Total dose of radiation
Oral hygiene and preradiation care	Presence of lymph node metastasis	Dose rate/day
Alcohol and tobacco abuse		Mode of radiation delivery
		Tumor surgery

27. What is the incidence of ORN?

The incidence of ORN ranges from 1%-44.2%, with an overall incidence of 11.8% in most studies published before 1968. Recent studies showed incidences of 5%-15%, with an overall incidence of 5.4%. ORN has a bimodal incidence, peaking at 12 months and again at 24-60 months. However, it can occur as long as 30 years later. It is often related to traumatic injuries, such as preirradiation extraction (4.4%), postirradiation extraction (5.8%), and denture trauma

(<1%). ORN may occur spontaneously (albeit rarely) due to progression of periapical or periodontal disease.

28. What is the difference in incidence between maxilla ORN and mandible ORN?

ORN is more common in the mandible than in the maxilla because of the lesser blood supply to the mandible and the compact bone structure of the mandibular bone. Another possible explanation is that the mandible is involved in the field of irradiation more often than the maxilla is in most oral cancers.

29. What is the effect of the anatomic site of the tumor on ORN incidence?

Oral cancers have the highest incidence of ORN, especially those of the tongue, retromolar region, and floor of the mouth. This is likely from the direct involvement of the mandible in the radiation field and the aggressive and radical surgical approach for resection of these tumors.

30. What is the effect of neck lymph node metastasis on the incidence of ORN?

There is no difference in incidence of ORN when the neck is N_1, N_2, or N_3. However, there is a significantly higher incidence of ORN when the neck is N_0. This paradoxical effect is probably because patients with N_0 tumors have a better prognosis and live longer than patients with cervical involvement and therefore are at higher risk to develop ORN later in life.

31. How does tumor size affect the incidence of ORN?

No difference in ORN incidence has been reported when the tumor size increases from T_1-T_3. However, there is a significant increase in incidence of ORN when the tumor size is T_4. This increase is likely caused by bone invasion and the patient being subjected to both surgery and radiation therapy.

32. Does the mode of radiation delivery affect ORN incidence?

There is positive correlation between increased risk of ORN and mode of irradiation. The majority of patients who develop ORN are radiated with an external beam source. This difference may be related to the fact that fewer patients are treated with implants or with external beam source plus an implant source.

33. What is the effect of total radiation dose on the incidence of ORN?

The incidence of ORN is uncommon when the total radiation dose is below 5000 cGy. When the total external radiation dose is between 6000 cGy and 7000 cGy, ORN occurs more frequently. When the total dose is above 7500 cGy, ORN is almost 10 times higher than for doses <5000 cGy. Dose of radiation is probably the most important factor affecting incidence of ORN of the jaws.

34. What is the pathophysiology of ORN?

There are two general hypotheses regarding the pathophysiology of ORN: the "older concept" put forward by Watson and Scarborough (1938) and Meyer (1970), and a more recent hypothesis by Marx (1983). For a long time it was believed that ORN developed after a triad of radiation therapy, local trauma, and infection of the irradiated bone. Watson and Scarborough and Meyer speculated the sequence of events leading to ORN to be radiation, trauma, and infection leading to radiation osteomyelitis.

The "new concept" of pathophysiology of ORN is based on findings of several studies that showed that ORN can occur without trauma or suppuration and that microorganisms are found with ORN in only rare instances, compared with the usual presence of deep organisms in osteomyelitis. Marx's theory holds that ORN is a radiation-induced, wound-healing defect. According to this hypothesis, the pathophysiologic sequence is (1) irradiation, (2) hypovascular, hypoxic, and hypocellular tissue (the "three H's"), (3) tissue breakdown, and (4) a nonhealing wound in which the tissues' metabolic demand exceeds supply.

35. What is the histopathology of ORN?
The most common histopathologic features of ORN, which includes acute cellular damage, endarteritis, hyalinization, and vascular thrombosis, are evident soon after radiation exposure. Fewer osteocytes are seen, along with marrow fibrosis and sequestrum formation. These changes are considered subclinical for 6 months. Hypovascularity and fibrosis are evident 6-12 months after radiotherapy.

36. What are the clinical features of ORN?
- Exposed bone, loss of soft tissue and bone
- Pain and dysesthesia/anesthesia
- Pathologic fracture and orocutaneous fistula
- Soft tissue necrosis
- Trismus

37. What are the radiographic features of ORN?
- Diffuse radiolucency without sclerotic demarcation is seen.
- Mottled osteoporosis and sclerotic areas can be identified after bone sequestra are formed.
- Computed tomography (CT) and bone scintigraphy can be used to evaluate the extension and behavior of ORN.

38. What are the methods of management of ORN?
Depending on the stage of the disease, the management is based either on a conservative approach or on use of an HBO-surgical approach.

39. What is the conservative management of ORN?
ORN can be managed without the need for HBO or major surgical intervention. This approach consists of:
- Daily local irrigation (saline solution, $NaHCO_3$, or chlorhexidine 0.2%)
- Systemic antibiotics
- Avoidance of irritants (tobacco, alcohol, and denture use)
- Good oral hygiene instructions
- Gentle removal of sequestrum in sequestrating lesions

40. What is the HBO protocol?
HBO therapy is an administration of 100% oxygen via head tent, mask, or endotracheal tube within a special chamber at 2.4 atmospheric absolute (ATA) pressure for 90 min each session ("dives"). The treatment should be delivered five times a week, once a day.

41. What is the mechanism of action of HBO therapy?
HBO has been shown to help induce tissue healing by:
- Angiogenesis
- Inducing fibroplasia and neocellularity
- Promoting survival of osteoprogenitor cells
- Promoting the formation of functional periosteum

42. What are the indications for HBO therapy in OMFS?
- Prophylaxis to prevent ORN when surgical procedures in the irradiated field are indicated after completion of radiation treatment
- Treatment of ORN
- Before bony and soft tissue reconstruction and before placement of dental implants in irradiated bone

- Treatment of necrotizing fasciitis, gas gangrene, and chronic refractory osteomyelitis

43. What are the general principles of use of HBO therapy and surgery in management of ORN?

HBO therapy alone or in conjunction with surgery (depending on the stage of the disease) is often used to treat ORN of the mandible or maxilla using the following guidelines:

- HBO and surgery are indicated when the lesion is symptomatic and did not respond to conservative measures alone.
- HBO with or without surgery is indicated for treatment of ORN. According to the Marx–University of Miami protocol, depending on the extent of the disease, combined surgery and HBO treatment consists of three treatment stages of advanced clinical severity: stages I, II, and III.
- HBO is indicated when surgery to remove the sequestrum or bony reconstruction is planned.

44. What is stage I treatment of ORN?

All patients who meet the definition of ORN should begin stage I treatment and receive 30 treatments of HBO along with rigorous wound care. After 30 treatments, the wound is reevaluated for definitive improvement, decreased exposed bone, resorption, spontaneous sequestration, and softening of exposed bone. If the wound shows any of these signs, then the patient receives another 10 treatments for a full course of 40 treatments. If no improvement is seen after 30 HBO treatments, the patient is considered a nonresponder to stage I treatment and is advanced to stage II treatment.

45. What is stage II treatment of ORN?

A patient with a chronic, persistent (nonprogressive) form of ORN that persists after 30 treatments of HBO is considered nonrespondent to stage I and should advance to stage II treatment. This stage consists of intraoral surgical debridement (transoral alveolar sequestrectomy) of all necrotic bone to a bleeding bone with primary closure of the wound in a layered fashion. If healing progresses after surgery and the wound remains closed, 10 additional treatments of HBO are given. If no improvement is seen after the surgical debridement and the wound breaks down leaving larger areas of exposed bone, the patient is a nonresponder to stage II treatment and is advanced to stage III treatment protocol.

46. Who is a candidate for stage III treatment of ORN?

A patient with an exposed bone in the field of radiation with one or more of the following features should be considered a candidate for stage III treatment.

1. No response to stage II therapy
2. Patient who presents initially or after previous treatment of ORN with one of the following:
   - Pathologic fracture of the mandible
   - Orocutaneous fistula
   - Radiographic evidence of osteolysis of the inferior border of the mandible
   - Soft tissue dehiscence and continuous bony exposure despite treatment with stage II protocol

47. What is stage III treatment of ORN?

Patients who are candidates for stage III treatment should have had 30 treatments of HBO before surgical intervention. This is followed by transoral resection of the mandibular bone to bleeding bone. The remaining segments of the mandible are stabilized with either extraskeletal pin fixation or maxillomandibular fixation. This is followed by 10 additional postresection treatments of HBO. Later, bony reconstruction may be carried out if the patient is a suitable candidate.

48. What are the possible complications of HBO treatment?

- Barotrauma
- TMJ rupture

- Oxygen toxicity
- Ear and sinus trauma
- Central nervous system and pulmonary reactions and myopia

- Pneumothorax and air embolism
- Fire, transient visual problems, claustrophobia

49. What are the contraindications to use of HBO?

Absolute Contraindications:	Relative Contraindications:
Optic neuritis	Seizure disorder
Untreated pneumothorax	Claustrophobia
Congenital spherocytosis	Pregnancy
Fulminate viral infections	Emphysema

50. What is the HBO protocol for prophylactic use before oral surgical procedures in irradiated patients?

This protocol consists of once-daily treatment 5 days/week. The patient should receive 20 consecutive treatments before extraction or before any other oral surgical procedure within the field of radiation. Ten additional treatments should be administered postoperatively.

CONTROVERSIES

51. Should extractions be performed with the use of prophylactic HBO?

Pro: This approach is based primarily on the randomized, prospective study by Marx et al. of 137 patients that compared a conservative protocol with that of HBO plus surgery. This study was updated in 1991 to include 300 patients. According to this study, the incidence of ORN in the non-HBO group was 30%, compared with 5.4% in the HBO group. Calculation of cost of ORN treatment was found to far exceed the cost of prophylactic HBO. Accordingly, most authors argue that HBO is very cost effective.

Con: Authors against the use of prophylactic HBO for extractions argue that the incidence of loss of continuity of the mandible after mandibular extractions in irradiated mandible due to ORN is generally low (2.5%-4.5%). Considering that HBO is 80% effective in prevention of ORN, the rate of ORN with the use of HBO will be reduced to 0.5%-1.0%. Therefore, at best, HBO may preserve 2-3 mandibles while unnecessarily treating 97-98. Accordingly, these authors argue that HBO is not cost effective.

52. Should prophylactic HBO therapy be instituted before dental implants in the irradiated jawbone?

Pro: Animal and clinical studies showed improved soft tissue wound healing and decreased dehiscence after implants with HBO. These studies also showed improved torque removal forces of implants in irradiated bone with HBO and significantly greater quantity of bone-implant contact in irradiated rabbit tibias treated with HBO compared with implants placed without prior HBO treatment. Furthermore, some authors argue that the previously reported high success rate of dental implants in irradiated bone without prior HBO is explained by the low radiation dose used and the placement of implants outside the field of radiation.

Con: The argument against the placement of dental implants with HBO in irradiated patients is based on the high success rate of integration of implants in humans and improved integration of implants in the animal model without the use of HBO, especially if longer integration time is allowed. Accordingly, the potential benefit of HBO therapy balanced against its cost and potential complications does not justify its use in an irradiated mandible before placement of dental implants.

53. What is the protocol for HBO therapy when used before implant placement in the irradiated patient?

This protocol is advocated by some authors and consists of:

- Strict oral hygiene regimen before and after implant placement
- Use of the longest and widest implant type and the maximum number of implants possible
- Implant surgery delayed until 6 months after irradiation
- Thorough informed consent
- Cessation of smoking
- Preoperative HBO (increase integration time by 3 months)
- Overengineered implant-supported prosthesis
- A similar protocol for implants in irradiated maxilla and mandible
- Previously integrated implants should be buried before irradiation and subjected to 20 HBO treatments before uncovering.

54. What is bisphosphonate-related osteonecrosis (BRON) of the jaw?

This is a condition of painful exposure of bone in the mandible and maxilla of patients receiving bisphosphonate pamidronate.

55. What are the most commonly used bisphosphonates that cause this condition?

Most studies have shown that the largest number of patients reported to have BRON are those receiving pamidronate intravenously (Aredia [Novartis Pharmaceuticals, East Hanover, NJ]) and those receiving zoledronate (Zometa [Novartis]), and the fewest are those receiving alendronate (Fosamax; Merck, West Point, Pa).

56. What other factors are comorbidities of BRON of the jaw?

According to one study, the mandible was affected 68% of the time, the maxilla was affected 27.7% of the time, and both the maxilla and the mandible were affected simultaneously 4.2% of the time. The presentation is painful exposed bone approximately 70% of the time and painless exposed bone 31% of the time. The mean duration of time during which patients took the medications was 14.3 months, with a range of 9.4 months–3 years. Approximately 27% of the patients were smokers. Other comorbidities include periodontal disease and carious lesions of the teeth.

57. What are the indications for bisphosphonate use?

Bisphosphonates are commonly used by millions of postmenopausal women to stabilize bone loss caused by osteoporosis. It acts by inhibiting resorption by osteoclasts. The more potent form of the drug is delivered intravenously to stabilize metastatic cancer (mainly breast and prostate cancer) in bone and treat multiple myeloma and severe hypercalcemia.

58. What is the treatment for BRON?

When exposed bone in the jaw is identified in patients receiving bisphosphonates, the patient should be referred to an oral and maxillofacial surgeon who can inform him or her of the nature of the problem and coordinate treatment with the oncologist. No attempt should be made to debride or recontour the bone or to cover the exposed bone with flap. HBO treatment is of no benefit. Discontinuation of medications should be done only by the oncologist and, in fact, it has no immediate impact on the disease process. Therefore the treatment should be conservative and directed toward elimination or control of the pain and prevention of progression of the disease. If the exposed bone is secondarily infected, then long-term antibiotics such as penicillin V-K, 500 mg four times a day, and 0.12% chlorhexidine (Peridex; Proctor and Gamble, Cincinnati, Ohio) are recommended. Prevention of the disease is more effective and consists of 0.12% chlorhexidine, dental cleaning, and fluoride carriers. Extraction should be avoided at all costs in patients receiving or who have received bisphosphonates. In these patients, root canal treatment and tooth amputation should be considered as an alternative to extraction.

BIBLIOGRAPHY

1. Chapman L: Management of dental extractions in irradiated jaws: a protocol without hyperbaric oxygen therapy. J Oral Maxillofac Surg 55:275-281, 1997.
2. Curi MM, Laura L: Osteoradionecrosis of the jaws: a retrospective study of the background factors and treatment in 104 cases. J Oral Maxillofac Surg 55:540-544, 1997.
3. Epstein J, Meij VD, McKenzie M et al: Postradiation osteonecrosis of the mandible. A long-term follow-up study. Oral Surg Oral Med Oral Pathol Oral Radiol Endod 83:657-662, 1997.
4. Johnson R, Marx RE, Buckley SB: Hyperbaric oxygen. In Worthington P, Evans JR (eds): Controversies in Oral and Maxillofacial Surgery. Philadelphia, 1994, Saunders.
5. Keller EE: Placement of dental implants in the irradiated mandible: a protocol without adjunctive hyperbaric oxygen. J Oral Maxillofac Surg 55:972-980, 1997.
6. Lambert PM, Intrieve N, Eichstaedt R: Management of dental extractions in irradiated jaws: a protocol with hyperbaric oxygen. J Oral Maxillofac Surg 55:268-274, 1997.
7. Larsen PE: Placement of dental implants in the irradiated mandible: a protocol involving adjunctive hyperbaric oxygen. J Oral Maxillofac Surg 55:967-971, 1997.
8. Marx RE: A new concept in the treatment of osteoradionecrosis. J Oral Maxillofac Surg 41:351-357, 1983.
9. Marx RE, Johnson RP, Kline SN: Prevention of osteoradionecrosis: a randomized prospective clinical trial of hyperbaric oxygen versus penicillin. J Am Dent Assoc 111:49-54, 1985.
10. Marx RE, Sawatuari Y, Fortin M et al: Bisphosphonate-induced exposed bone (osteonecrosis/osteopetrosis) of the jaws: risk factors, recognition, prevention and treatment. J Oral Maxillofac Surg 63:1567-1575, 2005
11. Meyer I: Infectious diseases of the jaws. J Oral Surg 28:17-26, 1970.
12. Parker SL, Tong T, Bolden S et al: Cancer statistics, 1996. CA Cancer J Clin 46:5-27, 1996.
13. Rosenberg SW, Arm RN: Management of patient receiving antineoplastic and radiation therapy. In: Clinician's Guide to Treatment of Common Oral Conditions, 4th ed. Baltimore, 1997, American Academy of Oral Medicine.
14. Ruggerio SL, Mehrotra B, Rosenberg TJ et al: Osteonecrosis of the jaw associated with the use of bisphosphonates: a review of 63 cases. J Oral Maxillofac Surg 62:527-534, 2004.
15. Wang JK, Wood RE, McLean M: Conservative management of osteoradionecrosis. Oral Surg Oral Med Oral Pathol Oral Radiol Endod 84:16-21, 1997.
16. Watson WL, Scarborough JE: Osteoradionecrosis in intraoral cancer. Am J Roentgenol 40:524-534, 1938.

45. ORAL AND MAXILLOFACIAL RECONSTRUCTION

Vincent J. Perciaccante, DDS, and Jeffrey S. Jelic, DMD, MD

1. What is an autograft? An allograft? A xenograft?

An *autograft* is transplanted from one region to another in the same individual. An *allograft* is a transplant from one individual to a genetically nonidentical individual of the same species. A *xenograft* is a transplant from one species to another.

2. What do the terms *osteoinduction, osteoconduction,* and *osteogenesis* mean?

Osteoinduction refers to new bone formation from the differentiation of osteoprogenitor cells, derived from primitive mesenchymal cells, into secretory *osteoblasts*. This differentiation is under the influence of bone inductive proteins or bone morphogenic proteins (BMPs)—agents from bone matrix. *Osteoinduction* implies that the pluripotential precursor cells of the host will be stimulated or induced to differentiate into osteoblasts by transplanted growth factors and cytokines. Such grafts help produce the cells that are necessary to produce new bone.

Osteoconduction is the formation of new bone from host-derived or transplanted osteoprogenitor cells along a biologic or alloplastic framework, such as along the fibrin clot in tooth extraction or along a hydroxyapatite block. Osteoconductive grafts provide only a passive framework or *scaffolding*. These grafts are biochemically inert in their effect on the host. The grafted material therefore does not have the ability to actually produce bone. This type of graft simply conducts bone-forming cells from the host bed into and around the scaffolding.

Osteogenesis is the formation of new bone from osteoprogenitor cells. *Spontaneous osteogenesis* is the formation of new bone from osteoprogenitor cells in a wound. *Transplanted osteogenesis* is formation of new bone from osteoprogenitor cells placed into the wound from a distant site. Osteogenic grafts include the advantages of osteoinductive and osteoconductive grafts, in addition to the advantage of transplanting fully differentiated osteocompetent cells that will immediately produce new bone. Autogenous bone is the only graft that possesses all these properties.

3.   What is bone morphogenic protein (BMP)?

BMP is a protein complex responsible for initiating osteoinduction. BMP is part of the cytokine family of growth factors, which occurs in the organic portion of bone called the bone matrix. BMP is osteoinductive: It acts on progenitor cells to induce differentiation into osteoblasts and chondroblasts. The target of BMP is the undifferentiated perivascular mesenchymal cell. BMP may be the main signal regulating skeletal formation and repair; is known to induce bone formation de novo, following the same pathways as endochondral ossification; and is responsible for ectopic bone formation by certain tumor cells, epithelial cells, and demineralized bone.

BMPs appear to be stored within bone matrix and released with resorptive activity. This is why cortical bone, which carries the largest proportion of the total bone matrix, is mixed with cancellous bone to elevate the concentration of BMP in the graft. Recombinant technology has now made purified BMP readily available as a commercial product. As many as 14 BMPs have been identified. Two in particular, rBMP-2 and rBMP-7 (also called osteogenic protein or OP-1), are particularly efficacious and may induce bone formation even without an autogenous bone carrier graft.

4.   What other growth factors and cytokines are present in bone matrix?

Transforming growth factor-beta (TGF-β), insulin-like growth factor (IGF), interleukins (IL-1, IL-6), platelet-derived growth factor (PDGF), colony-stimulating factors (CSFs), heparin-binding growth factors (HBGFs), tumor necrosis factor-alpha (TNF-α), prostaglandins (PGs), and leukotrienes.

5.   Which contains more BMP: cortical or cancellous bone?

Demineralized cortical bone has been shown to contain more BMP than demineralized cancellous bone.

6.   What is platelet-rich plasma?

Platelet-rich plasma is an autologous source of PDGF and TGF-β1 and TGF-β2. These factors have been shown to increase bone graft maturation rates and bone density. The platelet-poor plasma byproduct produced in the process can be used for fibrin glue, which can be placed in the donor site, such as the ilium, obviating the need for the use of products such as Avitene. Fibrin glue also can be used to help mold the particulate bone and cancellous marrow (PBCM) bone graft at the recipient site.

7.   What are the steps in bone induction?

The steps during bone induction mimic the steps of endochondral bone formation:

1. Chemotaxis of mesenchymal progenitor cells to the area

2. Synthesis of type III collagen
3. Differentiation of chondroblasts
4. Conversion of connective tissue into cartilage (type II collagen)
5. Invasion by capillaries
6. Calcification
7. Synthesis of type IV collagen
8. Synthesis of type I collagen
9. Ossification

8.   What is creeping substitution?
Creeping substitution describes the process by which a wave of osteoclasts, and subsequently a wave of osteoblasts, systematically remove nonviable bone and then replace it with viable bone.

9.   Where are osteoprogenitor cells found?
Osteoprogenitor cells are found within bone marrow, endosteum, and the cambium layer of periosteum.

10.   What is the prevalence of mesenchymal stem cells in the bone marrow of an adult?
At birth, prevalence is 1 in 10,000 marrow cells. The prevalence diminishes with age, and by teenage years it drops tenfold to 1 in 100,000. At age 35, the prevalence of mesenchymal stem cells is 1 in 250,000 marrow cells. Later in life, it continues to diminish to 1 in 400,000 at age 50 and 1 in 2,000,000 by age 80.

11.   What is the piezoelectric effect? How does it affect grafted bone?
It is phenomena that explains Wolff's law, which states that form follows function. In 1957, Fukada and Yasuda discovered that when a bone is deformed by mechanical stress, an electric charge is generated. Bone deposition occurs in areas of **electronegativity,** whereas bone resorption is associated with **electropositivity.** The separation of charge is attributed to the piezoelectric effect. Clinically, when a bone is flexed, concave surfaces undergo compression and become electronegative, and bone is deposited onto them. In contrast, convex surfaces are placed under tension and become electropositive, and bone is resorbed from these surfaces. The piezoelectric effect transforms the weak, chaotic architecture of grafted bone into an organized tissue capable of withstanding functional loads.

12.   What are the advantages and disadvantages of *cancellous* bone grafts?
Advantages are mostly based on its rich cellular capability: (1) Cancellous bone grafts provide an immediate reserve population of viable bone-forming cells, as well as a population of progenitor cells that are capable of differentiating into osteoblasts; (2) the porous microstructure of cancellous grafts allows ingrowth of endothelial buds and provides a large surface area for osteoblastic/osteoclastic activity. The result is an immediate increase in graft density and rapid graft incorporation. These qualities also make the graft more resistant to infection and sequestration if soft tissue coverage is compromised.
Disadvantages arise from the fact that cancellous bone grafts do not possess any macroscopic structural integrity. Thus the graft cannot be rigidly fixed and will deform, migrate, or resorb if placed under tension or compressive functional forces.

13.   What are the advantages and disadvantages of *cortical* bone grafts?
Advantages of the cortical graft are due to its structural capabilities: (1) Its rigid lamellar architecture does not deform with compression or tension, allowing rigid fixation of the graft and its use in load-bearing or structural applications; (2) cortical bone also has a higher concentration of BMP, and cortical chips incorporated into cancellous bone grafts enhance osteoinductive potential of the graft.

Disadvantages are also due to the lamellar architecture: (1) Cortical bone does not carry a large population of osteocompetent cells, and the tenuous haversian system does not allow diffusion of nutrients to maintain the few viable osteoblasts or osteoprogenitor cells that are transplanted; (2) lamellar bone provides little surface area for remodeling activity, so that graft density initially decreases, and the graft weakens as osteoclasts begin a very slow process of incorporation; (3) lamellar bone makes the graft more susceptible to infection and complete graft loss if soft tissue cover is compromised.

14. **What do the terms *phase I* and *phase II* refer to when describing physiology of bone graft healing?**

Axhausen proposed the two-phase theory of osteogenesis. During **phase I,** bone is formed from cells that have been transplanted with the graft. These cells often have survived transplantation, proliferated, and formed new osteoid. This phase is most active within 4 weeks of transplanting the graft and is responsible for immediate increase in graft radiopacity. However, phase I bone is randomly oriented and easily resorbed.

Phase II involves bone production from cells in the recipient bed of the host. Phase II bone is formed either by the osteoblasts existing in host bone or by recipient bed progenitor cells that have been induced to become osteoblasts. This phase also involves resorption and remodeling of the immature bone that was produced in phase I into mature lamellar bone. Phase II bone production begins at about 2 weeks and peaks around 6 weeks, but the remodeling process continues indefinitely.

Phase I determines the *quantity* of bone that the graft will form. During phase II, reorganization of bone from phase I into *quality* lamellar bone occurs. Although phase II bone healing does not contribute to the total volume of bone produced by the graft, if phase II bone is not produced, the phase I bone will resorb.

15. **How does a surgeon determine how much bone will be adequate to reconstruct a particular bony defect?**

In general, for most oral and maxillofacial defects, 10 cc of noncompacted corticocancellous bone is required for every 1 cm of linear defect to be reconstructed.

16. **What are the different sources of autogenous bone? How much bone can be harvested from each?**

The **anterior iliac crest** can be used to harvest a maximum of 25-50 cc of PBCM or a corticocancellous block of 2×6 cm.

The **posterior iliac crest** can provide up to 75-100 cc corticocancellous bone, or a 5×5 cm block (2-2.5 times the bone harvested from the anterior ilium can be harvested from the posterior ilium on the same individual).

The **proximal tibial metaphysis** can provide 25 cc of cancellous bone, but such bone is generally of low quality because of the fatty marrow at this site.

The **rib** can provide 12-18 cm length bone segment (with up to 1 cm cartilage cap). This bone is generally more useful for condylar reconstruction and for orbital or zygomatic onlay grafting. The rib can also be used as a carrier for corticocancellous bone harvested from other sites.

The **calvarium** can offer a larger amount (5-6 strips of 3×1 cm) of bone from the parietal site, although it is also mostly cortical bone type.

Intraoral sites to obtain bone graft have also been used and include the mandibular symphysis, external oblique ridge, and maxillary tuberosity. The mandibular symphysis offers ease of harvesting, but only 10 cc or less of mostly cortical bone can be obtained. The external oblique ridge also provides mostly cortical bone and of limited amount.

Note that graft volumes and dimensions reported in the literature vary widely with factors such as patient age, gender, and body habitus, as well as the degree of graft compaction.

17. Should maxillofacial defects from cancer ablative surgery be reconstructed immediately, or is delayed reconstruction preferred?

Generally, these defects should be reconstructed *immediately* or *as soon as possible*, preferably within the first year after resection. Early reconstruction limits scar contracture, facial deformity, and oral dysfunction and has been demonstrated to promote the fastest and most uneventful return to a normal lifestyle. Most recurrences and second primary tumors begin at the defect site as mucosal lesions, and radiographs are as efficacious as clinical exam for identifying these lesions. For this reason, recurrence is more frequently identified—and earlier—in reconstructed patients. Additionally, salvage surgery and radiation treatments are just as effective in reconstructed as in unreconstructed defects.

Some authors advocate a *3- to 5-year waiting period* before reconstruction because reconstruction would mask recurrence and inhibit tumor surveillance, and the reconstruction would be lost due to the resection. Such masking and inhibition is especially problematic in cases of malignant lesions or tumors that have a high incidence of recurrence. These lesions often can grow substantially within the inherent space in this region before symptoms become apparent and the recurrence is detected. For this reason, standard postoperative waiting periods for tumor control may be prolonged before undertaking maxillary reconstruction to ensure a tumor-free state.

18. What are the criteria for a successful mandibular bone reconstruction?

The ultimate goal for any reconstruction procedure is to achieve restoration of the reconstructed organ and functional rehabilitation of the patient. In regard to reconstruction of the mandible, success is:

- **Restoration of mandibular continuity,** to allow greatest restoration of oral functions, aesthetics, and mechanical advantage, and to provide normal contours/appearance and foundation for future restoration
- **Restoration of alveolar bone height,** to allow placement of a denture or other prosthetic rehabilitation devices
- **Restoration of osseous bulk,** to allow an adequate volume of tissue to achieve a strong prosthetic base and to prevent fracture and failure under function
- **Maintenance of osseous content for at least 18 months.** Grafts, which are stable after 18 months, usually remain functional. Late graft resorption, which occurs between 6 and 18 months, is directly related to diminished vascularity of recipient soft tissue bed (phase II contribution) or diminished graft cellularity. It is likely to be unrelated to rigid fixation or degree of function.
- **Restoration of acceptable facial form,** which is necessary to the patient's self-image and allows a return to normal social activities
- **Acceptability of endosseous implants.** The successful bone graft accommodates placement of a dental implant and therefore the gamut of restorative dental techniques.
- **Recoverable, nondebilitating donor site surgery.** Even with achieving the other six goals, if the patient sustains permanent donor site morbidity, the reconstruction cannot be considered a completely successful procedure.

19. What are the major considerations in repair of large mandibular defects?

Soft tissue coverage, amount of bone replacement, stabilization of the graft, and future occlusal rehabilitation.

20. What can be used to hold PBCM grafts in place during mandibular reconstruction?

Several materials have been used to contain PBCM grafts at the recipient site. These include alloplasts such as titanium mesh, stainless steel, Teflon, and Dacron-urethane trays. Allogenic bone cribs such as rib, ilium, and mandible also have been used because they are better tolerated by thin or irradiated tissue and are bioresorbable. The recent availability of fibrin glue as a byproduct of plasma-rich platelets has allowed the use of a reconstruction plate as another modality for holding PBCM in place during mandibular reconstruction.

21. Is the following statement true or false? The most difficult defect of the mandible to reconstruct is one that crosses the midline.

True. The reason for this difficulty is due to the need in this area for hard tissue support of the chin's soft tissue as well as suspension of the extrinsic tongue musculature.

22. What is the protocol for preparing the recipient bed for mandibular reconstruction in a previously irradiated site?

Irradiated tissues are hypovascular, hypocellular, and hypoxic. Patients who have received more than 5000 cGy of radiation to the tissue bed before mandibular reconstruction often require a **qualitative improvement** to this tissue. If the tissue bed is sufficient quantitatively, consider hyperbaric oxygen (HBO) therapy. The protocol consists of 30 preoperative HBO dives at 2.4 atmospheres for 90 min and 10 postoperative HBO dives at 2.4 atmospheres for 90 min. If the tissue is lacking in quantity, use a myocutaneous flap or free microvascular flap to provide tissue bulk.

23. What are the boundaries of the compartment that is harvested in anterior iliac crest bone graft?

The iliac crest has two thick segments, which are suitable for corticocancellous bone harvesting. The anterior and posterior sites are separated by an intervening marrowless segment approximating the sacroiliac joint. The anterior third of the iliac crest contains a marrow compartment, which begins 1 cm behind the anterior superior iliac spine (ASIS). In adults, the anterior ilium at this location averages 1.3 cm in thickness. The tubercle is located approximately 6 cm posterior to the ASIS. The tubercle is the thickest portion of the crest and averages 1.7 cm in the average adult. The posterior boundary of the anterior marrow compartment is actually located 1-2 cm posterior to the tubercle. The marrow space of the anterior ilium only extends 2 cm inferior to the iliac crest. A maximum of 25 cc of compacted corticocancellous bone can be safely harvested from the anterior hip of the average adult.

24. What is the surgical approach to harvesting bone graft from the anterior iliac crest?

Place a sand bag under the sacral spine to display the landmarks of the iliac crest and allow surgical access. A second sandbag is recommended under the shoulder to prevent overrotation of the spine. Palpate and mark the ASIS. Identify and mark the tubercle 5-6 cm posterior to the ASIS. Before actually marking the incision line (and at the time of incision), the assistant should press on the skin just above the iliac crest to roll this skin superiorly. In this manner, the postoperative scar will be located below the crest and below the belt line.

Start the skin incision at least 1 cm posterior to the ASIS to prevent damage to the lateral femoral cutaneous nerve, which provides sensation to the lateral thigh. The incision will parallel the iliac crest for approximately 5 cm. It should not extend more than 2 cm beyond the tubercle, to limit the possibility of damaging the lateral cutaneous branch of the iliohypogastric nerve.

Incise the periosteum within the white line that represents the approximation of abdominal wall muscles and gluteal muscles. After reflection of the periosteum and overlying musculature from the medial side of the ilium, use an osteotome or a saw to harvest the medial cortex of 3-5 mm of cancellous bone, with the appropriate dimensions desired for reconstruction. It is often possible to harvest additional cancellous bone after removal of the medial cortex. Achieve adequate hemostasis before closure of the wound. Close the wound in layers, and apply pressure dressing with or without suction drain.

25. What is the best storage media to maintain harvested bone cell viability?

The ideal storage medium for a bone graft is tissue culture media. The solution is balanced and buffered to a pH of 7.42 and contains essential organic and inorganic cell nutrients. In studies comparing bone cell turnover, tissue culture media has shown a significant increase over saline. However, saline is currently the most commonly used storage medium for bone grafting today, because it is inexpensive and still has graft cell viability of 95% at 4 hr. The disadvantage of saline is that it causes washing of the harvest bone and therefore loss of growth factor after several hours of immersion. This loss may lead to a decrease in overall graft ossicle size.

Note that antibiotics and blood are cytotoxic, and sterile water is hypotonic and has the potential to lyse cells.

26. What are the advantages and disadvantages of the posterior ilium approach over the anterior ilium for autogenous bone harvest in major jaw reconstruction?

The **advantages** of the posterior ilium approach include the ability to harvest more bone; fewer complications, including less postoperative pain; and less disturbance in ambulating, with possible reduction in postoperative hospitalization. These differences from the anterior ilium approach are mostly related to differences in soft tissue and osseous anatomy.

Disadvantages of the posterior approach include increased operating time and increased hazards in moving the patient during anesthesia.

27. What are the possible complications to the donor site associated with harvest of anterior iliac crest bone graft?

Possible complications can be acute or chronic, and major or minor. **Acute major complications** include superior gluteal artery or sciatic nerve injury, pain, infection, ileus, herniation at the donor site, seroma, hematoma, pelvic fracture, and perforation of the peritoneum. **Chronic major complications** include long-term, disabling pain; paresthesia and anesthesia of the skin of the lateral thigh and/or lateral hip and buttocks; gait disturbances; hernia; hip click; and scar at the incision site. Minor complications include transient nerve injury, superficial wound infection, minor drainage, and temporary dysthesia.

28. What are the possible complications associated with harvest of posterior iliac crest bone graft?

Nerve injury is possible, including dysesthesias and paresthesias of the buttocks due to injury to the superior and middle clunial nerves, which are cutaneous sensory nerves. The superior nerve passes over the superior portion of the crest and travels inferiorly to supply sensation over the posterior buttocks. The middle nerve emerges medially through foramina in the sacrum and travels laterally to supply sensation to the medial buttocks.

Hemorrhage may occur due to transsection of the superior gluteal artery and may require a laparotomy to prevent exsanguinations.

Dislodging of the endotracheal tube can occur during repositioning from prone to supine position, but can be prevented with careful repositioning.

Loss of lower extremity motor functions, though rare, may occur due to injury to the motor enervation to the lower extremity by the sciatic nerve. The sciatic notch and sciatic nerve are 6-8 cm inferior to the posterior iliac crest.

Fractures of the pelvis also are rare complications when proper technique is followed.

29. Which nerves are most commonly injured in the anterior ilium bone harvest approach?

The incision can affect two peripheral sensory nerves: the **lateral cutaneous of the subcostal nerve** (T12) and the **lateral cutaneous branch of the iliohypogastric nerve** (L1). Both nerves cross the anterior iliac crest from medial to lateral between the tubercle and the anterior iliac spine. Both nerves provide sensory innervation to the skin overlying the gluteus medius and gluteus minimus muscles. Transection or retraction injury to these nerves may result in anesthesia or paresthesia in this area.

The lateral femoral cutaneous nerve of the thigh (L2 and L3) runs approximately 1 cm below the anterior iliac spine and courses on the medial aspect of the ilium and iliacus and almost always below the inguinal ligament; thus it is protected from surgical injury. However, perforation of the muscle may injure this nerve, causing similar symptoms to the skin over the upper and middle thigh below the level of the acetabulum.

30. What is the average incidence of neurosensory deficit following anterior ilium harvest?
In a study by Marx and Morales, 19 of 50 patients had an average neurosensory deficit of 45 cm^2.

31. What is the incidence of neurosensory deficit following posterior ilium harvest?
Marx and Morales found that 10 of 50 patients had an average neurosensory deficit of 16 cm^2. The superior cluneal nerves (L1, L2, L3) and the middle cluneal nerves (S1, S2, S3) are involved. An oblique incision parallel to the course of the superior cluneal nerves may affect them less frequently or to a lesser degree.

32. What are the seven anatomic structures that attach to the anterior iliac crest?
The fasciae latae, inguinal ligament, tensor fasciae latae, sartorius, iliacus, and the internal and external abdominal oblique muscles attach to the anterior iliac crest.

33. What are the surgical options for total temporomandibular joint (TMJ) replacement?
- Alloplastic fossa and condyle (custom design and stock design)
- Free vascularized (fibula, ileum, second metatarsophalangeal joint, and scapula)
- Autogenous (costochondral, clavicle, ileum)
- Allogeneic cadaveric/ banked bone

34. What are the *indications* for alloplastic reconstruction of the TMJ?
- Ankylosis or reankylosis with severe anatomic abnormalities
- Failed autogenous graft
- Failed previous alloplastic reconstruction
- Resorption of autograft by foreign body reaction (e.g., Proplast-Teflon)
- Severe inflammatory joint disease
- Patient with multiple previous operations and compromised vascular bed

35. What are the *contraindications* for TMJ reconstruction with an alloplastic prosthesis?
- Young age, because of the limited longevity of the prosthesis and the potential need for a second surgery, and because of skeletal immaturity and lack of growth potential
- Compromised immune system, because such nonvascularized grafts may increase the risk for infection
- Presence of an active infection (acute or chronic)
- Allergy to the materials used for manufacturing of the prosthesis

36. What are the *advantages* of alloplastic TMJ reconstruction?
- There is no need for maxillary-mandibular fixation or mandibular immobilization.
- Physical therapy can begin immediately.
- There is no donor site morbidity.
- Surgery time is decreased.
- An alloplastic prothesis can be easily designed to accommodate irregular anatomy (e.g., destructive lesions or growth asymmetries).
- It offers reliable/predictable control of occlusion and occlusal correction.
- It is resistant to autoimmune destruction.

37. What are the *disadvantages* of alloplastic TMJ reconstruction?
- Cost
- Mechanical longevity is less—intrinsic implant failure due to material fatigue.
- Biologic longevity is less—failure due to break down of tissue-implant interface (e.g., loose

screws or cements) or possible tissue reactions.
• The implant has no growth potential.

38. What length of cartilage should be harvested with a costochondral graft used for TMJ reconstruction?

To decrease the lever arm and risk for separation at the bone-cartilage interface, the length of the cartilage harvested should be minimized: 3-5 mm of cartilage is sufficient for TMJ reconstruction. Leaving a periosteal-perichondral sleeve helps reinforce this junction.

39. Which donor rib is the most preferable for costochondral graft reconstruction?

Because the sixth rib harvest lends itself to a cosmetic incision at the inframammary crease, and the dissection in this area can be carried out between the terminal extent of the pectoralis major and rectus abdominus muscles, the **right sixth rib** is the best rib for harvest. Harvesting from other ribs on the right side, although acceptable, may cause a more unaesthetic scar, and the dissection may increase the chances of hemorrhage, pain, and pneumothorax.

Note that when rib harvest is performed on the left side, it is important to differentiate postoperative pain from cardiogenic pain.

40. What are the possible donor site complications in rib harvest?

Complications associated with rib and costochondral graft harvest include pain, scar, paresthesia or anesthesia of the lateral chest wall, tear of the pleura leading to a pneumothorax, and atelectasis. The incidence of pneumothorax is higher when harvesting a costochondral graft than with rib harvest because of the relatively greater difficulty in reflecting the perichondrium off the cartilage compared with reflecting the periosteum off the bone when harvesting rib without cartilage. Most of the complications associated with rib and costochondral graft harvest are, however, transient and resolve within a few days to weeks. Also, in most instances of pleural perforation, it can be managed without the need for insertion of a chest tube.

41. What are the different flap classification methods?

There are many methods for classifying tissue used for reconstruction, but the most common are:

Tissue composition—cutaneous, muscle, fasciocutaneous, myocutaneous, osteocutaneous, and innervated (sensate) cutaneous

Source of blood supply—in *axial flaps* (also called direct), the blood supply is provided by a known vessel that runs within the base of the flap. The artery usually runs along the longitudinal axis of the flap, and perforators extend directly between the skin and this artery. In *random flaps* (also called indirect), a distributing artery gives rise to multiple unnamed perforating arteries. These multiple unnamed perforating arteries then enter the base of the flap in a random pattern. These unnamed perforators not only supply the tissue comprising the base of the flap but also contribute multiple, random, cutaneous perforators to the dermal plexus. Thus the blood supply to the skin takes an indirect route through a hierarchy of arterioles.

Method of transfer to donor site—*local* transfer occurs via advancement, rotation, and interpolation. *Distant* transfer occurs via direct, tube, free (i.e., split-thickness skin graft, iliac crest bone graft, cartilage), and free vascularized.

42. What are the most commonly used regional flaps for maxillofacial reconstruction?

Flaps that have proved to be predictable, single-stage soft tissue transfers, with known axial and random vascular patterns, are the **sternocleidomastoid flap, temporalis muscle, pectoralis major, trapezius, latissimus dorsi, and platysma flaps.** These have elevated maxillofacial soft tissue reconstruction to new level. Other less commonly used flaps include masseter muscle, deltopectoral, and forehead flaps. These can be used as isolated muscle flap or in combinations with other tissues such as the skin, fascia, or bone.

43. What are the major sources of blood supply to these flaps (Table 45-1)?

Table 45-1	*Blood Supply to the Flaps*
FLAP	DOMINANT BLOOD SUPPLY
Pectoralis major myocutaneous	Thoracoacromial artery
	Superior and lateral thoracic arteries contribute
Deltopectoral skin	Perforators from internal mammary artery
Temporalis muscle	Anterior and posterior deep temporal arteries
Platysma myocutaneous	Submental branch of facial artery
Trapezius myocutaneous	Transverse cervical artery
Latissimus dorsi myocutaneous	Thoracodorsal artery
Sternocleidomastoid myocutaneous	Branches of occipital and superior thyroid arteries

44. Which factors most affect aesthetics and function following reconstruction with local flaps?

Using the physical characteristics of tissue can lead to better functional and aesthetic results after reconstruction with local flaps. Such characteristics include integration of relaxed skin tension lines, taking into consideration the cosmetic units of the face, and better use of the physical properties of the skin.

45. What are pedicle flap failure and free flap failure?

Pedicle flap failure tends to show distal necrosis. This occurs when the design of the flap prevents the random cutaneous vascular supply from adequately perfusing the peripheral tissue, or because of external causes of vascular occlusion such as hematoma or compression. *Free flap failure* is classically described as an all-or-none survival pattern (although segments of distal necrosis are possible), mostly caused by intrinsic intraluminal vascular occlusion at the level of the anastomosis.

46. How can a flap be monitored postoperatively?

Although not always reliable, clinical observation of skin color, skin temperature, capillary refill, and dermal puncture bleeding are the most useful methods to monitor a flap in the postoperative period. Cool and pale tissue suggests arterial (inflow) problems. Venous (outflow) problems are characterized by a congested, bluish appearance, with brisk capillary refill and puncture bleeding. More advanced monitoring methods include intravenous injection of fluorescein dye, conventional or laser Doppler flowmetry, surface temperature probe, transcutaneous tissue oxygen tension, tissue pH, and radioactive tracer clearance.

47. Are there any measures that can prevent microvascular flaps from failing?

Emergent exploration of the anastomosis may be necessary to salvage free flaps (note that, overall, free flap survival is 95% or better). Unfortunately, close observation is often the only means of treatment available, because venous congestion is the most common intrinsic reason for failure of technically correct flaps (pedicle or free). Some surgical techniques and postoperative maneuvers, however, increase the chances for flap survival:

- Use noncrushing instruments when handling the flap, as well as noncompressive tissue manipulation and noncompressive dressings.
- Obtain absolute surgical hemostasis, and use drains to avoid hematomas and seromas.
- Prevent graft mobility by adequate suture anchorage and by immobilizing the donor site.

- Sutures should be tension-free and parallel to blood vessels. Promptly remove compromising sutures when necessary.
- Control the initial swelling phase with cooling compresses and liberal use of steroids.
- Use appropriate antibiotics.
- Avoid vasoactive drugs such as caffeine and nicotine.
- In appropriate circumstances, HBO therapy, topical nitroglycerine, lidocaine, papaverine, aspirin, dextrans, and surgical leaching are often used for salvage of free flaps.

48. What is the difference between random pattern flaps and axial pattern flaps?

Random pattern flaps consist of skin, subcutaneous tissues, and, possibly, muscle. The blood supply is from the dermal and subdermal plexuses. Axial pattern flaps derive their blood supply from dominant vessels within the flap that can be identified during the dissection.

49. What are the boundaries for the largest possible buccal mucosa grafts?

Buccal mucosa grafts can be harvested from the pterygomandibular raphe to the commissure, and then closed primarily without functional deficits. Grafts wider than 2 cm in a vertical dimension, however, may cause trismus.

50. What is the difference between full-thickness and split-thickness skin grafts?

Split-thickness skin grafts (STSGs) are 0.30-0.45 mm thick. The skin is sectioned below the papillary dermis so it will only contain the epidermis and a portion of the upper reticular dermis. Because the skin adnexa (hair follicles and associated sebaceous glands, eccrine and apocrine sweat glands) originate in the midreticular dermis or in the subcutaneous fat layer (hypodermis or panniculus adiposis), they are generally not included in STSGs.

In **full-thickness skin grafts** (FTSGs), the dermis is not split. The plane of cleavage is designed to separate the subcutaneous fat from the dermis. The actual thickness of an FTSG is extremely variable and depends on the location on the donor site and the sex, age, and health of the patient.

The eyelid and supraclavicular and postauricular skin are the thinnest on the body, whereas the palms, soles, and trunk are the thickest. Women have thinner skin. The dermis is very thin in children, increases until age 50, and then atrophies. Conditions such as malnutrition, chronic steroid therapy, and insulin-dependent diabetes mellitus also affect dermal thickness. Be aware of these variables when planning graft harvesting.

51. What are primary and secondary contractions?

Primary contraction refers to the immediate shrinkage of a harvested graft as it is cut free. This form of contraction is due to elastic fibers within the dermis. More dermis means more elastic fibers, so FTSGs have more primary contraction than STSGs. *Secondary contraction,* or wound contraction, is the more significant concern clinically. This type of contraction is caused by the myofibroblasts located in the donor site and is characteristic of the healing of all open wounds. Secondary contraction predominates during the first 2 weeks of healing but peaks at 8 days.

52. What percentage of contraction can be expected from STSGs and FTSGs?

Generally, the exact percentage of contraction of skin graft cannot be predicted simply on the basis of whether the skin graft is an FTSG or STSG. In relation to *primary contraction,* the proportion of the skin graft harvested, compared with the skin's total thickness, is important in determining the amount of primary wound contracture. If STSGs of identical thickness are harvested from various regions of the body, the grafts harvested from thick skin will contract more than those from thinner areas. Thus **the thickness of the graft relative to donor skin thickness** is the most important factor in determining primary wound contraction.

In *secondary contraction,* the thickness of a graft is not as important as **the percentage of the dermis being transplanted**. The larger the percentage of dermis that is grafted, the less secondary contraction can be expected. A wound covered with a three-quarter STSG may contract less than a wound covered with one-quarter STSG. A half-thickness STSG, if taken from an area with thin skin, may perform clinically more like an FTSG.

53. What are the advantages and disadvantages of STSGs?

Advantages: STSGs tolerate less vascularity than FTSGs and may survive in less than ideal conditions. Because blood vessels arborize as they ascend into the dermis, STSGs have a higher number of blood vessels on the undersurface of the graft. This higher potential for vascularity gives STSGs a large capacity to absorb nourishment from the underlying bed. In addition, nutrient fluids have shorter distances to diffuse, and thinner grafts have fewer cellular elements requiring nourishment. STSGs therefore can be applied to any vascular surface or any surface where healthy granulation tissue exists.

STSG donor sites heal spontaneously. Epithelial cells migrate from adnexal structures to reepithelialize the harvested site. In addition, if necessary, the same donor can be used to reharvest skin in the future. Also, meshing STSGs greatly increases the surface area that can be reepithelialized, and therefore a larger defect can be covered with a smaller graft.

Disadvantages: significant amount of contracture; inability of the graft site to accommodate growth well in children; abnormal pigmentation at both harvest and donor site; and poor mechanical strength.

54. What are the advantages and disadvantages of FTSGs?

Advantages: FTSGs are the ideal choice for epithelial coverage. They are much more resistant to contracture than STSGs, grow in children, have a texture and pigmentation that is more similar to normal skin, and are functionally more durable.

Disadvantages: Because of thickness and limited exposure of the microvasculature, it is difficult for simple diffusion to maintain cell viability throughout the graft. Therefore FTSGs can be placed only in very clean, highly vascular donor sites. For this reason, harvesting is limited to sites such as palpebral, postauricular, supraclavicular, and dorsal pedal skin. Because the donor site can only be harvested once and the graft cannot be meshed and expanded, FTSGs provide much more limited coverage.

Problems associated with intraoral use of FTSG intraskin grafts include possible hair growth, disagreeable color and odor, and a tendency to excessive keratinization when placed under a denture base.

55. What is STSG healing?

During the ischemic phase 0-48 hr postoperatively, the graft appears pale. During this phase, nutrition and excretion are by exudation and diffusion. During the period 24-72 hr postoperatively, the graft gains a pinkish tint as reanastomosis between tissue surface vessels of the graft and those of the host bed is established. At 3-6 days postoperatively, the graft becomes cherry red, with demonstrable capillary refill if neovascularization occurs. Endothelial buds grow into the graft from the host bed and reestablish the microcirculation.

Note that these phases may be longer in thicker grafts and/or may only occur in the deeper regions of thicker grafts, with the superficial layers sloughing off.

56. What are the most common causes of STSG failure?

- Inadequate recipient site (poor vascularity)
- Hematoma under the graft
- Graft mobility
- Infection
- Technical errors (e.g., placement over epithelium or necrotic tissue, placed upside down, cut too thick or too thin)
- Poor storage of graft

57. What changes occur in FTSGs placed in the oral cavity?

In general, no surface tissue changes occur after placement of FTSGs in the oral cavity. Mucosalization of a skin graft does not occur. There may be a thinning of the keratin layer, but transplanted skin maintains most of its original characteristics.

58. What are the disadvantages associated with intraoral use of mucosal and palatal tissue grafts?

Oral mucosa is certainly the preferred tissue for intraoral grafting, but it does present some difficulties. Disadvantages of buccal mucosa grafts are poor load-bearing qualities, technical difficulties in obtaining and handling thin grafts, and limited surface available for harvest.

Disadvantages of palatal mucosa are technical difficulty procuring split-thickness grafts of any size, limited availability, and rugated surface texture. Full-thickness palatal grafts are technically easier to obtain, but they have protracted, painful, and often unsatisfactory healing at the donor site.

59. What are the important aspects of lateral canthus reconstruction?

The goal of lateral canthus reconstruction is mobilization of the lateral canthal soft tissue complex, which includes mobilization of the ligament periosteum and orbicularis muscle. This soft tissue complex can be approached by a variety of incisions, including hemicoronal, lateral canthotomy, and brow, or via existing lacerations and/or incisions. The lateral canthus area is undermined subperiosteally until the complex can be elevated without resistance. The confluence of tissue then can be reattached to the lateral orbital rim by either plate or screw fixation through a hole secured with suture or wire, or to the periorbital tissue when the correction is for only a minor deformity. The canthopexy should be positioned superiorly approximately 3-4 mm above the medial canthal ligament. An inferior tilt of the lateral canthus usually is unaesthetic. This type of canthal deformity is called antimongolian and is often seen in certain craniofacial abnormalities, such as Treacher Collins syndrome, or in traumatic cases associated with residual, inferior, displaced zygomatic fractures.

Soft tissue revisions of the canthal region should be the final phase of posttraumatic orbital reconstruction. To optimize aesthetic results after reconstruction, it is important to develop revisions so that the bulk of the scar falls within the relaxed skin tension lines. This can be achieved by using fusiform excision, Z-plasty, W-plasty, and geometric excisions.

60. What is the pathophysiology of enophthalmos? How it is corrected?

Loss of bone and ligament support allows posterior displacement of the globe by gravity and scar contracture, leading to enophthalmos. Enophthalmos may also result from fat necrosis, tethering of orbital contents, and neurogenic conditions. Clinically, enophthalmos is not evident until at least a 4-mm change occurs in the position of the globe when measured in an anteroposterior plane from the lateral orbital rim to the zenith of the cornea.

Enophthalmic corrections involve accurate restoration of the shape and size of the bony orbit.

61. What are the different approaches to surgical access of the orbit?

For extensive reconstructive procedures involving the nasoethmoidal region, the **hemicoronal or coronal approach** has been used successfully. Incisions placed through scars from **previous incisions or lacerations** can also be used, although they may require some lengthening. Circumvestibular, subciliary, lower lid crease, transconjunctival, and inferior orbital rim incisions are used to approach the inferior orbital rim and orbital floor. However, the **inferior orbital rim approach** generally is avoided because it may leave some unfavorable scarring. The **circumvestibular incision** may be used with a facial degloving procedure, although with some difficulty. The **subciliary and inferior lid crease incisions** provide excellent access and favorable healing characteristics. The **transconjunctival incision** provides excellent cosmesis and superior lateral orbital rim exposure, especially when the lateral canthotomy incision is added. There is an increased risk of lid deformity (especially entropion) if the wound is not reapproximated properly. The lateral orbital rim is best approached through hemicoronal, brow, or **lateral canthotomy** approaches. Scarring from the **brow approach** can be minimized by keeping the incision beveled parallel to the hair follicles or making the incision above or below instead of within the brow, thereby avoiding the possibility of alopecia.

62. When performing a tongue flap, what determines whether it should be an anteriorly or posteriorly based flap?

The location of the defect determines where a tongue flap is based. For defects of the soft palate, retromolar region and posterior buccal mucosa, a posteriorly based flap is used. Anteriorly based flaps are used for hard palate defects, defects of the anterior buccal mucosa and anterior floor of the mouth or lips.

63. Which skin donor site for nasal defect grafting provides the best type and quality match of nasal skin?

The best donor site for grafting of small defects of the nose is the nose itself. When bilobe advancement flaps cannot be used, the next best site for color and texture match is the preauricular skin between the tragus and hair-bearing sideburns. The next most commonly desired site is the supraclavicular skin, followed by the posterior upper arm.

Denuded nasal cartilage may be perforated to increase blood supply to the skin graft of the nose. Larger lateral nose and alar defects are best matched with nasolabial flaps. Forehead flaps will supply enough skin to cover all nine nasal cosmetic units.

64. What is the blood supply to a paramedian forehead flap?

The axial blood supply to the paramedian forehead flap is by an arcade of vessels supplied by the supraorbital, supratrochlear, infratrochlear, dorsonasal, and angular branches of the facial artery.

65. When is a paramedian forehead flap divided?

The paramedian forehead flap can be divided as early as 2 weeks, but most advocate 3 weeks. Often a contouring procedure is done at this time by elevating the flap at an intermediate operation, creating a bipedicle flap that extends from the brow to the columellar inset. The flap can be defatted and thinned and repositioned on the nose with peripheral and quilting sutures. The pedicle is not transected. Three weeks later the pedicle can be divided.

66. Bilobed flaps are a good choice for what type of nasal defects?

Bilobed flaps are a good choice for nasal tip and alar defects.

67. What are the size and orientation for bilobed flaps?

The first lobe is equal to the size of the defect, and the diameter of the second lobe is decreased to facilitate closure. The total arc of a bilobed flap can be up to 100 degrees, with the maximum rotation of each lobe limited to 50 degrees.

68. What size of lip defect can be closed primarily?

Defects of approximately one third of the lower lip and one quarter of the upper lip can be closed primarily without resulting in a significant microstomia.

69. What are some flaps that can be used for lip reconstruction?

Some of the local flaps used for closure of lip defects include the Abbe flap, the Abbe-Estlander flap, and the Karapandzic flap.

70. What type of defect can be reconstructed with a nasolabial flap?
Defects of the upper and lower lips, commissure, buccal mucosa, and floor of mouth and nasal defects may be reconstructed with appropriate inferior or superior based nasolabial flaps.

71. What are some options for lower eyelid reconstruction?
- **Direct closure**—can be used in full-thickness defects of up to 30% of the lower eyelid in a young patient and up to 45% in an elderly patient.
- **Tenzel semicircular rotational flap**— can be used for defects of up to 60% of the lid.
- **Hughes tarsoconjunctival flap**—can be used for defects of more than 50% of the lower lid. This upper lid to lower lid sharing technique requires a secondary stage to separate the flap.
- **Mustardé cheek flap**—can be used for very large defects up to the entire lower lid.

72. What are some options for upper eyelid reconstruction?
- **Direct closure**—can be used in full-thickness defects of up to 33% of the lower eyelid in a young patient and up to 40% in an elderly patient.
- **Tenzel semicircular rotational flap**—can be used for defects of up to 60% of the lid.
- **Sliding tarsoconjunctival flap**—can be used on defects of the upper lid that are too large for direct closure by horizontally sliding a section of tarsus from the remaining lid to close the defect and placing a skin graft.
- **Cutler-Beard (bridge) flap**—can be used to repair full-thickness upper lid defects of more than 60% up to defects of the entire upper lid. This procedure requires a secondary stage and an inset ear cartilage graft to reconstruct the tarsus.

73. What are advantages of using stereolithographic models in mandibular tumor surgery?
Decreased surgical time, preoperative planning, and accuracy of plate contouring.

BIBLIOGRAPHY

1. Axhausen W: Die Knochenregeneration-ein zweiphasisches Geschehen. Zentralbl Chir 77:435-442, 1952.
2. Banwart JC, Asher MA, Hassanein RS: Iliac crest bone graft harvest donor site morbidity Spine 20:1055-1060, 1995.
3. Bardach J: Local flaps and free skin grafts in head and neck reconstruction. St Louis, 1992, Mosby.
4. Bloomquist DS, Turvey TA: Bone grafting in dentofacial deformities. In Bell WH (ed): Modern Practice in Orthognathic and Reconstructive Surgery. Philadelphia, 1992, Saunders.
5. Buchbinder D, St-Hilaire H: Tongue flaps in maxillofacial surgery. Oral Maxillofacial Surg Clin North Am 15:475-486, 2003.
6. Carlson ER: Regional flaps in oral and maxillofacial reconstruction. Oral Maxillofac Surg Clin North Am 5:667-685, 1993.
7. Carlson ER: Mandibular bone grafts: techniques, placement, and evaluation. OMFS Knowl Update 1:35, 1994.
8. Chen WP: Oculoplastic Surgery: The Essentials. New York, 2001, Thieme.
9. Cunningham LL, Madsen MJ, Peterson G: Stereolithographic modeling technology applied to tumor resection. J Oral Maxillofac Surg 63: 873-878, 2005.
10. Cutting CB, McCarthy JG, Knize DM: Repair and grafting of bone. In McCarthy JG (ed): Plastic Surgery. Philadelphia, 1990, Saunders.
11. Ferraro N, August M: Reconstruction following resection for maxillofacial tumors. Oral Maxillofac Clin North Am 5:355-383, 1993.
12. Gerard DA, Hudson JW: The Christensen Temporomandibular Prosthesis System: an overview. Oral Maxillofac Clin North Am 11:61-72, 2000.
13. Hall MB, Vallerand WP, Thompson D et al: Comparative anatomic study of anterior and posterior iliac crest as donor sites. J Oral Maxillofac Surg 49:560-569, 1991.
14. Haug RH, Buchbinder D: Incisions for access to craniomaxillofacial fractures. Oral Maxillofac Surg Clinic North Am 1:1-29, 1993.

15. Manson PN, Clifford CM, Su CT et al: Mechanisms of global support and posttraumatic enophthalmos: I. The anatomy of the ligament sling and its relation to intramuscular cone orbital fat. Plast Reconstr Surg 77:203-214, 1986.
16. Marx RE: Physiology and particulars of autogenous bone grafting. Oral Maxillofac Surg Clin North Am 5:599-613, 1993.
17. Marx RE, Morales MJ: Morbidity from bone harvest in major jaw reconstruction: a randomized trial comparing the lateral anterior and the posterior approaches to the ileum. J Oral Maxillofac Surg 48:196-203; 1988.
18. McCarthy JG, Lorenc ZP, Cutting C et al: The median forehead flap revisited: the blood supply. Plast Reconstr Surg 76:866-869, 1985.
19. McCord CD, Codner MA: Eyelid Surgery: Principles and Techniques. Philadelphia, 1995, Lippincott-Raven.
20. Mercuri LG: The TMJ concepts patient-fitted total temporomandibular joint reconstruction prosthesis. Oral Maxillofac Surg Clin North Am 1:73-91, 2000.
21. Rudolph R, Ballantyne DL: Skin grafts. In McCarthy JG (ed): Plastic Surgery. Philadelphia, 1990, Saunders.
22. Schmidt BL, Dierks EJ: The nasolabial flap. Oral Maxillofacial Surg Clin North Am 15 487-495, 2003.
23. Skouteris CA, Sotereanos GC: Donor site morbidity following harvesting of autogenous rib graft. J Oral Maxillofac Surg 47:808-812, 1989.
24. Zitelli JA: The bilobed flap for nasal reconstruction. Arch Dermatol 125:957-959, 1989.

46. FACIAL COSMETIC SURGERY

Vincent B. Ziccardi, DDS, MD

1. What considerations should soft tissue envelope assessment take into account in the planning of facial cosmetic surgery?

First and foremost is the overall health of the skin and the degree of actinic damage. Healing capacity will be adversely affected by highly damaged skin, which must be discussed with the patient preoperatively. Any lesions that are present should be evaluated, documented, and possibly biopsied before surgery. Other factors include the general elasticity and recoil quality of the skin. This is especially important when considering lower eyelid blepharoplasty and cervicofacial liposuction. The amount of subcutaneous tissue affects the overall aesthetic result of surgical rejuvenative procedures. Some patients may require soft tissue augmentation in the lips, cheeks, or natural folds. Finally, the facial animation of a patient during speech and laughter and while at rest should be assessed. In some cases, overactive mimetic muscles of facial expression may create wrinkles and folds that the patient finds objectionable. These may be considered for treatment with botulinum toxin type A injections.

2. What are the objectives of rhytidectomy?

Rhytidectomy ("face lift") removes the lax and redundant skin of the face and neck, including the prominent nasolabial folds, jowls, and submental region, that contribute to the aged appearance of the face. During the aging process, the elastic fibers of the dermis and the superficial musculoaponeurotic system (SMAS) layer begin to undergo degeneration and are replaced by fibrous connective tissue. The SMAS should be addressed during the face-lift operation to assist in the maintenance of this surgical procedure. Factors that contribute to the aging process include genetics, ultraviolet light damage, gravity, and tobacco use. As gravity causes the skin to sag, the lines of fascial attachment between the skin and mimetic muscles become accentuated. Most face-lift operations involve a skin-flap technique with some manipulation of the SMAS involving either plication or imbrication.

3. What are some potential complications of the rhytidectomy procedure?

Anticipated sequelae of rhytidectomy include swelling, discomfort, paresthesia, and ecchymosis. The clinically significant complications involve sloughing of the flap due to a compromised blood supply or facial nerve injury. Active smokers should not undergo face-lift operations due to compromised vascular supply. Hematoma formation, if it occurs, can also result in loss of the skin flap due to elevation of the skin off the vascular bed, which can be managed by pressure dressing, drain placement, achievement of surgical hemostasis, or evacuation of hematoma when clinically evident. Injury to the facial nerve is a significant complication that may be minimized by understanding the anatomy and identifying the SMAS surgical plane during dissection. Infection is another potentially significant complication that rarely occurs following use of prophylactic antibiotic coverage. Other potential complications may include unfavorable scarring and earlobe deformities due to placement of incision design and retraction upon healing.

4. What characteristics make the ideal surgical candidate for submental liposuction?

The ideal candidate for submental liposuction is a patient with distinct supraplatysmal fat deposits and skin with good recoil that allows for postoperative draping of the soft tissue envelope. Traditionally, patients older than age 40 have been excluded; however, it is better to make the assessment on an individual basis. Because the procedure is carried out through one or more small skin incisions, there is no excision of excess skin. Therefore a patient with excessively redundant skin or very poor recoil would have an unpredictable and less desirable outcome with nonuniform skin redraping. Ideally, the fat that is manually removed by the tumescent cannula technique is located in the supraplatysmal plane. Any fat located below the platysma muscle is best approached by an open approach under direct vision to avoid vascular injury or development of cobra neck deformity. The platysma muscle could be plicated at that point, if indicated, as well as part of a localized anterior neck lift procedure.

5. At what anatomic plane is submental liposuction safely performed?

Submental liposuction is performed at the supraplatysmal plane, a distinct layer of subcutaneous fatty tissue located below the dermis at which the procedure is safely performed in a near-bloodless field. The area treated from the submental incision is bounded by the anterior border of the sternocleidomastoid muscle, inferior border of the mandible, and superior border of the thyroid.

6. What is the tumescent technique, and what purpose does the tumescent fluid serve in liposuction?

The tumescent technique is a local anesthetic technique that allows submental liposuction to be readily and safely performed. The tumescent fluid is essentially a tenfold-diluted local anesthetic that provides for profound anesthesia and wound hemostasis during surgical manipulation. Using either a spinal needle or multiport injector, the tumescent fluid is injected into the appropriate surgical plane; 100 mL or more of tumescent fluid can be easily used in the submental region. After injection of the tumescent fluid, adequate time is allowed for the onset of anesthesia and analgesia, at which time the region may take on a blanched appearance. The liposuction cannulas are then inserted into this already established plane, which has been previously hydrodissected by the tumescent fluid.

7. By what mechanisms does submental liposuction achieve its results?

Submental liposuction achieves its results on several levels. First, there is the physical removal of fat from the supraplatysmal plane. The amount of fat removed varies depending on the patient and operator, but ranges between 5 and 25 mL on average. The creation of multiple tunnels radiating from the entry port creates a potential dead space that is then compressed with the postoperative pressure dressing. Additionally, scar contracture of the fatty tissue develops during healing. Most important, however, is the compression and redraping of the soft tissue envelope afforded by the pressure dressing. Patients must understand the importance of the pressure dressing. It is an absolute contraindication to perform the surgery if a patient will not be compliant with the postoperative management. The author's protocol includes 72 hr of continuous pressure dressing (except while bathing), followed by 4 weeks of wearing the dressing for 12 hr/day. Pressure garments are commercially available for this purpose; however, 3-inch-wide Ace bandages may be used alternatively.

8. What are some other surgical options available to improve the esthetics of the submental region?

A relatively significant improvement in the draping of tissues can be achieved with chin augmentation using either alloplastic implants or osteoplastic osteotomy techniques. This will improve the neck-chin angle and more aesthetically drape the tissues in the submental region. Additional methods to improve the submental region aesthetics include skin excision, platysma muscle plication, and neck-lifting procedures. Many of these techniques can be incorporated to create a comprehensive treatment plan. The disadvantage to most of the adjunctive techniques is that they require additional surgery and external skin incisions with higher incidence of potential complications, compared with closed syringe cervicofacial liposuction surgery.

9. What complications are associated with submental liposuction, and how are they best prevented and treated?

Submental liposuction is a relatively safe procedure; however, several surgical complications are possible that must be discussed with the patient preoperatively. Expected postoperative sequelae include bruising, swelling, pain, and numbness in the skin overlying the surgical site. Patients must be informed of additional complications, including contour abnormality or inadequate fat removal that might require treatment by repeat surgery. Infection can occur in any surgical wound but is minimized with sterile technique and at least prophylactic antibiotic coverage. Bleeding resulting in a hematoma can occur due to the potential dead space created, which can be minimized by the postoperative pressure dressing that should be worn up to 1 month after surgery at least 12 hr/day. In addition, the use of a pressure dressing enhances the recontouring of the submental region during the healing process. Facial nerve injury may occur to the marginal mandibular branch if the operator is overzealous in the region above the inferior border of the mandible when approached from the submental portal. This may be prevented by strict adherence to the appropriate plane of dissection and keeping the cannulas below the inferior border of the mandible. Finally, all patients must have realistic expectations of the procedure and an understanding that it is not a substitute for neck-lifting or rhytidectomy procedures.

10. In which circumstances is lipoinjection or fat transfer a useful adjunctive aesthetic procedure?

Lipoinjection or fat transfer is a useful adjunctive technique for soft tissue augmentation of the face. It is widely used in the augmentation of the lips, nasolabial fold, and contracted scar augmentation. Microinjections have been described for use in acne scar rejuvenation. The fat is autologous and well tolerated by the patient; however, it has a somewhat unpredictable resorption pattern that must be overcontoured intraoperatively to offset some of the anticipated resorption. Patients may require repeat fat injections in the future. Alternative materials include collagen injections into the dermis or the use of alloplastic materials.

11. What are the advantages and disadvantages of the open rhinoplasty technique?

The major disadvantage of an open rhinoplasty technique is the transcolumnellar incision, which could be potentially problematic if unfavorable scarring occurs. In addition, prolonged edema of the nasal tip may take several months to resolve. Paresthesia of the nasal tip also persists for a variable period. The surgical procedure is more time consuming, and there is the potential for skin loss or slough. The advantages of an open technique, however, include direct visualization of the structures to be modified, precise surgical manipulation of exposed elements, and an excellent teaching modality to clearly demonstrate the effects of surgical techniques. For significant nasal deformities such as cleft lip patients, some surgeons opt to use the open approach due to the significance of the preexisting deformity.

12. What aesthetic changes result from performing a cephalic excision from the lower lateral cartilage?

The cephalic or upper-edge excision of the lower lateral cartilage in rhinoplasty is a common surgical manipulation. The purpose of this procedure is to reduce the bulk of the nasal tip width along with some cephalic elevation of the nasal tip. It is critical to preserve at least 5-7 mm of residual lower lateral cartilage after cephalic excision to prevent elimination of some nasal tip support. Overresection will give the appearance of a pinched and elevated tip that is not aesthetically pleasing.

13. Why are intradomal sutures used in nasal surgery?

The intradomal region is located at the nasal tip where the lower lateral crura curve to form the medial crura. This defines the nasal tip, which is seen externally on the nasal skin as two light reflexes approximately 5 mm apart. An individual with thick skin may not have a well-defined tip and a unilateral broad light reflex may be noted. In narrowing and redefining the nasal tip region, some surgeons will use an intradomal suture to narrow and cephalically elevate the nasal tip. This is generally done in conjunction with other surgical manipulations such as cephalic trimming of the lower lateral cartilage or placement of a nasal tip shield graft.

14. Why is dorsal nasal reduction usually accompanied by lateral osteotomies?

Reduction of the nasal dorsum usually results in the creation of an open roof deformity. This deformity results from the roof being taken off the nasal dorsum with two lateral bony struts and a central septal strut. If this open roof defect is not collapsed upon itself with the lateral osteotomies, a broad and irregular deformity will result from the adaptation of the soft tissues into the broad dorsum, creating the open roof deformity.

15. What is one of the most important considerations in evaluating patients before performing lower eyelid blepharoplasty?

The assessment of lower lid laxity should be undertaken by all surgeons before lower lid blepharoplasty. In general, the lower lid is pulled away from the eye and the time for recoil to occur is observed. A young person will have a "snap" as the lid quickly recoils in place, whereas an elderly person may demonstrate an ectropion, which slowly returns to normal position. The patient with moderate to severe lid laxity will be at risk for postoperative ectropion or eversion of the lower eyelid. These patients must have detailed informed consent about the possible ramifications of lower eyelid surgery and the possible need for additional procedures, such as lateral lid shortening or canthoplasty.

16. What are the common surgical approaches used for lower eyelid blepharoplasty?

One of the most commonly used approaches for lower eyelid blepharoplasty is the skin-orbicularis muscle flap technique. The excess skin and herniated orbital fat, along with any hypertrophic orbicularis muscle, can be excised by this technique. This is a relatively easy approach in an avascular plane above the orbital septum. In this surgical technique, the incision is created approximately 1.5 mm below the lash line and extended approximately 1 cm laterally in the lateral canthal region following the natural creases. The incision is started with a scalpel, and the area of the lateral canthal region is undermined below the orbicularis muscle above the orbital retinaculum and then extended along this plane at the level of the subciliary incision. Blunt dissection may be assisted with the use of cotton tip applicators. Once the dissection is complete, the orbital fat pads are identified and the septum is incised over the designated region while applying some gentle pressure on the globe to allow for the extrusion of orbital fat. The fat is clamped, cut, and cauterized before releasing to prevent retrobulbar hemorrhage. The skin-muscle flap is rolled laterally and superiorly while the patient looks upward and the excess tissue is excised with scissors. Additional orbicularis muscle may be excised if the patient tends to have a hypertrophic orbicularis bulge.

Alternatively, many surgeons prefer the transconjunctival approach when no skin or muscle excision is required. In this technique, the lower eyelid is everted and an incision is created above the fornix. Blunt dissection is used to dissect out the orbital fat pads. After thorough hemostasis, the surgical site is irrigated and closure of the conjunctiva with resorbable ophthalmic gut sutures can be performed, depending on the surgeon's preference. The incidence of lid retraction and ectropion is reduced with the transconjunctival approach compared with the subciliary approach.

17. How many fat pads are encountered during the upper and lower eyelid blepharoplasty procedures?

The upper eyelid has two fat pads, including the nasal and middle pad. The nasal pad is the smaller of the two. The lacrimal gland is located laterally and should not be mistakenly excised during upper lid blepharoplasty. The lower eyelid has three fat pads: nasal, middle, and temporal. The nasal fat pad is the smallest, and the fat generally has a white appearance. The middle fat pad is the largest of the three and is separated from the nasal pad by the inferior oblique muscle. The temporal pad is of variable size and may have more than one compartment. Any blood vessels that traverse the fat pads must be thoroughly cauterized to prevent postoperative retrobulbar bleeding.

18. What other facial anatomic structures should be assessed before performing upper eyelid blepharoplasty?

In conjunction with the evaluation of the upper eyelids before blepharoplasty, assessment of the brow should also be undertaken. In many cases, the brow will be ptotic and worsen the appearance of the upper eyelids. If the upper lid blepharoplasty was performed without correction of the brow, the result would be less than desirable and, possibly, more eyelid skin would be removed than required. Male patients generally have a straight and relatively flat brow, whereas females should have a laterally elevated brow. The distance from the pupil center to the brow is approximately 20 mm. When assessing these patients, the brow should be elevated with the examiner's hand to determine the effect of concomitant brow lifting and the contribution to the upper eyelid deformity.

19. What is the Mustardé technique of otoplasty?

The Mustardé otoplasty technique is primarily designed to produce a cartilaginous fold in the antihelical area through the use of horizontal mattress sutures. The site of the proposed antihelical fold is marked with methylene blue after an elliptic strip of skin is removed from the posterior aspect of the ear. This is determined by bending the ear toward the head and observing where the fold develops. Three to five horizontal mattress sutures are introduced equidistant from the predetermined location of the fold and tightened to establish the desired contour of the antihelical fold. Abrasion or scoring of the cartilage can be used to weaken the cartilage in a patient with a very thick cartilaginous ear structure.

20. What are some of the advantages and disadvantages of alloplastic implants for facial augmentation?

Alloplastic implants are frequently used in facial rejuvenation surgery. The desirable features of these implants include their ease of placement through intraoral incisions, availability off the shelf, and the large number of anatomic sizes and shapes commercially available. Most implants can be secured with a screw for immediate stabilization. The alloplastic implants obviate the need for a donor surgical site with its concomitant morbidity. The downside to the use of alloplastic materials is that they are foreign bodies that are usually encapsulated with fibrous tissue capsules upon healing. They are susceptible to infection because there is no true tissue ingrowth and vascularization, and they may migrate, causing local morbidity. Silicone chin implants have been shown to cause underlying bone resorption after many years. The most critical component to the successful use of alloplastic facial implants is maintaining adequate soft tissue coverage. Implants should only be placed where they can be situated under well-vascularized tissues. If an implant becomes infected, the prognosis for maintaining it is very poor. Some local morbidity is associated with the removal of implants, including scar contracture and associated soft tissue deformities, which may require secondary augmentation procedures.

21. What surgical techniques are useful for the revision of facial scars?

The simplest procedure for scar revision is the fusiform or elliptic excision, which is used for scars that fall within the resting skin tension lines of the face. Scar repositioning techniques are used to move scars located near facial landmarks or better align the scar with the resting skin tension lines. Included within the category are the Z-plasty, W-plasty, and geometric revision procedures. The Z-plasty is most commonly used near the commissure of the mouth, lateral alar region of the nose, and periorbital region. The W-plasty is used in most other areas of the face or when the scar diverges from the resting skin tension lines by more than 35 degrees. Dermabrasion is a useful adjunct for scar camouflage, allowing the blending of scar margins with the surrounding skin. It may be performed as the initial procedure for scar revision or as a secondary procedure on a scar that has previously undergone excision or revision surgery.

22. What is dermabrasion best suited for today?

The crater type of acne scar is suitable for dermabrasion because of the gradual blending of the edges into the surrounding tissue, leaving less of a shadow cast by the crater ridge. The remodeling of the region results in a smoothing of the depressed defects of the skin and a less noticeable scar. Removal of tattoos and the blending of scars are other important uses of the dermabrasion procedure. A number of other dermatologic conditions traditionally have been treated with dermabrasion, such as the removal of fine rhytids, but these may be better managed with laser resurfacing or chemical peeling. Dermabrasion may be carried out to the level of the reticular (deep) or papillary (superficial) dermis, depending on the desired result. The author's preference for dermabrasion is for facial scars that may have undergone excision or revision procedures but require additional treatment for final camouflage. This is performed with diamond fraises or wire brushes using local anesthesia with or without conscious sedation. Wire brushes tend to gouge the skin if not properly used; therefore diamond fraises may be better for the less experienced surgeon. The surgery may be completed using either spray refrigeration or application of skin tension. Pinpoint bleeding denotes the level of the papillary dermis. Wounds are covered with antibiotic ointment, sterile petrolatum, or nonadherent dressings. Patients must observe strict adherence to sun avoidance for up to 6 months after surgery to prevent pigmentary changes.

23. What is the pretreatment protocol for chemical peeling?

Preparing the skin for chemical peeling is an important aspect of chemical rejuvenation. Retin-A (0.025%-0.1%) is applied daily for at least several weeks before peeling in order to reduce healing time. Alternatively, some surgeons advocate use of an alpha-hydroxy acid for this purpose. Either agent will thin the stratum corneum and allow a more uniform penetration of the peeling agent. Use of a bleaching agent such as hydroquinone (2%-4%) may be indicated for patients at risk of developing postinflammatory hyperpigmentation. A prepeel skin regimen requires daily application of products, which could identify noncompliant patients who would not be good candidates for skin peeling. Patients should be prescribed a broad-spectrum antibiotic, such as a cephalosporin, antiviral, and antifungal medication, to take orally the day before skin peeling and up to 10-14 days postpeel in addition to their topical home care.

24. What are the advantages of trichloroacetic acid (TCA) as a chemical peeling agent?

TCA is a popular agent used for superficial and medium-depth peels. Advantages of TCA include no systemic toxicity: inexpensive; stable; no need to neutralize agent once applied; and endpoint indicated by the intensity of skin frosting after application.

25. What surgical techniques are available to perform a brow lift?

A number of techniques are available for a surgeon to select from to perform a brow lift. A direct brow lift is performed by placing the incision within the eyebrow parallel to the hair follicles, which provides 1:1 lift. This is useful in older patients with thick brows in which most of the deformity is laterally located. Alternatively, a midforehead lift is used in older patients with prominent horizontal furrows. This is the least cosmetic result, as the incision lies within the visible portion of the forehead. Classically, a coronal brow lift was performed using a coronal incision. This allowed complete control and direct visualization of the musculature with excision of skin to the predetermined level. This would result in an alteration of the hairline and would require more time with associated blood loss compared with other techniques. The procedure performed most often today is an endoscopic brow lift, which allows the surgeon to selectively elevate various segments of the eyebrows and modify musculature accordingly. It has been described using three to five entry portals contained within the hair-bearing area and retention of the lift using burr holes, screws, and recently barbed sutures. This procedure requires specialized equipment, including the use of an endoscope.

BIBLIOGRAPHY

1. Aiach G, Levignac J: Aesthetic Rhinoplasty. Edinburgh, 1991, Churchill Livingstone.
2. Epker BN: Aesthetic Maxillofacial Surgery. Philadelphia, 1994, Lea & Febiger.
3. Hupp JR (ed): Atlas of the Oral and Maxillofacial Surgery Clinics of North America: Esthetic Surgery for the Aging Face, 6th vol. Philadelphia, 1998, Saunders.
4. Johnson CM, Wyatt CT: A Case Approach to Open Structure Rhinoplasty. Philadelphia, 2005, Saunders.
5. Putterman AM, Warren LA: Cosmetic Oculoplastic Surgery, 3rd ed. Philadelphia, 1999, Saunders.
6. Rubin MG: Manual of Chemical Peels: Superficial and Medium Depth. Philadelphia, 1995, J.B. Lippincott.
7. Thomas JR, Holt GR: Facial Scars: Incision, Revision, and Camouflage. St Louis, 1989, Mosby.

47. DENTAL IMPLANTS

Frank P. Iuorno, Jr., DDS, MS, and Kenneth J. Benson, DDS

1. What are the different dental implant categories?

Dental implants are divided into three categories based on their relationship to the oral tissues:
1. Subperiosteal
2. Endosteal
3. Transosseous

Endosteal implants are subdivided into root-form implants and plate-form or blade implants. Root-form implants can be smooth, threaded, perforated, and solid or hollow, vented, coated, or textured. Currently, the most commonly used implants are root-form implants. Only endosseous and transosseous implants are considered true osseointegrated implants.

2.   What is osseointegration?
    Several definitions have been proposed over the years to describe a successful dental implant in the human jaw. However, the most inclusive definition to date describes osseointegration as "a process whereby clinically asymptomatic rigid fixation of alloplastic materials is achieved and maintained in bone during functional loading."[2]

3.   What criteria were used to determine the success of an implant before 1986?
    Before 1986, the criteria for a successful implant were different from those used today. According to the 1978 Harvard–National Institutes of Health (NIH) consensus conference on implantology, an implant was considered successful despite the presence of one or more of the following clinical features:
*   Mobility of <1 mm in any direction
*   Bone loss of no more than one third of the vertical height of the implant
*   Gingival inflammation amenable to treatment
*   Absence of symptoms, such as infection, numbness, pain, or maxillary sinus or nasal symptoms
*   Implant functional for 5 years in 75% of cases

4.   What became the criteria for successful implants after 1986?
    In 1986, with the introduction of osseointegration, the criteria for successful implants were revised:
*   Implant clinically immobile
*   No radiographic evidence of any peri-implant radiolucency
*   Vertical bone loss of <0.2 mm after the first year of function
*   Absence of any symptoms, such as pain, infection, numbness, or maxillary sinus or nasal symptoms
*   Success rate of 85% after 5 years and 80% after 10 years

5.   When are dental implants indicated?
    Dental implants are used to achieve rehabilitation of the oral and facial tissue after tooth loss with and without bone loss, after jaw bone loss due to tumor resection, after tooth loss from trauma, and for partially or completely congenitally missing teeth. More specifically, implants are used to achieve one of the following purposes:
*   Fixed restoration of single or multiple teeth in a partially edentulous jaw
*   Retention of removable prosthesis in a partially edentulous jaw
*   Retention of a prosthesis in a completely edentulous jaw
*   Retention of fixed prosthesis in completely edentulous maxilla or mandible
*   Retention of maxillofacial prosthesis after loss of jawbone from trauma or after tumor resection
*   As a fixture for orthodontic tooth movement when conventional anchorage is not feasible or is cumbersome

6.   What are Brånemark's surgical principles for ensuring osseous integration of implants?
    Brånemark established a set of surgical principles based on animal and human research that, if followed during implant placement, ensures osseointegration of the dental implants:
*   The implant should be placed in direct contact with the bone.
*   Implants should be inserted in bone in a surgically prepared site, using a graded series of drills followed by a tap rotating at 15 rpm.
*   Absolute temperature control at the surgical site should not exceed 47° C to minimize thermal necrosis of bone adjacent to implant.

- The mucosa should remain sutured over the newly inserted implant, and the implant should remain functionless for 3-6 months.
- At a second stage (3-6 months later), the implant is exposed and an abutment and the implant are connected to the prosthesis. Consequently, loading of the implant is done only after the implant is osseointegrated. This last principle has changed in the last few years by successfully loading implants immediately after placement with no impact on the success rate.

7. How much space is needed between implants for successful integration?

Imagine that a square box is drawn around the implant. In the buccal-lingual dimension, a minimum of 0.5 mm of bone is required around the implant. Therefore for a standard 3.75-mm implant, the operator would need approximately 5 mm of bone in this dimension. Mesiodistally, for implant survival, the same 0.5 mm is required for implant survival. Prosthodontically, at least 3 mm is necessary on both sides of the implant to create the proper emergence profile of a restoration. Consequently, the recommendation for distance between implants for single-tooth restoration is 7 mm from the center of one implant to the other.

8. How much space is observed between implant and bone in an osseointegrated titanium implant?

The chemical properties and the interface chemistry are determined by the oxide layer and not by the metal of the implant. Therefore the dense oxide film of a titanium implant, for example, is about 100 angstroms (Å) thick.

9. Can an implant be placed in an extraction site? What is the prognosis for such a procedure?

Limitations to placing immediate implants include lack of bone to gain initial stability and inability to cover the site with soft tissue when using a two-stage system. Provided no acute infection is present and adequate bone for initial stability (usually found in the apical one third to two thirds) is available, the soft tissue defect may be overcome using a "bio-col" technique. This is a technique whereby a membrane is used to prevent soft tissue ingrowth at the implant-bone interface in conjunction with a collagen plug to ensure watertight closure.

10. Can an implant be placed into grafted bone?

Implants can be placed into grafted bone immediately if native bone is adequate for initial stability of the implant or if the graft was done 3-6 months earlier. Successful placement of implants into bone graft using either alloplastic or autogenous material has been reported.

11. How much is the surface area of an implant increased by increasing the diameter of an implant compared with increasing its length?

For each 0.25-mm increase in implant diameter, there is a 10% increase in surface area. Therefore a 1-mm increase in diameter increases surface area by 40%. Studies have shown that for implants larger than 15-18 mm, there is no further significant biomechanical advantage, regardless of implant diameter.

Some authors have shown that increasing the length of an implant to more than 18 mm provides no additional mechanical advantage and possibly increases the incidence of failure rate because of the difficulty of adequately irrigating during the preparation of the site.

12. What major anatomic structures in the maxilla and mandible can affect implant placement? How can these problems be overcome?

In the posterior maxilla, a pneumatization of the maxillary sinus can result in a decrease in the available bone in this region. This deficiency can be overcome by bone grafting of this region. If the interarch space is adequate for restoration (implant-to-crown ratio), a sinus-lift bone graft procedure is indicated. However, if there is an excessive interarch space, onlay bone graft with or without sinus-lift procedure is a better choice. Distraction osteogenesis both to increase the bone height and to close the interarch space is another option when there is an increased interarch space.

In the anterior maxilla, bony defects are occasionally observed on the buccal surface, caused either by traumatic extraction or by buccal concavity around the apical one third of the root. These defects must be treated before or during implant placement. Angulation of the implant to engage existing bone often will result in an implant that is unable to receive a direct axial load and will be more prone to failure after a restoration is placed.

In the posterior mandible, the inferior alveolar nerve is one of the most common impediments to implant placement. Frequently, there is insufficient bone height to place even an 11.5-mm implant in the posterior mandible without the risk of nerve injury. Remedies for this problem depend mostly on restoration length and available interarch space. As in the maxilla, if there is sufficient interarch space, the nerve must be surgically repositioned (lateralized) to gain adequate bone length to achieve a proper crown-to-root ratio and anchorage for the implant. If there is excessive interarch space, onlay bone grafting or distraction osteogenesis should be considered to gain vertical bone height and decrease the interarch space before implant placement.

The lingual concavity of the mandible in the posterior and anterior regions is another anatomic area to be considered during placement of mandibular implant. Computed tomography (CT) or plain tomography should be considered if there is any question as to whether an implant can be placed without perforating the concavity and risking implant failure or damage to the lingual nerve.

13. What is the ideal fixture depth in relation to the adjacent tooth?

To gain proper emergence profile, a single tooth restoration should be placed 3-4 mm apical to the cementoenamel junction of the adjacent tooth. This will allow for tissue covering of any metal margins and provide more natural emergence of the implant from the soft tissue. At the same time, the dental papilla will be able to grow between the natural tooth and restoration, and the patient will find it easier to maintain the implant.

14. Is it necessary to have attached gingiva when placing implants?

Ideally, implants are more easily maintained if an adequate cuff (1-2 mm) of attached tissue is left around the restoration. This does not mean, however, that attached tissue is necessary at the time of placement. In the edentulous mandible, there is often a paucity of attached tissue at the time of placement, and most patients have high mentalis muscle attachments that extend to the crest of the remaining alveolus. At the time of placement, or at a later time but before uncovering the implant in a two-stage implant system, measures can be taken to lower these muscle attachments (lip-switch or other vestibuloplasty procedures) to gain immobile tissue.

15. How do you test for osseointegration at the time of implant uncovering?

Torque testing can be done to test for osseointegration at the time of implant uncovering. Ideally, one should be able to place a force of 10-20 Ncm without unscrewing an implant if it is successfully osseointegrated. Other clinical subjective signs of integration are percussion and immobility when placing a fixture mount or impression coping on the implant. When a lateral force of 5 lb is applied, no movement should be seen. Horizontal mobility of >1 mm or movement <500 g of force indicates a failed implant.

16. What methods are used to uncover implants? Can a laser or electrocautery be used?

Conventional uncovering is done with a blade. If there is a minimal band of keratinized tissue, an incision is made to split this band and the tissue is sutured to either side of the healing abutment. If there is adequate attached immobile tissue, a punch biopsy can be used after localization of the implant with a needle. Lasers can also be used, but care must be taken to avoid reflecting energy off the implant to the adjacent bone, which will cause irreversible thermal damage. Electrocautery can also be used carefully without touching the fixture to avoid transmitting heat throughout the socket.

17. Can bone be grafted to a failing implant?
If an implant is mobile, it must be removed as soon as possible to prevent further bone resorption. If the implant is integrated and has a bony fenestration or dehiscence, then guided tissue regeneration or bone grafting procedures may be performed. However, a dehiscence or fenestration must be significant and growing before considering grafting.

18. What are the radiographic signs of implant failure?
The most useful radiographic sign of implant failure is loss of crestal bone. Early crestal bone loss is a sign of stress at the perimucosal site. At least 40% of the trabecular bone must be lost to be detected radiographically. Rapid progressive bone loss indicates failure. This will usually be accompanied by pain on percussion or function.

19. What preoperative radiographs are necessary for adequate work-up before implant placement?
Panoramic and periapical radiographs are helpful and necessary, although they offer no information regarding the internal anatomy of the alveolar process or residual ridge. In addition, they do not permit accurate three-dimensional superimposition of a clinically verified radiopaque template, which can be used as a surgical guide. Multiplanar reformatted CT can be used to obtain this information if it cannot be obtained easily by a combination of conventional radiographic techniques and clinical exam.

20. How many implants are adequate for support of mandibular removable prosthetic replacement in an edentulous mandible?
In general, a minimum of two implants is necessary for support of an implant-retained, tissue-supported prosthesis. It is best to place these as far apart on the ridge as possible while avoiding the mental nerve. For an implant-supported and implant-retained prosthesis, at least three implants should be used, with the length of the cantilever being 1.5 times the distance between the most anterior and posterior implants, as measured in the horizontal plane.

21. Are magnetic resonance imaging (MRI) or CT scans contraindicated in a patient with dental implants?
MRI and CT scans are not contraindicated in patients with pure titanium implants. Most CT scanners can subtract titanium and other metals from the image and eliminate the scatter images.

22. Are there any absolute contraindications to implant placement?
No. However, because smoking affects the healing of bone and overlying tissue, it should be considered a relative contraindication to implant placement. Similarly, in patients with uncontrolled systemic diseases such as diabetes, immunocompromised patients, and patients with bleeding disorders, implant placement should be considered with extreme caution.

23. What are the most common reasons for endosseous dental implant removal?
- Lack of integration
- Lack of bone support
- Loss of bone
- Surgical malposition
- Psychiatric reasons

24. What are the possible complications of endosseous dental implants?
The most commonly reported reasons for dental implant failure are:
- Infection
- Perforation of the maxillary sinus and nasal cavity

- Loss of implant
- Bone resorption around implant
- Nerve injury and numbness
- Cost and long-term treatment period
- Fracture of the mandible

25. What is the long-term success rate of endosseous implants?

The 5-year combined success rate of maxillary and mandibular dental implants is 94.6%. Albrektsson et al. reported maxillary implants with a success rate of 84.9% for 5-7 years. For irradiated maxilla, the success rate of implants is 80%; in grafted maxilla, the success rate is 85%.

In large, long-term studies of mandibular and maxillary endosseous implants, the success rate ranges from 84%-97%. Specifically, the maxillary implant success rate after 1 year is 88% and is 84% after 5-12 years. In the mandible, the 1- to 2-year success rate is 94%-97%, the 5- to 12-year success rate is 93%, and the 15-year success rate is 91%. The success rate in the mandible posterior region is 91.5% and in the maxillary posterior region is 82.9%, whereas the success rates are higher in the anterior mandible, in the 94%-97% range.

26. What is the success rate of endosseous implants placed in an autogenous bone graft site?

In a study by Keller et al., 248 commercially pure titanium endosseous implants were placed in 54 consecutive patients who required bone grafting. Types of grafts included cortical, corticocancellous, and particulate bone. All 74 antral sites received a block graft. Endosseous implant success over the 12-year period was 878 and bone graft success reached 100%. A higher loss of implants occurred in the Le Fort I fracture groups compared with other grafting approaches.

27. Can endosseous implants be successfully placed in an irradiated bone?

Many studies indicate successful integration of endosseous implants in irradiated fields even without the use of hyperbaric oxygen (HBO) therapy. A study by Anderson et al. demonstrates a success rate of 97.8% for endosseous implants placed into an irradiated field. This study evaluated 90 implants placed in 15 patients for treatment of malignancies in the maxillofacial region with radiation doses ranging from 44 cGy–68 cGy. Other studies show similar rates of success without the use of HBO.

28. When is a transmandibular implant (TMI) indicated?

A TMI can be placed in a totally edentulous mandible of any bone height. However, a TMI works particularly well in the prosthetic restoration of a severely atrophic mandible (<12 mm of bone vertically).

29. After seating a single-tooth implant with an insertion force of 45 Ncm, is hand tightening of an abutment acceptable for immediate provisionalization?

The short answer is "yes." However, hand tightening, although acceptable, has a very high incidence of screw loosening. To decrease the number of emergency patients with loose restorations, use of a calibrated mechanical torque wrench is advised to apply appropriate tightening.

30. How tight does an abutment screw need to be to decrease the incidence of loosening?

In the above case, most authors recommend applying 35 Ncm to tighten the abutment. In general, following individual manufacturers specifications will decrease loosening and decrease those emergency calls.

31. What are three key features for successful implant treatment for single-tooth edentulism?

1. Primary stability
2. Oxidized implant surfaces
3. Light centric occlusion only and removal of lateral excursives on the restoration

32. If an implant is placed into an immediate extraction site, when can an immediate loading be carried out?

- Implants firmly engaged into socket walls provide primary stability.
- Oxidized surfaces will speed up osseointegration for good secondary stability.
- Natural high regenerative potential of the socket
- Light centric contact on a restoration

33. Which type of implant surface has shown better bone healing response? Machine or oxidized surface implants?

Multiple studies show an increased response of bone to oxidized surfaces. This implant feature has allowed quicker secondary stability because osseointegration is quicker.

34. What methods improve primary stability of implants placed in fresh extraction sites?

Careful preoperative measurements and surgically stepped drilling sequences are critical to ensure engagement of the implant surface with extraction socket walls. Also, if anatomic considerations allow, preparing 2-3 mm of the implant osteotomy apical to the socket apex will allow excellent stability with implant delivery.

35. What considerations should be made for implants in an irradiated patient?

As with any other dentoalveolar procedure, one must know the irradiated field and dose, anatomic considerations with amount of bone available, and time period the radiation was delivered. Dose is a big factor, with 55 Gy and greater being an amount that is traditionally the level at which treatment should be given with the most caution (particularly in the mandible).

36. How can one approach implant rehab for a patient who had 55 Gy of radiation delivered for a right-sided posterior floor of mouth tumor?

Many would consider HBO as an adjunctive treatment for implant rehab. Using standard HBO protocol (20 dives before implant surgery and 10 dives postimplant) will provide improved bone healing and turnover with improved angiogenesis in the irradiated tissues. Also, one must know where the radiation was delivered, because some areas ultimately have less radiation delivered than others and treatment can be planned accordingly, with more implants delivered in a less radiated area of the mandible/maxilla.

37. What is a zygoma implant?

A zygoma implant is an extended-length (30-52.5 mm) machined titanium fixture that is placed through the crestal (slightly palatal) aspect of the resorbed posterior maxilla transantrally into the compact bone of the zygoma. These implants are usually used when the existing osseous structures do not allow standard implant placement. Zygoma implants are used for cross-arch stabilization in conjunction with two to four standard implants in the anterior maxilla.

38. What osseous cortices provide the initially stability for zygoma implants?

In addition to two to four conventional fixtures in the anterior maxilla, the initially stability of zygoma implants is assured by its contact with four cortices:

1. The ridge crest
2. The sinus floor
3. The roof of the maxillary sinus
4. The superior border of the zygoma

39. What are the indications for zygoma implants?

Zygoma implants are most often used in cases of moderate to severe atrophy. They provide an alternative for treatment of the patient with extreme resorption of the edentulous maxilla or large pneumatized sinus without the need for bone grafting. They should also be considered for any patient in need of posterior maxillary implant support with and without significant atrophy.

BIBLIOGRAPHY

1. Adell R, Lekhholm U, Rockller B et al: A 15-year study of osseointegrated implants in treatment of the edentulous jaw. Int J Oral Surg 18:387-416, 1981.
2. Albrektsson CJ, Sennerby L: What is osseointegration? In Worthington P, Evans JR (eds): Controversies in Oral and Maxillofacial Surgery. Philadelphia, 1997, Saunders.
3. Albrektsson T, Brånemark P-I, Hansson HA et al: Osseointegrated titanium implants. Requirements for ensuring a long-lasting, direct bone-to-implant anchorage in man. Acta Orthop Scand 52:155-170, 1981.
4. Albrektsson T, Dahl E, Enbom L et al: Osseointegrated oral implants. A Swedish multicenter study of 8139 consecutively inserted Nobelpharma implants. J Periodontol 59:287-296, 1988.
5. Anderson G, Andreasson L, Bjelkengren G: Oral implant rehabilitation in irradiated patients without adjunctive hyperbaric oxygen. Int J Oral Maxillofac Implants 13:647-654, 1998.
6. Becker W, Becker BE, Alsuwyed H et al: Long-term evaluation of 282 implants in maxillary and mandibular molar positions. A prospective study. J Periodontol 70:896-901, 1999.
7. Bosker H, Jordon R, Sindet-Pedersen S et al: The transmandibular implant: a 13-year survey of its use. J Oral Maxillofac Surg 49:482-492, 1991.
8. Brånemark P-I: Precision, Predictability. Gothenburg, Sweden, 1990, Institute for Applied Biotechnology.
9. Brånemark P-I: Introduction to osseointegration. In Brånemark P-I, Zarb G, Albrektsson T (eds): Tissue Integrated Prostheses. Chicago, 1985, Quintessence.
10. Keller EE, Eckert SE, Tolman DE: Maxillary antral and nasal one-stage inlay composite bone graft: preliminary report on 30 recipient sites. J Oral Maxillofac Surg 52:438-448, 1994.
11. Noack N, Willer J, Hoffmann J: Long-term results after placement of dental implants: longitudinal study of 1964 implants over 16 years. Int J Oral Maxillofac Implants 14:748-755, 1999.
12. Schliephake H, Schmelzeisen R, Husstedt H et al: Comparison of the late results of mandibular reconstruction using nonvascularized or vascularized grafts and implants. J Oral Maxillofac Surg 57:944-950, 1999.
13. Schow SR, Parel SM: The zygoma implant. In Miloro M, Larsen P, Ghali GE et al (eds): Peterson's Principles of Oral and Maxillofacial Surgery, 2nd ed. Hamilton, Ontario, 2004, B.C. Decker.
14. Steinemann SG, Eulenberger J, Maeusli PA et al: Adhesion of bone to titanium. Adv Biomater 6:409, 1986.
15. Zarb G, Albrektsson T: Osseointegration: a requiem for the periodontal ligament? [editorial]. Int J Periodontal Rest Dent 11:88, 1991.

48. PREPROSTHETIC SURGERY

Vincent J. Perciaccante, DDS

1. How does the blood supply of the edentulous mandible differ from that of the dentate mandible?

As edentulous bone loss (EBL) progresses, there is a change in the blood supply to the mandible. The inferior alveolar vessels become smaller. The primary blood supply to the dentate mandible moves **centrifugally** from the inferior alveolar artery. The primary blood supply to the edentulous mandible flows **centripetally** from the periosteum. Elevation of the periosteum on mandibles that have had severe bone loss could compromise blood supply. Therefore, during surgical procedures, elevation of the periosteum should be done judiciously in the edentulous atrophic mandible.

2. Does alveolar bone resorb more quickly in the mandible or in the maxilla?

EBL in the maxilla is usually more rapid and severe. This may be due to the lack of muscle attachments to the maxilla and, therefore, the lack of functional stimulus after tooth loss.

3.   **What skeletal relationship results from EBL?**
      The skeletal relationship that results from EBL is **pseudo Class III.** Most EBL in the maxilla takes place on the lateral and inferior aspects of the ridge; therefore, the crest moves posteriorly and superiorly. As the height and width of the mandibular ridge deteriorate, the crest moves further anteriorly. As vertical dimension collapses, the mandible autorotates forward as well.

4.   **How are edentulous alveolar ridges classified (Table 48-1)?**

Table 48-1 *Classification of Edentulous Ridges*	
CLASS	DEFINITION
Kent Classification of Edentulous Ridges (1986)	
I	Alveolar ridge is of adequate height but inadequate width, with lateral deficiencies or undercut areas
II	Alveolar ridge deficient in both height and width, with a knife-edge appearance
III	Alveolar ridge has been resorbed to the level of basilar bone, producing a concave form in the posterior areas of the mandible and sharp ridge form with bulbous, mobile soft tissues in the maxilla
IV	Resorption of the basilar bone, producing a pencil-thin, flat mandible or maxilla
Caywood Classification of Edentulous Ridges (1988)	
I	Dentate
II	Immediately postextraction
III	Well-rounded ridge form, adequate in height and width
IV	Knife-edge ridge form, adequate in height but inadequate in width
V	Flat ridge form; inadequate in height and width
VI	Depressed ridge form, with some basilar loss evident

5.   **What is combination syndrome?**
      Combination syndrome is excessive resorption of the edentulous alveolar ridge of the anterior maxilla, caused by the forces generated by opposition of natural mandibular anterior teeth.

6.   **When and how are torus mandibularis and torus palatinus treated?**
      Mandibular tori usually need to be removed when a mandibular denture is being planned. The denture flange typically will impinge on these exostoses of bone. Palatal tori often do not need to be removed. Dentures often can be constructed over them. However, if a palatal torus is extremely large and fills the vault, extends beyond the dam area, has traumatized mucosal coverage, has deep undercuts, interferes with speech, or poses a psychologic problem for the patient, it should be removed.
      The tissue over mandibular tori is extremely thin and friable. Great care should be taken when elevating it. This tissue can be "ballooned" out by injecting some local anesthesia directly under it. The incision should be crestal or lingual circumdental. No releasing incisions should be made. After careful elevation of tissues, a groove can be cut along the intended line of removal with a fissure burr. Mallet and osteotome may be used to cleave the torus in this plane. After the bone has been smoothed and the area thoroughly irrigated, the wound can be closed. Gauze should be placed under the tongue to minimize the chance of hematoma.

Before removing a palatal torus, a stent should be fabricated. This should be done on a study cast that has had the exostosis removed. A double-Y incision should be made over the midline of the torus. After careful elevation of the flaps, the torus should be scored multiple times in the anterior, posterior, and transverse dimensions. An osteotome can be used to remove each of these small portions. This decreases the risk of fracturing into the floor of the nose. A large burr or bone file is used to smooth the area. After thorough irrigation, the wound is closed with horizontal mattress sutures, and the stent is placed.

7. How can an abnormal frenum be excised?
- Z-plasty
- V-Y advancement
- Diamond excision

8. What is epulis fissurata, and how is it treated?
Epulis fissurata is submucosal fibrosis secondary to chronic denture irritation. The denture must first be relieved in the area to treat inflammation and irritation. The denture can then be lined with tissue conditioner and left out as much as possible. After maximum resolution has occurred, surgical excision or cryosurgery removes the epulis fissurata.

9. What is papillary hyperplasia, and how is it treated?
Papillary hyperplasia of the palate is of unknown etiology and is seen in patients with ill-fitting dentures. It presents as numerous papillary projections that cover the hard palate. Initially, the ill-fitting denture should be removed or relined with tissue conditioner. The tissue can be removed using a large curette, electrocautery, mucoabrasion, acrylic burr, or cryosurgery.

10. In denture reconstruction, how much space is needed between the crest of the tuberosity and the retromolar pad?
At the correct vertical dimension, the distance from the crest of the tuberosity to the retromolar pad should equal at least 1 cm.

11. What can be done if there is inadequate intermaxillary distance at the tuberosity?
A tuberosity reduction can be performed to remove excess tuberosity. An elliptic incision is made over the tuberosity and carried down to bone. This wedge is resected. The buccal and palatal tissues are undermined subperiosteally. Submucous wedges are removed from each flap and the wound is closed. This decreases the vertical and horizontal dimensions of the tuberosity.

12. What can be done for supererupted but healthy maxillary posterior teeth that interfere with a restorative plan?
Over time after loss of mandibular posterior teeth, maxillary teeth may supererupt into the edentulous mandibular space. This impinges on the room needed for mandibular restoration as well as freeway space. Often, these teeth are healthy and periodontally sound. They may be planned as abutments for a maxillary prosthesis. In these cases, extraction may not be the best choice, and the amount of supereruption may be too great for crown preparation and full coverage. The maxillary posterior segmental osteotomy can be used to reposition these segments superiorly.

13. What is the average size of the maxillary sinus?
The average size of the maxillary sinus is 14.75 cc, with a range of 9.5-20 cc. On average the width is 2.5 cm; height, 3.75 cm; and depth, 3 cm.

14. How should tears of the sinus membrane be managed during sinus lift?
Tears over corticocancellous grafts will heal. Particulate grafts may be lost if they migrate through perforations. Small tears may not pose a problem because the membrane folds over itself as it is lifted. Larger tears should be patched with a material such as Surgicel or Collatape.

15. How much native bone is required for immediate placement of implants with sinus lift?
A minimum of 4-5 mm of alveolar bone.

16. What is the proper size of the window for a sinus lift?
The window for a maxillary sinus lift begins at the anterior aspect of the sinus and continues inferiorly to several millimeters above the sinus floor. The window extends posteriorly approximately 20 mm. The superior osteotomy is approximately 10-15 mm above the inferior osteotomy.

17. What is guided tissue regeneration?
Different cell types migrate into a wound at different rates during repair. Membranes can be used to hinder the migration of undesirable cell types (fibrous connective tissue). This will allow repopulation of the wound with the desirable cell type (bone).

18. What is the goal of anterior maxillary osteoplasty?
In situations where implants are desired in a maxilla with adequate height but inadequate width, an anterior maxillary osteoplasty may provide the solution. It is used to widen the crest of the ridge. An incision is made labial to the vestibule, and a submucosal dissection is carried down to the crest of the ridge. At the crest of the ridge, the periosteum is incised, and the dissection continues palatally in the subperiosteal plane. A vertical bone cut is made obliquely from the crest of the ridge to the floor of the nose. The labial segment is mobilized, and an interpositional bone graft is placed.

19. What is a visor osteotomy?
A visor osteotomy is a procedure to increase the vertical height of the mandible by vertically splitting the anterior portion of the mandible (anterior to the mental foramen) and repositioning the lingual segment superiorly in relation to the buccal segment.

20. What is the sandwich osteotomy?
The sandwich osteotomy horizontally splits the mandible, the cranial fragment is repositioned superiorly, and an interpositional bone graft is placed. There also is a modification called the sandwich-visor osteotomy, which is a combination of these two techniques.

21. What is the desired thickness of a split-thickness skin graft (STSG)?
STSGs can be of varying thickness. An STSG is composed of the epidermis layer and part of the dermis layer. The STSG can be classified as thin, intermediate, or thick, based on the amount of dermis included. STSGs are between 0.010 and 0.025 inch.

22. Which types of skin grafts contract the most? The least?
The thinner a skin graft, the more the contraction. A thin STSG contracts more than an intermediate STSG, which contracts more than a thick STSG. Full-thickness skin grafts hardly contract at all.
Primary contraction is caused by elastic fibers in the skin graft as soon as it has been cut. This can be overcome when a graft is sutured in place. Secondary contraction begins about postoperative day 10 and continues for up to 6 months.

23. What is plasmic imbibition?
Plasmic imbibition is the process by which a skin graft absorbs a plasmalike fluid from its underlying recipient bed. It is absorbed into the capillary network by capillary action. This process is the initial means of survival for a skin graft and continues for approximately 48 hr.

24. Does grafted skin most resemble the donor site or the recipient site?
Grafted skin maintains most of its original characteristics, except that sensation and sweating more closely resemble the recipient site.

25. What are the goals of vestibuloplasty?

Vestibuloplasty, skin grafting, and floor of the mouth lowering increase the depth of the sulcus, which helps control lateral displacement of a denture. The skin graft also provides attached tissue, which will not be elevated by movement of the lip, cheeks, and tongue, providing a stable denture seating area. Skin grafts provide more comfortable load-bearing tissue than mucosa. The mandibular resorption rate beneath skin is probably slower.

26. What are the possible graft donor sites for vestibuloplasty?
- Skin
- Palatal mucosa
- Buccal mucosa

27. What are the advantages of using a stent to secure a graft in place for a vestibuloplasty?

A stent can be used to adapt the skin with accuracy to any contour in the labiobuccal area and undercuts in the lingual area. A stent also provides additional graft stabilization and protects the graft from food in the oral cavity.

28. What are the advantages of suturing a graft in place for a vestibuloplasty?

Patients are more comfortable without the stent. Stent construction and adaptation materials are not necessary.

29. What is the lip-switch procedure?

The lip-switch procedure is a transpositional flap vestibuloplasty. An incision is made in the labial mucosa. A thin mucosal flap is elevated, continuing into a supraperiosteal dissection on the anterior aspect of the mandible to the crest of the ridge. The mucosal flap is sutured to the depth of the vestibule covering the anterior aspect of the mandible, and the denuded tissue on the inner surface of the lip heals by secondary intention. A modification transposes the lingually based mucosal flap with an inferiorly based facial periosteal flap.

30. What is a submucous vestibuloplasty?

Submucous vestibuloplasty can be used for improvement of the maxillary vestibule in situations in which the alveolar ridge resorption is not severe but mucosal and muscular attachments exist near the crest of the ridge. Through a midline incision, submucosal and subperiosteal dissections are performed. The tissue between these two tunnels is cut and allowed to retract. A splint is relined and secured in place for 7-10 days.

31. How is floor of the mouth lowering performed?

An incision is made on the lingual aspect of the alveolus. A supraperiosteal dissection is carried inferiorly, and the mylohyoid and genioglossus muscles are sharply dissected from their insertions. No more than half the superior aspect of the genioglossus muscle should be released. The mucosal margins are then sutured to the new depth, either with sutures passed externally or in a circummandibular fashion.

32. What is the minimum distance from the inferior border that the mentalis must remain attached, during vestibuloplasty, to prevent a sagging chin?

A minimum of 10 mm of muscular tissue must remain attached to the vestibular periosteum in order to avoid a sagging chin.

33. What is a tuberoplasty?

Tuberoplasty is hamular notch deepening. The hamular notch occurs where the posterior border of the maxillary denture rests. The posterior palatal seal is placed in the deepest portion of the notch. Patients with decreased vertical height of the tuberosity may have an inadequate notch. In tuberoplasty, a curved osteotome is used to fracture the pterygoid plates free from the tuberosity and displace them in a posterior direction. The tissue is then sutured to the depth of the area, creating a new notch. This procedure has limited predictability of success.

34. What procedures can be done to augment a severely atrophic maxilla with a good palatal vault?
In the severely resorbed maxilla that still retains an adequate palatal vault, the Le Fort I osteotomy with anterior-inferior repositioning and interpositional bone graft can be used.

35. What procedures can be done to augment a severely atrophic maxilla with a poor palatal vault?
In a severely resorbed maxilla with a poor palatal vault, onlay grafting may be useful. This can be accomplished with onlay grafting of rib or horseshoe-shaped corticocancellous ilium. Implants may or may not be placed at this time, depending on the residual maxillary bone. Soft tissue procedures are often needed secondarily.

BIBLIOGRAPHY

1. Davis WH, Sailer HF: Preprosthetic surgery. Oral Maxillofac Surg Clin North Am 6:4, 1994.
2. Fonseca RJ: Oral and Maxillofacial Surgery, 7th vol. St Louis, 2000, Saunders.
3. MacIntosh RB: Autogenous grafting in oral and maxillofacial surgery. Oral Maxillofac Surg Clin North Am 5:4, 1993.
4. Marx RE, Carlson ER, Eichstaedt RM et al: Platelet-rich plasma: growth factor enhancement for bone grafts. Oral Surg Oral Med Oral Pathol Oral Radiol Endod 85:638-646, 1998.
5. Marx RE, Morales MJ: Morbidity from bone harvest in major jaw reconstruction: a randomized trial comparing the lateral anterior and posterior approaches to the ilium. J Oral Maxillofac Surg 48:196-203, 1988.
6. Peterson LJ, Indresano AT, Marciani RD et al: Principles of Oral and Maxillofacial Surgery. Philadelphia, 1992, J.B. Lippincott.

49. SLEEP APNEA AND SNORING

Kenneth J. Benson, DDS

1. How is *snoring* defined?
Snoring is a partial airway and pharyngeal flow obstruction that does not awaken the individual. Movement of air through an obstructed airway creates the snoring sound.

2. Does snoring always indicate the presence of obstructive sleep apnea syndrome (OSAS)?
No. Although patients who have OSAS are typically loud snorers, and snoring usually indicates some degree of obstructed breathing, not all people who snore have OSAS. In fact, about 25% of adult males snore, and this number increases with age, reaching about 60% at age 60 years. Most snoring, however, is not pathologic and may be reduced or prevented by lifestyle changes.

3. Can a snoring patient with excessive daytime somnolence but without other classic symptoms have OSAS?
Yes. The lack of other classic symptoms of OSAS does not mean the diagnosis of OSAS can be ruled out. Because snoring is an indication of partial airway obstruction, understanding the potential of the process to worsen over time is important.

4. **What is the surgical management of snoring?**

    Laser-assisted uvulopalatoplasty (LAUP) and Bovie-assisted uvulopalatoplasty (BAUP) are the most commonly used procedures for treatment of snoring. Both procedures involve amputation of the uvula and creation of a 1-cm trench in the soft palate on either side of the uvula. After healing, the soft palate stiffens, reducing its ability to vibrate, and thus reduces snoring. Occasionally the procedure is repeated to resect more tissue without causing velopharyngeal insufficiency. The procedure is usually done under local anesthesia in the office. The advantage of LAUP over BAUP is the prevention of deeper tissue damage and possibility of less postoperative pain, but both procedures are equally effective.

5. **What is obstructive sleep apnea (OSA)?**

    OSA is repetitive, discrete episodes of decreased airflow (hypopnea) or frank cessation of airflow (apnea) for at least a 10-sec duration in association with >2% decrease in oxygen hemoglobin saturation.

6. **Is there a difference between OSA and OSAS?**

    Yes. These are not the same processes. OSA is an objective lab finding. OSAS involves sleep apnea with signs and symptoms of disease.

7. **What are the differences between apnea and hypopnea?**

    Apnea is the cessation of airflow lasting for more than 10 sec. *Hypopnea* refers to a greater than two thirds decrease in tidal volume. Both show a decrease in oxygen saturation of at least 2%.

8. **How many sleep stages are there in normal sleep patterns?**

    There are five sleep stages: one rapid eye movement (REM) stage and four non-REM stages.

9. **During which sleep stages do most obstructive events occur?**

    Stages III and IV and the REM stage, which are the deeper stages of sleep. Pharyngeal wall collapse is more common during these stages because the muscles are most relaxed.

10. **What factors may contribute to OSA events?**

    Anything that effectively causes patient drowsiness may contribute to OSA. Alcohol, sedatives, and narcotics are good examples. Weight gain can also potentiate OSA events, as can allergies and upper respiratory infections.

11. **What is the primary symptom of OSAS?**

    Excessive daytime sleepiness.

12. **What other symptoms of OSAS may be present?**

- Morning headache
- Restless sleep and frequent arousal at night
- Impotence
- Hypertension

13. **What are the important elements of the physical exam of a patient suspected of having OSA?**

    A thorough head and neck exam should be performed in any patient who presents with possible OSA. Exam should include the nose for signs of obstruction or septal deviation, hypertrophic turbinates, and allergic rhinitis. The oral cavity should be examined for large tonsils, redundant soft palate and uvula, redundant lateral pharyngeal walls, macroglossia, and retrognathia. The neck exam should evaluate for thick neck and laryngeal obstruction. The patient should also be examined for signs of cor pulmonale and hypertension.

14. What is the main objective test for diagnosing OSAS?

Polysomnography is the most commonly performed evaluation for diagnosis of OSAS. It comprises the following tests:

- Electroencephalography (EEG)
- Electrooculography (EOG)
- Chin and leg electromyography (EMG)
- Electrocardiography (EKG)
- Nasal and oral airflow
- Thoracic and abdominal efforts
- Pulse oximetry
- The less formal home sleep study and multiple sleep latency tests (MSLTs) may also be included.

15. What is the respiratory disturbance index (RDI)?

The RDI represents the number of obstructive respiratory events per hour of sleep. The RDI along with oximetry is the primary clinical indicator in the diagnosis of OSAS.

16. How is RDI calculated?

$$RDI = apnea + hypopnea/total \ sleep \ time \times 60$$

An RDI of 5 is the upper limit of normal.

17. What is the modified Mueller technique?

While undergoing a fiberoptic nasopharyngoscopy, the patient performs an inspiratory effort against a closed mouth and nose. The examiner observes any oropharyngeal or hypopharyngeal obstruction.

18. How are lateral cephalograms used in evaluation of patients for OSAS?

Cephalometric analysis helps confirm physical exam and fiberoptic nasopharyngoscopy exam results. The following are normal measurements of the cephalogram:

- Sella nasion A point (SNA): 82
- Sella nasion B point (SNB): 80
- Posterior airway space (PAS): 11 mm
- Posterior nasal spine-palate (PNS-P): 35 mm
- Mandibular plane-hyoid (MP-H): 15 mm

19. What is Fujita's classification of upper airway obstruction?

Type I Fujita—upper pharyngeal obstruction including palate, uvula, and tonsils; normal base of tongue

Type II Fujita—type I obstruction plus base of tongue obstruction

Type III Fujita—obstruction at tongue base, supraglottis, and hypopharynx; normal palate

20. What are the classes of sleep apnea?

Obstructive, central, and mixed.

21. What is the difference between OSA and central sleep apnea?

With OSA, there is a normal inspiration effort, but upper airway obstruction causes intermittent cessation of airflow. Central sleep apnea is marked by a lack of inspiratory effort secondary to failure of respiratory centers in the central nervous system to provide the phrenic nerve with appropriate afferent information to activate the diaphragm.

22. Who usually treats central sleep apnea?

Neurologists and sleep specialists.

23. How is OSA classified?

The combination of RDI and oxyhemoglobin desaturation (SaO_2) is a good parameter for scoring OSA severity (Table 49-1).

Table 49-1	*Classification of OSA*	
	RDI	SaO_2
Mild OSA	10-30	>90%
Moderate OSA	30-50	<85%
Severe OSA	>50	<60%

OSA, Obstructive sleep apnea; *RDI,* respiratory disturbance index.

24. What are some systemic complications associated with OSAS?
- Cor pulmonale
- Daytime somnolence
- Death
- Depression
- Hypertension
- Hypoxia
- Polycythemia vera
- Stroke

25. What are the criteria for cure of OSAS?
The surgical cure should have respiratory and sleep results equal to the second night of continuous positive airway pressure (CPAP) titration.

For patients on CPAP, a nonsurgical treatment, cure is determined as:
- A postoperative RDI reduction of at least 50% with a maximum of 20 (i.e., an RDI of 26 should be reduced to 13, and an RDI of 80 should be reduced to 20)
- Postoperative SaO_2 that is normal or with only a few brief falls below 90%
- Normalization of sleep architecture

26. What are the nonsurgical treatment methods for OSAS?
Nasal CPAP is the most effective nonsurgical treatment for OSAS. It consists of an airtight mask held over the nose by a strap wrapped around the patient's head. CPAP is maintained by a machine that is similar to a ventilator. Although nasal CPAP is nearly 100% effective in relieving OSAS, it is very poorly tolerated. Even when it is initially successful, many patients (30% or more) eventually stop using it because of the discomfort.

Tongue-retaining devices and mandibular positioning devices are other nonsurgical methods of treating OSAS. These devices open the airway by holding the tongue or mandible forward during sleep. As with CPAP, discomfort and poor compliance are major problems.

Behavioral modifications, such as weight loss and avoidance of alcohol and sedatives, may also reduce OSAS. Again, patient compliance is a major stumbling block.

27. What are the potential complications of CPAP?

Mask Related:	Pressure/Airflow Related:
Skin rash	Rhinorrhea
Conjunctivitis from air leak	Nasal dryness/congestion
	Chest discomfort
	Sinus discomfort
	Tympanic membrane rupture (rare)
	Massive epistaxis (rare)
	Pneumothorax (rare)

28. What are the surgical options for management of OSAS?
- Tracheotomy
- Uvulopalatopharyngoplasty (UPPP)
- LAUP
- Mandibular osteotomy with genioglossus advancement
- Hyoid suspension

- LA-UPPP
- Tongue reduction
- Maxillary and mandibular advancement

29. What is a "U-triple-P"?

UPPP is a surgical procedure performed to enlarge the oropharyngeal airway in an anterior-superior and lateral direction. The tonsils are removed (if they have not been removed previously), along with the posterior edge of the soft palate, including the uvula. The tonsillar pillars are then sewn together, and the mucosa on the nasal side and oral side of the cut edge of the soft palate are sewn together. This is the most common surgical procedure performed for treatment of OSAS.

30. What are the results of UPPP in treatment of OSAS?

UPPP offers promising results to many patients suffering from OSAS, but success rates vary:
- Elimination of snoring in 80%-100% of cases
- Subjective decrease and improvement in excessive daytime somnolence in 80%-100% of cases
- Measured RDI decrease by approximately 50% in 50% of patients

Despite having an approximate 50% reduction in RDI, a patient may still have significant OSA; therefore UPPP may not improve an OSA patient enough to decrease mortality. CPAP and tracheostomy are still the gold standards to decrease OSA mortality rates.

31. What are the potential complications of UPPP?

Bleeding is the most common postoperative complication. Velopharyngeal insufficiency occurs in 5%-10% of patients but is rarely permanent. Nasopharyngeal stenosis is rare but can be a complication. Other minor complaints include dry mouth, tightness in the throat, and an increased gag reflex.

32. What is the role of LAUP in OSAS?

LAUP is highly effective in the treatment of snoring, with successful results in 85%-90% of patients. However, the effectiveness of LAUP in the treatment of OSAS has not been well established. Snoring and OSAS probably represent a continuum of a similar pathology, but it is still difficult to determine where LAUP is effective and where it is not. Therefore the current recommendation is that all patients should undergo a sleep study before surgery for snoring or OSAS. Additional research is still needed to support the use of LAUP in the treatment of OSAS.

33. What is an appropriate phase I surgical treatment plan for an OSAS patient with an oropharyngeal site of obstruction?

UPPP is excellent for snoring but has only a 40% success rate with OSAS at this obstruction site.

34. What phase I treatment would be appropriate for OSAS in the presence of oropharyngeal and hypopharyngeal obstruction?

UPPP and genioglossus advancement. A modified hyoid myotomy may also be used in phase I surgical treatment.

35. What is the next step after phase I treatment?

CPAP treatment is continued for 6 months, at which time the patient is reevaluated with polysomnography. If phase I treatment is unsuccessful, then phase II surgery would be appropriate. Phase II surgery involves orthognathic surgery, which consists of combined maxillary and mandibular advancement.

36. What is the most effective surgical management of OSAS?

Tracheostomy.

37. What is the success rate of maxillomandibular advancement (MMA) in the treatment of OSAS?

Many consider MMA the most promising surgical alternative to tracheostomy. Although there are currently no long-term studies, recent evidence suggests 100% effectiveness of MMA based on the polysomnographic data. MMA is very effective because it increases upon airway space.

BIBLIOGRAPHY

1. Davila DG: Medical considerations in surgery for sleep apnea. Oral Maxillofac Surg Clin North Am 7:205-217, 1995.
2. Hausfeld JN: Snoring and sleep apnea syndrome. In: American Academy of Otolaryngology—Head and Neck Surgery Foundation: Common Problems of the Head and Neck. Philadelphia, 1992, Saunders.
3. Munoz A: Sleep apnea and snoring. In Jafek BW, Stark AK (eds): ENT Secrets. Philadelphia, 1996, Hanley & Belfus.
4. Nelson PB, Riley RW: A surgical protocol for sleep disordered breathing. Oral Maxillofac Clin North Am 7:345-356, 1995.
5. Nimkam Y, Miles P, Waite P: Maxillomandibular advancement surgery in obstructive sleep apnea syndrome patients: long-term stability. J Oral Maxillofac Surg 53:1414-1418, 1995.
6. Prinsell J: Maxillomandibular advancement surgery: a site-specific treatment approach for obstructive sleep apnea in 50 consecutive patients. Chest 116:1519-1520, 1999.
7. Riley R, Troll R, Powell N: Obstructive sleep apnea syndrome: current surgical concepts. Oral Maxillofac Surg Knowl Update 2:79-97, 1998.
8. Riley RW, Powell NB, Guilleminault C: Maxillofacial surgery and obstructive sleep apnea: a review of 80 patients. Otolaryngol Head Neck Surg 101:353-361, 1989.
9. Sher AE: Obstructive sleep apnea syndrome: a complex disorder of the upper airway. Otolaryngol Clin North Am 23:593-605, 1990.
10. Tina B, Waite P: Surgical and nonsurgical management of obstructive sleep apnea. Principles Oral Maxillofac Surg 3:1531-1547, 1992.

50. FACIAL ALLOPLASTIC IMPLANTS: BIOMATERIALS AND SURGICAL IMPLEMENTATION

Steven G. Gollehon, DDS, MD, FACS, and
John N. Kent, BA, DDS, FACD, FICD

1. What is alloplast? What advantages do alloplastic materials offer today's surgeon?

The term *alloplastic* is synonymous with *synthetic*. This indicates that the material is produced from inorganic sources and contains no animal or human components. Alloplastic materials offer a prepackaged solution to common reconstructive surgical problems without the need for autogenous grafting and donor site morbidity. Moreover, they may greatly decrease operative time and the complexity of surgical procedures.

2. How does biocompatibility factor into the choice of alloplastic augmentation materials?

The success of any alloplastic material depends on its biocompatibility with surrounding host tissues. Material biocompatibility is influenced by the chemical and physical characteristics of the implant material itself, the surgical technique involved, tissue site of implantation, and host reaction to the implant. These complex interactions between the human body and implant explain why so few safe and effective biomaterials exist despite the tremendous advances that have been made in biomaterial development and engineering over the past half century.

3. In the final healing stages after placement of an alloplastic implantable material, what "barrier protection" is essential for long-term implant success?

The final stage of healing after placement of an alloplastic material requires the formation of an encapsulating fibroconnective tissue scar. The formation of this end-stage tissue is initiated by the surgical placement of the alloplast, which produces an initial acute inflammatory response of the adjacent tissues. The response becomes chronic, and the tissue begins to granulate to form an encapsulating foreign body reaction that evolves into the enveloping fibrotic scar. This resulting barrier protects the "foreign" alloplastic material from "self" tissues. In some form, all alloplastic implants will develop fibrous encapsulation. Several features, especially the implant's surface characteristics, have been shown to influence the degree and composition of this capsule.

4. What tissue characteristics are essential for successful placement of an alloplastic material?

The composition of the alloplastic material implanted clearly has an impact on biocompatibility, but the anatomic location and the surgical technique used for alloplast placement exhibit an equal and often greater impact on long-term clinical success. Ensuring that the biomaterial is appropriately matched to the tissue plane within which it will be implanted is ultimately the responsibility of the treating surgeon.

The tissue quality of the area in which the implant is to be placed must be carefully scrutinized for vascularity and soft tissue coverage. Patients with previous irradiation of the area in question may not be candidates for implant placement because the resulting decrease in vascularity impedes the ability of the body to mount an adequate inflammatory response to microbial invasion should the implant become inoculated or secondarily infected.

Tissue overlying an implant should be as thick as possible. Implanting material under thin tissue significantly increases the chances of wound dehiscence, implant exposure, and extrusion in the postoperative period. Implants placed immediately under the dermis or under a thin, subcutaneous tissue layer may eventually cause further thinning, especially if the implant lacks sufficient flexibility or if it is placed in an area of significant tissue mobility. In all cases, the overlying dermis of the skin thins from the pressure of the underlying avascular implant.

5. What are the sequelae of placing alloplastic materials in inflamed or chronically infected tissue?

Placement of alloplasts in or through a contaminated or infected tissue bed greatly increases the chances of implant infection and subsequent failure. Because many implants are unable to tolerate host tissue vascular ingrowth, the lack of vascular supply added to the surface affinity of many alloplasts for bacterial adhesion creates an intolerable environment for alloplast materials. Nothing less than optimum aseptic technique and clean tissue planes are required for alloplast placement.

6. What are the characteristics of an ideal alloplastic implant material?

Kent et al. defined the requirements for an ideal facial implant material:

1. The material is readily available in block and precarved forms and can be carved easily.
2. It can be steam-autoclaved repeatedly.
3. It can be bent or molded to improve bone interface and overlying facial contour.
4. It should be low modulus, permitting deformation to clinical requirement, but not have "memory" characteristics that may lead to mobility, extrusion, or resorption.
5. It should have surface porosity for rapid tissue ingrowth and immediate stabilization on bone and surrounding soft tissue.

6. Deformation or resorption of bone beneath implants from soft tissue and muscle tension should not be clinically significant.
7. Redistribution of soft tissue overlying the face of implant materials should be minimal so that the clinician can determine implant size predictably.
8. The healed tissue implant matrix should have gross physical characteristics approaching bone with supple overlying soft tissue and skin.
9. The material should be osteoconductive or osteophilic to satisfy the clinical requirement of calcified tissue ingrowth and stabilization.
10. The material should have no objectionable color characteristics when used in areas with less than ideal skin coverage.
11. The material should be excised easily if the surgical result is not satisfactory.
12. The material should permit additional augmentation when necessary.
13. The material should be highly biocompatible, exerting no local or distant cytotoxic effects.

Although no single implant material satisfies all the requirements for craniofacial augmentation, several polymers and ceramics satisfy many clinical requirements (Table 50-1).

7.   What special techniques should be used when handling alloplastic materials in the operating room?

Patients undergoing alloplastic biomaterial placement should receive an intravenous antibiotic infusion during placement and an oral course of antibiotics after surgery. Coverage for *Staphylococcus* or *Streptococcus* infection (depending on the path of insertion)—1 g of a first-generation cephalosporin or 600-900 mg of clindamycin—should be given. No other specific antibiotic amount or duration of administration has been shown to be of superior clinical advantage. Because of the hydrophilic nature of some implants, additional antibiotic coverage can be achieved by washing or soaking the implant before intraoperative insertion. Finally, the implant should be kept in its sterile packing until ready for placement. Clean instruments should be used to handle the implant; handling the implant with the gloved hand should be kept to a minimum. Some authors even advocate donning fresh sterile gloves if the implant is to be handled. Contact with the surrounding skin, soft tissues, and oral cavity should be kept to a minimum to prevent bacterial inoculation onto the implant's surface. Currently, no studies confirm that this treatment has a significant effect on preventing postoperative infections. However, these precautions will limit contamination and therefore improve implant success and survival.

8.   What are the advantages of dimethylsiloxane (silicone) implant materials?

A combination of bulk and preformed silicone rubber implants with or without polymer fabric has been used to augment frontal, zygomatic, nasal, chin, parasymphyseal, paranasal, orbital, maxillary, malar, nasal dorsum, columella, ear, and mandible deficiencies. Their history of clinical acceptance is the longest of all facial implant materials. Despite recent criticism stemming from the breast implant controversy, silicone implants have been used since the 1950s. Preformed silicone is available commercially for many facial applications, and room temperature, vulcanizing silicone may be used to customize implant shapes for specific deformities. Because implant migration and extrusion remain a major problem, other advantages are the ease of intraoperative modification with scalpel or scissors and the stability with screw or suture fixation. The material's "memory" demands adaptation to bone contour in the relaxed state because bending may lead to extrusion or bone resorption. Silicone implants are easily sterilized by steam autoclave or irradiation without damage to the implant composition. In addition, silicone is widely used throughout the medical and surgical community because of the lack of adverse tissue reactivity; only a thin to moderate fibrous tissue capsule forms without ingrowth, and tissue reactions are acceptable if there is adequate soft tissue coverage and bony stabilization. Porous silicone implants and silicone bonded to Dacron with Silastic Medical Grade Adhesive Type A (Wright Dow Corning) have been used to enhance stability. Porous silicone can be used successfully only where functional load and tissue movement will not induce implant tearing and fracture.

Table 50-1   Commonly Used Facial Alloplasts: Clinical Considerations

	SOLID SILICONE RUBBER	PMMA	POROUS PMMA	HA PTFE	EXPANDED PTFE	MESHED POLYMER	POROUS POLYETHYLENE	DENSE HA	POROUS HA
Surface porosity	−	−	+	+	−	+	+	−	+
Modules of elasticity	−	−	−	+	−	+	−	−	−
Memory	−	±	±	+	−	+	±	±	±
Adaptability	+	+	+	+	+	+	−	−	−
Color	+	+	+	+	+	+	+	+	+
Ease of removal	+	+	−	+	+	−	−	+	−
Osteophilic	−	−	−	+	−	−	−	+	+
Displacement	−	−	+	+	±	+	−	+	+
Bone resorption	−	−	−	−	+	±	+	+	+
Soft tissue reaction	+	−	−	+	+	−	±	+	+
Degradation	+	+	+	+	+	−	+	+	+

+, Advantages; −, disadvantages; *PMMA*, polymethylmethacrylate; *HA*, hydroxyapatite; *PTFE*, polytetrafluoroethylene.

9.   What has been the evolution of the use of polytetrafluoroethylene (PTFE)?

PTFE was originally marketed as Proplast in the 1980s. The FDA withdrew Proplast from the market because of material fragmentation and subsequent foreign body reactions due to mechanical loading as a glenoid fossa replacement in temporomandibular joint (TMJ) reconstruction. It has reappeared as GORE-TEX, an expanded microporous polymer of PTFE that is useful in the subcutaneous augmentation of bony and soft tissue contour defects associated with craniofacial deformities.

GORE-TEX is available in 1-, 2-, and 4-mm sheets that can be trimmed easily and placed subcutaneously by a variety of open and closed techniques. GORE-TEX, as demonstrated in several animal model studies, produces minimal foreign body reaction and elicits a delicate fibrous encapsulation. The microporous nature of this material allows minimal soft tissue ingrowth, which stabilizes the alloplast but allows easy removal if indicated. It was approved by the FDA as an implant material for facial applications in 1994 and has been used for subdermal implantation in the lip, nasolabial folds, glabella, nasal dorsum, and other subcutaneous facial defects. In addition, it has gained popularity for bony augmentation of the midface, malar, and mandibular areas. The fibrillar composition results in noninterconnected surface openings with pore sizes between 10 and 30 μm. This allows for microvascular ingrowth and minimal fibroconnective tissue encapsulation.

10.   Why has the use of polyethylene increased recently?

Polyethylene (Medpor) is a nonresorbable, porous (pore size: 125-250 μm) material that possesses high tensile strength. This biocompatible alloplast can be carved, contoured, and adapted three-dimensionally in the reconstruction of facial deformities. Animal studies demonstrate minimal foreign body response to the thin, fibrous capsule that forms around the polyethylene implant. In addition, this encapsulation is not associated with significant contraction. The porosity of Medpor allows rapid tissue and vascular ingrowth, but it is hard, difficult to sculpt, and not truly osteoconductive (although some limited bony ingrowth may occur). This material currently is being used in applications such as temporal contour reconstruction and midfacial and mandibular augmentation.

11.   What are the disadvantages of polymethylmethacrylate (PMMA) as an implant material?

Acrylic biomaterials are derived from polymerized esters of either acrylic or methylacrylic acids. With a long history of use in orthopaedic surgery as a bone cement for joint prostheses, PMMA resin is fabricated intraoperatively by mixing a liquid monomer with a powdered polymer to create a rigid, nearly translucent plastic. Unfortunately, PMMA has some downsides:

- PMMA has an offensive odor when mixed.
- Its fumes are teratogenic, so female personnel who are pregnant or who are planning to become pregnant must leave the operating room.
- The exothermic reaction created as the two polymers cure (8-10 min) can reach as high as 80° C. Cool irrigation is necessary to prevent adjacent tissue damage secondary to this high curing temperature.
- Bacteria have a high affinity for adherence to the surface of the material. Therefore it cannot be placed in areas where indigent opportunistic microbes reside, such as the oral cavity or the paranasal sinuses.

12.   How can PMMA's disadvantages be bypassed?

- Preoperative wax-up models can be fabricated and subsequent impressions can be reproduced in stone. From this model, an accurate acrylic implant can be fabricated, gas-sterilized, and brought to the operating room for placement, ensuring accurate fit, decreased operative time, and the absence of tissue damage from the heat of polymerization.
- Antibiotics can be combined with the acrylic mixture to further reduce the incidence of microbial inoculation and implant failure.

- Although PMMA is rigid, the adjunctive use of metal mesh reinforcement decreases the risk of fracture on impact and more closely approximates the strength of cranial bone.

13. What are the most common uses of PMMA today?

PMMA is used most often in forehead contouring and cranioplasty procedures for full-thickness skull defects.

14. What is HTR-PMI?

Hard tissue replacement (HTR) is a composite of PMMA and polyhydroxyethyl-methacrylate that has significant strength, interconnected porosity, significant hydrophilicity, and a calcium hydroxide coating that imparts a negative surface charge. Although it has a long clinical history of use in dentistry and jaw implantation as a granular bone replacement material, it is also available as a preformed craniofacial implant that is custom manufactured to the patient's defect from a computed tomography (CT) scan (HTR-PMI; Walter Lorenz Surgical, Jacksonville, Fla). It is useful as a replacement for large, full-thickness defects involving the cranial, frontal, and orbital regions where sufficient autologous material may not be available or where there is significant morbidity with the size of the donor defect.

15. What are the major advantages and disadvantages of calcium phosphate ceramic implantable materials?

Hydroxyapatite and related calcium materials interact with and may ultimately become an integral part of living bone tissue. All current calcium phosphate biomaterials can be classified as **polycrystalline** ceramics. Either porous or dense ceramic forms can serve as a permanent bone implant, because they show no tendency to bioresorb. Limitations of calcium phosphate implant materials subtend their mechanical properties. These materials are brittle, with low-impact resistance and relatively low strength. Biocompatibility of calcium phosphate ceramics is excellent and body response is characteristic, whether solid or porous. They appear to become directly bonded to bone by natural bone-cementing mechanisms; bone is deposited without intervening fibrous tissue. A great advantage of these alloplasts is their ability to osteoconduct with actual tissue ingrowth and incorporate into the surrounding tissue.

Unfortunately, these alloplasts offer no osteoinductive potential. Hydroxyapatite granules became available in the early 1980s for maxillofacial reconstruction, particularly alveolar ridge augmentation. Block forms (Interpore, CeraMed) of these alloplasts have been successful as interpositional grafts in facial osteotomies; however, because of their potential for fracture or fragmentation, they should not be used in load-bearing areas. Nonceramic hydroxyapatite is available in powder and liquid forms. Either form may be mixed intraoperatively and used to fill bony defects. Within 10-15 min after placement, the substance undergoes direct crystallization to form pure hydroxyapatite. Currently, two forms of calcium carbonate cement are available: Bone Source and CRC. The current thinking is that these cements will develop significant bony ingrowth and the alloplast will eventually need to be replaced. Prospective studies will need to be done to see if this is true.

16. What is the difference between intraoral and extraoral access in the placement of alloplastic facial implants?

Adequate native or transplanted covering without excessive tension is necessary to ensure the acceptance of any graft or facial implant. The extraoral approach for facial augmentation offers the advantages of accurate placement and ease of access. The intraoral approach has the advantage of no visible scar but carries a higher rate of infection.

17. What perioperative and intraoperative techniques help ensure consistent success of facial alloplasts?

Implants should lie in healthy tissue away from regions of excessive scarring or areas of irradiation. The implant should be buried as deeply as possible in a supraperiosteal pocket or placed directly on bone if the implant is porous or osteophilic. Preoperatively determined landmarks, measurements, facial moulage, or three-dimensional imaging should be used to ensure accurate placement. Frequent scalpel blade changes are required when carving the implant to feather edges that would otherwise be palpable. A broad, firm contact of the implant with underlying closures is preferred, particularly with intraoral techniques. Compression of implant pores should be avoided. Appropriate antibiotic protocol should be followed before and after surgery, and a porous implant should be soaked in antibiotic or vacuum impregnated upon implantation. The implant should be sutured, wired, or screwed into position firmly and further supported with a compressive dressing to minimize dead space and hematoma formation.

18. What information should patients understand about alloplastic augmentation materials and surgery in order to give true informed consent?

The success of implants is dependent on physical characteristics, biologic response, proper preparation and handling, clinical experience, surgical technique, and postoperative patient management. Patient compliance, ensured through proper selection and thorough explanation, is extremely important. Potential complications include:

- Infection
- Untoward reaction to medication, anesthesia, or surgical procedures
- Poor wound healing
- Hematoma
- Seroma
- Motor or sensory nerve damage or irritation
- Neuralgia

- Loss of sensation
- Intolerance to any foreign implant
- Unremitting previously established symptoms
- Changes in surrounding tissue
- Implant migration
- Extrusion or structural failure
- Additional surgical intervention

19. Which intraoral or extraoral approaches should be used for the placement of alloplastic materials in the mandibular symphysis, ramus, or inferior border?

These deficiencies are either vertical or lateral and may be corrected by either an intraoral or extraoral approach. Preformed and carved alloplasts can be constructed to exact specification using facial three-dimensional CT or moulage. Autogenous bone or hydroxyapatite grafts can be fashioned to correct these contour defects as well. The **intraoral approach** requires a standard genioplasty incision and dissection of the mandibular symphysis; a vertical vestibular incision similar to that used for ramus osteotomy through periosteum and a subperiosteal dissection is completed along the lateral surface of the angle and ascending ramus. Curved elevators facilitate release of the soft tissue attachments along the inferior border and posterior ramus. An appropriately contoured ramus angle implant is inserted into the subperiosteal pocket, and bone screws are used to secure the implant to the lateral cortex of the mandible.

The **extraoral technique** for angle and inferior border augmentation involves the standard submandibular approach. A modified Risdon incision is made, preferably in an existing rhytid through subcutaneous fat down to the platysma muscle. The platysma is then divided segmentally with blunt hemostats. A nerve tester set at 2 mA is used to test selectively for the cervical and marginal mandibular branches of the facial nerve as they dip below the inferior border of the mandible. Once divided, the platysma is retracted superiorly and inferiorly in the surgical field, exposing the superficial layer of the deep cervical fascia. Great care must be taken because the facial nerve lies in this layer. Once encountered, the nerve is selectively freed and retracted superiorly. In addition, anteriorly, the facial artery and vein are usually encountered near the submandibular lymph node. These vessels must be ligated if they become an obstacle in the proper placement of the implant. Should they become breached during the surgical procedure, the likelihood of a postoperative hematoma is extremely great and will adversely affect the successful integration of the implant without infection or need for repeat surgery. After the nerve and vessels have been addressed, careful dissection of a pocket along the posterolateral border of the mandibular angle under the pterygomasseteric sling is done, and atraumatic placement of the implant and subsequent fixation can be done with ease. The site is irrigated with copious amounts of antibiotic-impregnated saline, and a careful layered closure is achieved with resorbable suture. Placement of a Jobst jaw bra with 4- × 4-inch dressings over the mandibular angles for 48 hr achieves good postoperative stability and minimizes swelling. Most patients tolerate this postoperative regimen extremely well because they can resume their normal activities within 1-2 days.

20. How are asymmetric mandibular excesses corrected?
Vertical inferior border excesses and outward bowing of the mandible in patients with condylar hyperplasia may require reduction by either an inferior border resection or a horizontal wedge osteotomy procedure, usually through an intraoral vestibular approach. Inferior border leveling by this technique also provides autogenous bone, which may be required for augmentation of the contralateral angle ramus or inferior border. A horizontal wedge osteotomy procedure relocates the inferior border and its soft tissue attachments superiorly but requires difficult repositioning of the inferior alveolar nerve.

21. What implant considerations must be made before augmentation of the chin in a vertical vs. horizontal dimension?
The versatility of the sliding horizontal osteotomy of the mandibular symphysis is well documented and is used to correct asymmetries of the chin by reducing or increasing the vertical height of the chin or its anterior and posterior projection. Hydroxyapatite blocks and autogenous grafts are most suitable for lengthening, whereas silicone rubber and other polymer implants have been used successfully in the correction of parasymphyseal contour deficiencies (either lateral or anterior), occasionally in conjunction with a horizontal osteotomy.

22. Which access is best for augmentation of the mandibular symphysis? What methods of fixation of osteotomies or implants are indicated?
The osteotomy or alloplast implant placement is accomplished most easily by an intraoral approach through a mucosal incision anterior to the depth of the mucobuccal fold through the underlying mentalis muscle. The symphysis and inferior border soft tissue are degloved for placement of the implant to advance soft tissue; the soft tissue remains attached to the symphysis when a horizontal osteotomy is performed. Implants are stabilized with screws or sutures, and the osteotomized symphysis is stabilized with screws or bone plates.

23. What is the difference between use of zygomatic complex osteotomies vs. the placement of zygomatic implants to correct malar deficiencies?
Residual depression or flattening of the malar eminence is noted before or, more clearly, after conventional osteotomies to correct the maxillary and mandibular deformities. Occasionally, the correction of malar deficiency is significant enough to warrant zygomatic complex osteotomies. The use of autogenous tissues for onlay grafting sometimes is unpredictable secondary to variable resorption. Alloplasts are used to correct these problems.

24. What implant materials could be considered for placement of malar implants?
Particulate hydroxyapatite may be used, but preventing migration of hydroxyapatite from the desired augmentation site during placement is a technically demanding procedure. Block forms of hydroxyapatite have been used successfully for infraorbital augmentation; however, their brittle nature makes lateral malar augmentation difficult. The use of polyethylene (Medpor) makes augmentation of this aspect of the facial skeleton much more simple and predictable.

25. What surgical approach is indicated for the placement of malar implants? How are they stabilized?
For the intraoral approach to zygomatic augmentation:
1. A standard horizontal vestibular incision is made above the maxillary canine and premolar teeth through the small facial muscles overlying the anterior maxilla and zygomatic bone.

2. A subperiosteal dissection extending from the medial infraorbital rim across the body of the zygoma is completed.
3. The infraorbital nerve is identified and isolated, thus preventing inadvertent injury.
4. The implant is carved to fit into the preformed soft tissue pocket, over the zygomatic arch, and stabilized with screws, sutures, or wires.

26. How are alloplastic materials used in the correction of saddle nose deformities in the nasal dorsum?

In a saddle nose deformity, the nasal dorsum lacks adequate ventral projection. The condition is occasionally congenital but more often results from trauma, infection, or excessive resection of the septum. The saddle formation may affect the bone or the cartilaginous nasal dorsum in isolation or include both structures. The guideline for correction includes the outer deformity in addition to a thorough analysis of the function of the internal nasal airway. The collapse of the nasal dorsum is always associated with impairment of nasal airflow, which becomes greater as the saddle formation extends further caudally. Alloplastic implants are readily available, preformed, and easy to use for these purposes. They do not deform and are negligibly resorbable. Conversely, there remains the lifelong risk of extrusion or infection because of their anatomic location.

27. What is the role of alloplastic implants in the correction of craniofacial defects?

Alloplasts have done very well in recent years in improving the long-term results of craniofacial defect reconstruction. These defects usually are approached through a coronal incision, exposing the defect in a subperiosteal plane. The temporal branches of the facial nerve are avoided through careful dissection lateral and superior to the supraorbital ridges beneath the deep layer of the superficial temporal fascia. Once the defect is exposed, the underlying dura is thoroughly neurosurgically evaluated, with repair, if necessary, using pericranium or lyophilized dura. Various alloplastic augmentation materials may be used, including PMMA and the newer calcium carbonate cements. Once fixed or set, the contours of these materials may be adjusted with burrs to achieve an acceptable aesthetic result. Reinforcement with titanium mesh to achieve optimum postoperative strength and stability can be done easily and offers extra protection and comfort to the patient.

BIBLIOGRAPHY

1. Artz JS, Dinner MI: The use of expanded polytetrafluoroethylene as a permanent filler and enhancer: an early report of experience. Ann Plast Surg 32:457-462, 1994.
2. Bessette RW, Casey DM, Shatkin SS et al: Customized silicone rubber maxillofacial implants. Ann Plast Surg 7:453-457, 1981.
3. Chisholm BB, Lew D, Sadasivan K: The use of tobramycin-impregnated polymethylmethacrylate beads in the treatment of osteomyelitis of the mandible: report of three cases. J Oral Maxillofac Surg 51:444-449, 1993.
4. Eppley BL: Alloplastic implantation. Plast Reconstr Surg 104:1761-1783, 1999.
5. Eppley BL, Prevel CD, Sadove AM: Resorbable bone fixation: its potential role in craniomaxillofacial trauma. J Craniomaxillofac Trauma 2:56-61, 1996.
6. Kent JN, Craig MA: Secondary autogenous and alloplastic reshaping procedures. Atlas Oral Maxillofac Surg Clin North Am 4:83-105, 1996.
7. Kent JN, Misiek DJ: Biomaterials for cranial, facial, mandibular and temporomandibular joint reconstruction. In Fonseca R, Walker R (eds): Oral and Maxillofacial Trauma, 2nd vol. Philadelphia, 1991, Saunders.
8. Kent JN, Misiek DJ, Kinnebrew MC: Alloplastic materials for augmentation in cosmetic surgery. In Peterson L (ed): Principles of Maxillofacial Surgery, 3rd vol. Philadelphia, 1992, J.B. Lippincott.
9. Lacey M, Antonyshyn O: Use of porous high-density polyethylene implants in temporal contour reconstruction. J Craniofac Surg 4:74-78, 1993.
10. Lin PH, Hirko MK, von Fraunhofer JA et al: Wound healing and inflammatory response to biomaterials. In Chu CC, von Fraunhofer JA, Greisler HP (eds): Wound Closure Biomaterials and Devices. New York, 1997, CRC Press.

11. Maas CS, Gnepp DR: Expanded polytetrafluoroethylene (GORE-TEX soft tissue patch) in facial augmentation. Arch Otolaryngol Head Neck Surg 119:1008-1017, 1993.
12. Park JB, Lakes RS: Polymeric implant materials. In Park JB, Lakes RS (eds): Biomaterials: An Introduction. New York, 1992, Plenum.
13. Ripamonti U, Petit JC, Moehl T et al: Immediate reconstruction of massive cranio-orbito-facial defects with allogeneic and alloplastic matrices in baboons. J Craniomaxillofac Surg 21:302-308, 1993.
14. Rubin JP, Yaremchuk MJ: Complications and toxicities of implantable biomaterials used in facial reconstructive and aesthetic surgery: a comprehensive review of the literature. Plast Reconstr Surg 100:1336-1356, 1997.
15. Schoenrock LD, Reppucci AD: Correction of subcutaneous facial defects using GORE-TEX. Facial Plast Surg Clin North Am 2:373-389, 1994.
16. Silver FH, Maas CS: Biology of facial implant materials. Facial Plast Surg Clin North Am 2:241-254, 1994.
17. Szabo G, Suba Z, Barabas J: Use of Bioplant HTR synthetic bone to eliminate major jawbone defects: long-term human histologic examinations. J Craniomaxillofac Surg 25:63-68, 1997.
18. Yukna RA: Clinical evaluation of HTR polymer bone replacement grafts in human mandibular class II molar furcations. J Periodontol 65:342-349, 1994.

51. APPLICATION AND INTERVIEW PROCESSES FOR ORAL AND MAXILLOFACIAL SURGERY RESIDENCY PROGRAMS

Esther S. Oh, DDS

1.   What should I do if I am interested in oral and maxillofacial surgery (OMFS)?

Because an OMFS residency is a long-term commitment, the decision is a major one. Dental students consider an OMFS career at different stages during their dental school education and after, but it is never too early to speak to an oral and maxillofacial surgeon (faculty or private practitioner) about your interest and concerns. Try to get as much experience as possible through dental school rotations, observing in the operating room, externships, and volunteering in a private practice. The more exposure you have to the OMFS field, the more likely you will be able to either confirm or change your choice.

2.   What is the difference between PASS and Match?

PASS, which stands for Postdoctoral Application Support Service, acts as a centralized clearing house for all applicants to postdoctoral dental education programs. This organization allows you to complete and send a single standardized application to multiple schools with the click of a button. In addition, it allows dental programs to receive uniform information on all its applicants. Usually the application is available around mid-May of each year, then invitations for interviews are given for October through December.

Match is short for Postdoctoral Dental Matching Program, sponsored by National Matching Services, Inc., and is a separate organization that places applicants into first-year dental residency training programs. Besides OMFS, other residencies that participate include Advanced Education in General Dentistry (AEGD), General Practice Residency (GPR), Orthodontics, and Pediatrics. After applying to and interviewing at OMFS programs, you will rank the interviewed programs in order of preference of where you would like to attend. You are not required to rank all the programs interviewed, only the ones you would consider attending if you are "matched" there. The OMFS programs that interview you follow the same guidelines. Once the rank lists are submitted, a computer generates the results based on "the game theory" and matches you to one program, to which you are bound by contract to attend. The match list usually is due early January, and the results are given at the end of January.

Almost all OMFS programs participate in both PASS and Match, and therefore you need to apply to both. Be sure to check the website for relevant information and dates and apply as early as possible: www.adea.org/pass.

3.   To how many and to which OMFS programs should I apply?

Most OMFS applicants apply to an average of 16 programs, so be prepared for a costly investment. Several versions of OMFS residencies are offered, including dental school–based or hospital-based programs, and those that offer additional degrees for additional years, such as an MD, PhD, or MS programs. Those that offer the MD degree are 6 years long and are either MD-integrated (medical school is imbedded within the 6 years of training) or MD-optional (medical school is completed after the 4 years of OMFS training). Successful completion of the USMLE (United States Medical Licensing Examination) is required for the MD programs and consists of steps 1, 2, and 3 taken at different points during your training.

Another consideration includes the program's location. If possible, try not to rule out programs based on geography; there are many top-quality training centers in not-so-ideal locations that would make the sacrifice well worth it. Consult the OMFS faculty and residents for guidance on where to apply based on your expectations and preferences. The American Student Dental Association (ASDA) offers an OMFS Postdoctoral Program Guide that may be purchased from their website: www.asdanet.org.

4.   Should I do the 4- or 6-year program?

About half the OMFS programs offer 4-year OMFS certificates, half offer 6-year MD degrees, and a few offer both 4- and 6-year tracks. Although this is a controversial topic within the OMFS field, neither is superior to the other, and the decision as to which to choose is a personal one. For example, many applicants who plan to pursue private practice usually opt for the 4-year track, whereas some common reasons to pursue the 6-year degree include the desire to attend medical school, plans to apply for a fellowship, entering academics (although an MD is not required to teach), or the desire to use the MD degree as an extra marketing tool in private practice. Some applicants apply to both 4- and 6-year programs, but most have a preference before applying. Your opinion on this topic is sure to be asked during your interviews, so be prepared to have a definitive answer!

5.   What is the difference between an externship, internship, and fellowship?

During an **externship,** a dental student visits a program voluntarily for a short period (usually 1-4 weeks) to gain additional exposure to OMFS. Ideally, you should do an externship where you plan to apply, and therefore it is imperative to work hard and get along with the residents. You should consult your OMFS faculty and residents for their recommendations. Usually, externships are done during the third year of dental school and are a good way to put a face to your application. Because an interview exposes you to people who are on their best behavior during a short period, an externship will allow you to see the inner workings of that program.

In an **internship,** a dental school graduate participates for 1 year at a program that has a similar schedule as for a first-year OMFS resident. Graduates choose this option either to gain additional experience and confirm their decision to pursue OMFS or to improve their application for the next PASS/Match cycle. Usually, internship applications are not through the Match program and can take place before or after the results of the Match are posted.

In a **fellowship,** graduates of an OMFS residency choose to pursue further training and focus on an area of interest within the specialty of OMFS. Common fellowships include craniofacial surgery, cosmetic surgery, oncology and reconstructive surgery, microneurosurgery, and orthognathic surgery. These programs are offered in the United States and overseas, and many prefer the applicant to have a 6-year MD degree.

6. **What are AAOMS, ROAAOMS, ABOMS, and JOMS?**

AAOMS is the American Association of Oral and Maxillofacial Surgeons. It is a nonprofit professional organization that helps address the public and professional needs of the specialty through education, research, and advocacy. For more information, go to www.aaoms.org.

ROAAOMS is the Resident Organization of the American Association of Oral and Maxillofacial Surgeons. It was established in 1994 to provide a forum and support network for residents' issues. If you are enrolled in an accredited OMFS residency, your membership in the ROAAOMS is automatic.

ABOMS is the American Board of Oral and Maxillofacial Surgeons, which is the professional organization that governs the specialty. It offers an oral and written board examination that challenges the knowledge and clinical competence of the oral and maxillofacial surgery residency graduate. The written examination can be taken the year of graduation from a residency program or thereafter. The oral portion of the examination is usually taken a few years after successful completion of the written examination. A surgeon is a "diplomate" or "boarded" when he or she has successfully passed both the oral and written examinations. Only graduates of accredited American or Canadian oral and maxillofacial surgery programs are eligible to take the examination. Although optional, most surgeons choose to go through this process for quality assurance and as a marketing tool. For more information, visit www.aboms.org.

JOMS stands for the Journal of Oral and Maxillofacial Surgery. It is the monthly publication of the AAOMS. This journal is peer reviewed and publishes scientific and clinical articles related to the OMFS specialty, new products, and innovations within the OMFS field. For more information, visit www.joms.org.

7. **How important is research for the application to OMFS residency? How important is the essay?**

Although research is not required, it is highly recommended, even if the topic is not within the scope of OMFS. Most applicants will have done research, and therefore the experience will help keep you on an even playing field. In addition, it will show your ability to move beyond the required curriculum to enhance your critical thinking skills.

The essay has different priorities for different programs, but the reviewers probably will appreciate that you keep it short and to the point. Mostly they will make sure you can read and write English. Therefore it is imperative not to have spelling or grammar errors. Inevitably, most essays will sound the same, so just make sure you do not stick out in a bad way.

8. **Who should I ask for recommendation letters?**

PASS requires four letters of recommendation: one from the institution's dean, and then three evaluators of your choice. Some programs may allow additional letters to be sent to them directly. Ideally, you should ask only oral and maxillofacial surgeons, because they will have the most clout when explaining to their colleagues why you have what it takes to make a contribution to their field. Big names always help, but the reader of the evaluation will know if the writer is a stranger to you. Try to give a minimum of 1 month for the person to write the recommendation for you, and be sure to provide them with your curriculum vitae, address of where to send the letter, required postage, any additional specifications, and your contact information for any further questions.

9. **How should I prepare for interviews?**

After submitting your applications, the most difficult part is waiting. You can occupy your time by preparing a professional-looking suit, comfortable shoes for a fair amount of walking, and a less formal outfit for dinner (remember it is always safer to overdress rather than underdress). You also can read different journals to monitor the latest trends in the OMFS field, as well as familiarize yourself with the details of your own research project(s). Ask OMFS faculty and residents at your school to conduct a mock interview, during which you can practice your handshake and eye contact; going through the process will put you more at ease during the real thing.

Once you start getting interview invitations, that's when the fun begins. If they have not provided the information already, ask about the closest airport and recommended hotels, itinerary, specific names of the interviewers, expected weather, and the dress code for dinner. You can "Google" the program and the individual interviewers to familiarize yourself with their research/interests and any other well-known facts. Reading about and possibly visiting the city's main attractions may be helpful in your final decision as well.

You may get multiple interviews for similar timeframes, so book plane tickets no earlier than 2-4 weeks in advance to avoid having to cancel or rebook flights. Try to capitalize on frequent flyer miles, and use a credit card that will give you additional miles. Regardless of the travel day, booking airline tickets on a Tuesday seems to be less expensive than other days. Reserving an aisle seat near the front will allow for easy access to the bathroom and exit off the plane. Because this is not the ideal time for the airline to lose your luggage, try to pack so you don't have to check any bags. You can save money by coordinating with other applicants to share hotel rooms or car rentals. Also, now is the time to get your school requirements in order so you can be as flexible as possible for your interviews.

10. What should I do if interview dates conflict?

Because most programs offer only one date, this conflict is inevitable. You may try to ask the program administrators if they can be flexible, but most likely you will have to make a choice. Each program averages only 15-20 interviewees for two or three spots. Therefore try to extend the courtesy of notifying the program of your cancellation as soon as possible so they can offer the opportunity to another hopeful applicant. If you have difficulty deciding which program to go to and which interviews to cancel, ask the OMFS faculty and residents at your school to help you decide.

11. What is involved in an interview?

Often the day begins with breakfast and a presentation of the program's curriculum and highlights. A dinner outing is occasionally offered by the program before or after the main interview day. The actual interview with the faculty and residents will be conducted one-on-one or two-on-one, or you may be faced with a panel of about 10 interviewers at once. Some common questions they will ask include, "Why OMFS?" "Do you want to do a 4- or 6-year program, and why?" and "Do you have any questions for us?" Some programs may ask difficult questions, or they may have you perform a task in front of them (i.e., read a computed tomogram, apply a suture, or place an arch bar). Don't worry if you do not have the correct response; usually they are just trying to gauge how you handle stressful situations. It is okay to acknowledge your deficiency and show them you are teachable.

12. What kinds of questions should I ask?

Try to maintain a delicate balance between academic and personal questions. Make sure you do not ask questions that can be found on the program's website, and save questions such as the amount of vacation you get until an appropriate time. You should maintain a positive tone, even if asking about something negative. For example, instead of, "What's bad about this program?" you could say, "What would you change?" Or if you want to ask, "Do you have a life outside of residency?" you could instead inquire, "What do you do in your free time?" Some questions are designated for the faculty (i.e., ABOMS pass rate, curriculum structure, where graduates go afterward, if a surgical anatomy course is offered), and some are geared more toward the residents (i.e., are they happy, would they do it again, amount of implant and outpatient anesthesia experience, how often is an attending present, what percent of surgeries do the residents cut [vs. faculty or fellow]). Some information can be gathered through casual conversation (i.e., number of residents who are single vs. those who are married/kids, relationship with the Otolaryngology/Plastic Surgery/Periodontics departments, or affiliation with a GPR).

13. What are they looking for when they interview me?

The main focus of the interview is to see who will be the best fit for their program. Faculty may look for someone who is humble and teachable as well as articulate, well informed about the profession, and who can represent their program well. Residents also have input in the decision and usually look for someone who is a "team player" and who they want to be around for the next 4-6 years. Therefore you should try to balance your time between the residents and the other interviewees. Most likely you will see many of the same people at multiple interviews, and they may become your future co-residents. You may want to keep their contact information to keep a professional and personal network, as well as stay updated on where everyone matches.

Try not to be too talkative and annoying, or too quiet and unmemorable. In addition, do not be weird or arrogant/insecure; remember that your academic qualifications got you the interview, but it is your personality that will seal the deal. Although it may be tempting to carry around a notepad, avoid looking too nerdy; keep mental notes instead. Again, the key is not to stick out in a bad way. With all that said, try to smile, be yourself, and enjoy the privilege of meeting new people and seeing new places.

14. What should I do after interviews?

Once you have returned home from an interview, send a personal thank-you note within a week. Also, you should review your experience and write down details that will help you rank the programs. One possible strategy is to list several significant categories and write notes in each column for each program. Some topics may include: city/social life, cost of living, current residents (especially the upcoming chiefs) and their personality/chemistry, faculty, staff, caseload, salary, tuition, benefits, call schedule, vacation, extramural rotations offered, other unique traits, and your gut feeling.

Do not play the game of ranking the programs based on whether that program will rank you high. Instead, be honest with yourself and rank the list in order of your true preference. Also, do not rank programs where you know you will not be happy. If you do, you are creating the possibility of being stuck and miserable there for the next 4-6 years. Some programs may go against the Match policy and call or write you to offer "hints," but these promises are neither safe nor guaranteed until Match day, when all will be revealed. You can keep in touch with the other applicants directly, or participate in the discussion forums on www.studentdoctor.net or www.asdanet.org.

Index

A

AAC (antibiotic-associated colitis), 313
AAOMS (American Association of Oral and
    Maxillofacial Surgeons), 438
ABCD mnemonic, for injury evaluation, 115,
    120-121, 134
Abdomen
    evaluation of traumatic injury to, 137
    preoperative exam of, 18, 20
    radiographic evaluation of, 54
ABOMS (American Board of Oral and
    Maxillofacial Surgeons), 438
Abrasions, soft tissue, 283
Abscess
    cellulitis vs., 296
    defined, 295
    drug of choice for, 320
    revealing in tomography scan, 62
Absorption, laser, 376
ACE (angiotensin-converting enzyme) inhibitors
    as congestive heart failure treatment, 171
    as hypertension treatment, 162
    hypertension treatment, 167
Acetaminophen
    as Class B analgesic, 224
    contraindicated in renal disease, 189, 191
    metabolized by liver, 185
Acetylcholinesterase inhibitors, 89
Achondroplasia, 354
Acid-base disorders
    classifications of, 46-47
    signs of, 98
Acid-fast stains, 49
Acne, dermabrasion for, 409
Acquired immunodeficiency syndrome. See AIDS
    (acquired immunodeficiency syndrome)
ACT (activated clotting time), 38
ACTH (adrenocorticotropic hormone), 199
Actinomycosis, 315, 317
Activated clotting time (ACT), 38
Acute renal failure. See ARF (acute renal failure)
Acyclovir, formulations, 308
Adenoid cystic carcinoma, of salivary glands, 4,
    363
Adenoma
    nonsecreting chromophobe, 196
    pleomorphic, 4, 363
    as type of MENS, 195
Adenosine, resuscitation dosage, 133

ADH (antidiuretic hormone). See also SIADH
    (syndrome of inappropriate antidiuretic
    hormone)
    known as vasopressin, 192
    production of, 193
    release of, 193
    TBW maintenance, 93
Admission orders, surgical notes, 11
Adrenal crisis, 195
Adrenal insufficiency, 192, 195
Adrenal medulla, epinephrine release from, 205
Adrenergic inhibitors, treating hypertension,
    168-169
Adrenocorticotropic hormone (ACTH), 199
Adult respiratory distress syndrome (ARDS), 177
Advanced cardiac life support, 120-133
Advanced Education in General Dentistry
    (AEGD), 436
Advanced glycosylation end-products (AGE), 201
Advanced trauma life support, 134-140
AED (automated external defibrillator), 117-118
AEGD (Advanced Education in General
    Dentistry), 436
Aerobes
    found in oral cavity, 292
    in odontogenic infections, 294
A-fib, 125
A-flutter, 125
AFP (alpha-fetoprotein), as cancer marker, 50
Age, induction agent dose and, 80
AGEs (advanced glycosylation end-products), 201
AIDS (acquired immunodeficiency syndrome)
    chest radiographs in, 54
    clinical manifestations of, 211-212
    drug therapy, 212
    salivary glands disease associated with, 361
Aiming beam, 378
Air conduction, vs. bone, 15
Airway
    assessing in trauma patient, 134
    in basic life support, 115
    categories of obstructions to, 116
    clearing foreign bodies from, 117
    clearing with cricothyrotomy, 140-141
    clearing with tracheostomy, 141-147
    maneuvers for establishing, 118-119, 140
    preoperative evaluation of, 20-21
    sudden cardiac death and restoration of, 131
    viewing films of, 57

441

Alanine aminiotransferase (ALT) liver function
test, 42, 183
Alar cartilages, 228
Albright's syndrome, 356
Albumin
evaluating in immunocompromised patients,
210
in liver disease, 41-42, 134, 184
Alcoholism, orofacial features in chronic, 186
Aldosterone, 192
Alfentanil (Alfenta), 1, 79
Alkaline phosphatase (ALP), as liver disease
indicator, 42, 184
Allergies
to latex, 71
to local anesthetics, 71, 74
Allodynia, 256
Allogenic bone grafts, 273
Allografts, 389
Alloplastic facial implants, 427-435
biocompatibility and, 427-428
chin augmentation complications, 339-340
commonly used, 430-432
ideal materials, 428-429
informed consent for, 433
in nerve conduits, 260
operating room handling of, 429
perioperative/intraoperative considerations,
432-433
placement of, 428, 432-434
pros and cons, 408-409
reconstructing orbital floor, 273
TMJ reconstruction, 396-397
Alloplastic materials, defined, 427
ALP (alkaline phosphatase), as liver disease
indicator, 42, 184
Alpha-fetoprotein (AFP), as cancer marker, 50
Alpha-glucose inhibitors, 205
Alpha-hydroxy acid, prepeel skin regimen, 409
Alpha receptors, hypertension and, 164
ALT (alanine aminiotransferase) liver function
test, 42, 183
Alveolar bone
controlling bleeding after surgery on, 250
resorbtion in mandible vs. maxilla, 417
Alveolar disease
defined, 52
Alveolar fractures, treating, 266-267
Alveolar grafts, in cleft repair, 349
Alveolar nerve. *See* IAN (inferior alveolar nerve)
Alveolus
embryonic formation of anterior maxillary, 341
Ambu bag
managing hypoxic events, 91

Ambulatory surgery
management for patient taking NPH insulin, 204
Ameloblastomas
treating, 368
American Association of Oral and Maxillofacial
Surgeons (AAOMS), 438
American Diabetes Association, 202
American Society of Anesthesiologists (ASA)
physical status classification, 14
use of fresh frozen plasma, 38
use of platelets, 38
Amide local anesthetics
defined, 66
mechanism for metabolizing, 184
metabolizing, 1
Amine group, local anesthetics, 67
Amino acids
insulin lowering blood levels of, 198
Aminoglysides, 315
Aminophylline
drugs interfering with, 176
Amiodarone
defined, 123
resuscitation dosage, 132
AMIs (acute myocardial infarctions)
lab tests for, 47
Amoxicillin, 160
antimicrobial spectrum of, 310
formulations, 307
pediatric and adult dosages, 309
profile of, 312
Amoxicillin-clavulanate
antimicrobial spectrum of, 310
formulations, 307
pediatric and adult dosages, 309
Ampicillin, 160
antimicrobial spectrum of, 310
formulations, 307
pediatric and adult dosages, 309
Amylase levels, evaluating pancreas, 44-45
ANA (antinuclear antibody)
collagen vascular diseases, evaluating, 48
Anabolism
in TMJ synovium and articular disc, 323-324
Anaerobes
found in oral cavity, 292
in odontogenic infections, 294
Analgesia
anesthesia vs., 256
Analgesics
metabolized primarily by liver, 185
postsurgical and chronic pain in TMJ disorders
and, 330
pregnancy and OMFS, 223-224

Anastomose
  defined, 260
Anatomy
  applied orofacial. *See* Orofacial anatomy,
    applied
Anemia
  causes of iron deficiency, 180
  CRF-induced, 190
  defined, 180
  diagnosing/classifying with RBCs, 34-35
  pernicious, 180
  sickle cell, 180
Anesthesia
  analgesia vs., 256
  inferior alveolar nerve block, 249
  inhalational. *See* Inhalational anesthesia
  intravenous sedation. *See* Intravenous sedation
  local anesthetics. *See* Local anesthetics
  malignant hyperthermia from, 2
  in orbital floor fractures, 273
  in patients with ischemic heart disease, 156
  postoperative dysuria from, 7
  when to avoid in soft tissue injuries, 284
Anesthesia, preoperative evaluation
  ASA physical status classification, 14
  diabetic patients, 22
  goals, 14
  obese patients, 22
  resulting in changes, 21
  URIs and general guidelines for, 21-22
Anesthesia dolorosa
  defined, 256
Anesthetics
  pregnancy and OMFS, 224
  renal disease and, 189
  symptoms of MH during, 148
Angina, Ludwig's, 3
Angina pectoris
  overview of, 154
Angiography
  oral and maxillofacial surgeons using, 60
Angiotensin-converting enzyme (ACE)
    inhibitors
  as congestive heart failure treatment, 171
  hypertension treatment, 162, 167
Angiotensin I
  produced in kidneys, 193
Angiotensin II
  causing increase in blood pressure, 193
  produced in kidneys, 193
Angle of Louis
  defined, 15
ANH (atrial natriuretic hormone), TBW
    maintenance, 93

Animal bites
  bacteria causing infection in, 5, 316
  treating, 317
Anion gap, 100
Anisocoria, 1, 18
Anisocytosis, 36
Ankylosis, 278
Antagonists
  benzodiazepine, 78-79
  opioid, 79-80
Anterior cord syndrome, 138
Anterior pituitary tumors, 195-196
Anteroposterior (AP) mandibular deficiencies,
    333
Antibiotic-associated colitis (AAC), 313
Antibiotics
  in alloplastic biomaterial placement, 429
  antimicrobial spectrum of, 310-311
  bacterial resistance to, 309
  causes of failure, 313
  in chemical peels, 409-410
  in chemotherapy, 211
  combinations vs. single agent, 320
  commonly used, 307-308, 311-312
  in dental and oral surgical procedures,
    160-161
  effect of long-term therapy, 179
  in epistaxis in emergency department, 271
  in facial lacerations, 290
  formulations for, 307-308
  generations of, 319
  in joint replacement patients, 219
  metabolized by liver, 185
  in orofacial infection, 291-322
  pediatric and adult dosages, 309
  penicillin as choice, 311
  in pregnancy, 223
  principles of use, 306
  prophylactic administration, 311, 319-321
  in prosthetic joint patients, 221-222
  in renal disease, 189
  in SSI, 321
  triple, 320-321
  unnecessary, 311
  when to use, 311
  in wound infections from bites, 5
Anticentromere, 48
Anticholinergics, 80
Antidiuretic hormone. *See* ADH (antidiuretic
    hormone); SIADH (syndrome of
    inappropriate antidiuretic hormone)
Anti-DNA collagen vascular diseases, 48
Antifungal agents, 317
Antigen-specific systemic immunity, 208

Antihypertensive agents
  categories and classes of, 164-165
  pharmacology of, 165-167
  sympathetic nervous system receptors of, 64
Antimicrosomal collagen vascular diseases, 48
Anti-SCL, 70, 48
Antithrombin III, 39-40
Antithymocyte globulin, in HIV, 318
Antiviral agents, 317
Anulus of Zinn, 8, 244
Aorta, in chest films, 53
Aortic insufficiency, 157
Aortic stenosis, 157
AP (anteroposterior) mandibular deficiencies, 333
Apert's syndrome, 351, 352
Apex, in chest films, 53
Apnea. *See* Sleep apnea and snoring
Apopneurosis, 236
Appendix, location of, 18
Application process, OMFS residency, 436-440
Applied orofacial anatomy. *See* Orofacial
    anatomy, applied
ARDS (adult respiratory distress syndrome), 177
ARF (acute renal failure)
  defined, 187-188
  major classes of, 188
  peritoneal dialysis for, 190
Arnold's nerve, 230
Aromatic group, local anesthetics, 67
Arrhythmia
  dysrhythmias vs., 31
  in elderly person with hyperthyroidism, 197
  electric-shock related, 122
  principal bradyarrhythmias, 126-127
  with prolonged QT interval, 30
  tachyarrhythmias, 123-124
Arterial blood gas analysis, 225
Arterial catheters, 157
Arterial desaturation, 90
Arthography, 59
Arthoscopic surgery, TMJ
  advantages of lasers in, 326
  overview of, 325
  stages of osteoarthritis, 327-328
Arthrocentesis, TMJ, 325
Arthroplasty, 328
Articaine, 66, 69
Articular disc, TMJ
  anabolism/catabolism in synovium and,
    323-324
  internal derangement of, 329-330
  properties of, 322-323
  surgery and, 325
Articulated arm lasers, 377
Artifacts, on ECG monitors, 31

ASA (American Society of Anesthesiologists)
  physical status classification, 14
  use of fresh frozen plasma, 38
  use of platelets, 38
Ascher's syndrome, 357
Aspartate aminotransferase (AST) liver function
    test, 42, 47, 183
Aspiration
  management of, 177-178
  patients predisposed to, 105, 106
  as pneumonia cause, 109
  preoperative evaluation and, 21
  preventing, 111
Aspirin
  as anticoagulant, 36, 37, 179, 182
  contraindication in renal disease, 189-190
  metabolized by liver, 185
AST (aspartate aminotransferase) liver function,
    42, 47, 183
Asthma
  clinical manifestations of, 176
  N_2O-O_2 sedation contraindication, 84
Asymmetric mandibular excesses, 434
Asystole
  causing pulseless condition, 130
  ECG sign of, 30
  overview of, 129
  treating, 130, 132
  verifying flat-line rhythm as, 129-130
Atelectasis
  defined/managing, 176
  postoperative, 109, 113-114
  tracheostomy-related, 146
  treating with incentive spirometry, 113
Atrial fibrillation, 27
Atrial flutter, 27, 123
Atrial natriuretic hormone (ANH), TBW
    maintenance, 93
Atrophic mandible fractures, 268-269
Atropine
  administering, 8, 131
  resuscitation dosage, 132
Attitude, positive, 10
Auditory canal, external, 240
Auditory exam, preoperative evaluation, 15, 20
Auer bodies, 36
Auricular hematoma, 287
Auricular nerve, locating, 260
Autogenous bone grafts, 273, 392
Autografts, 389
Automated external defibrillator (AED), 117-118
AV (atrioventricular node)
  intrinsic firing rate of, 23
  normal route of conduction, 24
Avandamet, 205-206

Avulsed teeth
managing primary and secondary, 267
media for transporting, 251
reimplantation not indicated for primary, 251
splint time, 252
Avulsion injuries
of ears, 287
of lips, 289
as soft tissue injury, 283
Axial flaps, 397
Axial pattern flaps, 399
Axial plane, orbital fractures, 272
Axis of cardiac impulse, in ECGs, 25
Axonotmesis, 256
Axons, forward growth of injured, 8, 258
Azathioprine, 318
Azithromycin, 160
Azotemia, 193

B

Babinski sign, 18
Bacteremia, 220-221
Bacteria
antibiotic resistance of, 306, 309
Gram staining and, 292-294
morphologic findings and, 295
Bacterial infections
causes of odontogenic, 291, 293, 294, 296
cellulitis vs. abscess, 295-296
in diabetics, 207
diagnosing odontogenic, 297
orofacial, 291, 296
penicillin's mechanism of action on, 3
of prosthetic joints, 219-220
treating odontogenic, 297-306
Bacterial parotitis, 361, 362
Barbiturates, 75-76
Barium swallow (esophagram), 54
"Barrel chest," 176
Barrier protection, and alloplastic materials, 428
Basal cell nevus syndrome (Gorlin's syndrome)
clinical features of, 356
mandibular prognathism associated with, 4
Basal rate, 206
Basic life support (BLS), 115-120
Basilar skull fracture, 280
Basophil count, 34
Basophilic stippling, 36
Battle's sign, 280
BAUP (Bovie-assisted uvulpalatoplasty), 423
B-cell testing, 208
Benzocaine, as methemoglobinemia cause, 69
Benzodiazepines
affecting CNS, 77-78
amnestic effect of, 1

Benzodiazepines *(Cont'd)*
antagonist for, 78-79
clinical uses of, 77
most commonly used, 78
as preoperative medication, 78
Beta blockers
abrupt withdrawal of, 154
as congestive heart failure treatment, 171
as hypertension treatment, 162
in perioperative period, 154
Beta lactam group of antibiotics, 307-308
Beta receptors, hypertension and, 164
Bicarbonate, serum concentration of, 45-46
Bicoronal incisions, 274
Bifid uvula, 345
Biguanide, 204
Bilateral sagittal split osteotomy. *See* BSSO
(bilateral sagittal split osteotomy)
Bile acids, as liver disease indicator, 42
Bilirubin, 42
Bilobed flaps, 402
Binder's syndrome (nasomaxillary dysplasia), 354
Binocular diplopia, 275
Biocompatibility, of alloplastic materials, 427-428
Biological barriers, against microbiologic
invasion, 283
Biopsy. *See also* FNA (fine-needle aspiration)
biopsy
incisional vs. excisional, 254
on lesions in transplant patients on
immunosuppression, 206
liver, 185
paralleling lines of muscle tension, 254
Bisphosphonate-related osteonecrosis (BRON) of
jaw, 6, 388
Bisulfite allergies, 71
Bite block, in mandibular tooth removal, 248
Bite wounds, 284-285
Bladder, postoperative overextension of, 110
Bleeding
controlling after surgery on alveolar bone, 250
postoperative dental extractions, 250
Bleeding disorders
causes of, 182
liver disease and, 185
preventing/managing in renal failure patients,
191
Blepharoplasty, 407-408
Blind finger sweeps, contraindicated in pediatric
patients, 117
Blindness, surgery for zygomatic fractures and,
278
Blood
classifying flaps by supply of, 397, 398
heart sounds of, 16

Blood *(Cont'd)*
  normal volume of, 100, 136
  pregnancy affecting volume of, 224
  to scalp, 236-237
Blood chemistry test, 40
Blood coagulation
  acceptable preoperative platelet count, 37
  affect of aspirin, 179
  affect of heparin, 39-40, 179
  aspirin acting against, 37
  clotting factors synthesized in liver, 37
  DIC, 39
  discontinuing warfarin before surgery, 179
  liver disease patients and, 186
  pathways of, 180
  platelet count and, 36
  pregnancy affecting, 225
  types of tests, 37-38
  vitamin K deficiency affecting, 37, 178-179
Blood gas measurements
  acid-base abnormalities, 46-47
  overview of, 45-46
  oxygenation, 47
Blood glucose, monitoring levels, 45
Blood oxygen tension (Po$_2$), 46, 47
Blood pressure
  Angiotensin II causing increase in, 193
  hypertension and. *See* Hypertension
  measuring, 17-18
Blood smears, 32, 36
Blood transfusion
  acquiring hepatitis C through, 49
  acquiring HIV through, 211
  causing decreased reticulyte count, 35
  causing hypocalcemia, 97
  Hgb and Hct readings and, 35
  for immunocompromised patients, 210
  indications for fresh frozen plasma, 38
  indications for platelets, 37, 38
  as possible etiology for low platelet count, 36
Blowout fracture, of orbit, 275
BLS (basic life support), 115-120
BMP (bone morphogenic protein), 390
Body fluid osmolality, 94
Body temperature, heart rate and, 7
Bolus, 206
Bone
  articulated by zygoma, 246
  conduction, 15
  effect of radiation on, 381
  external nasal skeleton, 228
  growth factors and cytokines in, 390
  nose, 246
  orbital, 231, 245
  reconstructing, 5, 389-404

Bone grafts
  alveolar cleft repair, 349
  autogenous, sources of, 392
  cancellous, 391
  cortical, 391-392
  with dental implants, 412, 414
  harvesting iliac crest, 394
  healing of, 392
  reconstructing orbital floor, 273
  recurrence of tumors, 366
  with sinus lift implants, 419-420
  storing harvested cells, 394-395
Bone induction, 390-391
Bone loss, as sign of implant failure, 6
Bone marrow, mesenchymal stem cells of, 391
Bone morphogenic protein (BMP), 390
Bone scan, 55, 373
Bovie-assisted uvulpalatoplasty (BAUP), 423
Bowel sounds
  preoperative evaluation, 20
Bowstring test
  overview of, 275
Bradyasystolic
  PEA rhythm, 128
Bradycardia
  defined, 25, 126
  ECG signs of, 31
  management of, 127
  sinus, 30
  types of, 126-127
Bradypnea
  defined, 175
Brain injuries
  classifying with Glasgow Coma Scale, 137-138
  epidural vs. subdural hematomas in, 137
Branchial cysts, in older patients, 367
Brånemark's surgical principles for dental
    implants, 411-412
Breathing
  determining presence or absence of, 116
  normal rate of, 175
  primary and secondary ABCD surveys, 120-121
  rescue, 115-116
Brevital (methohexital), 76
Bridge flap, upper eyelid reconstruction, 403
BRON (bisphosphonate-related osteonecrosis) of
    jaw, 6, 388
Bronchial carcinoma, 174-175
Bronchitis, radiographs in chronic, 53
Brow approach, in surgical access to orbit, 401-
    402
Brow lifts, 410
BSSO (bilateral sagittal split osteotomy)
  dysfunction of inferior alveolar nerve
      following, 3

BSSO (bilateral sagittal split osteotomy) *(Cont'd)*
  possible complications of, 337
  treating isolated mandibular deficiency with, 3, 333
Buccal fascial space, 298
Buccal mucosa grafts, 399
Buccal nerve, long
  injury to, 8, 257
  as local anesthetic injection site, 73
Buccinator muscle, 249
BUN, renal function, 44
Burns, thermal, classification of, 139
Burr cells, 36
Byetta (exanatide), 206

C

CA 125, screening for cancer, 50
Café au lait spots, 355
Caffey's disease, 318
Calcifying epithelial odontogenic tumor (CEOT), 365-366
Calcitonin, 192
  as aneurysmal bone cyst treatment, 366
Calcium. *See also* Hypercalcemia; Hypocalcemia
  metabolism of, 43
  postoperative care scenarios, 101-103
  tests for, 25, 43, 48, 97
Calcium channel blockers
  as congestive heart failure treatment, 171
  dose, mechanism of action and complications of, 167
  as hypertension treatment, 162
Calcium chloride or gluconate, 133
Calcium phosphate ceramic facial implants, 432
Calories, 107
Calvarium, as bone graft source, 392
Cancellous bone grafts, 391
Cancer. *See also* specific types of cancer
  antithrombin III decrease in, 39-40
  bronchial, 177
  oral, 370-376, 380
  radiation therapy for head and neck, 380-389
  risk in transplant patients, 209
  screening and testing for, 50, 55
Cancer antigen 19-9 (CA 19-9), 50
Canine fascial space infections, 298
Carbapenem, first clinical use of, 308
Carbohydrate requirements, 107
Carbon dioxide, 41, 83-84
Carbon dioxide (CO_2) lasers
  basic tissue interaction used in, 377
  coagulation necrosis surrounding wound, 378
  skin resurfacing with, 5
  used in OMS, 376
Carbon dioxide response curve, 86

Carcinoembryonic antigen (CEA), 50
Carcinoma in situ
  defined, 5
  vs. invasive, 370-371
Cardiac angiography, 157
Cardiac arrest
  diagnosing, 121
  emergency services at scene of, 118
  with injury, 118
  mechanisms of, 121
  in pediatric patients, 139, 149
  signs of, 118
Cardiac arrhythmias
  vs. dysrhythmias, 31
  in elderly person with hyperthyroidism, 197
  postoperative, 110, 112
Cardiac catheterization
  valvular heart disease evaluation, 157
Cardiac ischemia, 121
Cardiac life support, advanced, 120-133
Cardiac output
  effect of PEEP on, 173
  pregnancy-related increase in, 224
Cardiac risk index, 163-164
Cardiac scans, 55
Cardiac tamponade, 131
Cardiogenic pulmonary edema, 130-131
Cardiogenic shock, 135
Cardiopulmonary resuscitation, 115-120
Cardiovascular diseases, 153-172
  congestive heart failure, 169-171
  hypertension, 161-169
  ischemic heart disease, 153-158
  myocardial infarction, 153-158
  valvular heart disease, 153-158
  valvular heart disease, perioperative considerations for, 158-161
Cardioversion, synchronized, 124, 131
Caries
  as adverse effect of radiation of oral tissues, 373
  before radiation therapy, 382
Carotid arteries
  external branches of, 234
  as nasal blood supply source, 228-229
Carotid sheath, 233-234
Cartilage
  of external nasal skeleton, 228
  main function of, 322
  rhinoplasty and, 407
  in TMJ reconstruction, 397
Catabolism, 323-324
Cat bites
  organisms from, 284, 316
  other traumatic injuries vs., 289
  treating, 284, 316

Cat scratch disease, 315
Catheters, maxiumum rate of fluid through, 135
Cavernous sinus, 316
Cavitary lesions, lung masses, 54
Caywood classification of edentulous ridges, 418
CBC (complete blood count), 32-33, 51
CD4 counts, indicator of HIV infection, 49-50
CD4+ lymphocyte, and AIDS patients, 211-212
CEA (carcinoembryonic antigen), 50
Cefaclor
    antimicrobial spectrum of, 311
    formulations, 307
    pediatric and adult dosages, 309
Cefadroxil, 160, 312
Cefazolin
    antimicrobial spectrum of, 311
    formulations, 307
    pediatric and adult dosages, 309
Cefoxitin
    antimicrobial spectrum of, 311
    formulations, 307
    pediatric and adult dosages, 309
Cell-mediated immunity, 208
Cellulitis
    abscess vs., 296
    defined, 295
Central antiadrenergics, 166
Central cord syndrome, 138
Central DI, 95, 194
Central line, 131-132
Central nervous system (CNS)
    benzodiazepines and, 77-78
    lidocaine toxicity in, 72
    local anesthetic toxicity in, 74
Central sleep apnea, 424
Centrifugal movement of blood supply, 417
Centripetal movement of blood supply, 417
CEOT (calcifying epithelial odontogenic tumor),
        365-366
Cephalexin
    antimicrobial spectrum of, 311
    formulations, 307
    pediatric and adult dosages, 309
    profile of, 312
Cephalic excision, from lower lateral cartilage,
        407
Cephalometric bony analysis
    common systems of, 338
Cephalosporins, 189, 315, 319
Cephradine
    antimicrobial spectrum of, 311
    formulations, 307
    pediatric and adult dosages, 309
Cervical lymph node metastasis, in squamous cell
        carcinoma, 375

Cervical lymphoepithelial (branchial) cysts, 367
Cervical ranula, 362
Cervical spine, radiographic evaluation of, 57
Cervical spine fractures, with mandibular
        fractures, 9, 264
Cervicofacial necrotizing fasciitis, 313-314
Charcot-Bouchard aneurysm, 169
Cheek, through-and-through lacerations of, 289
Chem 7 test, 40
Chemical peeling, 409-410
Chemotherapy
    effect on immune system, 210-211
    for oral cancer, 373
    for salivary gland tumors, 364
    using prophylactic antibiotics with, 211
Chest compressions
    complications of, 120
    for infants, 7
    overview of, 116-120
Chest pain, ischemic, 121
Chest x-rays
    of AIDS patients, 54
    of chronic bronchitis, 53
    of congestive heart failure, 170
    of COPD, 52
    diagnostic value of PA, 52-54
    lateral, 52-53
    of lung masses, 54
    of oral cancer, 373
    patterns of disease on, 52
    of pneumothorax, 52, 54
    types of, 52-53
    of valvular heart disease, 157
Cheyne-Stokes breathing, 16
CHF (congestive heart failure), 169-171
Chief complaint, 9, 13
Chin augmentation, 406, 434
Chloramphenicol
    antimicrobial spectrum of, 310
    formulations, 308
    pediatric and adult dosages, 309
Chloride, 41
Chondromalacia, TMJ dysfunction and, 332
Christmas disease, 179
Chromophere, 379
Chromosomal abnormality, in Down syndrome,
        358
Chronic bronchitis, 53
Chronic myelogenous leukemia, 181
Chronic obstructive pulmonary disease (COPD),
        52, 83-84
Chvostek's sign, 2, 98
Circulation, 120-121
Circumoral numbness, in local anesthetic toxicity,
        69

Circumvestibular incision, 401
Cirrhosis, affect on drug metabolism, 183-184
Cis-astracurium, 3, 184
CK (creatinine kinase)
    as acute myocardial infarction indicator, 47
    as malignant hyperthermia indicator, 147
Clarithromycin, 160
Clavicle
    in chest films, 53
    first rib lying under, 16
Cleft lip and cleft palate patient, 341-350
    ages for, 4, 349-350
    anatomy of, 341-345
    repair of, 345-349
    unrepaired, 348
Cleft palate team, 345
Clindamycin
    antimicrobial spectrum of, 310
    as excellent antibiotic, 311
    formulations, 308
    pediatric and adult dosages, 309
    profile of, 312
    prophylactic regimen for, 160-161
Closed-mouth block, 73
Clostridium difficile, causing antibiotic-associated
    colitis, 313
Clotrimazole, 308, 310
Clotting factors
    FFP replacing deficiencies in, 2
    produced by liver, 185
    synthesized in liver, 1, 37
CNS (central nervous system)
    benzodiazepines and, 77-78
    lidocaine toxicity in, 72
    local anesthetic toxicity in, 74
Coagulase, defined, 291
Coagulation. *See* Blood coagulation
Coagulation necrosis
    overview of, 377
Cocaine, adverse drug effects of, 70
Codeine
    histamine release effect of, 1
    liver diseases and, 135
Coherent light, 378
Colitis, antibiotic-associated, 313
Collagen vascular diseases, 47-48
Colloid resuscitation fluids, 132
Coloboma, 352
Combination syndrome, 418
Compartment syndrome, 138-139
Complete blood count (CBC), 32-33, 51
Complete cleft lips, 344
Complete clefts, 344
Computed tomography. *See* CT (computed
    tomography)

Condylar fractures, 264-266, 268
Condylar hyperplasia, mandibular, 334
Cone beam imaging, vs. CT scan, 1, 60
Congestive heart failure (CHF), 169-171
Consensual light reflex, 19
Continuous feeding, 106
Continuous positive airway pressure (CPAP),
    425-426
Contraction, in skin grafts, 399, 420
Contusions, as soft tissue injury, 283
COPD (chronic obstructive pulmonary disease),
    52, 83-84
Corneal reflex, 19
Coronal approach, in nasoethmoidal
    reconstruction, 401
Coronary angiography, for ischemia, 155
Coronary artery disease
    ECG findings in, 121-122
    epinephrine and levonordefrin dosage for,
        69-70
Coronectomy (partial odontectomy), on impacted
    mandibular molar, 255
Cortical bone grafts, 391-392
Corticotropin-releasing hormone (CRH), 199
Cortisol, 199
Cosmetic surgery, facial
    lasers used in skin resurfacing, 377
    overview of, 404-410
Costochondral graft, for TMJ reconstruction, 397
Costophrenic angles, in chest films, 53
Coumadin. *See* Warfarin (Coumadin)
CPAP (continuous positive airway pressure),
    425-426
CPR (cardiopulmonary resuscitation), 115-120
Cranial nerves
    function and foramina of, 238-240
    passing through cavernous sinus, 316
Craniofacial defects, and alloplastic implants, 435
Craniofacial disjunction, Le Fort III fracture, 279
Craniofacial dysostosis (Crouzon's syndrome),
    351, 353
Craniosynostoses, 354
Cranofacial syndromes, 350-359
C-reactive protein (C-RP) test, 48
Creatinine
    as glomerular filtration rate indicator, 2, 187
    as renal function indicator, 44
Creatinine kinase (CK)
    as acute myocardial infarction indicator, 47
    as malignant hyperthermia indicator, 147
Creeping substitution, 391
Crestal bone loss, and implant failure, 6
CREST syndrome, 48
CRH (corticotropin-releasing hormone), 199
Cricothyrotomy, 140-141

Crocodile tears, 8, 233
Crouzon's syndrome (craniofacial dysostosis), 351, 353
Crystalloid resuscitation fluids, 132
C-spine CT scan, 57
CT (computed tomography)
   vs. cone beam, 1, 60
   contrast indicated/contraindicated for, 57
   of cysts and benign jaw tumors, 60
   dental implant treatment planning, 60
   of frontal sinus fractures, 281
   of head and neck, 57
   of invasive squamous cell carcinoma, 371
   of mandibular fractures, 61
   of maxillary sinus neoplasm, 373
   of maxillary sinus pathology, 61
   of midfacial fractures, 61
   not contraindicated in patients with titanium implants, 6
   of orbital fractures, 272
   orbital ZMC fractures, 277
   for patients with dental implants, 414
   plain film tomography vs., 57
   of salivary gland tumors, 361
Cutler-Beard (bridge) flap, upper eyelid reconstruction, 403
Cyclophosphamide, 318
Cyclosporine
   drug interactions of, 216-217
   for HIV-infected persons, 318
   oral manifestations of, 216
Cysts, oral and maxillofacial
   diagnostic imaging of, 60
   overview of, 365-369
Cytokines, bone matrix, 390

D
D₅W (5% dextrose in water)
   in fluid resuscitation, 2
   in postoperative care, 96
   in symptomatic hypernatremia, 99
Danger space, 296-297
Dantrolene sodium, 149
Darwin's tubercle, 15
D-dimer assay, 39
Deafferentation pain, 257
Debridement, of bite wounds, 289
Decamethonium, as malignant hyperthermia trigger, 148
Decannulation of tracheotomy, 146
Deep venous thrombosis (DVT), 7, 109-110
Defibrillation
   basic life support services, 115
   primary and secondary ABCD surveys, 120-121
   treating V-fib with, 123

Deficiency in complement, 209
Deformities. See also Cleft lip and cleft palate patient
   craniomaxillofacial, 350-351
   nasal, associated with cleft lip, 343
   nasal fracture, 270
   saddle nose, 271, 435
Delayed nerve repair, 259
Delayed-type hypersensitivity (DTH) skin testing, 208
Delivery systems, for lasers, 377
De novo cancer, 209
Dense HA (hydroxyapatite), as facial alloplast, 430
Dental cartridges, of local anesthetics, 65-66
Dental implants
   attached gingiva and, 413
   Brånemark's principles for, 411-412
   categories of, 410-411
   CT scan for planning, 60
   endosseous, 414-415
   failure of, 6, 414
   history of, 411
   indications for, 411
   in irradiated patients, 416
   osseointegration of, 6, 411, 413
   oxide layer in, 6
   placement of, 412, 414
   problems in maxilla and mandible, 412-413
   prophylactic HBO therapy before/after, 387-388
   radiographs for, 414
   at site of extraction, 412, 416
   surface area of, 412
   uncovering, 413-414
   zygoma implants, 416
Dentoalveolar fractures, treating, 266-267
Dentoalveolar surgery, 248-256
Dentofacial abnormalities, 333-341
Depolarizing NMB (succinylcholine [SCh]), 88
Dermabrasion, 409
Dermoid cysts, 5
Desflurane
   delivery of, 82
   known to trigger MH, 2
   minimal alveolar concentration of, 84
   partition coefficients for, 87
   wake-up potential of, 87
Diabetic ketoacidosis (DKA), 200
Diabetic patients, 198-207
   chronic complications of, 201
   contraindications for metformin in type 2, 197
   defined, 198
   diabetes insipidus, 94-95, 194
   diabetes mellitus, 199, 202, 316

Diabetic patients *(Cont'd)*
monitoring glucose levels, 45
preoperative evaluation of, 22
using blood glucose to diagnose, 45
Diagnostic imaging, 52-63
Diagnostic peritoneal lavage (DPL), 136-137
Diagnostic positive aspiration (DPA), 136
Dialysis
peritoneal vs. hemodialysis, 190
preoperative considerations, 191
surgery with renal disease and, 190
Diaphragm
in chest films, 53
effect on heart of, 16
Diazepam, 78
Dibucaine number, 90
DIC (disseminated intravascular coagulation)
defining, 38-39, 182
diagnosing, 39
potential in postsplenectomy patients, 218
treating, 39
Dicloxacillin
antimicrobial spectrum of, 311
formulations, 307
pediatric and adult dosages, 309
Diffusion hypoxia, 87
Digastric muscle, 247
Digitalis
as congestive heart failure treatment, 171
signs and symptoms of toxicity, 30, 171
Dimethylsiloxane (silicone), for facial implants, 429
Diplopia
defined, 274
incidence after zygomatic fracture, 278
monocular and binocular, 275
orbital floor complication, 273
orbital fractures and, 272
Dipyridamole thallium imaging, in ischemia, 155
Direct closure, lower/upper eyelid reconstruction, 403
Direct light reflex, 19
Disruptions, craniomaxillofacial, 351
Disseminated intravascular coagulation. *See* DIC (disseminated intravascular coagulation)
Distant transfer, reconstruction tissue, 397
Distilled water, 248
Diuretics
as antihypertensive agent, 162, 164
as congestive heart failure treatment, 171
dose, mechanism of action and complications of, 165
loop vs. thiazide, 95
DKA (diabetic ketoacidosis), 200
Dobutamine, 132-133

Dog bites
organisms from, 284, 316
other traumatic injuries vs., 289
treating, 284, 316
Döhle's inclusion bodies, 36
Dopamine, 132
Dorsal nasal reduction, 407
Down syndrome, 358
Doxycycline, 312
DPA (diagnostic positive aspiration), 136
DPL (diagnostic peritoneal lavage), 136-137
Drainage
of abscesses, 320
with lacrimal system, 231, 286
lymphatic nose, 305
of odontogenic infections, 305, 306
paranasal sinus, 230
Drooling, 5, 364
Drowning, 118
Drug overdose, 118
Dry socket (localized osteitis), 251
DTH (delayed-type hypersensitivity) skin testing, 208
Ductoplasty, 315
Duodenum, UGI studying, 54
DVT (deep venous thrombosis), 7, 109-110
Dynamic compression, in rigid fixation, 267
Dysesthesia, 256, 258
Dysrhythmias, 31
Dystopia, ocular, 273
Dysuria, postoperative, 7
Dyursia, postoperative, 110-111

E

Ear exam, preoperative, 15
Ears
classifying injuries to, 287
hematoma, 287
lacerations of, 288
nerves supplying, 230
EBL (edentulous bone loss), 417, 418
Eccentric dynamic compression, in rigid fixation, 267
ECF volume, 93-94, 98
ECG (electrocardiogram), 23-32
analyzing rhythms, 25-32
calcium and potassium affecting, 25, 97
components of, 23-24
in congestive heart failure, 170
in coronary artery disease, 121-122
determining heart rate from, 24
flat-line tracings, 7, 129-130
inaccurate diagnoses, 31
in ischemic heart disease, 30, 121, 154-156
lead placement, 25, 30-31

Echocardiography
  congestive heart failure evaluation, 170
  ischemic heart disease evaluation, 155
  valvular heart disease evaluation, 157
Ectropion, orbital fracture incisions, 274
Edema
  acute cardiogenic pulmonary, 131-131
  defined, 97
  subglottic, tracheostomy-related, 146
Edentulism, single-tooth implants, 415
Edentulous alveolar ridges, 418
Edentulous bone loss (EBL), 417, 418
Edentulous mandible fractures, 268
Effective osmolality, 94
Eikenella, 5
Elderly patients, and intravenous anesthetics, 80
Electrocautery, in dental implantation, 414
Electrocution, arrythmias following, 122
Electrolyte disturbances, 40-41, 93-104
Electronegativity, piezoelectric effect, 391
Electropositivity, piezoelectric effect, 391
ELISA (enzyme-linked immunosorbent assay)
      test, 49, 211
Elliptic excision, in facial scar revision, 409
Ellis–van Creveld syndrome, 352
Emergency medical services. See EMS
      (emergency medical services)
EMLA cream, 69
Emphysema
  barrel-chest appearance in, 176
  radiographic views of, 33
  subcutaneous, 136, 146
  using inhalational anesthetics, 83-84
EMS (emergency medical services)
  advanced cardiac life support, 120-133
  advanced trauma life support, 134-140
  basic life support, 115-120
  tracheostomy and cricothyrotomy, 140-147
Endocarditis, 159, 160
Endocrine diseases, 192-198
Endosseous dental implants, 414-415
Endotracheal intubation
  basic life support using, 119
  drugs administered through, 8, 131
  harvesting posterior iliac crest bone and, 395
  pregnancy and, 224
  in trauma patients, 134
End-stage renal disease, 101
Energy density (fluence), 377
Enflurane, as malignant hyperthermia trigger, 2,
      82
Enophthalmos, 273-275, 401
Enteral nutrition, 105, 107-108
Enzyme-linked immunosorbent assay (ELISA)
      test, 49, 211

Enzymes, liver, 42
EOA (esophageal obturator airway), 119
Eosinophils, 34
Epidermoid cysts, 5
Epidural hematomas, 137
Epinephrine
  administering via endotracheal tube, 8, 131
  adverse effects of, 70
  adverse effects of, combined with halothane,
      86
  coronary heart disease dose, 69-70
  effect on plasma glucose levels, 199
  for hypertensive patients, 163
  with lidocaine, adult dosage, 65-66
  as local anesthetic adjunct, 69
  metabolic effects of, 72, 199
  narcotic sedation of, 66
  release from adrenal medulla, 207
Epistaxis
  emergency management of, 271
  in nasal intubation, 119
  in nasoorbital-ethmoidal fracture, 271-272
  in orbital zygomatic fractures, 277
Epstein-Barr virus, 317
Epulis fissurata, 419
Erb's point, 1, 15
Er:YAG lasers, 5, 377
Erysipelas, 3, 313
Erythromycin
  antimicrobial spectrum of, 310
  avoiding in renal disease patients, 2, 189
  formulations, 307
  interfering with aminophylline, 176
  pediatric and adult dosages, 309
  profile of, 312
  scrutinizing other medicines patient is on when
      using, 185
Esophageal obturator airway (EOA), 119
Esophagram (barium swallow), 54
ESR (erythrocyte sedimentation rate) test, 48
Essay requirements, for OMFS residency, 438
Ester anesthetics
  allergic potential of, 71
  allergies to Novocain and, 74
  metabolizing, 1
  overview of, 66-67
Estrogen, role in TMJ dysfunction, 331
Etomidate, 77, 80
Excisional biopsy, 254
Exenatide (Byetta), 206
Exercise ECG, for ischemia, 155
Exercise thallium scintigraphy, for ischemia, 155
Exophthalmos, 273, 275
Expanded PTFE (polytetrafluoroethylene), as
      facial alloplast, 430

Externship, OMFS residency program, 437
Extraconal fat, 246
Extraction
  dental implants at site of, 412, 416
  evidence of bone formation at site of, 254
  posteroperative bleeding, 250, 254
  before radiation therapy, 382
  recommended sequence of, 249
  sectioning through mandibular molars, 250
  using prophylactic HBO during, 387
Extraocular muscles
  anatomy and physiology of, 231-233
  function of, 244
  traumatic injury to, 276
Extraoral blocks, 73
Extremities
  assessing in trauma patients, 138-139
  complications when harvesting posterior iliac
    crest bone, 395
Eyebrows
  lifting, 410
  shaving when repairing facial lacerations, 290
Eyelids
  anatomy of, 231-233
  injuries to, 286
  interval between open, 230
  performing blepharoplasty on, 407-408
  reconstruction of, 403
  sebaceous and sweat glands of, 8, 233
Eyes
  anatomy of, 231-234
  crocodile tears, 8, 233
  preoperative evaluation, 1, 18-20

F
Face
  alloplastic implants, 427-435
  cosmetic surgery, 404-410
  lacerations of, 288-290
  plain film views of, 55
Facial muscles, of expression, 241
Facial nerve
  locating during parotid surgery, 364
  overview of, 240-243
  paralysis of, 242, 288
Factor IX deficiency, 179
Fascial muscles, receiving innervation, 8
Fascial spaces, 298-305
  buccal, 298
  canine, 298
  lateral pharyngeal, 302-303
  masseteric, 300
  primary vs. secondary, 296
  pterygomandibular, 300-301
  retropharyngeal, 303-304

Fascial spaces *(Cont'd)*
  sublingual, 298-299
  submandibular, 299
  submental, 299-300
  temporal, 301-302
  typical sites of incision and drainage, 305
Fasciitis, cervicofacial necrotizing, 313-314
FAST (focused assessment sonography), 136
Fasting, preoperative, 21
Fat pads, in facial cosmetic surgery, 408
Fat requirements, 107
Fat transfer (lipoinjection), in cosmetic surgery,
    406
Favorable fracture, of mandible, 262-263
FDPs (fibrin degradation products), 39, 40
Fellowship, OMFS residency program, 437
Fentanyl (Sublimaze)
  causing histamine release, 1
Fetus (human embryo)
  development milestones for, 223
  development of cleft lips/palates, 342-345
  number of pharyngeal arches in, 341
  sensitivity to radiation, 2
Fever
  defined, 112
  effect on heart rate, 110
  in Hodgkin's disease, 1, 14
  postoperative, 108-114
  quotidian, 14
  remittent vs. intermittent, 1, 14
FFAs (free fatty acids), effect of insulin on, 198
FFP (fresh frozen plasma) transfusions
  indications for, 38, 180
  replacing deficiencies in factors II, V, VII, and
    IX, 2
  treating bleeding diathesis from liver disease,
    185
Fiberoptic guide, for lasers, 377
Fibrillation
  atrial, 27
  ECG signs of, 31
  ventricular. *See* V-fib (ventricular fibrillation)
Fibrin degradation products (FDPs), 39, 40
Fibrinogen, 2, 38-40, 48
Fibrinogen assays, 40
Fibrin split products (FSPs), 40
Fibroblastic phase of wound healing, 285
Fibroma, ossifying, in children, 367
Fibrous dysplasia, 368
Fine-needle aspiration biopsy. *See* FNA (fine-
    needle aspiration) biopsy
Firing rate, of sinus node, 23
First-degree burns, 139
First-degree heart block, 28, 127
Flap design, 249

Flaplike lacerations, 283
Flaps. *See also* Skin grafts
    aesthetics and function of, 398
    classification of, 397
    in dentoalveolar surgery, 250
    for maxillofacial reconstruction, 397
    Millard rotation-advancement, 346-347
    mucoperiosteal, 250
    repositioning over sound bone, 251
    tongue, 5-6, 402
    Vomer, 348
Flat-line tracings, ECG, 7, 129-130
Floating ribs, 15
Flow murmurs, 16-17
Fluid and electrolyte management, 2, 93-104
Flumazenil, 78-79
Fluothane, 70
Flutter, ECG signs of, 31
FNA (fine-needle aspiration) biopsy
    in benign intraosseous lesions, 368
    in salivary gland pathology, 4, 360
    in thyroid pathology, 196
Focal infections, 320
Focused assessment sonography (FAST), 136
Foreign body airway obstruction, 117, 119
Free fatty acids, effect of insulin on, 198
Free flap failure, 398-399
Free thyroxine index (FTI), 48
Frenum, excising abnormal, 419
Fresh frozen plasma transfusions. *See* FFP (fresh
        frozen plasma) transfusions
Frey's syndrome, 356-357
Frontal sinus fractures, 281-283
Frontonasal process, anatomy of, 228
FSPs (fibrin split products), 40
FTSGs (full-thickness skin grafts), 285-286,
        399-401
Fujita's classification of upper airway obstruction,
        424
Full-thickness mucoperiosteal flaps, 250
Full-thickness skin grafts (FTSGs), 285-286,
        399-401
Fungal infections
    affecting head and neck, 317
    antifungal agents, 317
    risk in immunocompromised patients, 209
Fusiform excision, for facial scars, 409

G

G-6-PD (glucose-6 phosphate dehydrogenase),
        181
GABA (gamma-aminobutyric acid) receptor, 1
Gag bite, 264
Galea of scalp, 236, 237
Gallium scan, 55

Gamma-aminobutyric acid (GABA) receptor, 1
Garré's osteomyelitis, 317-318
GCS (Glasgow Coma Scale), 18-19, 137-138
Gelatin sponge (Gelfoam), 250
General Practice Residency (GPR), 436
Genetics, in cleft deformities, 345
Genioplasty, 339, 340
Geriatric patients, and local anesthetic toxicity, 69
Gestational diabetes, 199
Gestation time, normal, 222
GFR (glomerular filtration rate)
    creatinine used as measurement of, 2, 187
    kidney dysfunction and, 44
GGT, in liver disorder, 42
Giemsa stain, 49
Gilbert's syndrome, 185
Gingiva
    bleeding, with mandibular lesion, 366
    dental implant success and, 411, 413
    effect of radiation therapy on, 381
    in Papillon-LeFèvre syndrome, 358
Glanders, 315
Glands of Moll, 8, 233
Glands of Zeis, 8, 233
Glasgow Coma Scale (GCS), 18-19, 137-138
Glomerular filtration rate. *See* GFR (glomerular
        filtration rate)
Glossopharyngeal nerve, 230, 341
Glucagon, 199, 207
Glucocorticoids, treating HIV-infected persons, 318
Glucose
    breakdown into sorbitol, 201
    growth hormone regulating, 199
    insulin facilitating uptake of, 198
    metabolism of, 198, 199
    monitored by lab, 45
    physiologic effect of decrease in plasma, 207
    release of epinephrine affecting, 207
    tissue transport of, 201
Glucose-6 phosphate dehydrogenase (G-6-PD),
        181
Glucovance, 206
Glycopyrrolate, 82
Glycosylation of platelets, 202
Goals, of preoperative evaluation, 13-14
Goldenhar's syndrome, 353
Goldman Cardiac Risk Index, 163-164
GORE-TEX, as facial alloplast, 431
Gorlin's syndrome (basal cell nevus syndrome),
        4, 356
GPR (General Practice Residency), 436
Graft-vs.-host disease, in organ transplants, 218
Gram-negative cocci, 292, 294-295
Gram-negative rods, 292, 294-295
Gram-positive cocci, 292, 294-295

Gram-positive rods, 292, 294-295
Gram stain, 292-295
Granulomatous infections, head and neck
  manifestations of, 314-315
Grid method of heart rate determination, 24
Grodinsky and Holyoke, 296-297
Growth factors, of bone matrix, 390
Growth hormone, in glucose regulation, 199
Guided tissue regeneration (GTR), 414, 420
Gustatory sweat auriculotemporal syndrome,
  356-357

H

H&P (history and physical exam), taking surgical
  notes, 11-12
H$_2$ blockers, for obese patients with difficult
  airways, 81
Haemophilus influenzae infection, causing
  sinusitis, 316
Hallermann-Streiff syndrome, 352
Halothane
  adverse effects of, 70
  combined with epinephrine, 86
  as malignant hyperthermia trigger, 2
  minimal alveolar concentration of, 84
  partition coefficient of, 87
Hammular notch deepening, 421-422
Hand tightening, in dental implants, 415
HA PTFE (hydroxyapatite
  polytetrafluoroethylene), as facial
  alloplast, 430
Hard tissue replacement (HTR-PMI), 432
Harris-Benedict equation, 107
Hashimoto's thyroiditis, 48
HAV (hepatitis A virus), 185
HBO (hyperbaric oxygen) therapy
  controversies over, 387-388
  in osteoradionecrosis, 385-387
  with radiation therapy, 380
HBV (hepatitis B virus), 185-186
HCO$_3^-$, in blood gas measurement, 45-47
Hct (hematocrit), 33-35
HCV (hepatitis C virus), 186
HDV (hepatitis D virus), 186
Head
  CT scan, 57, 61-62
  necrotizing fasciitis of, 314-315
  patients irradiated for cancer in, 380-389
Headache
  with nasal fractures, 271
  with obstructive sleep apnea syndrome, 423
  with some hypertension drugs, 168
  with viral parotitis infection, 4, 361
Health care workers, exposed to HIV, 212, 215
Hearing tests, 15

Heart
  axis of electrical impulse of, 25
  block, 127-128
  failure. *See* Congestive heart failure (CHF)
  murmurs, 16-17
  muscle relaxants and, 89
  orthotopic transplant of, 31
  point of maximum impulse, 16
  preoperative evaluation, 16, 17, 19
  signs of local anesthetic toxicity in, 74
  testing for acute myocardial infarction, 47
  viewing chest films, 53
  wide-complex beats, 31
Heart rate. *See also* Bradycardia; Tachycardia
  body temperature and, 7
  ECG-based determination of, 24
  fever-related increase in, 110
Heart sounds
  causes of, 16
  fetal, 223
Heart valves, prosthetic, as bacterial endocarditis
  risk factor, 159
Heerfordt's syndrome, 357
Heimlich maneuver, 117
Hematocrit (Hct), 33-35
Hematogenous prosthetic joint infections, 219
Hematology, 178-183
Hematoma
  auricular, 287
  epidural, 137
  nasal septal, 270, 271
  retrobulbar, 275
Hemicoronal approach, in nasoethmoidal
  reconstruction, 401
Hemifacial microsomia, 353
Hemimandibular hypertrophy, 334-335
Hemodialysis, 190
Hemodynamic effects, of volatile anesthetics, 85
Hemoglobin
  bilirubin abnormalities in, 42
  in blood gas measurement, 46-47
  complete blood count, 33
  cyanosis-related reduction of, 1, 16
  determining anemia, 34-35
  methemoglobinemia-related reduction of, 69
  nonenzymatic glycosylation of, 201
  normal range of, 35
  not useful as blood loss indicator, 35
  in trauma patients, 134
  using RBC clinically, 34-35
Hemophilia A, 181-182
Hemophilia B
  as factor IX deficiency, 179
  hemophilia A vs., 181-182
  replacement therapy for, 182

Hemorrhage
  blood volume in pregacy protecting from, 224
  causing shock in trauma patients, 136
  classes of, 136
  decreased Hct and Hgb-related, 35
  diagnosing with angiography, 60
  in facial cosmetic surgery, 408
  left shifts increasing likelihood of, 32
  posterior iliac crest bone graft–related, 395
  retinal, in hyphema, 276
  subarachnoid, 50
  subconjunctival, 277
  tracheostomy-related, 143
  valvular heart disease–related, 159
Hemostasis
  in hypovolemic shock, 131
  phases of, 179
Heparin
  effect on blood coagulation, 179
  features of, 2
  low-molecular-weight, 182
  overview of, 39-40
  reversal of, 179
Hepatitis, tests for, 49
Hepatitis A virus, 185
Hepatitis B virus, 185-186
Hepatitis C virus, 186
Hepatitis D virus, 186
Hepatitis E virus, 186
Hering-Breuer reflux, 18
HEV (hepatitis E virus), 186
Hgb. *See* Hemoglobin
High mandibular plane angle
  mandibular deficiencies, 333
Hilium, in chest films, 53
Histamine, opioid-stimulated release of, 1
HIV (human immunodeficiency virus) infection
  anti-viral therapy for, 318
  categories of patients with, 3, 211
  drug interactions in, 213-214
  features of, 3
  health care workers exposed to, 212, 215
  sicca-syndrome–like condition in, 362
  testing for, 211
  type of virus in, 211
Hodgkin's disease, 14, 181
Hollow wave guide technology, lasers, 377
Homans' sign, 7, 19, 110
Homeostasis, 250
Hormones, ketogenic, 207
Horner's syndrome, 276, 358-359
Hotline, malignant hyperthermia, 150-151
Howell-Jolly bodies, 36
HTR (hard tissue replacement)-PMI, 432

Hughes tarsoconjunctival flap, lower eyelid
    reconstruction, 403
Human bites
  organisms from, 285, 316
  other traumatic injuries vs., 289
  treating, 285, 317
  wound infections from, 5
Human embryo. *See* Fetus (human embryo)
Human immunodeficiency virus. *See* HIV (human
    immunodeficiency virus) infection
Humoral immunity, deficiency of, 208
Hydrogen ion (acidosis), 129
Hydroquinone, prepeel skin regimen, 409
Hydroxyapatite, as facial alloplast, 430
Hydroxyapatite polytetrafluoroethylene, as facial
    alloplast, 430
Hyoid pharyngeal arch, 341
Hyperaldosteronism, 196
Hyperalgesia, 256
Hyperbaric oxygen therapy. *See* HBO (hyperbaric
    oxygen) therapy
Hypercalcemia
  causes of, 43
  mnemomic for symptoms of, 98
  treating symptomatic, 196
Hypercapnia
  as postoperative hypertension cause, 110
  respiratory failure–related, 175
Hyperdontia, syndromes of, 355
Hyperesthesia, 256, 257
Hyperkalemia
  causes, signs and symptoms of, 97
  causing pulseless electrical activity, 129
  effect on ECG, 25
  postoperative care and, 103
Hyperlipidemia, effect on plasma sodium
    measurement, 100
Hypernatremia, 96-100
Hyperosmolar nonketotic coma, 200-201
Hyperparathyroidism, secondary, renal
    failure–related, 188
Hyperpathia, 257
Hyperpnea, 16
Hypersegmentation, 36
Hypertension, 161-169
  alpha and beta receptors in, 164
  categories of, 161
  classifying, 162
  defined, 161
  Goldman Cardiac Risk Index for, 163-164
  modifying behavior to treat, 162
  oral hypertensive agents for, 164-169
  pharmacology for, 162-163
  postoperative, 110

Hypertension *(Cont'd)*
  primary vs. secondary, 161
  recording highest mean arterial pressure, 161
Hypertensive emergencies
  parenteral drugs for, 168-169
  vs. urgency, 161
Hyperthermia. *See* MH (malignant hyperthermia)
Hyperthyroidism
  in elderly persons, 197
  screening for, 48
Hyperventilation, 16
Hyperventilation (respiratory alkalosis)
  causing acid-base disorders, 47
  diagnosing, 174
Hyphema, 276
Hypoalbuminemia, 97-98
Hypocalcemia
  causes of, 43, 97
  Chvostek's and Trousseau's sign in, 2
  effect on ECG, 25
  hypoalbuminemia causing, 97-98
  postoperative care and, 103
Hypodontia, 355
Hypoesthesia, in orbital floor fractures, 273
Hypoglossal nerve, in submandibular triangle, 235
Hypoglycemia, 202-204
Hypokalemia
  causing pulseless electrical activity, 129
  effect on ECG, 25
  severe, 94
  signs and symptoms of, 97
Hyponatremia
  in hospitalized patients, 96
  hypoosmolar, 96
  low serum sodium concentration as artifact of
    measurement, 100
  postoperative care and, 102, 104
Hypoosmolar hyponatremia, 96
Hypoparathyroidism, 194
Hypopnea, vs. apnea, 423
Hypotension, postoperative, 110
Hypothermia, ECG manifestation of, 30
Hypothyroidism
  postoperative complications of subclinical, 197
  screening for, 48
Hypotonic saline solutions, 98
Hypoventilation (respiratory acidosis)
  causing acid-base disorders, 46
  causing cardiac arrest in pediatric patients, 139
  diagnosing, 174
  postoperative care and, 98-99
Hypovolemia
  causing pulseless electrical activity, 129
  ketamine for, 80
  signs and symptoms of, 131

Hypoxia
  causing cardiac arrest in pediatric patients, 139
  causing pulseless electrical activity, 129
  managing, 90
Hysterical dysphagia, 358

I
IAN (inferior alveolar nerve)
  axons and fascicles in, 257
  bilateral split osteotomy-related deficits of, 3
  free nerve grafts and, 260
  injury during removal of third molars, 8, 257
  location of, 249
  managing hypoxic events, 253
  overview of, 8
  relationship with mandibular third molar roots,
    252
  repairing, 259-261
  in surgical ablation of cysts and tumors,
    367-368
Iatrogenic, defined, 31
Idiopathic condylar resorption, 337-338
Iliac crest
  anterior, 5, 392, 394-395
  harvesting bone from, 394-396
  posterior, 392, 395
IMF (intermaxillary fixation), 265
Imipenem, 308
Immune system, effects of
    chemotherapeutic/immunosuppressant
    drugs, 210-211
Immunocompromised surgical patients, 208-219.
    See also AIDS (acquired
    immunodeficiency syndrome); HIV
    (human immunodeficiency virus) infection
Immunodeficiency, causes and types of, 208
Immunosuppressant therapy
  causes of, 208
  effect on immune system, 210-211
  in graft-vs.-host disease, 218
  for HIV-infected patients, 318
  with tacrolimus, 217
  in transplant patients, 209, 215, 216
Incentive spirometry, treating atelectasis, 113
Incisional biopsy
  indications for, 4
  of parotid gland, 362-363
Incisions
  bicoronal, 274
  circumvestibular, 401
  inverted-U entrance, 143
  lateral brow, 274
  orbital fracture, 274
  subciliary lower eyelid, 274
  in surgical access to orbit, 401-402

Incisions *(Cont'd)*
  transconjunctival, 274, 401-402
  typical sites of drainage and, 305-306
Incomplete cleft lips, 344
Indium 111 white blood cell scans, detecting
  osteomyelitis, 55
Infarction, ECG signs of, 30
Infections. *See also* Bacterial infections; Fungal
    infections; Odontogenic infections; Viral
    infections
  antibiotic use and, 291-322
  deep-space, 112, 293
  diabetes mellitus as risk factor for, 207
  IV catheter–related, 109
  local anesthetics often ineffective at area of, 72
  possible complication of transplant patients,
    209
  prosthetic joint, 219-222
  urinary tract, 113
  wounds prone to, 112, 113
Inferior alveolar nerve. *See* IAN (inferior alveolar
    nerve)
Inferior alveolar nerve blocks
  buccinator muscle pierced by, 249
  clinical revelance of, 68
  delivery into nerve sheath, 74
  V-shaped landmark for, 249
Inferior head, lateral pyterygoid muscle, 227
Inferior lid crease incision, 401
Inferior orbital rim approach, 401
Infestation, vs. infection, 319
Inflammation
  diagnostic imaging of jaw, 61
  impeding onset of local anesthesia, 72
Informed consent
  in preoperative evaluation, 14
  using alloplastic materials with, 433
Infratemporal fossa, managing displaced tooth in,
    253
Inhalational anesthesia
  known to trigger MH, 2
  maintaining hepatic blood flow, 184
  overview of, 82-91
Inital lag phase, in wound healing, 285
Injury, ECG signs of, 30
Innervation, of fascial muscles, 8
INR (international normalized ratio), 38, 178
Insensible fluid loss, 95, 103
Insulin
  dietary protein response, 207
  effect on free fatty acids, 198
  facilitating glucose uptake, 198
  hormonal interactions of, 207
  lowering amino acid levels, 198
  lowering plasma glucose, 198

Insulin *(Cont'd)*
  pumps, 206
  stimulating release of, 203
  surgery for patient taking, 203-204
  tissues not requiring, 201
  types of, 203
Intense pulsed light (IPL), 378-379
Intercostal angle, 16
Interleukin, of bone matrix, 390
Interleukin-1, in osteoarthritis, 327
Intermaxillary fixation (IMF), 265
Intermaxillary segment, merger with medial nasal
    process, 341
Intermittent fever, 1
Internal laryngeal branch, 230
International normalized ratio (INR), 38, 178
International Sensitivity Index (ISI), 178
Internship, OMFS residency program, 437
Interstitial pattern of disease, 52
Interview process, OMFS residency, 438-440
Intracellular cations, 93
Intraconal fat, 246
Intradomal region, sutures in nasal surgery, 407
Intranasal packing, 270
Intraoperative frozen-section evaluation of
    salivary tumors, 363
Intraoral approach, orbital fracture surgery, 274
Intraoral ranula, 362
Intraoral sites
  as bone graft source, 392
  placing alloplastic facial implants, 432-433
Intraorbital fracture, 272-273
Intraosseous salivary tumors, 363
Intravenous catheter sites, frequency of changing,
    109
Intravenous contrast, patients with previous
    allergy to, 57
Intravenous drug abuse, as valvular heart disease
    cause, 157
Intravenous pyelogram (IVP), 54, 55
Intravenous sedation, 75-82
Intrusion injuries to teeth, 251
Inverted-U entrance incisions, 143
IPL (intense pulsed light), 378-379
Iron deficiency anemia, 180
Irradiation mucositis, 381, 383
Irrigation
  distilled water use in, 248
  preventing infection of bite wounds, 289
  preventing infection of wounds, 248
Ischemic heart disease
  ECG signs of, 30
  management of chest pain, 121
  overview of, 153-158
  for patients with acute, 122

ISI (International Sensitivity Index), 178
Isoflurane
  hepatic effects of, 184
  as malignant hyperthermia trigger, 2
  minimal alveolar concentration of, 84
  partition coefficients for, 87
IV catheter sites, frequency of changing, 109
IV contrast agents
  anaphylactic reactions to, 57
  indicated/contraindicated for head and neck CT
    scans, 57
IV drug abuse, as valvular heart disease cause,
    157
IVP (intravenous pyelogram), 54, 55
IVRO (internal vertical ramus osteotomy), 339
Ivy method, platelet count, 36

J
Jacobson's nerve, 230
Jarisch-Herxheimer reaction, 317
Jaw. *See* Cleft lip and cleft palate patient
  bisphosphonate-related osteonecrosis of,
    388
  cysts and tumors of, 365-369
  diagnostic imaging modalities for, 60-61
  inflammatory disorders of, 61
  malignant diseases of, 60-61
  osteomyelitis of, 318-319
Joints
  indications for total reconstruction of in TMJ,
    326
  replacements, 219-222
JOMS (Journal of Oral and Maxillofacial
    Surgery), 438

K
Kent classification of edentulous ridges, 418
Ketamine, 77, 80
Ketoconazole
  as antifungal agent, 317
  formulations, 308
  pediatric and adult dosages, 310
Ketogenic hormones, 207
Ketones, 22
Kidneys
  effects of myoglobinuria on, 149
  fluid balance in, 94
  functions of, 187
Kiesselbach's plexus
  anterior epistaxis involving, 271
  nosebleeds and, 229-230
  overview of, 8
Klinefelter's syndrome, 4
Korotkoff sounds, 17
KUB radiographic view, 54

Kussmaul breathing, 16
Kwashiorkor, 105

L
Laboratory tests, 32-51
  acid-based abnormalities in, 46-47
  AMI, 47
  bilirubin abnormalties, 42
  blood chemistry, 40
  blood gas, 45-46, 47
  blood glucose, 45
  bone disease, 48
  calcium, 43
  cancer, 50
  CBCs, 32, 50
  cell-mediated deficiency, 208
  chronic salivary gland infections, 315
  coagulation, 37-38
  collagen vascular diseases, 47
  C-RP, 48
  CSF, 50
  diabetes, 202
  DIC, 39
  electrolyte disturbance, 40-41
  ESR, 48
  FDPs, 40
  fresh frozen plasma transfusions, indications
    for, 38
  FSPs, 40
  hematocrit, 35
  hemoglobin, 35
  heparin, 39-40
  HIV, 49-50, 211
  immunocompromised patients, preoperative lab
    studies, 210
  left shifts, 32
  liver, 37, 41-42
  odontogenic infections, 297
  oral cancer, 373
  pancreas, 44-45
  pathology specimens, 48-49
  platelets, 36-39
  primary adrenal insufficiency, 195
  prothrombin time, 39
  RBC, 34-35
  renal function, 44
  reticulocyte count, 35
  sick euthyroid syndrome, 197
  smears, 36
  thyroid screening, 48
  urinalysis, 44, 50
  viral hepatitis, 49
  WBC, 32-34
Lacrimal bone, 245
Lacrimal drainage system, 231, 286

Lacrimal gland
  autonomic innervation of, 231
  traumatic transection of, 288
Lactated Ringer's solution, 135
Lactating patients, local anesthetic use in, 73
Laryngeal nerve, tracheostomy-related injury to, 146
Larynx, sensory innervation of, 230
Laser-assisted uvulopalatoplasty (LAUP), 423, 426
Lasers
  in arthroscopic surgery, 326
  carbon dioxide, 5, 376-378
  in oral and maxillofacial surgery, 376-379
  uncovering implants using, 413-414
  use in uvulopalatoplasty, 423, 426
  YAG, 377-379
Lateral brow incisions, 274
Lateral canthotomy, in surgical access to orbit, 402
Lateral canthus reconstruction, 401
Lateral cephalograms, 424
Lateral chest projection, 52-53
Lateral pharyngeal fascial space infections, 302-303, 305
Lateral pyterygoid muscle, 227, 247
Latex allergies, 71
Latissimus dorsi flaps, 397-398
LAUP (laser-assisted uvulopalatoplasty), 423, 426
LDH levels, AMI test, 47
LE (lupus erythematosus), 48
Leads, placing ECG, 25, 30-31
L-E-A-N mnemonic, 8, 131
Learning deficiency
  syndromic children and, 351
  Treacher Collins syndrome and, 351-352
Le Fort fractures, 278-279
Le Fort I osteotomy, 336-337, 339
Left shifts, 32-34
Leishmaniasis, 315
Leprosy, 315
Lesser's triangle, 235
Leukemia, 181
Levonordefrin, 69-70
Lidocaine
  administering via endotracheal tube, 8, 131
  dosages of, for adults, 65-66
  dosages of, for resuscitation, 133
  dosages of, pediatric patients, 66
  effects of toxicity, 72
  important data about, 74
  narcotic sedation of, 66
  as refractory ventricullar fibrillation treatment, 123
Life support, basic, 115-120

Light reflexes, in ear examination, 15
Limbs, craniofacial syndromes affecting, 354
Lingual nerve
  anatomic relationship to Wharton's duct, 234-235
  injury during removal of third molars, 8, 257
  location in relation to mandibular third molar, 254
  success rate for repair to, 261
Lip
  carcinoma of, 371
  embryonic formation of upper, 341
  reconstruction of, 5, 402-403
  treating avulsive injury to, 286, 289
  treating through-and-through laceration of, 286
Lip adhesion procedure, in cleft lips, 346
Lipase levels, evaluating pancreas, 44-45
Lipid solubility, 1, 71
Lipoinjection, 406
Liposuction, submental, 6, 405-406
Lip-switch procedure, 421
Liver
  clotting factors synthesized in, 37
  location of, 18
  synthetic function of, 41-42
Liver disease
  biopsy, 185
  enzymes, 42
  lab trends in, 42
  muscle relaxants for patients with, 3
  overview of, 183-187
  tests for, 41
Liver-spleen scan, 55
Liver transplant patients, surgical considerations in, 186-187
LMWH (low-molecular-weight heparin), 182, 255
Lobule, 228
Local anesthetics
  lipid solubility of, 1
  metabolization of, 1
  not using with vasoconstrictor for postoperative hemorrhage, 250
  overview of, 65-74
  properties of, 72
Localized osteitis (dry socket), 251
Local transfer, in reconstruction tissue, 397
Lockwood's suspensory ligament, 275-276
Long buccal nerve injury, during removal of third molars, 8, 257
Long-term enteral feedings, 106
Loop diuretics
  defined, 95
  dose, mechanism of action and complications of, 165
  postoperative care, 103

Lorazepam, 78
Lordic chest radiographs, 54
Lower lip pits, syndrome associated with, 358
Low mandibular plane angle, mandibular
    deficiencies, 333
Low-molecular-weight heparin (LMWH), 182,
    255
Ludwig's angina
    defined, 3, 313
    postoperative care, 102
    treating, 313
    treating patient with low potassium, 95
Lung
    Hering-Breuer reflux, 18
    radiographic imaging of, 53-54
    ventilation-perfusion lung scans, 55
Lupus erythematosus (LE), 48
Lymphangiomas, treating cervicofacial, 368
Lymphatic drainage, of nose, 229
Lymph nodes, 20
    metastatic involvment of, 362, 368, 370-371
    sentinel node of, 5
    superior cervical chain of, 15
Lymphocytes, 34
Lymphoepithelial lesion, benign, 357

M

MAC (minimal alveolar concentration), 85
MAC (mycobacterium avium complex), in AIDS
    patients, 212
Macroangiopathy, diabetic, 201
Macroglossia, 353
Macules, 15
Madibulectomy, 373-374
Magnesium
    in calcium metabolism, 43
    during cardiac resuscitation, 133
Magnesium sulfate, for refractory V-fib/pulseless
    VT, 123
Magnetic resonance imaging. *See* MRI (magnetic
    resonance imaging)
Major extracellular cation
    defined, 93
Malar complex fracture, 276
Malar implants, 434-435
Malformations, craniomaxillofacial, 350-351
Malignancy, salivary gland, 359
Malignant hyperthermia (MH)
    defined, 2
    inhalational anesthetics known to trigger, 2
    overview of, 147-151
Mallampati classification of oropharynx, 21
Malnutrition, 2, 105-107
Mandible
    alveolar bone resorption in, 417

Mandible *(Cont'd)*
    ameloblastoma of, 365
    condylar hyperplasia of, 334
    deficiencies of, 3, 333, 337
    in dental implantation, 412-413
    dentate, blood supply of, 417
    edentulous bone loss in, 417-418
    excess of, asymmetric, 434
    giant cell lesions of, 337
    hemimandibular hypertrophy of, 334-335
    idiopathic condylar resorption in, 337
    implants for removable prosthetic replacement,
        414
    metastatic bronchiogenic carcinoma of, 175
    osteoradionecrosis, 384
    radiographs of, 55, 262
    reconstruction of, 393-394
    resection of, 244
    teeth, removing posterior, 248
    teeth, removing using bite block, 248
    trauma to, 61, 262-269
Mandible, cysts and tumors of
    diagnostic imaging of, 60
    metastatic, 175
    surgical ablation of, 367-368
Mandible fractures
    associated injuries with, 9, 264
    bilateral parasymphyseal, 264
    in children vs. adults, 263
    complications of, 264
    CT scan for evaluation of, 57
    radiographs for, 262
    surgical management of, 265
    tension band for managing, 264
    treating mandibular angle fractures, 265-266
Mandibular process, merger of, 342
Mandibular prognathism
    features/treatment of, 334
    procedures for correcting, 337
    syndromes associated with, 4, 354-355
Mandibular symphysis
    augmentation of, 434
    as bone graft source, 392
Mandibulectomy, marginal, 373-374
MAP (mean arterial pressure) readings, recording
    perioperatively, 161
Marasmus, 105
Marcus Gunn pupil, 272
Marfan's syndrome, 4
Marginal mandibular branch, facial nerve, 241
Markings, ECG, 24
Masseteric fascial space
    surgical intervention, 300
    typical sites of incision and drainage, 305
Masseter muscle, 244, 246

Mastication, muscles of, 227, 246-247
Masticatory myalgia, 329
Match (Postdoctoral Dental Matching Program), 436
Maturation phase, in wound healing, 285
MaxFace CT scan, 57
Maxilla
  alveolar bone resorption in, 417
  anterior osteoplasty of, 420
  AP deficiency of, 336
  atrophic, augmentation of, 422
  cysts and tumors of, diagnostic imaging, 60
  cysts and tumors of, metastatic, 175
  in dental implantation, 412-413
  edentulous bone loss in, 417-418
  fractures of, 9, 263-264, 278-280
  osteoradionecrosis (ORN), 384
  removal of teeth, 249, 254
  restoration of posterior teeth, 419
  shift rule for impacted cuspids, 249
  transverse expansion of, relapse rate in, 4
  vertical deficiency of, 336
  vertical excess of, 335-336
Maxillary processes, of external nose, 228
Maxillomandibular advancement (MMA), treating OSAS, 427
Maxillomandibular fixation (MMF)
  in condylar fractures, 266, 268
  overview of, 265
McCune-Albright syndrome, 355
Mean arterial pressure (MAP) readings, recording perioperatively, 161
Mean corpuscular hemoglobin concentration (MCHC), 34-35
Mean corpuscular volume (MCV), 34-35
Mechanical barriers, against microbiologic invasion, 283
Mechanical ventilation, 175
Medial canthal incisions, 274
Median cleft, malformation syndromes of, 355
Medical emergencies
  advanced cardiac life support in, 120-133
  advanced trauma life support in, 134-140
  basic life support in, 115-120
  malignant hyperthermia in, 147-151
  tracheostomy and cricothyrotomy in, 140-147
Medical history, 13
Medpor (polyethylene), 430, 431
Meglitinides, 204-205
Melkersson-Rosenthal syndrome, 357-358
MENS (multiple endocrine neoplasia syndrome), 195
Mentalis, in preprosthetic surgery, 421
Mental space, 21
Meperidine (Demerol), 1

Mepivacaine
  adult dosages, 65
  pediatric dosages, 66
  properties of, 72
Mesenchymal stem cells, 391
Meshed polymer, as facial alloplast, 430
Metabolic acidosis, 47
Metabolic alkalosis, 47
Metabolic equivalent demands (METs), 20
Metabolic test, 40
Metaglip, 205-206
Metastatic neck disease, 362
Metformin (Glucophage)
  contraindications to, 197, 204
  as oral hypoglycemic, 204
Methemoglobinemia, 69
Methicillin, 315
Methohexital (Brevital), 76
Methylparaben allergies, 71
Metoclopramide, 82
Metronidazole
  antimicrobial spectrum of, 311
  formulations, 308
  pediatric and adult dosages, 309
  penicillin used with, 311
  profile of, 312
METs (metabolic equivalent demands), 20
MH (malignant hyperthermia)
  defined, 2
  inhalational anesthetics known to trigger, 2
  overview of, 147-151
MI (myocardial infarction), 153-158
  conditions mimicking acute, 131
  diagnosing, 112
  perioperative, 154
  risk factors for, 155-156
MIC (minimal inhibitory concentration), of antibiotics, 307
Microbiologic invasion, protection from, 283
Microvascular disease, in glycosylation of platelets, 202
Midazolzam, 78
Midface deficiency, malformation syndromes of, 355
Midfacial fractures, 269-280
  diagnostic imaging modalities, 61
  maxillary, 278-280
  nasal, 269-272
  orbital, 272-276
  zygomatic, 276-278
Mid-lid incisions, 274
Midzolam, 78
Mikulicz's disease, 357
Millard rotation-advancement flap, 346-347
Minimal alveolar concentration (MAC), 84, 85

Minimal inhibitory concentration (MIC), of antibiotics, 307
Mitral regurgitation, 157
Mitral stenosis, 157
Mixed motor nerves, suturing, 8
MMA (maxillomandibular advancement), treating OSAS, 427
MMF (maxillomandibular fixation)
in condylar fractures, 266, 268
overview of, 265
Möbius' syndrome (congenital occlusofacial paralysis)
muscles affected in, 358
overview of, 358
Modified Mueller technique, 424
Modified radical neck dissection (MRND), 374
MOIST 'N DAMP mnemonic, 170-171
Molars, mandibular
coronectomy for impacted, 255
in facial space infections, 300-302
fracture incidents in, 262
Garré's osteomyelitis of, 317-318
in metastatic bronchiogenic carcinoma, 175
Molecular genetic testing, in malignant hyperthermia, 150
Monocular diplopia, 275
Monocyte counts, 34
Morphine
contraindication in renal disease, 189
histamine release effect of, 1
Motor nerves
of nose, 229
of scalp, 237
suturing, 8
Motor response, in Glasgow Coma Scale, 19
Mouth. *See also* Oral cavity
common sites for oral cancer, 5
embryonic formation of, 341
lowering floor of, 421
Movement disorders, extraocular, trauma-related, 276
MPD (myofascial pain dysfunction), 329
MRI (magnetic resonance imaging)
for cysts and benign jaw tumors, 60
indications/contraindications for, 6, 59-60
for infections in head and neck, 61-62
for invasive squamous cell carcinoma, 371
for malignant jaw diseases, 61
for patients with dental implants, 414
for salivary gland tumors, 361
for TMJ, 58-59
MRND (modified radical neck dissection), 374
Mucoceles, 361-362
Mucoepidermoid carcinoma, 4, 363
Mucoperiosteal flaps, 250

Mucous membrane, protecting from microbiologic invasion, 283
MUD PILES mnemonic, 98
Mueller technique, modified, 424
Mueller's muscle, 276
Multiple endocrine neoplasia syndrome (MENS), 195
Muscle relaxants
as NMBs. *See* Neuromuscular blocking agents (NMBs)
for patients with liver dysfunction, 184
Muscles
affected in Möbius' syndrome, 358
associated with malignant hyperthermia, 147
etiology of pain in, 329
involved in displacing mandibular fractures, 263
of mastication, 227, 246-247
orofacial, in cleft lip and palate, 342-343
Mustardé otoplasty technique, 403, 408
Mycobacterium avium complex infection (MAC), in AIDS patients, 212
Myocardial infarction. *See* MI (myocardial infarction)
Myocardial injury, ECG signs of, 122
Myocardial ischemia
angina as symptom of, 154
detecting intraoperatively, 156
ECG signs of, 23
mitral regurgitation in, 158
pathophysiology of, 153
as sign of shock, 130
treating acute, 122
Myocardium, oxygen supply and demand of, during MI, 153
Myofascial pain, temporomandibular disorders, 329
Myofascial pain dysfunction (MPD), 329
Myoglobinuria, malignant hyperthermia–related, 149

N
Naloxone, 79-80
Narcan, administering via endotracheal tube, 8, 131
Narrow-complex tachycardia, 123-125
Nasal bones
fractures of, 269-272
overview of, 228
radiographic evaluation of trauma to, 55
Nasal epistaxis, 229-230, 271
Nasal intubation, vs. oral, 119
Nasal packing, 270
Nasal process, medial, merger with intermaxillary segment, 341

Nasal septum
  hematoma of, 271
  overview of, 228
Nasoduodenal intubation, for enteral nutrition,
  105
Nasofrontal duct fractures, 282
Nasogastric tube (NGT)
  contraindications in midface fractures, 272, 279
  indications for, 106
Nasolabial angle, 338
Nasolabial flaps, 403
Nasolacrimal duct, 8, 231
Nasomaxillary dysplasia (Binder's syndrome),
  354
Nasoorbital-ethmoidal (NOE) fracture
  bowstring test in, 275
  clinical findings in patient with, 271-272
  defined, 274
  surgical approach to, 274
Nausea, postoperative, 7, 111
Nd:YAG laser, 379
Neck
  anatomic zones of, 289
  cancer of, 374-375, 380-389
  cosmetic surgery to lift, 406
  CT scan of, 57, 61-62
  metastatic lymph node of, 362, 367, 370
  necrotizing fasciitis of, 313-314
  penetrating trauma to, 289
  soft tissue infection in, 61-62
Necrosis
  acute tubular, 193
  coagulation, 377, 378
  distal, 398
  soft tissue, 385
Necrotizing fasciitis, 313-314
Neoplasms
  in AIDS patients, 212
  common salivary gland, in children, 363
Nephrogenic DI, 95, 194
Nephropathy, diabetic, 188, 201
Nephrotic syndrome, 40-41, 44
Nerve blocks, from onset of anesthesia, 68
Nerve conduits, alloplastic, 260
Nerve grafts, 260
Nerve impulse transmission, local anesthetics
  affecting, 67-68
Nerve injury
  classifications of, 256
  closed, 258-259
  open, 258
  pathophysiology of, 256
  posterior iliac crest bone grating–related,
    395
  repair of, 259, 260

Nerves
  supplying ears, 230
  supply to scalp, 236-237
Neurapraxia, 256
Neurilemoma (schwannoma), 356
Neurogenic shock, 135
Neurologic abnormalities, in AIDS patients, 212
Neuromuscular blocking agents (NMBs), 89-90
Neurons, orofacial, 331
Neuropathy
  diabetic, 201
  peripheral, in end-stage renal disease, 188
Neurosensory deficits, ilium bone graft
    harvest–related, 396
Neurotmesis, 256
NGT (nasogastric tube)
  contraindications in midface fractures, 272, 279
  indications for, 106
Nitrous oxide
  contraindications for, 83, 226
  delivery of, 83
  as diffusion hypoxia cause, 87
  minimal alveolar concentration of, 84
  partition coefficient of, 87
  second gas effect in, 84
Nitrous oxide–oxygen sedation
  in asthma patients, 84
  in chronic obstructive pulmonary disease
    patients, 83-84
  in obstetric patients, 87
NMBs (neuromuscular blocking agents), 88-90
Nodular pattern of disease, 52
Nodules, 15
NOE (nasoorbital-ethmoidal) fracture
  bowstring test in, 275
  clinical findings in patient with, 271-272
  defined, 274
  surgical approch to, 274
Noncavitary lesions, lung masses, 54
Nondepolarizing NMBs, 88-89
Nonenzymatic glycosylation of hemoglobin, 201
Non-Hodgkin's lymphoma, 181
Non-REM stages of sleep, 423
Nonspecific immunity, 208
Nonsteroidal antiinflammatory drugs. *See*
    NSAIDs (nonsteroidal antiinflammatory
    drugs)
Nonsupparative osteomyelitis, 318
Normal route of conduction, 24
Nose
  bones of, 228, 246
  cosmetic surgery for, 406-407
  deformities, associated with cleft lip, 343
  deformities, saddle nose, 271, 435
  external, anatomy of, 228

Nose *(Cont'd)*
external, embryonic formation of, 341
fractures of, 269-272
lymphatic drainage of, 229
mapping nerve supplies to, 229
paranasal sinus drainage of, 230
reconstruction of, 402-403
vascular supply to, 228-229
Nosebleeds
Kiesselbach's plexum and, 229-230
managing in emergency, 271
in midface fracture, 279
Notes, surgical, 10
Novocaine allergy, 71, 74
NPH insulin, 203-204
NSAIDs (nonsteroidal antiinflammatory drugs)
effect on renal function, 189
hypertension medications and, 163
inhibiting platelet aggregation, 36
inhibiting prostaglandin synthesis, 2
risk in pregnancy, 226
Nuclear scans, 55
Nurses, getting along with, 10
Nutritional support, postoperative care, 105-108
Nystagmus, 19
Nystatin, 308, 309, 312

O

Obese patients
intravenous sedation in, 81
medical and anesthetic problems in, 22
Oblique muscles, 6, 276, 396
Oblique ridge, as bone graft source, 392
Obstetric anesthesiologists, 74
Obstructive salivary gland disease, viewing on
sialogram, 58
Obstructive sleep apnea. *See* OSA (obstructive
sleep apnea)
Obstructive sleep apnea syndrome. *See* OSAS
(obstructive sleep apnea syndrome)
Ocular dystopia, 273
Oculocardiac reflex, 19
Odontogenic infections
anatomy of, 293
bacteria responsible for, 291, 294
diagnosing, 292, 297
drainage of, 306
factors influencing spread of, 296
follow-up appointments after, 306
principles of therapy for, 297
progression of, 295
severity of, 306
Odontogenic jaw tumors, benign, 60
Odontogenic keratocysts, 5, 366
OGT (orogastric tube), 107

Olfactory placode, of nose, 228
Onset time
decreasing muscle relaxant, 89-90
of local anesthetics, 71-72
Open joint surgery, of temporomandibular joint,
325
Open rhinoplasty, 406-407
Operative notes, 13
Opioids
antagonists, 79-80
as choledochuduodenal sphincter spasm cause,
184
clinical uses of, 79
as intravenous induction agent, 7
pharmacogologic effects of, 79
types of, 79
Oral cancer, 370-376
cervical lymph node metastasis in, 375
effects of radiation therapy, 373, 381
evaluating and diagnosing, 373-374
sentinel node biopsy in, 374-375
signs of, 375
squamous cell carcinoma in, 370-371
staging system for, 370-372
treatment modalities for, 372-373
types of neck dissections in, 374
Oral glucose tolerance test, 202
Oral intubation, vs. nasal, 119
Oral mucosa
disadvantages of intraoral grafting, 401
effects of radiation on, 381
Orbit
fractures of, 272-276
surgical access to, 401-402
volume of, in orbital trauma, 275-276
Orbital apex syndrome, 275
Orbital cavity, anatomy of, 245
Orbital contents entrapment, 273
Orbital fat, 246
Organic heart murmurs, 16-17
Organogenesis, 223
Organ space SSIs, 112
ORN (osteoradionecrosis)
effects of, 380
incidence of, 6
overview of, 383-387
pathophysiology of, 6
Orofacial anatomy, 227-248
Orogastric tube (OGT), 107
Oropharynx airway exam, 20-21
Orthotopic heart transplantation, changes in ECG
readings, 31
OSA (obstructive sleep apnea), 7, 423-425
OSAS (obstructive sleep apnea syndrome)
complications of, 425

OSAS (obstructive sleep apnea syndrome)
  (Cont'd)
  diagnosing, 424
  OSA vs., 423
  pickwickian syndrome in, 22
  snoring and, 422
  symptoms of, 423
  treatment of, 425-426
Osseointegration, of dental implants, 6, 411, 413
Osseous genioplasty, complications of, 340
Osseous surgical margins, 366, 367
Osteoarthritis, TMJ
  chondromalacia in, 332
  disc displacement and, 323
  pathogenic pathway in, 324
  primary vs. secondary, 332
  stages of, 326-328
Osteoconduction, 390
Osteogenesis, 4, 390
Osteoinduction, 389
Osteomyelitis, 55, 317-319
Osteoprogenitor cells, 391
Osteoradionecrosis (ORN). *See* ORN
    (osteoradionecrosis)
Osteotomy
  bilateral sagittal split, 3, 333, 337
  in chin augmentation, 406
  in fibrous dysplasia, 368
  as hemimandibular hypertrophy treatment,
    335
  internal vertical ramus, 339
  lateral, in dorsal nasal reduction, 407
  Le Fort I, 336-337, 339
  for mandibular excess correction, 434
  for mandibular symphysis augmentation, 434
  sandwich, 420
  transoral vertical, 334
  visor, 420
  of zygomatic complex, vs. zygomatic implants,
    434
Otoplasty, Mustardé technique of, 403, 408
Otoscopic exam, 20
Outpatient anesthesia, propofol for, 80
Oxacillin
  antimicrobial spectrum of, 311
  formulations, 307
  pediatric and adult dosages, 309
Oxidized regenerated cellulose (Surgicel), 250
Oxidized surfaces, in dental implant healing, 416
Oxygen. *See also* Nitrous oxide–oxygen sedation
  delivery of, 82-83
  evaluating blood gas for, 47
  in hypoxic events, 91
  in pulse oximeter readings, 87
  resuscitation using, 132

Oxyhemoglobin dissocation curve, 80-81, 172
Oxyhemoglobin saturation, 90

P
PA (posteroanterior) chest films, 52-54
Pain
  after local anesthetic injection, 68
  in bisphosphonate-related osteonecrosis of jaw,
    6
  caused by irradiation mucositis and xerostomia,
    383
  chest, 121-122, 125, 127, 155, 176
  evaluating abdominal, 20, 54-55
  evaluating cervical spine, 57
  facial, 331-332
  in salivary gland malignancy, 4
  in superficial incisional infection, 112
  in temporomandibular disorders, 329-331
  thermal burn, 139
  using succinylcholine for, 88
  using tramadol for chronic, 2, 81
Palatal clefts, 344
Palatal mucosa grafts, for vestibuloplasty, 401
Palpable nodules, within thyroid gland, 196
Palpation, abdominal, 20
Palpebral fissure (rima), 230
Pancreatic disease, laboratory tests for, 44-45
Panoramic radiography, 60-61, 267-268
Panorex radiograph, anatomic landmarks on, 56
Papillary hyperplasia, 419
Papillon-LeFèvre syndrome, 358
Papule, 15
Paralysis, facial nerve, 242-243
Paramedian forehead flaps, 402
Paranasal sinuses, 230
Parasymphyseal fractures, 264, 268
Parathyroid gland, resection of, 194
Parenteral nutrition, 101, 102, 108
Paresthesia, 257
Parkes Weber syndrome, 358
Parotidcomasseteric fascia, relationship of facial
    nerve to, 241
Parotid duct, 286-287
Parotidectomy, facial nerve location during,
    241
Parotideomasseteric fascia, 237, 238
Parotid gland
  diagnosing acute bacterial parotitis, 362
  facial nerve location during surgery on, 364
  facial nerve paralysis and, 359
  incisional biopsy for diagnosing, 4, 362-363
  infection of, 315
  sarcoidosis of, 361-362
  tumors of, 363-364
Parotitis, viral vs. bacterial, 361

Paroxysmal supraventricular tachycardia (PSVT), 123-125

Partial odontectomy (coronectomy), on impacted mandibular molar, 255

Partial pressure of oxygen, 90, 134

Partial-thickness (second-degree) burns, 139

Partial thromboplastin time. *See* PTT (partial thromboplastin time)

Particulate bone and cancellous marrow (PBCM) grafts, in mandibular reconstruction, 393-394

Partition coefficients, in inhaled anesthetics, 86-87

PASS (Postdoctoral Application Support Service), 436, 438

Passavant's ridge, 343

Passive plating, in rigid fixation, 267

Pasteurella multocida, 5

PBCM (particulate bone and cancellous marrow) grafts, in mandibular reconstruction, 393-394

Pco$_2$
in blood gas measurement, 45
postoperative care scenario, 101

PDA closure, NSAIDs and, 226

PE (pulmonary embolus)
origination of, 109
postoperative management of, 178
signs and diagnosis of, 177

PEA (pulseless electrical activity)
causes of, 129
causing pulseless condition, 130
sudden cardiac death and, 131
treating, 129, 132
types of, 128

Pectoralis major flaps, 397-398

Pediatric patients
in acute malignant hyperthermia, 149
antibiotic dosages for, 309-310
cardiac arrest cause in, 139
chest compressions in, 7, 116-117
clearing foreign body airway obstructions in, 117
cysts in, 5, 367
frontal sinus fractures in, 283
lidocaine or mepivacaine drug dosages, 66
local anesthetic toxicity in, 69
mandibular fractures in, 263
methemoglobinemia risk in, 69
narcotic sedation effects in, 66
normal volume of blood in, 136
postoperative care of, 21, 102, 111
postponing elective surgery in children with URIs, 21-22
rescue breathing for, 115-116

Pediatric patients *(Cont'd)*
resuscitation efforts for, 118
salivary gland diseases in, 361, 363
tumors in, 367

Pedicle flap failure, 398-399

PEEP (positive end-expiratory pressure), 173-174

Pel-Ebstein fever, 1, 14

Pell and Gregory impacted mandibular third molar classifications, 255

Pelvis fractures, posterior iliac crest bone grafting–related, 395

Penicillin
action mode of, 3, 309
excellence of, 311
G and V types, 309-310, 312
third-generation antibiotics and, 319
use in salivary gland infection, 315

Pentothal, 76, 80

Periodontium, effects of radiation on, 381

Periosteal thickening, conditions associated with, 318

Peripheral ameloblastoma, 368

Peripheral antiadrenergics, 166

Peripheral facial nerve paralysis, 359

Peripheral nerve blocks, at onset of anesthesia, 68

Peripheral parenteral nutrition (PPN), 108

Peripheral sensitization, 331

Peritoneal dialysis, 190

Pernicious anemia, 180

PERRLA (pupils equal, round, and reactive to light and accommodation), 15

PET scans, salivary gland tumor diagnosis, 361

Pfeiffer's syndrome, 353

pH
in acid-base disorders, 46
anesthesia induction and, 71-73, 76, 78
in blood gas analysis, 45, 47
causing risk of aspiration in obese patients, 22
in compartment syndrome, 138
in dissociation curve shifts of respiratory disorders, 172-173
in respiratory acidosis, 174
in respiratory alkalosis, 98-99, 174
in respiratory failure, 175
for storing harvested bone cells, 394
in Type I diabetes, 200
of urine, 44

Pharyngeal arches, 341

PHD mnemonic, for asystole etiology, 129

Philadelphia chromosome, 181

Phlebitis, postoperative, 109

Phone fast rule, 118

Phone-first rule, 115, 118

Phosphorus, in calcium metabolism, 43

Photoablative reaction, in lasers, 376

Photothermal reaction, in lasers, 376
Physical examination, 14
Pickwickian syndrome, 22
Pierre Robin sequence/syndrome, 354
Piezoelectric effect, 391
Pinguecula, 15
Pituitary tumors, anterior, 195-196
Plain angles, mandibular, 333
Plain film tomography, 57
Plasma
    osmolarity of, 100
    platelet-rich, 390
Plasma cholinesterase (pseudocholinesterase), 2,
    90
Plasmic imbibition, 7, 420
Platelets
    in complete blood count, 33
    function assessment of, 37-39
    glycosylation of, 202
    plasma rich in, 390
    vitamin K deficiency affecting, 37
Plating, passive, in rigid fixation, 267
Platysma flaps, 397-398
Pleomorphic adenoma, 4, 363
Pleural effusion, 176
Plummer-Vinson syndrome, 181, 358
Plunging ranula, 362
PMI (point of maximum impulse), of the heart,
    16
PMMA (polymethylmethacrylate) alloplastic
    facial implants, 430-432
Pneumocystitis carinii, 54, 212
Pneumomediastinium, as tracheostomy
    complication, 146
Pneumonia
    AIDS-related, 54, 212
    aspiration, 107-109, 111, 177
    bacterial, postoperative, 108
    diabetes-related, 207
    postoperative, 108-109, 111-112
    tracheostomy-related, 146
Pneumothorax
    radiographic appearance of, 52, 54
    signs of, 176
    tracheostomy-related, 146
    treating, 176
Pocket principle, in ear injury, 287
Poikilocytosis, 36
Point of maximum impulse (PMI), of the heart,
    16
Polycrystalline ceramics, 432
Polyethylene (Medpor), 430, 431
Polyhydroxyethylmethacrylate, 432
Polymethylmethacrylate alloplastic facial
    implants, 430-432

Polyostotic fibrous dysplasia, 357
Polyphagia, diabetes mellitus–related, 200
Polysomnography, for obstructive sleep apnea
    diagnosis, 424
Polytetrafluoroethylene (PTFE), as facial
    alloplast, 430, 431
Polyuria
    diabetes insipidus–related, 95, 194
    diabetes mellitus–related, 200
    hypercalcemia-related, 98
    severe hypokalemia-related, 94
Porous HA (hydroxyapatite), as facial alloplast,
    430
Porous PMMA, as facial alloplast, 430
Porous polyethylene, as facial alloplast, 430
Positive attitude, maintaining, 10
Positive end-expiratory pressure (PEEP), 173-174
Positive pressure ventilation, effect on hepatic
    blood flow, 184
Postdoctoral Dental Matching Program (Match),
    436
Posterior nasal packing, 270
Posteroanterior chest films, 52-54
Postmaxillectomy, 373
Postoperative care
    in acute MH attacks, 149
    in diabetes, 203
    fluids and electrolytes in. *See* Fluid and
        electrolyte management
    in liver transplant patients, 186-187
    monitoring flaps in, 398
    nutritional support in, 105-108
    in patients with TMJ dysfunction, 330
    thrombotic events in pregnant patient, 225
    in tracheostomies, 146
Postoperative complications, 108-114
    aspiration pneumonia, 109
    atelectasis, 109, 113
    bleeding, 110
    cardiac arrhythmias, 110, 112
    cleft palates, 348
    deep-space SSIs, 112
    dentoalveolar surgery, 250
    DVT, 110
    dysuria, 7, 110-111
    emboli, 109
    fevers, 108-109, 110, 112-114
    Homans' sign, 110
    hypertension, 110
    hypotension, 110
    infection at IV catheter sites, 109
    infection at wound site, 113
    myocardial infarction, 112
    nausea and vomiting, 111
    phlebitis, 109

Postoperative complications *(Cont'd)*
  pneumonia, 111
  preventing aspiration, 111
  respiratory complications, 109
  seromas, 111
  subclinical hypothyroidism, 197
  superficial incisional SSIs, 112
  surgical wound infections, 112
  tracheostomy, 146
  urinary tract infections (UTIs), 113
  Virchow's triad, 109
Postsplenectomy patients, 218
Posttraumatic enophthalamos, 274
Potassium
  of 70-kg man, 98
  in bone disease evaluation, 48
  causing electrolyte disturbance, 41
  effect on ECG, 25, 97
  interaction with aldosterone, 192
  Ludwig's angina treatment, 95
  postoperative care scenarios, 100, 103-104
Potassium hydroxide (KOH) stain, 49
Power density, in irradiation, 377
PPN (peripheral parenteral nutrition), 108
Pramlintide (Symlin), 206
Pregnant patients. *See also* Fetus (human embryo)
  fetal sensitivity to radiation, 2
  local anesthetics used in, 73
  nitrous oxide sedation unsafe for, 87
  overview of, 222-226
  PMMA implants toxic for, 431
Premature atrial contractions, ECG signs of, 26
Premature ventricular contractions (PVCs)
  ECG signs of, 29
  in postoperative cardiac arrhythmia, 110
Preoperative 12-lead, ECG, 30-31
Preoperative evaluation, 13-23
Preoperative notes, 13
Prepalatal clefts, 344
Preprosthetic surgery, 417-422
Preradiation patients, 381-382
Prerenal azotemia, 193
Pressure-volume loops, 157
Prilocaine
  dosage of, 65
  as methemoglobinemia cause, 69
Primary ABCD survey, 120, 134
Primary adrenal failure, 195
Primary contractions, in skin grafts, 399, 420
Primary fascial spheres, secondary vs., 296
Primary immunodeficiency, 208
Primary maxillary central incisor, injuries of, 251
Primary palate, 342
Priming technique, for inhalational anesthetics, 90

PR interval, of ECG, 23
Procainamide, as ventricular tachycardia
    treatment, 123
Procaine
  allergic potential of, 71
  metabolism of in liver disease, 184
Proplast, 431
Propofol (Diprivan)
  combined with volatile anesthetics, 85
  effect on intracranial pressure, 80
  as outpatient anesthetic, 80
  pharmacologic effects of, 76
Prostaglandins
  in bone matrix, 390
  NSAIDs inhibiting synthesis of, 2, 226
  in osteoarthritis, 327
Prostate-specific antigen (PSA), 50
Prosthetic joint patients, 3, 219-222
Protein
  binding, as liver disease indicator, 184
  binding, in local anesthetic duration, 71
  dietary, increasing for perioperative liver
      disease, 186
  dietary, response of insulin and glucagon to,
      207
  metabolism of in diabetic patient, 198
  as nutrition component, 105, 107
Proximal nasal bones, fracture of, 269
PSA (prostate-specific antigen), 50
Pseudocholinesterase, 2, 90
Pseudo-EMD, PEA rhythm, 128
PSVT (paroxysmal supraventricular tachycardia),
    123-125
PT (prothrombin time) test, 178
  clotting factors measured by, 180, 186
  in disseminated intravascular coagulation
      diagnosis, 39
  in immunocompromised patients, 210
  in international normalized ratio, 178
  as liver disease indicator, 41, 185
  measuring intrinsic and common pathways
      with, 38
  in postoperative pulmonary embolus
      management, 178
  in renal failure patients, 190
  in warfarin monitoring, 178-179
Pterygoid muscle, medial, 247
Pterygomandibular raphe
  buccal mucosa grafts harvested from, 399
  in fascial space infections, 298, 301
PTFE (polytetrafluoroethylene), as facial
    alloplast, 430, 431
Ptosis, traumatic, 276
PTT (partial thromboplastin time)
  clotting factors measured by, 180, 186

PTT (partial thromboplastin time) *(Cont'd)*
   in immunocompromised patients, 210
   as liver damage indicator, 185
   measurements of, 180
   overview of, 37-38
   in renal failure patients, 190
   for use of low-molecular-weight heparin, 255
Pulmonary artery wedge pressure, as myocardial
      ischemia indicator, 156, 157
Pulmonary embolus (PE)
   origination of, 109
   postoperative management of, 178
   signs and diagnosis of, 177
Pulp necrosis, 251
Pulse, in rescue breathing, 116
Pulseless conditions, 123, 130
Pulseless electrical activity. *See* PEA (pulseless
      electrical activity)
Pulse oximetry, 90
Pulse pressure, defined, 17-18
Pupils
   autonomic nerve supply to, 233
   equal, round, and reactive to light and
      accommodation (PERRLA), 15
PVCs (premature ventricular contractions)
   ECG signs of, 29
   in postoperative cardiac arrhythmia, 110
P wave, ECG, 23
Pyramidal disjunction, Le Fort II fracture, 279
Pytergium, 15
Pyterygomandibular raphe, muscles of, 227

Q

QRS complex, ECG, 23
Q-switching, 379
Qualitative platelet disorders, 36
Quantitative platelet disorders, 36
Quotidian fever, 14

R

Rabies prophylaxis, for animal bite wounds, 289
Raccoon eyes, 280
Radiation therapy
   dental implants and, 416
   dosage of, 6
   endosseous implants and, 415
   fetal sensitivity to, 2
   for head and neck cancer, 380-389
   for malignant salivary gland tumors, 364
   mandibular reconstruction after, 394
   for marginal mandibulectomy, 373-374
   in oral cancer, 372, 373, 381
   types of, 380
Radical neck dissection (RND), 374
Radioactive tracers, in bone scans, 55

Radionuclear ventriculography, 170
Radionuclide scanning, 61, 361
Radionuclide scintigraphy, 60
Ramsay Hunt syndrome, 357
Random flaps, 397
Random pattern flaps, 399
Ranulae, 362
Rapid eye movement (REM) stage, of sleep, 7,
      423
RBCs (red blood cells)
   diagnostic peritoneal lavage and, 136-137
   using clinically, 34-35
RDI (respiratory disturbance index), 424
Rebound, 18
Recommendation letters, OMFS residency, 438
Reconstruction, oral and maxillofacial
   bone required for, 5
   overview of, 389-404
Red blood cells (RBCs)
   diagnostic peritoneal lavage and, 136-137
   using clinically, 34-35
Reflection, laser, 376
Reflexes, testing deep tendon, 18
Reiter's syndrome, 357
Releasing incisions, 250
REM (rapid eye movement) stage, of sleep, 7,
      423
Remittent fever, 1, 14
Renal disease
   drugs to be avoided in, 2
   overview of, 187-192
   testing for, 44
Residency programs, OMFS, 436-440
Resident Organization of the American
      Association of Oral and Maxillofacial
      Surgeons (ROAAOMS), 438
Respiration
   normal rate of, 175
   postoperative complications, 109
   pregnancy changing, 224-225
   preoperative evaluation, 16, 20-21
Respiratory acidosis (hypoventilation)
   causing acid-base disorders, 46
   causing cardiac arrest in pediatric patients, 139
   diagnosing, 174
   postoperative care and, 98-99
Respiratory alkalosis (hyperventilation)
   causing acid-base disorders, 47
   diagnosing, 174
Respiratory center, 174-175
Respiratory disorders, 172-178
Respiratory disturbance index (RDI), 424
Respiratory failure, acute, 175
Resuscitation, of trauma victims, 132, 135
Reticulocyte count, 35

Retin-A, prepeel skin regimen, 409
Retinopathy, diabetic, 201
Retromandibular approach, 242
Retromolar region
    cancer of, 384
    in denture reconstruction, 419
    using posteriorly-based flap for defects of, 384
Retropharyngeal fascial space infections, 303-304
Rheumatoid arthritis
    temporomandibular joint dysfunction
        associated with, 331-332
    testing for, 47
Rheumatoid factor, 47
Rhinoplasty, 406-407
Rhytidectomy (face lift), 404, 405
Ribs
    as bone graft source, 392
    in costochondral graft reconstruction, 397
    preoperative evaluation of, 15-16
RIF (rigid internal fixation), 265, 267-268
Rigid internal fixation (RIF), 265, 267-268
Ringer's solution, 101, 290
Rinne hearing test, 15
RND (radical neck dissection), 374
ROAAOMS (Resident Organization of the
        American Association of Oral and
        Maxillofacial Surgeons), 438
Rule of Tens, in cleft lip repair, 345
R wave, reading ECG, 24

S
Saddle nose deformity
    correction of, 435
    overview of, 271
Saline, for cleaning lacerations, 290
Salivary gland diseases
    antibiotics treating, 315
    in children, 361, 363
    classifications of, 314
    evaluating chronic, 315
    overview of, 359-365
    tumors, 4
Sandwich osteotomy, 420
Sarcoidosis, of parotid gland, 361-362
Scalp
    blood and nerve supply to, 236-237
    layers of, 236
Scalp proper, 236
Scar revision
    amount of time lapsing before, 291
    dermabrasion, acne-related, 409
Scatter, laser, 376
SCh (succinylcholine), 2
Schistocyte, 36
Schwannoma, 356

Scleroma, 315
SCM (sternocleidomastoid muscle), blood and
        nerve supplies for, 227
Sebaceous glands, of eyelids, 233
Secondary ABCD survey, 120-121, 134
Secondary avulsed teeth, 267
Secondary contractions, in skin grafts, 399
Secondary diabetes, 199
Secondary fascial spheres, primary vs., 296
Secondary immunodeficiency, 208
Secondary palate, 342
Second-degree (partial-thickness) burns, 139
Second-degree heart block
    identifying in ECG, 28
    overview of, 127-128
    treating, 128
Second gas effect, 84
Sedation drugs
    metabolized by liver, 185
    pregnancy and OMFS, 224
Selective neck dissection (SND), 374
Sensory nerves
    of nose, 229
    of scalp, 237
    suturing, 8
Sentinel node, 5, 374
Sentinel node biopsy (SNB), 374
Septal hematomas, acute, 270
Seromas, 111
Serum calcium, 101
Sesamoid cartilages, 228
Severe obstructive sleep apnea, 425
Sevoflurane
    as malignant hyperthermia trigger, 2
    minimal alveolar concentration of, 84
    partition coefficient of, 87
    wake-up potential of, 87
Shift rule, 249
Shock
    cardiogenic, 135
    hypovolemic, 131
    neurogenic, 135
    in trauma patients, 135
    types of, 130
SIADH (syndrome of inappropriate antidiuretic
        hormone)
    vs. diabetes insipidus, 94
    diagnosing, 194
    overview of, 193-194
    in postoperative care, 102
    treating, 194
Sialadenitis, 315
Sialoendoscopy, 360
Sialography, 57-58
Sialolithiasis, 360

Sick euthyroid syndrome, 197
Sickle cell anemia, 180
Sickle cells, 36
Signs, vs. symptoms, 14
Silicone, for facial implants, 429
Single-tooth edentulism, 415
Sinus bradycardia, 30
Sinuses
    ECG signs of, 25-26
    frontal fracture of, 281-283
    lift of, 419-420
    node, normal route of conduction, 24
Sinuses, maxillary
    anatomy of nasolacrimal duct, 8, 286
    average size of, 6, 419
    diagnostic imaging of, 56
    infections of, 316
    neoplasms of, 373
    pathology of, 61
    root or root tip displacement in, 253
Sinusitis, flora of, 316
Sinus rhythm, 26
Sinus tachycardia, 26
Sistrunk procedure, 5, 368
Sjögren's syndrome, 58, 361
Skin
    cosmetic facial surgery, 404-410
    cosmetic surgery lasers for, 377
    injuries to, 283-291
    layers of, 285
Skin grafts
    characteristics of, 420
    contraction in, 420
    full-thickness/split-thickness, 285-286, 399-400
    goals of, 421
    in oral and maxillofacial reconstruction, 389-404
    plasmic imbibition and, 420
    primary closure in, 290
    for traumatic wounds, 285-286
Sleep apnea. *See* OSA (obstructive sleep apnea);
    OSAS (obstructive sleep apnea syndrome)
Sleep stages, 423
Sliding tarsoconjunctival flap, upper eyelid
    reconstruction, 403
SMA 7 test, 40
SMAS (superficial musculoaponeurotic system)
    defining, 235-236
    extensions in neck, 238
    manipulating in face lifts, 404
    relationship of facial nerve to temporoparietal
    fascia and, 242
Smears, 36
Smoking
    dental implant placement and, 414
    increasing risk surgical wound infection, 321

SMP (sympathetically mediated pain), 257
SNB (sentinel node biopsy), 374
SND (selective neck dissection), 374
Snoring, 422-427
Sodium
    of 70-kg man, 98
    in electrolyte disturbances, 40-41
    interaction with aldosterone, 192
    in low serum concentration, 100
    as major extracellular cation, 93
Sodium bicarbonate, resuscitation dosage,
    133
Soft palate, muscles of, 247
Soft tissue
    cysts in children, 5
    effect of radiation therapy on, 380-381
    facial measurements, 338
    injuries, 283-291
    planning cosmetic surgery, 404
Solid silicone rubber, as facial alloplast, 430
Sorbitol, 201
Space 4 of Grodinsky and Holyoke, 296
Space infections, 296-304
Speech
    with unrepaired cleft palates, 348
    in velopharyngeal incompetence, 349
Sphenoid bone, 245
Spherocytes, 36
Spinal cord tracts, assessing, 138
Spironolactone, 166
Splenectomies, 218
Splinting, 251, 252
Split-thickness skin grafts. *See* STSGs (split-
    thickness skin grafts)
Spread routes, in oral carcinoma, 372
Squamous cell carcinoma, 370-372, 375
SRS (stereotactic radiosurgery), techniques of,
    373
SSI (surgical site infection), 7, 112
Stains
    Gram, 292-295
    for infectious agents, 48-49
Staphylococcal infections
    found in oral cavity, 291-292
    from human bites, 5
    odontogenic, 294
    producing coagulase, 291
    of prosthetic joints, 3
Stereotactic radiosurgery (SRS), 373
Sternocleidomastoid flaps, 397-398
Sternocleidomastoid muscle, blood and nerve
    supplies for, 227
Stethoscopes, using bell vs. diaphragm of, 17
Stickler's syndrome, 354
Strabismus, 20

Streptococcal infections
  in acute and chronic sinusitis, 316
  in erysipelas, 3
  from human bites, 5
  in oral cavity, 292
  odontogenic, 294
Stress fractures, preventing reoccurrence of, 367
Stridor, 16, 175
ST segment, in ECGs, 23, 30
STSGs (split-thickness skin grafts)
  contraction in, 7
  desired thickness of, 420
  overview of, 399-400
  varying thickness of, 7
Stylomastoid foramen, 238
Subciliary crease incisions, in surgical access to
      orbit, 401
Subciliary lower eyelid incisions, 274
Subcutaneous emphysema, tracheostomy-related,
      146
Subdural hematamas, vs. epidural, 137
Subglottic edema
  properties/adverse effects of, 79
  reducing intracranial pressure, 80
  tracheostomy-related, 146
Sublimaze (fentanyl)
  causing histamine release, 1
  properties/adverse effects of, 79
  reducing ICP, 80
Sublingual fascial space infections, 298-299
Submandibular approach, avoidance of facial
      artery in, 234
Submandibular fascial space infections, 299
Submandibular triangle
  hypoglossal nerves in, 235
  managing displaced roots or root tips in, 252
Submental fascial space
  infections, 299-300
  liposuction of, 6, 405-406
Submental region, 406
Submental vertex view, in radiographic studies,
      277
Submucous clefts, 344
Succinylcholine, 88
Sudden cardiac death, defined, 131
Sufentanil (Sufenta)
  causing histamine release, 1
  properties/adverse effects of, 79
Sulfa drug allergies, 71
Sulfonylureas, 204
Superficial incisional SSIs, 112
Superficial musculoaponeurotic system. *See*
      SMAS (superficial musculoaponeurotic
      system)
Superficial temporal fascia, 237

Superior alveolar artery, in Le Fort I incision, 339
Superior cervical chain lymph nodes, 15
Superior head, lateral pyterygoid muscle, 227
Superior orbital fissure syndrome, 245, 275,
      359-361
Superior pharyngeal constrictor muscle, 249
Superpulsing, 379
Supine abdominal radiographs, 54
Suprahyoid muscle group, 247, 339
Supraplatysmal plane, 405
Supraventricular origin, 31-32
Supraventricular tachyarrythmias, 124
Supraventricular tachycardia, 27
Sural nerve graft, 9
Surgery
  in HIV-infected persons, 212
  in pregnant patients, 223, 225-226
  principles of incision and drainage, 306
Surgery, readiness for, 9-13
Surgical intervention
  CEOT (calcifying epithelial odontogenic
      tumor), 365-366
  cleft palates, 346
  decreasing infection of surgical wounds, 321
  for drooling, 364
  frontal sinus fractures, 282
Surgical notes, 10-13
Surgical site infection (SSI), 7, 112
Surgical stress, in diabetic patients, 207
Sutures
  intradomal, in nasal surgery, 407
  materials used for, 285
  for nerve repair, 8, 260
  selecting for soft tissue injuries, 290
Sweat glands, of eyelids, 233
Symlin, 206
Sympathetically mediated pain (SMP), 257
Sympatholytics, as antihypertensive agent, 165
Symphyseal fractures, 268
Symptomatic hypercalcemia, 196
Symptomatic hypernatremia, 99
Symptoms
  listening and translating, 9
  physical signs vs., 14
Synchronized cardioversion, 124, 131
Syndromes
  affecting oromaxillofacial region, 350-359
  affecting salivary glands, 4, 361-362
  of inappropriate antidiuretic hormone. *See*
      SIADH (syndrome of inappropriate
      antidiuretic hormone)
Synovial clearance, in osteoarthritis, 327
Synovial joint cartilage, 322
Synovial membrane, preservation during
      arthoscopic procedures, 325

Synovitis, of temporomandibular joint, 324
Synovium, temporomandibular joint, 323-324
Syphilis, tertiary, 315
Systemic immunity, classes of, 208

T
Tachyarrhythmias, 123-124
Tachycardia
  cardioverting patients with, 124
  defined, 25
  identifying in ECG, 25
  narrow-complex, 123-125
  overview of, 123-124
  signs of, 31
  sinus, 26
  supraventricular, 27
  in trauma patients, 135
  ventricular, 30, 120
  wide-complex, 31, 126
Tachypnea
  defined, 175
Tacrolimus, 216-218
Tarsi, height of inferior/superior, 230
Taste sensory function, 244
TBG (thyroid-binding globulin), 48
TBW (total body water)
  of 70-kg man, 98
  hypoosmolar hyponatremia and, 96
  mechanisms maintaining, 93
  percentage and composition of, 93
TCA (trichlorrroacetic acid), as chemical peeling agent, 410
TCAs (tricyclic antidepressants), adverse drug effects of, 70
T-cell deficiency, risk in transplant patients, 209
T cells, graft-vs.-host disease and, 218
Tears of sinus membrane, during sinus lifts, 419
Teeth. *See also* Dental implants
  causing facial space infections, surgical approaches, 297-304
  causing space infections, 297
  effects of radiation on, 381
  extracting in line of fracture, 266
  managing avulsed primary and permanent, 267
  radiation caries in, 381
  treating avulsed or extruded primary, 251
  treating cyst-associated, 367, 368
Telecanthus, hypertelorism vs., 272
Temporal fascial space infections, 301-302, 305
Temporalis fascia
  below zygomatic arch, 237
  blood supply to, 238
Temporalis muscle
  blood supply to, 238
  defined, 247

Temporalis muscle *(Cont'd)*
  forming landmark for inferior alveolar nerve block, 249
Temporal pad fat, blood supply to, 238
Temporal region, 237-238
Temporomandibular joint. *See* TMJ (temoporomandibular joint)
Temporoparietal fascia
  defined, 237
  extension in face, 237
  relationship of facial nerve to SMAS and, 242
Tendons, testing deep reflexes, 18
Tennison-Randall method, 346
Tenon's capsule, 8, 245-246
Tension band, in treating mandibular fractures, 267
Tension pneumothorax, 129, 136
Tenzel semicircular rotational flap, lower/upper eyelid reconstruction, 403
Teratogenic malformation, in pregnant patients from radiation, 225
Termporalis muscle flaps, 397-398
Tetanus immunization, 5
Tetracycline
  contraindication in renal disease patients, 189
  metabolized by liver, 185
Thermal burns, 139
Thermal relaxation time, 377
Thiazide diuretics, 95, 165
Thiazolidinediones, 205
Thiopental sodium (Pentothal), 76, 80
Third-degree (full-thickness) burns, 139
Third-degree heart blocks, 29, 128
Third-generation cephalosporins, 319
Third molars
  cystic legions around impacted, 5, 366
  dislodged root tip from, 249
  displaced into infratemporal fossa, 253
  extraction of impacted mandibular, 252
  inferior alveolar nerve in relation to, 249, 252
  lingual nerve in relation to mandibular, 254
  mandibular fracture location and, 263
  removal of, 249-250, 257
Threshold potential, and local anesthetics, 68
Thrombocytopenia, 36, 38
Thrombosis
  causing pulseless electrical activity, 129
  cavernous sinus, 316
Through-and-through cheek laceration, 289
Through-and-through lip laceration, 286
Thyroglossal duct cysts, 5
Thyroid
  detecting Hashimoto's thyroiditis, 48
  managing palpable solitary nodule within, 196

Thyroid *(Cont'd)*
  screening tests for, 48
  testing for sick euthyroid syndrome, 197
Thyroid-binding globulin (TBG), 48
Thyroid stimulating hormone (TSH), 48
Thyroxine total, 48
Tibial metaphysis, as bone graft source, 392
Timing, of wound closures, 284
Tinel's sign, 8, 257
Tissue
  ablation of, 378
  adhesives for wounds, 290
  common maxillofacial reconstruction flaps,
    397
  reconstruction, 397
  regeneration of, 420
TMIs (transmandibular implants), 415
TMJ (temoporomandibular joint)
  alloplastic reconstruction of, 396-397
  anatomy of, 322-323
  ankylosis of, 328
  articular disc of, 323-324, 329-330
  blood and nerve supplies for, 227
  disorders and facial pain of, 329-333
  effect of radiation on, 381
  imaging of, 58-59
  in mandibular teeth removal, 248
  nonsurgical management of, 324
  osteoarthritis of, 323-324, 326-327
  pathophysiology of, 323-324
  reconstruction of, 396-397
  surgical treatment for, 324-328
TNM (tumor, node, metastasis) staging system,
    370-372
Tongue
  cancer, 5, 372
  flap, 5-6, 402
  lacerations of, 288
  lesions, 372
  obstructing airway in unconscious person, 115
Tonicity (effective osmolality), 94
Top 100 secrets, 1-9
Torque testing, 6
Torsades de pointes, 30
Torus mandibularis, 418
Torus palatinus, 418-419
Total avulsion, of ear, 287
Total body water. *See* TBW (total body water)
Total joint reconstruction surgery, TMJ, 326
Total parenteral nutrition (TPN), 106, 108
Toxic granulation, 36
Toxicity
  lidocaine, 72
  local anesthetic, 68-69, 74
  pediatric local anesthetic risks, 66

TPN (total parenteral nutrition), 106, 108
Tracheal stenosis, tracheostomy-related, 146
Tracheoesophageal fistula, tracheostomy-related,
    146
Tracheo-innominate fistula, tracheostomy-related,
    146
Tracheostomy
  for emergency airway in children, 2
  in obstructive sleep apnea syndrome, 426
  overview of, 140-147
Tramadol, 1, 81
Tranexamic acid, 182-183
Transconjunctival incisions, 274, 401-402
Transesophageal echocardiography, 156, 157
Transfusions
  fresh frozen plasma, 38
  indicators for blood, 35
Transient oral bacteremias, 220-221
Transmandibular implants (TMIs), 415
Transmaxillary fractures, Le Fort I fracture, 279
Transmission, laser, 376
Transplant patients
  graft-vs.-host disease in, 218
  immunosuppressive drug complications in, 209
  immunosuppressive drugs for, 215-216
Transverse expansion of maxilla, relapses from, 4
Transverse maxillary deficiency, 340
Trapezius flaps, 397-398
Trauma
  advanced life support for, 134-140
  intravenous sedation in major, 80
Treacher Collins syndrome, 351-352
Trichloroacetic acid (TCA), as chemical peeling
    agent, 84, 410
Tricyclic antidepressants (TCAs), adverse drug
    effects of, 70
Trigeminal nerve injury, 256-261
Trigeminal tract, 331
Triiodothyronine resin uptake, 48
Trimesters, pregnancy, 222, 223
Tripod fractures, 276-277
Troponin-I levels, AMI test, 47
Troponin-T levels, AMI test, 47
Trousseau dilator, 143
Trousseau's sign, 2, 98
Trypsin levels, 44-45
TSH (thyroid stimulating hormone), 48
Tuberculosis, 315
Tuberosity, in denture reconstruction, 419
Tubular necrosis, acute, 193
Tularemia, 315
Tumescent technique, in submental liposuction,
    405
Tumor, node, metastasis (TNM) staging system,
    371

Tumors
  cancer of oral cavity, 370-376
  degree of malignancy of, 372
  oral and maxillofacial, 365-369
  radiation therapy in head and neck cancer, 380-389
  of salivary glands, 4, 360-364, 361
Turberoplasty, 421-422
T waves, in ECG reading, 23, 30
(12-lead) ECGs, 30-31
Tympanomastoid fissure, finding facial nerve using, 364
Type 1 diabetes, 199, 200
Type 2 diabetes
  causing hyperosmolar nonketotic coma, 200-201
  defined, 199
  lab findings in, 207
  metformin contraindications, 204
  pathogenesis of, 200

U

UFH (standard unfractionated heparin), 182, 255
UGI (upper gastrointestinal series), 54, 55
Ultrapulsing, 379
Ultrasonography, 366, 373
Uncomplete clefts, 344
Unconscious patients, diagnosing entrapment of orbital contents in, 273
United States Medical Licensing Examination (USMLE), 437
Units of radiation, basic, 52
Upper respiratory infections
  nitrous oxide administration in, 83
  as obstructive sleep apnea risk factor, 424
Urinalysis, 44, 51
Urinary output
  in Class II hemorrhage, 136
  in infants, 102
  in malignant hyperthermia, 149
  in trauma patients, 135
Urinary tract infections (UTIs), as postoperative fever cause, 113
Urine specific gravity test, 44
URIs (upper respiratory infections)
  nitrous oxide administration in, 83
  as obstructive sleep apnea risk factor, 424
USED CARP mnemonic, 98
USMLE (United States Medical Licensing Examination), 437
UTIs (urinary tract infections), 113
U-triple-P. See LAUP (laser-assisted uvulopalatoplasty)
Uvulopalatopharyngolplasty. See LAUP (laser-assisted uvulopalatoplasty)

V

Vagus nerve, 230
Valvular heart disease
  overview of, 156-158
  perioperative considerations, 158-161
  risk of stenosis vs. regurgitation, 159
Vancomycin, 308-309, 311
Van der Woude's syndrome, 358
Varicella zoster virus infections, 209
Vasoconstrictors
  adverse effects of, 70, 250
  allergic potential of, 71
  calculating amount of, 72-73
  as local anesthetic adjunct, 69
  when to avoid in soft tissue injuries, 284
Vasolidators, as antihypertensive agent, 165, 167, 168
Vasopressin, 132, 192
Velopharyngeal incompetence (VPI), 349
Ventilation
  difficulties in obese patients, 22
  effect of volatile anesthetics on, 85-86
  indicator of effective, 116
Ventilation-perfusion lung scans, 55
Ventricles, intrinsic firing rate of, 23
Ventricular origin, 31-32
Ventricular tachycardia
  assessing in advanced cardiac life support, 120
  as ECG sign of digitalis toxicity, 30
Ventriculography, radionuclear, for congestive heart failure evaluation, 170
Verapamil, 133
Verbal response, Glasgow Coma Scale (GCS), 19
Vertical maxillary deficiency, 336
Vertical maxillary excess (VME), 3, 335-336
Vestibuloplasty, 421
V-fib (ventricular fibrillation)
  causing pulseless condition, 130
  defining, 122
  EMS and, 115
  following electrocution, 122
  overview of, 29-30
  sudden cardiac death and, 131
  treating, 123
Viral hepatitis
  presurgery precautions, 186
  testing for, 49
  types of, 185-186
Viral infections. See also specific viral infections
  AIDS. See AIDS (acquired immunodeficiency syndrome)
  HIV infection. See HIV (human immunodeficiency virus) infection
  risk in immunocompromised patients, 209
  viral parotitis infection, 4, 361

Virchow's triad
  deep venous thrombosis and, 110
  defined, 7, 109
  elements of, 225
Visor osteotomy, 420
Visual oximetry, 90
Vital signs, 14, 20
Vitamin K
  affecting platelet count, 37
  blood clotting factors dependent on, 178
  deficiency increasing prothrombin time, 39
  reversing action of warfarin, 179
VME (vertical maxillary excess), 3, 335-336
Volatile anesthetics
  defined, 82
  hemodynamic effects of, 85
  suitability for COPD patients, 83-84
  ventilatory effects of, 85
Volume depletion, 95, 96
Volume excess, postoperative care, 96
Vomer flap, 348
Vomiting, postoperative, 7, 111
Von Langenbeck operation, 346, 348
Von Recklinghausen's disease, 355, 356
Von Willebrand's disease, 181
VPI (velopharyngeal incompetence), 349
V-Y pushback repair, 346, 348

W

Waardenburg's syndrome, mandibular
    prognathism in, 4
Wake-up potential, volatile anesthetics, 87
Warfarin (Coumadin)
  effect on prothrombin time, 39
  monitoring test for, 178
  preoperative discontinuation of, 179
Waters view, in radiographs, 272, 277
Wavelengths, lasers with dual/multiple, 379
Wayson stain, 49
WBC (white blood cell count)
  diagnoses made using, 51
  diagnostic peritoneal lavage and, 136
  normal, 181
  overview of, 32-34
Weber hearing tests, 15
Weeping lubrication, 324
Wharton's duct, relationship of lingual nerve to,
    234-235
Whitnall's orbital tubercle, 231

Wide-complex tachycardias
  defined, 123
  types and treatment of, 126
  ventricles and, 31
Wolff-Parkinson-White (WPW) syndrome, 30,
    126
Wolff's law, 391
World Health Organization (WHO), on
    malnutrition, 2, 105
Wound closures
  overview of, 284-285
  tissue adhesives for, 290
Wound infections. *See also* Bacterial infections
  antibiotic prophylaxis for, 5
  bite wounds, 284-285
  as postoperative bleeding cause, 110
  as postoperative fever cause, 109
  prosthetic joints, 219
W-plasty, in facial scar revision, 409

X

Xenografts, 389
Xerostomia
  causes of, 362
  managing, 383
  radiation related to, 381
X-ray radiation, in fetus, 225
X-rays, chest. *See* Chest x-rays

Y

YAG lasers
  defined, 378
  Er:YAG laser, 377
  Nd:YAG laser, 379

Z

ZMC (zygomaticomaxillary complex) fractures,
    277
Z-plasty, 409
Zygoma
  anatomy of, 244
  fractures of, 276-278
  removal of maxillary first molar and, 249
Zygomatic arch
  danger zone for facial nerve as it crosses, 240-
    241
  temporalis fascia below, 237
Zygomatic bone, 246
Zygomatic implants, 416, 434